Emergencies of the Head and Neck

Emergencies of the Head and Neck

David W. Eisele, MD
Professor
Departments of Otolaryngology–Head and Neck Surgery
and Anesthesiology and Critical Care Medicine
The Johns Hopkins University School of Medicine
Baltimore, Maryland

Shelly J. McQuone, MD
Assistant Professor
Department of Otorhinolaryngology–Head and Neck Surgery
University of Pennsylvania Health System
Philadelphia, Pennsylvania

With Illustrations by
Michael Linkinhoker

Mosby
A Harcourt Health Sciences Company
St. Louis London Philadelphia Sydney Toronto

Mosby
A Harcourt Health Sciences Company

Library of Congress Catalog Card Number 00-041898

EMERGENCIES OF THE HEAD AND NECK ISBN 1–55664–470–1

Mosby, Inc.
A Harcourt Health Sciences Company
11830 Westline Industrial Drive
St. Louis, Missouri 63146

Printed in the United States of America.

Last digit is the print number: 9 8 7 6 5 4 3 2 1

Contributors

Steven G. Ashman, DDS, FACD
Assistant Professor, Otolaryngology–Head and Neck Surgery; Assistant Professor, Plastic and Reconstructive Surgery, The Johns Hopkins Medical Institutions, Baltimore, Maryland
Oral Cavity and Dental Emergencies

Hilary A. Beaver, MD
Assistant Professor of Clinical Ophthalmology, University of Iowa Hospitals and Clinics, Iowa City, Iowa
Ophthalmologic Emergencies

William R. Bell, MD, PhD
Professor, Medicine, Radiology and Nuclear Medicine, The Johns Hopkins University School of Medicine; Staff and Clinical Director, Hematology Department, The Johns Hopkins University Hospital, Baltimore, Maryland
Hematologic Emergencies

Michael S. Boyne, MD
Clinical and Research Fellow, Division of Endocrinology and Metabolism, The Johns Hopkins University School of Medicine, Baltimore, Maryland
Endocrine Emergencies

Mark T. Brown, MD
Private Practice, Austin, Texas
Flap Emergencies

Alyson D. Buckner, MD
Resident, Department of Otolaryngology–Head and Neck Surgery, The Johns Hopkins Hospital, Baltimore, Maryland
Hematologic Emergencies

Tamora Carter Bynoe, MD
Assistant Professor, Department of Anesthesiology, The Johns Hopkins School of Medicine, Baltimore, Maryland
Anesthetic Emergencies

Paul F. Castellanos, MD
Director, Voice and Swallowing Disorders Center, Division of Otolaryngology–Head and Neck Surgery, Maryland Shock Trauma Center, University of Maryland, Baltimore, Maryland
Acute Laryngeal Trauma

Richard E. Clatterbuck, MD, PhD
Fellow, Department of Neurosurgery, The Johns Hopkins University School of Medicine; Resident, The Johns Hopkins Hospital, Baltimore, Maryland
Intracranial Emergencies

Michelle Marie Cullen, MD
Director, The Sinus Institute, Duluth, Georgia
Nasal Emergencies

David W. Eisele, MD, FACS
Professor, Departments of Otolaryngology–Head and Neck Surgery and Anesthesiology and Critical Care Medicine, The Johns Hopkins University School of Medicine; Director, Division of Head and Neck Surgery, The Johns Hopkins Hospital, Baltimore, Maryland
Airway Emergencies; Penetrating Trauma of the Neck

Lee A. Fleisher, MD
Associate Professor of Anesthesiology; Joint Appointments in Medicine and Health Policy and Management, The Johns Hopkins School of Medicine; Clinical Director of the Operating Rooms, The Johns Hopkins Hospital, Baltimore, Maryland
Anesthetic Emergencies

Howard W. Francis, MD
Assistant Professor, Department of Otolaryngology–Head and Neck Surgery, The Johns Hopkins University School of Medicine, Baltimore, Maryland
Facial Nerve Emergencies

John L. Frodel, Jr, MD
Associate Professor, Division of Otolaryngology and Plastic Surgery, Department of Surgery, University of New Mexico Health Sciences Center, Albuquerque, New Mexico
Emergencies in Facial Cosmetic Surgery

Todd Gress, MD, MPH
Assistant Professor of Medicine, Department of Internal Medicine, Marshall University School of Medicine, Huntington, West Virginia
Medical Emergencies

Henry R. Halperin, MD, MA
Associate Professor of Medicine and Biomedical Engineering, The Johns Hopkins University, Baltimore, Maryland
Cardiopulmonary Resuscitation

Richard F. Heitmiller, MD, FACS
Associate Professor of Surgery, The Johns Hopkins University School of Medicine; Chief, Division of Thoracic Surgery, The Johns Hopkins Hospital, Baltimore, Maryland
Thoracic Emergencies

G. Richard Holt, MD, MSE, MPH
Executive Vice President, American Academy of Otolaryngology–Head and Neck Surgery Foundation, Alexandria, Virginia; Adjunct Faculty, Department of Otolaryngology–Head and Neck Surgery, The Johns Hopkins University School of Medicine, Baltimore, Maryland; Professor and Director, Division of Facial Plastic and Reconstructive Surgery, The Johns Hopkins Medical Institutions, Baltimore, Maryland
Penetrating Trauma of the Face

David M. Huchton, MD
Assistant Professor, Department of Otolaryngology–Head and Neck Surgery, The Johns Hopkins School of Medicine, Baltimore, Maryland
Foreign Bodies in the Upper Aerodigestive Tract

Stephanie Joe, MD
Fellow, Department of Otorhinolaryngology—Head and Neck Surgery, University of Pennsylvania Health System, Philadelphia, Pennsylvania
Emergencies in Facial Cosmetic Surgery

Alan Krasner, MD
Associate Medical Director, Pfizer Inc., Groton, Connecticut
Medical Emergencies

Paul W. Ladenson, MD
John Eager Howard Professor of Medicine; Professor of Pathology, Oncology, and International Health; Director, Division of Endocrinology and Metabolism, The Johns Hopkins Medical Institutions, Baltimore, Maryland
Endocrine Emergencies

Andrew G. Lee, MD
Associate Professor of Ophthalmology, Neurology, and Neurosurgery, University of Iowa Hospitals and Clinics, Iowa City, Iowa
Ophthalmologic Emergencies

Donald A. Leopold, MD
Professor and Chair, Department of Otolaryngology–Head and Neck Surgery, University of Nebraska Medical Center, Omaha, Nebraska
Nasal Emergencies

Charles J. Limb, MD
Resident, Department of Otolaryngology–Head and Neck Surgery, The Johns Hopkins University School of Medicine, Baltimore, Maryland
Otologic and Skull Base Emergencies

Pamela A. Lipsett, MD
Associate Professor of Surgery; Assistant Professor of Anesthesiology and Critical Care Medicine; Associate Professor of Nursing, The Johns Hopkins University; Attending Surgeon, Co-Director, Surgical Intensive Care Unit, and Surgical Critical Care Fellowship Director, The Johns Hopkins Hospital, Baltimore, Maryland
Shock

John P. Little, MD
Physician, East Tennessee Children's Hospital, University of Tennessee Medical Center, Knoxville, Tennessee
Pediatric Head and Neck Emergencies

Bernard R. Marsh, MD
Professor, Department of Otolaryngology–Head and Neck Surgery, The Johns Hopkins University School of Medicine, Baltimore, Maryland
Foreign Bodies in the Upper Aerodigestive Tract

Shelly J. McQuone, MD
Assistant Professor, Department of Otorhinolaryngology—Head and Neck Surgery, University of Pennsylvania Health System, Philadelphia, Pennsylvania
Penetrating Trauma of the Neck;
Neck Emergencies

Andrew J. McWhorter, MD
Resident, Department of Otolaryngology–Head and Neck Surgery, The Johns Hopkins University School of Medicine, Baltimore, Maryland
Otologic and Skull Base Emergencies

John K. Niparko, MD
Professor of Otolaryngology–Head and Neck Surgery and Director, Division of Otology, Neurotology, and Skull Base Surgery, The Johns Hopkins School of Medicine and Hospital, Baltimore, Maryland
Otologic and Skull Base Emergencies

Bert W. O'Malley, Jr., MD
Professor and Director, Division of Otolaryngology–Head and Neck Surgery, Johns Hopkins University School of Medicine, Baltimore, Maryland
Paranasal Sinus Emergencies

Charles N. Schoenfeld, MD, FACEP
Assistant Professor, Department of Emergency Medicine, The Johns Hopkins School of Medicine; Vice-Chair, Department of Emergency Medicine, The Johns Hopkins Bayview Medical Center, Baltimore, Maryland
Evaluation of the Emergency Patient

Rafael J. Tamargo, MD, FACS
Associate Professor of Neurosurgery, The Johns Hopkins University School of Medicine; Co-Director, Division of Cerebrovascular Neurosurgery, The Johns Hopkins Hospital, Baltimore, Maryland
Intracranial Emergencies

David E. Tunkel, MD, FAAP, FACS
Associate Professor of Otolaryngology–Head and Neck Surgery and Pediatrics, The Johns Hopkins University School of Medicine; Director of Pediatric Otolaryngology, The Johns Hopkins Hospital, Baltimore, Maryland
Pediatric Head and Neck Emergencies

Lesley Wong, MD
Associate Professor of Plastic Surgery, The Johns Hopkins University School of Medicine; Assistant Director, Baltimore Regional Burn Center, Baltimore, Maryland
Thermal Emergencies

Stephen C. Yang, MD, FACS
Assistant Professor of Surgery and Oncology, The Johns Hopkins University School of Medicine; Staff Surgeon, The Johns Hopkins Hospital and Johns Hopkins Bayview Medical Center; Director, Thoracic Oncology Program and Lung Transplantation Program, The Johns Hopkins Hospital, Baltimore, Maryland
Thoracic Emergencies

FOREWORD

Nothing has been more meteoric in change than technology as it is associated with the practice of medicine in the past quarter of a century. Advances in imaging, surgical intervention, and pharmacologic treatment provide seminal examples of this transition. This book, edited by Drs. David W. Eisele and Shelly J. McQuone, brings into focus the contemporary aspects of diagnosis and treatment of head and neck emergencies. Because of the multispecialty need for a *single* informational source, this effort should reside on the shelves of all who are exposed to emergencies of the head and neck.

Charles W. Cummings, MD
Andelot Professor and Chairman
Department of Otolaryngology–Head and Neck Surgery
The Johns Hopkins University School of Medicine

PREFACE

Emergencies of the head and neck can be life-threatening problems because of the potential for upper airway obstruction, severe hemorrhage from major blood vessels, or neurologic compromise. The successful care of the head and neck emergency patient requires a thorough understanding of head and neck anatomy and physiology and of head and neck problems and their management, and the ability to promptly intervene, both surgically and medically. Emergencies of the head and neck include emergencies related to primary problems of the head and neck such as upper airway compromise, trauma, and infections, as well as emergencies that arise during and after head and neck surgical procedures. For the purpose of this text we have defined "emergency" as any condition that requires evaluation and management of the problem within 24 hours of presentation. This book, although primarily intended for surgeons and other practitioners with the primary interest in head and neck disorders, is also intended for emergency physicians, family practitioners, internists, and other health care professionals who often care for patients with problems of the head and neck. We have attempted not only to be thorough in the coverage of head and neck emergencies, but also in the practical approach to these problems. Chapter authors have been chosen for their expertise, experience, and interest in the areas covered. We hope that this book will increase understanding of head and neck emergencies and that their prompt recognition and successful management will improve outcomes for patients.

David W. Eisele, MD

Shelly J. McQuone, MD

ACKNOWLEDGMENTS

We would like to thank each chapter author for his or her excellent contribution to this book. Special thanks go to Michael Linkinhoker for his superb illustrations, which wonderfully complement the text. We thank Brenda Emche for her administrative support. In addition, we would like to acknowedge Robert Hurley for his direction and support, as well as Stephanie Donley and Peter Faber, and the staff at Harcourt Health Sciences for their efforts.

David W. Eisele, MD

Shelly J. McQuone, MD

NOTICE

Medicine is an ever-changing field. Standard safety precautions must be followed, but as new research and clinical experience broaden our knowledge, changes in treatment and drug therapy become necessary or appropriate. Readers are advised to check the product information currently provided by the manufacturer of each drug to be administered to verify the recommended dose, the method and duration of administration, and the contraindications. It is the responsibility of the treating physician, relying on experience and knowledge of the patient, to determine dosages and the best treatment for the patient. Neither the publisher nor the editor assumes any responsibility for any injury and/or damage to persons or property.

THE PUBLISHER

Contents

CHAPTER 1

Evaluation of the Emergency Patient

Charles N. Schoenfeld, MD

The delivery of medical care in a hospital emergency department (ED) is unique in many ways. Numerous clinical, temporal, financial, and regulatory forces routinely impact the ability to care for patients in an ED.

The ED has no provision for scheduling patients and thus no reasonable ability to provide staff according to expected patient volume. This inability to predict patient loads often results in times when the clinical demand exceeds the ED's resources. This same lack of predictability occasionally results in excess capacity, but it is more common to be faced with overwhelming demand and limited resources.

The emergency medicine (EM) physician is responsible for every patient in the ED, whether in an examination room or in the process of triage and registration. This produces a tremendous pressure for situational awareness, the need to be aware of the clinical status of every patient in the ED. It also demands that the EM physician quickly recognize which patients are unstable. The willingness to listen to and rely on competent nursing and ancillary staff in such a situation is obvious.

In addition, EM physicians must be adept at multiple patient management. Whether preparing to evaluate a patient or awaiting diagnostic tests or the opinion of a consultant, the EM practitioner must constantly juggle the care of as many patients as are present in the ED.

One obvious effect of such demands is the need to maximize the speed and efficiency with which patients are moved through the ED. Neither the patients nor the ED is served by extensive evaluations unrelated to the stabilization or disposition of ED patients. Indeed, in a busy ED the priorities in patient care are first stabilization, then disposition, with or without a definitive diagnosis. A patient with upper airway obstruction, hypoxemia, and fever requires first, control of the life-threatening signs and symptoms and then, disposition to an appropriate inpatient service for definitive therapy and diagnosis. The ability to distinguish whether the patient has an obstructed airway caused by epiglottitis or a retropharyngeal abscess has minimal impact on the appropriate ED management of such a case. Immediate control of the airway is the emergent issue.

Triage is a concept unique to EM. Unlike an office or clinic setting, in which patients are seen according to the time they were scheduled, in an ED, patients are evaluated according to the severity of their presenting symptoms. The purpose of triage is to ensure that the most unstable patient is treated first, before one who is stable.

The concept of triage extends beyond assigning priorities for evaluation of the patients present. Triage is also applied in the evaluation of the individual patient. Prioritization in the injury and illness assessment, as well as in the order of intervention, is crucial in each patient. For example, a victim of a motor vehicle crash may display dramatic facial injuries, but information provided by emergency medical service personnel describes deformation of the steering wheel. In this patient, sternal tenderness or bruising may point to life-threatening injuries to the heart, lungs, or thoracic aorta that are not yet clinically evident. In such a case, the dramatic facial injuries, if not associated with signs or symptoms of impending airway compromise, are lower in priority than the chest trauma and must be triaged appropriately. The recognition of hidden illness or injury and the potential for clinical deterioration is critical to the evaluation of every patient in an ED. An EM physician cannot be distracted by impressive but noncritical injuries.

A critical component of any ED evaluation is historical information from peripheral sources. Accessing the medical record, the family, the police, or the emergency medical service providers to obtain information is often crucial. A patient involved in a serious automobile accident cannot provide a description of the starring of the windshield or the deformity of the steering wheel; such crucial data must be obtained from members of the emergency medical service. A patient intubated during a successful prehospital resuscitation cannot provide a history either; the family, coworkers, or medical record may be the only source of critical information in such a situation. The failure to obtain such information prior to the departure of those able to provide it is considered a significant error in ED protocol.

PRESENTATION

Patients presenting to the ED typically represent the entire spectrum of problems encountered by specialists in internal medicine, neurology, psychiatry, surgery, otolaryngology, orthopedics, obstetrics/gynecology, and pediatrics. Problems range from critical illness and injury to acute but noncritical conditions to primary care concerns. It is the task of the EM physician to determine where in this spectrum a given case falls and to provide appropriate resuscitation, evaluation, and disposition.

It is common for ED patients to present early in the course of evolution of their symptoms, especially when critically ill or injured. As a result, the EM physician is unable to rely on the natural history of a given process in order to establish a diagnosis. In addition, a given patient's signs and symptoms may evolve in the ED or after disposition, impacting the EM physician's initial decisions. For example, a hypertensive patient taking an angiotensin-converting enzyme (ACE) inhibitor who complains of mild tongue swelling for 1 hour must be recognized as being at risk for subsequent complete airway obstruction from angioedema. Although the incidence of angioedema among users of ACE inhibitors is only 0.1%,[1] its presence and potential for progression must be recognized. Assuming that a patient's complaints reflect a static condition is dangerous because the patient's condition could dramatically deteriorate.

Most often, patients presenting to the ED are new patients who are unknown by the treating physician. Although most EDs see some patients making repeat visits, they represent a minor percentage of total patient encounters. Thus the ability to temper the response to patients' complaints based on prior knowledge of previous behavior and clinical response is generally absent.

Patients may present with obvious conditions, either stable or critical, that allow rapid assessment, treatment, and disposition. They may also present with obscure but clearly life-threatening conditions that require immediate stabilization prior to diagnostic evaluation. Between these extremes lies an intermediate spectrum of complaints that allow a variety of levels of evaluation, depending on the patient's stability. For example, a 50-year-old hypertensive diabetic who is diaphoretic and complains of chest pain and whose electrocardiogram indicates an acute anterior myocardial infarction must be

BOX 1–1

Contraindications to Thrombolysis in Acute Myocardial Infarction

ABSOLUTE

Active internal bleeding
Uncontrolled hypertension (>200/120)
Pregnancy
Surgery or major trauma in the past 2 weeks
Head trauma in the past 1 month
Intracranial neoplasm
History of hemorrhagic stroke
Hemorrhagic retinopathy
CPR lasting longer than 10 minutes
Suspected pericarditis
Suspected aortic dissection

RELATIVE

Surgery or major trauma 2 to 6 weeks in the past
Stroke in the past 6 months
GI or GU bleed in the past 6 months
Active peptic ulcer disease
Bleeding disorder
Chronic hypertension with diastolic pressure >110

CPR, cardiopulmonary resuscitation; GI, gastrointestinal; GU, genitourinary.

rapidly stabilized and then assessed regarding contraindications to thrombolysis (Box 1–1). The primary goal of the EM physician here is first to ensure the patient's stability and then to preserve myocardium while avoiding catastrophic complications such as prescribing thrombolytics to a patient with a type I aortic dissection (Fig. 1–1).

At the opposite end of the spectrum is, for example, a 35-year-old patient with no known history of agonal respirations. Such a patient requires immediate control of the airway, ventilation with 100% oxygen, and assessment and support of the circulation. Only after the airway has been controlled, ventilation ensured, and the circulatory status stabilized (the typical ABC approach) can the physician investigate the hypoventilation's cause—opiate intoxication, reactive airway disease, acute myocardial infarction with pulmonary edema, or overwhelming sepsis. The experienced EM practitioner may elect to use parenteral naloxone first in a patient with evidence of recent venipuncture ("fresh tracks"), or 25 g of intravenous glucose (or 1 to 2 mg of parenteral glucagon) in a known diabetic with this presentation in order to avoid the risks of intubation. Such a decision may require transient support of the airway and breathing by bag-valve-mask, as dictated by the clinical circumstance and the patient's response. If this less invasive approach is selected, the EM physician must be prepared to change rapidly to a more aggressive approach if the patient's response is inadequate.

An example of a patient with an intermediate presentation is an elderly nursing home resident who presents febrile, with an acute change in mental status but with a stable clinical picture and stable vital signs. This patient is rapidly assessed to rule out meningitis (which is uncommon) and then evaluated for the more likely diagnoses of urosepsis or pneumonia.[2]

EVALUATION

Overview

One of the more challenging and anxiety-provoking aspects of EM is that data acquisition, whether historical or physical, is inversely proportionate to the stability of the patient. A patient presenting with agonal respirations, for example, clearly must have his or her airway

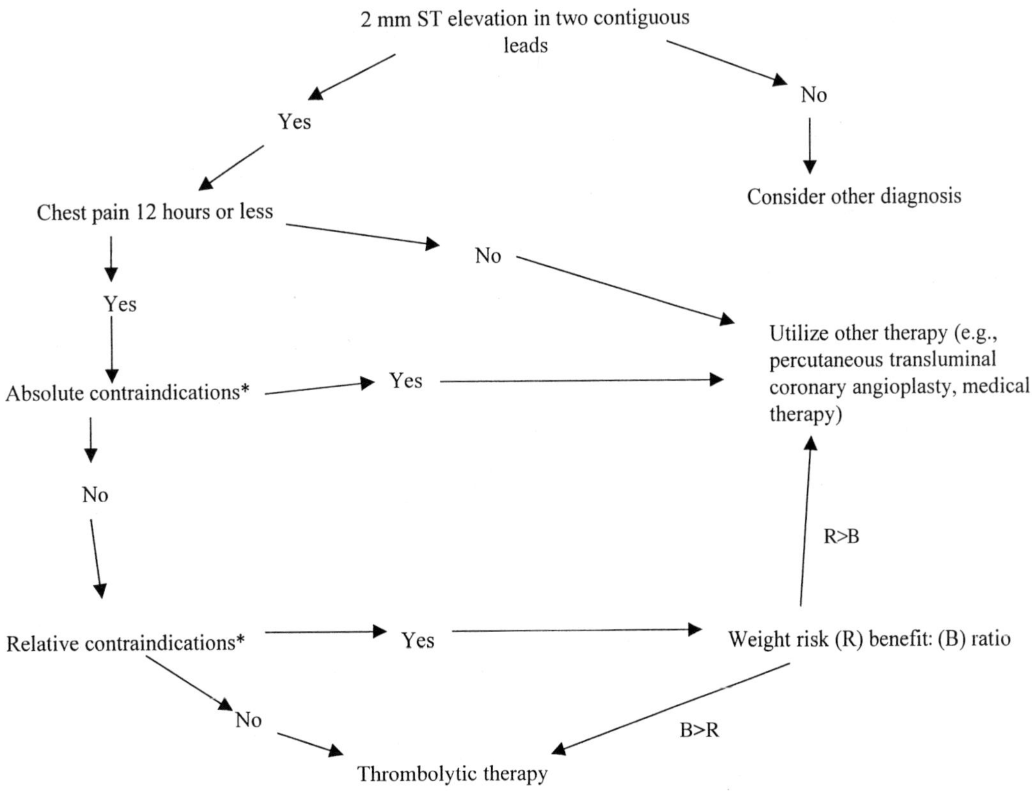

Figure 1–1. Algorithm for thrombolytic therapy in acute myocardial infarction. *See Box 1–1.

secured and breathing supported before the cause of respiratory failure is ascertained. In contrast, a patient presenting with dysphonia and dysphagia without respiratory embarrassment is approached in a more contemplative fashion, even if ultimately the need to establish an airway and provide ventilatory support is the same. The art of EM lies in the ability to decide which patients can be evaluated prior to therapy and which ones require treatment before a diagnosis is established. The distinction, though always crucial, is not always clear.

Further, the ED resources devoted to any patient must be in proportion to the illness. It is unnecessary to assign two nurses and an EM physician to the care of a stable patient with uncomplicated pneumonia, and it is disastrous to have only a patient aide and an EM physician caring for an unstable patient. It is imperative that ED resource allocation be determined by the instability of the patient. A useful method of maximizing the allocation of resources according to the needs of the patients is to use a team approach to define illness and injury. Experience has shown how many and what types of providers are required to care for specific conditions. A victim of major trauma, for example, requires a sufficient number of personnel to allow concurrent control of the airway and ventilatory support, intravenous access via large-bore catheters to support circulation, primary and secondary surveys to assess the severity of injury, and a dedicated individual to document the findings and the actions taken. Such personnel compose a trauma team; members should be chosen by those in the ED and trauma service. A similar approach is used in the case of a patient with an acute myocardial infarction: it must be determined how many and what type of caregivers are required to stabilize and evaluate the patient, then exclude contraindications and provide thrombolytic therapy, if appropriate, before the window of opportunity closes (see Box 1–1). Given the current potential for successful intervention in strokes, it may be reasonable to also create a stroke team that is activated as soon as a patient is recognized as a candidate for therapeutic intervention.

The composition of other teams, such as those responding to burns, epiglottitis, precipitate birth, or other defined clinical entities, should also be determined, with individuals and their responsibilities being defined in advance by members of the institution, the involved specialty service, and the portal of entry—the ED.

Head and Neck Emergencies

Given the high concentration of critical structures in the small anatomic area, it is imperative that the EM physician and consultants for head and neck (HN) emergencies pay particular attention to the ABCs in evaluating an HN emergency. Obstruction of the airway may be the presenting event in such situations, and aggressive efforts to establish a patent airway take precedence over other resuscitative efforts. Inability to breathe in HN emergencies (in the absence of upper airway obstruction) is usually caused by injuries to the cervical spine or by toxic metabolic crises such as drug overdose. Whatever the cause, aggressive airway control and artificial ventilation are key to a patient's survival. Circulatory collapse caused by blood loss may occur as a result of great vessel injury or of invasion by a contiguous tumor. More common is loss of the airway because of brisk bleeding; this degree of blood loss makes securing the airway a formidable task.

Beyond the ABCs, injury and illness involving the cervical cord, esophagus, facial structures, cervical fascia, and cerebral vessels all contribute to significant morbidity and mortality in HN emergencies. The majority of ED visits for HN emergencies are for such basic complaints as pharyngitis, otalgia, epistaxis, and isolated nasal fracture, but it is imperative that the ED practitioner or HN consultant recognize when such seemingly trivial presentations actually reflect more serious disease. Failure to recognize the potential complications of a parapharyngeal space abscess, malignant otitis externa in a diabetic, or posterior epistaxis, for example, invites catastrophe.

TRAUMATIC HEAD AND NECK EMERGENCIES

The full scope of traumatic HN emergencies is covered more fully in other chapters, but it is worthwhile to discuss some general management principles here. Of primary importance is the ability to recognize the need for protection of the airway and for ventilatory support. Secondarily, it is important to recognize the presence of other life-threatening injuries. The majority of trauma victims requiring airway management have no anatomic airway abnormalities, but intubating an acutely traumatized upper airway, in which active bleeding, traumatic distortion, or edema obscures landmarks, is a challenging process. The ability to create a medical (i.e., endotracheal tube) or surgical (i.e., tracheostomy or cricothyroidotomy) airway must be in the armamentarium of all EM practitioners and HN consultants. Further, the competent consultant should be aware of the capabilities of the particular ED. No HN consultant should attempt to manage a fragile airway in the ED without knowing what equipment and staff are available. All consultants who may be called upon to manage an unstable ED patient should visit the ED and critically assess the instruments and the assistance likely to be available before they are required to use them.

Another consideration in the evaluation of a traumatic HN emergency is the recognition that *all* head or facial injuries are associated with cervical spine injuries until proven otherwise. In such a circumstance, airway control must be performed with concomitant spinal immobilization. Manipulation of the head and upper airway can be performed only with simultaneous stabilization of the cervical spine. Further, it is mandatory that the EM and HN physicians realize that the radiologic absence of fracture does not exclude potentially unstable spinal ligamentous injury. Hardy reported a series of patients with cervical spine injuries that showed a 37% incidence of neurologic deficit without radiologic evidence of bony injury.[3] Another series demonstrated a 17% incidence of neurologic deficit in the absence of fracture.[4] In children, the spinal cord injury without radiographic abnormality (SCIWORA) syndrome has been described, usually in patients younger than 8 years.[5,6] One must assume ligamentous injury and instability in any patient with a diminished ability to sense or verbalize pain because of intoxication, significant closed head injury, other severe distracting injuries such as long bone or pelvic fractures, or the inability to communicate because of coma or intubation. In such circumstances, cervical spine immobilization is maintained by rigid cervical collar until ligamentous injury has been excluded. Such exclusion may be determined clinically by the absence of pain or tenderness and may require only the resolution of the symptoms of intoxication, intubation, or closed head injury or may require further radiographic evaluation. Radiologic imaging may be as simple as oblique or flexion/extension views of the cervical spine or as complex as computed tomography, or, preferably, magnetic resonance imaging.

NONTRAUMATIC HEAD AND NECK EMERGENCIES

By far, the most common HN complaints of ED patients are nontraumatic. Otalgia, throat pain, epistaxis, and otic or nasal foreign body are all familiar to ED physicians. Rarely do such presentations necessitate emergent evaluation by an HN consultant, although follow-up by such specialists is often recommended. However, patients with complaints that suggest imminent airway compromise, such as epiglottitis, stridor, or upper airway foreign body, or potential septic complications such as parapharyngeal abscess mandate early and appropriate intervention by an HN specialist. In addition, involvement of an HN consultant in seemingly trivial complaints may be warranted in select cases. A patient with pharyngitis who is unable to swallow liquids or with epistaxis that cannot be controlled in the ED requires hospitalization and inpatient treatment. Such circumstances clearly warrant HN consultation to prevent further deterioration of the patient's status.

PRIORITIES

In a busy ED, the priorities of patient care are first, stabilization, followed by evaluation and then by disposition, with or without a definitive diagnosis. An in-depth discussion of the priorities of evaluation and management of all emergencies is clearly impractical here, but it is reasonable to discuss a general approach and to highlight the priorities of managing commonly seen and life-threatening presentations. Specific issues involved in HN emergencies are discussed in subsequent chapters.

Usually, only a brief glance is required to identify critically unstable patients. An ashen, diaphoretic patient found to have hypotension, tachycardia, and tachypnea is obviously unstable. The EM physician must recognize that such a patient requires emergent stabilization and evaluation and that the sequence of stabilization followed by evaluation must be followed. It does not matter whether the patient's presentation is caused by a myocardial infarction or upper gastrointestinal bleeding; rapid and simultaneous assessment of the need to control the airway, support breathing, and provide adequate circulation is paramount. The concept of the "ABC's," although useful as a mnemonic, is followed only when a single provider is caring for the patient. Obviously, such a circumstance should not occur in an ED where a team approach is used.

The ED team must immediately evaluate the airway by ascertaining whether the patient is able to move air into and out of the lungs and whether the patient is able to protect his or her

Table 1–1. *Hemodynamic Parameters in Shock*

Type of Shock	Cardiac Output	Peripheral Vascular Resistance	Intravascular Volume
Cardiogenic	↓	↑	→
Septic	↑ or ↓	↓	→
Hypovolemic	↑	↑	↓
Neurogenic	↑	↓	→
Anaphylactic	↑	↓	→

own airway. At the same time, supplemental oxygen is provided while measures of adequate breathing are made (clinical estimations of tidal volume, pulse oximetry, or arterial blood gas). Supplemental oxygen may be provided by face mask in a patient with an open airway and adequate ventilatory drive or by bag-valve-mask in preparation for intubation. At the same time, other team members assess the adequacy of circulation and provide intravenous access. Adequate circulation is best evaluated in the ED by clinical monitoring of tissue perfusion; mentation and capillary refill are examined first, followed by measurement of urine output. The patient's blood pressure and pulse are crude but easily monitored markers as well. All hypoperfusing patients, in the absence of obvious cardiogenic shock, should first receive volume resuscitation. Vasopressor agents are used only after adequate volume resuscitation, as all causes of shock, other than cardiogenic, reflect inadequate volume relative to intravascular capacitance (Table 1–1). In specific clinical situations, the above sequence may be supplemented by disease-specific priorities. For example, in acute myocardial infarction, a major priority is to determine the patient's eligibility for thrombolytic therapy ("time is muscle" in this case). In institutions that use thrombolytic or other therapy for patients with acute strokes, the timeliness of determining a patient's eligibility for such intervention is equally important. In the case of major trauma, the need for a team approach is most critical. The cooperation of many disciplines is required, as EM, trauma surgery, radiology, nursing, laboratory (including the blood bank), and the operating room must work together to ensure the rapid assessment and disposition of the patient.

As previously mentioned, obvious opiate overdose or hypoglycemia may preclude the need for an aggressive ABC approach, as long as the patient's response is timely and appropriate to the therapy. Indeed, most EM physicians routinely order naloxone and D-50-W for unresponsive patients transported to the ED by emergency personnel.

OUTCOMES

In 1995, there were approximately 96,545,000 patient visits to EDs in the United States. Of these, 11% (approximately 10,628,000) required admission, and 17% of these admissions (approximately 1,822,000) were to critical care units, a reflection of the serious status of many ED patients. Slightly more than 1% (approximately 1,110,000) of patients presenting to EDs left prior to being evaluated by a physician. Only 0.3% (approximately 301,000) patients were dead on arrival or died in the ED. This contrasts with the approximately 697,082,000 office and clinic visits for complaints related to the ears, nose, and throat.[7] Given that in the same year, there were 71,000 practitioners devoted to the treatment of ear, nose, and throat disorders and 117,000 practicing EM physicians,[8] it is obvious that the vast majority of head and neck problems do not require emergent ED evaluation or consultation with HN specialists.

The best possible outcome for ED patients is obvious. They are triaged correctly, seen in a timely manner, stabilized, and evaluated without error, and they receive consultation and disposition appropriate to their clinical conditions. In a perfect scenario, they also receive a correct definitive diagnosis. This is the goal sought by all EM physicians.

However, every EM physician dreads hearing the phrase "Remember that patient you sent home?" The febrile child who initially looked well but returns with overwhelming meningococcemia and the car crash victim with neck pain whose unstable ligamentous injury was not recognized on initial presentation and who later develops a neurologic deficit serve to provide both a sense of humility and a reinforcement of the admonition "First, do no harm."

The ED represents a unique arena for patient care. Regulations, financial concerns, and unscheduled arrivals combine to produce pressures unlike those experienced in an office or clinic. The wide variety of patient types and the range of seriousness of the emergencies provide constant challenges to the EM practitioner. The early presentation of critically ill and injured patients often necessitates treatment prior to acquisition of objective data. The EM physician must be prepared to respond to changes in the evolving clinical picture. The detection and interpretion of subtle clues and the anticipation of potential causes of deterioration in patients remain challenging. Willingness to participate in and support a team approach to patient care is crucial.

Head and neck emergencies, because of their ability to produce significant morbidity and mortality, are prime examples of the clinical challenges faced in evaluating patients in the ED. They demonstrate the need to prioritize patient assessment and therapy as well as the importance of being aware of the potential for catastrophic clinical deterioration.

REFERENCES

1. Hawkins DW, Bussey HI: Hypertension in pharmacotherapy: A pathophysiologic approach. In DiPiro JT, ed. New York, Elsevier Science Publishing Co, 1989.
2. Marco CA et al. Fever among geriatric emergency patients: clinical features associated with serious illness. Ann Emerg Med 1995;26:18.
3. Hardy AG. Cervical spinal cord injury without bony injury. Paraplegia 1977;14:296.
4. Riggins RS, Krause JF. The risk of neurologic damage with fractures of the vertebrae. J Trauma 1977;17:126.
5. Pang D, Wilberger JE. Spinal cord injuries without radiographic abnormalities in children. J Neurosurg 1982;57:114.
6. Pang D, Pollack IF. Spinal cord injury without radiographic abnormality in children: the SCIWORA syndrome. J Trauma 1989;29:654.
7. Stussman BJ: National Hospital Ambulatory Medical Care Survey: 1995 Emergency Department Summary. Advance data from vital and health statistics; no. 285. Hyattsville, Mo, National Center for Health Statistics, 1997.
8. American Medical Association. Physician characteristics and distribution in the U.S., 1995.

ADDITIONAL READING

Advanced Cardiac Life Support (ACLS) Dallas, American Heart Association.

Advanced Trauma Life Support (ATLS). Chicago, American College of Surgeons Committee on Trauma.

Dailey RH. Approach to the patient in the emergency department. In Rosen P, Barkin RM, eds. Emergency Medicine Concepts and Clinical Practice, 3rd ed. 1992, Mosby, St Louis, Mo.

CHAPTER 2

Cardiopulmonary Resuscitation

Henry R. Halperin, MD, MA

More than 300,000 deaths are caused by cardiac arrest each year in the United States. For arrests that occur in the hospital, survival rates average around 15%.[1] For arrests that occur outside of the hospital, the survival rates are generally lower. A number of studies have shown that survival rates are related to the quality of resuscitative efforts.[2,3]

The goal of the Advanced Cardiac Life Support (ACLS) guidelines is to optimize the results of resuscitation by combining defibrillation, chest compression, drug therapy, ventilation, and other treatments. Because there are many possible causes and courses of cardiac arrest, the ACLS guidelines have become somewhat complicated so as to be comprehensive. The aspects of the guidelines that make the most difference in saving lives, however, are simple.

PRESENTATION AND EVALUATION

Cardiac arrest is the cessation of cardiac mechanical activity. It is a clinical diagnosis. In a nonanesthetized patient, it is confirmed by unresponsiveness, absence of a detectable pulse, and apnea or agonal respirations. In the setting of anesthesia or sedation, the presentation may be subtler, as the patient may not be responsive or breathing spontaneously. In the latter setting, constant monitoring of vital signs is imperative to determine when the patient (1) develops primary arrhythmias causing cardiac arrest; (2) is becoming hypotensive because of arrhythmias, volume changes, or drug reactions; or (3) is becoming hypoxic because of airway occlusion or pneumothorax. Hypotension or hypoxia can rapidly lead to cardiac arrest if uncorrected.

PRIORITIES

Defibrillation

The most important aspect of resuscitation after cardiac arrest in patients with ventricular fibrillation is early defibrillation. Numerous studies have shown that there is an inverse relationship between survival and the amount of time between onset of fibrillation and defibrillation (Fig. 2–1).[4] Delaying defibrillation even a few minutes can make the difference between survival and death. As most of the patients who survive are those who present with ventricular fibrillation, early defibrillation becomes even more important. Early defibrillation in a hospital setting may seem to be a given, but delays of 5 to 10 minutes are not uncommon.

Traditionally, small electrodes have been used for infants and children and are often labeled "pediatric" electrodes. This practice has been based primarily on the intuitive concept that smaller electrodes should be used for smaller patients. However, very small electrodes may result in excessively high transthoracic impedance and inadequate current flow.[5] Thus, the larger "adult" electrodes are likely to be more appropriate as soon as the electrode paddles fit completely on a child's thorax; for most children, this is possible at 1 year of age or 10 kg of weight. The flow of current is improved when adult electrodes are used in children.[6]

The electrodes should be placed in such a way as to locate the heart between the elec-

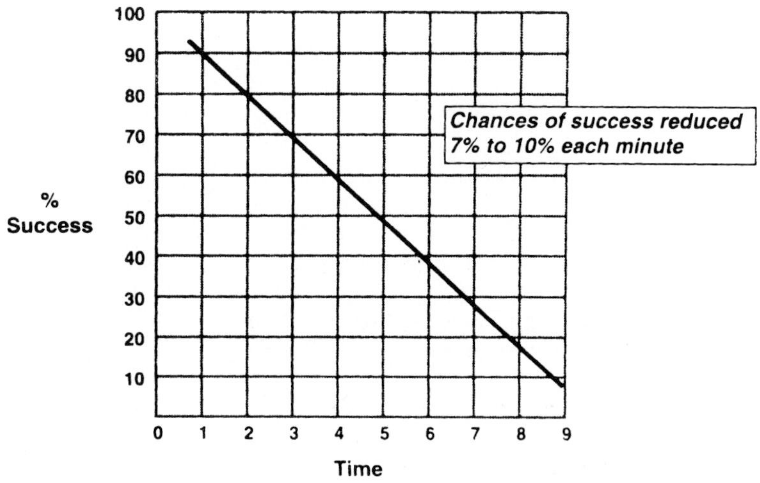

Figure 2–1. Resuscitation success vs. time. (From Cummins RO. From concept to standard of care? Ann Emerg Med 1989; 18:1269–1275.)

trodes (Fig. 2–2). The polarity of the paddles is unimportant.[7, 8] It is now understood that current does not take a straight line through the chest between electrodes, and a surprisingly small portion of the total current flow—only about 4%—actually traverses the myocardium during transthoracic defibrillation.[9] The most common electrode placement is the apex-anterior formation: one electrode is placed anteriorly to the right (the patient's right) of the upper sternum below the clavicle, and the second electrode is placed to the left of the nipple just outside the position of the normal cardiac apex. In female patients, it is generally recommended that the defibrillator paddles or self-adhesive pads not be placed directly on the tissues of the left breast. The breast should be elevated and the paddle or pad placed on the chest wall under or lateral to the breast, in the expectation that this reduces impedance and improves current flow.

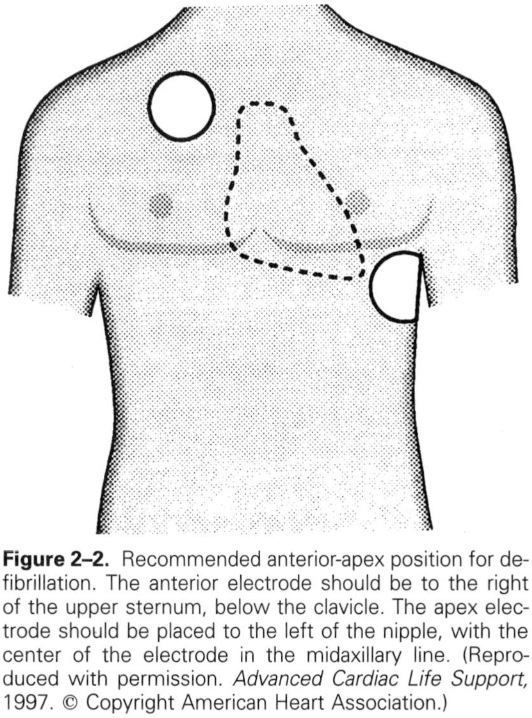

Figure 2–2. Recommended anterior-apex position for defibrillation. The anterior electrode should be to the right of the upper sternum, below the clavicle. The apex electrode should be placed to the left of the nipple, with the center of the electrode in the midaxillary line. (Reproduced with permission. *Advanced Cardiac Life Support,* 1997. © Copyright American Heart Association.)

Other electrode positions have been used successfully, too. In the anteroposterior position, one electrode is placed anteriorly over the left precordium and the other posteriorly in the right or left infrascapular position; in the apex-posterior position, the anterior paddle is placed over the cardiac apex and the posterior paddle in the right infrascapular location.[10] All of these positions appear to be satisfactory and to achieve equally high rates of terminating arrhythmia. In any individual patient, however, one position may be superior to others. In our experience, after several shocks have been administered unsuccessfully from one position, a shock occasionally achieves defibrillation when electrode positions are altered and a new position is used.

Shortening the current's pathway and, hence, the impedance, which improves success, may be achieved by using a more invasive defibrillation route. The most extreme examples of this technique include applying epicardial or endocardial electrodes either during open-chest resuscitation or by means of surgical insertion of specifically designed, implantable automatic defibrillators. In such situations, energy levels between 5 and 25 joules may be adequate.

Defibrillation can also be performed by using disposable, self-adhesive monitoring defibrillation pads that incorporate a conductive gel between the electrode and the skin surface.[10] This option is attractive, as the pads enhance operator safety by physically separating the operator from the patient. In elective situations (electrophysiologic studies, cardiac catheterization, elective cardioversion) they can be preplaced, facilitating optimal placement without the extreme stress that is present in an ongoing cardiac arrest. Transthoracic impedance is similar to that of standard hand-held electrodes.[10] Self-adhesive pads are routinely supplied with automatic external defibrillators and are used to detect the surface electrocardiogram, permit its analysis, and then deliver the defibrillating shock. Present recommendations for the size of pads used with these automatic external defibrillators state that the total area of the two electrodes should be at least 150 cm^2, and the minimal area of one pad should be at least 50 cm^2.[11]

Ventricular fibrillation can sometimes masquerade as asystole. True asystole does not terminate when electric shocks are applied. It has been suggested that the success rates for asystole (which are already dismal) may be further compromised by defibrillation.[12] However, occasionally the ventricular fibrillation vector may be perpendicular to the sensing electrode and hence be misinterpreted as asystole. The true incidence of ventricular fibrillation that mimics asystole is unknown. The prognosis for ventricular fibrillation depends primarily on the performance of defibrillation in a timely manner; if there is any doubt that ventricular fibrillation is being mistaken for asystole, defibrillation should be undertaken. It is also recommended that when asystole appears to be present, more than one lead position on the electrocardiographic monitor is checked before the final decision to avoid shocks is made.[13]

Chest Compression

The goal of cardiopulmonary resuscitation (CPR) by means of external chest compression after defibrillation fails or is not indicated is to maximize the generated coronary and cerebral blood flow.[14] Restoration of native cardiac activity and preservation of brain function are directly related to these flows.[15, 16] Cerebral and coronary flows should be maximized by optimizing the driving force of blood movement and the loading conditions.

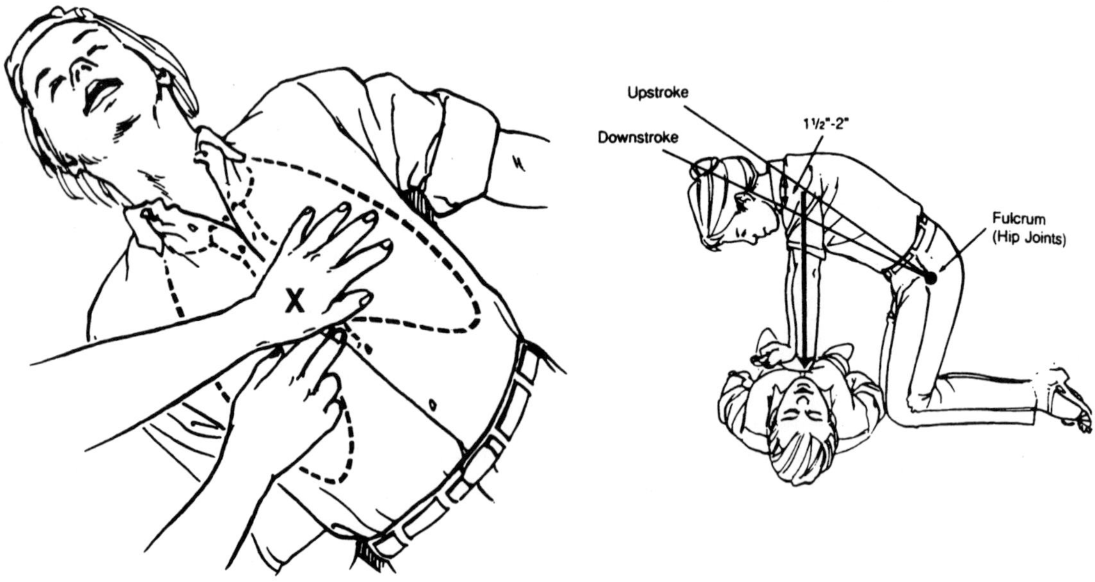

Figure 2–3. Recommendations for positioning and applying chest compression during CPR. Left: External chest compressions are applied by the rescuer, who places the heel of one hand over the lower half of the victim's sternum. The correct location is identified either by finding the xiphoid process at the lower tip of the sternum or by using the lower edge of the rib cage as a guide. Right: The second hand is placed on top of the first in such a way that the fingers do not touch the chest. Force is applied straight down, with the elbows locked and the shoulders in line with the hands. The goal is to displace the sternum 1.5 to 2.0 inches in the average-sized adult victim. (From the American Heart Association Guidelines for cardiopulmonary resuscitation and emergency cardiac care. JAMA 1992;268:2184–2198. Copyright 1992, American Medical Association.)

The ability of even properly performed chest compressions to generate adequate levels of flow is probably marginal; only about 15% of cardiac arrest victims survive. External chest compression is, however, the only technique for CPR that is widely available, and many lives are saved each year by standard CPR. Proper chest compression requires that the arms be locked and relatively straight and that the whole body be used in the compressions (Fig. 2–3). Often, just the arms are used for chest compression, which is extremely tiring and is not likely to generate sufficient compression force.

The mechanisms whereby blood moves during chest compression have been studied in order to determine ways of improving blood flow.[17, 18] Two major mechanisms have been identified: the cardiac compression pump and the intrathoracic pressure pump.

THE CARDIAC COMPRESSION PUMP

With the cardiac compression pump, it is postulated that chest compression does not cause intrathoracic pressure to rise. Instead, the heart and possibly some vascular structures are compressed between the sternum and the vertebral column (Fig. 2–4). It is presumed that blood is squeezed from the heart into the arterial circulation during chest compression, with the cardiac valves preventing retrograde blood flow. With release of chest compression, the heart would expand and fill with blood. Coronary and cerebral flow are presumed to occur in a fashion similar to that which occurs in intact circulation.

THE INTRATHORACIC PRESSURE PUMP

With the intrathoracic pressure pump, it is postulated that chest compression causes a rise in

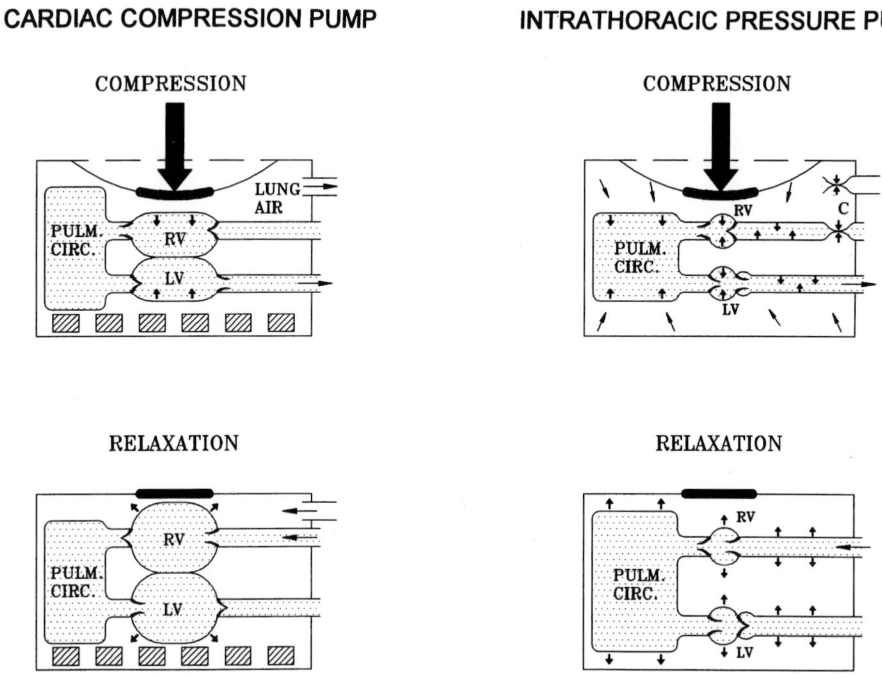

Figure 2–4. Left: Schematic representation of the cardiac compression pump. Right: Schematic representation of the intrathoracic pressure pump. With the cardiac compression pump, it is postulated that chest compression causes the left ventricle (LV) and possibly the right ventricle (RV) of the heart to be compressed between the sternum and the vertebral column. It is presumed that blood is squeezed from the heart into the arterial circulation during chest compression, when the cardiac valves prevent retrograde blood flow. It is also presumed that air moves freely out of the lungs, so that intrathoracic pressure does not rise, and that the pulmonary circulation (pulm. circ.) is not affected by chest compression. With chest relaxation, the heart would expand and fill with blood, and air would passively return into the lungs.

With the intrathoracic pressure pump, it is postulated that chest compression causes a rise in intrathoracic pressure (large arrows), which is transmitted to the intrathoracic vasculature. It is presumed that intrathoracic pressure can rise because of the collapse of airways (above the C), which reduces movement of air out of the lungs. All the intrathoracic structures are reduced in size, but not necessarily equally. There is also collapse of venous structures at the thoracic inlet (below the C), which helps prevent retrograde venous blood flow. With chest relaxation, there would be a fall in intrathoracic pressure and return of venous blood from the periphery into the thoracic venous system.

intrathoracic pressure that is transmitted to the intrathoracic vasculature (see Fig. 2–4). Intrathoracic arterial pressure is transmitted fully to extrathoracic arteries. Intrathoracic venous pressure is not, however, transmitted to the extrathoracic veins because of the large extrathoracic venous compliance and because of the closure of venous valves. This differential transmission of intrathoracic pressure to the extrathoracic vasculature produces extrathoracic arterial–venous pressure gradients, which cause blood to flow out of the thorax. With the release of chest compression, there would be a fall in intrathoracic pressure and a return of venous blood from the periphery into the thoracic venous system. Coronary flow, which is entirely inside the thorax, appears to be dependent on the extrathoracic arteries. As intrathoracic pressure rises during chest compression, blood moves from intrathoracic arteries to extrathoracic arteries. As intrathoracic pressure falls during chest relaxation, it appears that some blood from the extrathoracic arteries flows retrogradely into the intrathoracic arteries to perfuse the coronary arteries.

For intrathoracic pressure fluctuations, the amount of thoracic volume reduction produced by chest compression seems to be critical. According to Boyle's law, the more the chest volume is reduced, the more the intrathoracic pressure rises. In current clinical practice, chest volume is reduced by using the standard anteroposterior sternal displacement technique, although other techniques are being studied that may prove to be more effective.[19–21] For maximizing cardiac compression, however, the amount of thoracic volume reduction is probably not important. The major determinant of cardiac compression is probably the amount of anteroposterior chest displacement, although the exact determinants of cardiac compression are unknown. Whether the driving force for blood movement is intrathoracic pressure fluctuation or direct cardiac compression, the amount of chest compression is a critical determinant of flow (Fig. 2–5), and the quality of chest compression is likely to be a major factor in the effectiveness of CPR.

The amount of chest compression force, or displacement, appears to be a major determinant of the level of generated vascular pressure,[22, 23] but chest compression also has to be applied at the optimal rate and duration. Blood flow caused by intrathoracic pressure fluctuations should be insensitive to rate over a wide range but dependent on the duration of compression.[23–26] If direct compression of the heart plays a major role, however, flow should depend on rate. Above a specific threshold, flow should be insensitive to compression duration. The current recommendation of a rate of 80 to 100 compressions per minute probably maximizes blood flow from either pump. At that rate, the compression duration tends to be about 50% of the compression cycle,[27] which is optimal for moving blood by means of intrathoracic pressure fluctuations.[25] The rate of 80 to 100 compressions per minute is near the maximum that can be administered for any length of time by a rescuer and maximize the number of stroke volumes delivered to the circulation by a cardiac compression pump.[25]

The Use of Epinephrine

Numerous studies have shown that vascular pressures are improved and blood flow to the heart muscle and brain is increased with the use of vasoconstrictors.[28–31] This increased flow appears to be mediated through α-adrenergic agonism,[32–34] which increases peripheral resistance and decreases run-off of blood to the periphery. Decreased run-off slows the decay of arterial pressure during the release phase of chest compression, thereby raising aortic pressure, myocardial perfusion pressure (aortic minus right atrial mean release phase pressure), and cerebral perfusion pressure (carotid minus intracranial mean pressure).

The vasoconstrictor used most commonly today is epinephrine, which has both α- and β-agonist effects. It is clear that the α-agonist effects are responsible for the improvement in flow in vital organs. The utility of the β-agonist effects, however, is controversial. Some investigators believe that β-agonism is detrimental because it increases myocardial work,[28, 32] whereas others believe that β-agonism is beneficial because it increases inotropy.[32] The efficacy of epinephrine as compared with other vasoconstrictors remains to be determined.

There is currently much interest in using increased doses of epinephrine to augment vital organ flow during CPR, especially later in resuscitation when tissue acidosis, hypoxia, and ischemia may be more profound. The exact role of high-dose epinephrine has not been determined because of conflicting clinical and laboratory data.[35–39] Increased doses of epinephrine, which increase peripheral resistance, can increase blood flow to the heart muscle and brain.[30, 40] Increased doses of epinephrine may, however, have direct toxic effects on tissues and

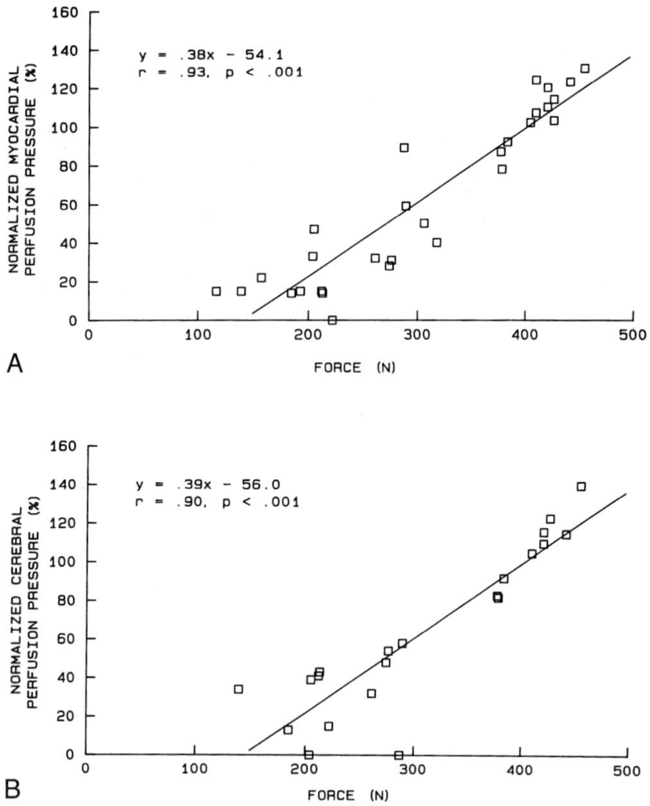

Figure 2–5. A: Correlation between normalized myocardial perfusion pressure and applied sternal force for manual CPR in a dog. The perfusion pressures for each dog are expressed as a percentage of the perfusion pressure obtained at an applied sternal force of 400 newtons (N) for that dog. B: Correlation between cerebral perfusion pressure and applied sternal force for manual CPR. Normalization was performed. There is a strong correlation ($p < .001$) between normalized perfusion pressures and applied force. (From Halperin HR et al. Determinants of blood flow during CPR. Circulation 1986;73:539–550.)

may exacerbate ischemic damage to other tissue by shunting blood away from them. The utility of high-dose epinephrine in favorably altering the loading conditions during external chest compression CPR is, therefore, questionable.

In contrast to its ability to increase blood flow to the myocardium and brain, increased peripheral resistance can reduce total cardiac output. Cardiac output is reduced because the increases in peripheral resistance are greater than the increases in generated vascular pressures.[30, 41] This decreased cardiac output can explain the observation that end-tidal carbon dioxide can decrease with increased doses of epinephrine.[30] End-tidal carbon dioxide has been studied as a noninvasive method of determining the adequacy of resuscitation because it appears to correlate with cardiac output and resuscitation success in some circumstances.[42]

In addition to the effects of vascular resistance and compliance on blood flow during CPR, it appears that the volume status contributes independently. If excessive volume is present in the vascular spaces during CPR, the venous pressures tend to be elevated during the release phase of chest compression, which can reduce the coronary perfusion pressure.[43] This finding strongly suggests that excessive volume should not be infused during resuscitation. If insufficient volume is present, however, forward flow appears to be compromised because arterial collapse is induced. Selective arterial infusion does appear to be of potential value in reversing this arterial collapse.[44]

Ventilation

If hypoxia resulting from an obstructed airway is the cause of cardiac arrest, it is obvious that the airway must be cleared for the patient to be successfully resuscitated. Even when cardiac arrest is not due to hypoxia, emergency ventilation has been considered an essential component of CPR. There are few studies and little direct evidence, however, that ventilation affects outcomes of cardiac arrest in nonhypoxic cardic arrest, although it has been assumed to be crucial for resuscitation. Recommendations for ventilation were based on studies performed in the 1950s and 1960s in living humans with normal cardiac output.[45–47] These studies assumed that the goal of ventilation during CPR was to achieve near normal tidal volumes and minute ventilation. Substantially less ventilation may be sufficient for gas exchange during CPR, however, because cardiac output and pulmonary blood flow are only 10% to 15% of normal during manual chest compression. As a consequence, the amount of hemoglobin passing through the pulmonary bed is reduced, and the amount of oxygen necessary to saturate hemoglobin is also reduced if the ventilation-perfusion mismatch is not large. Because venous return—and, thus, the quantity of carbon dioxide delivered to the lungs—are decreased, the amount of ventilation necessary to remove carbon dioxide is, presumably, reduced.

The amount of time before ventilation must be initiated during CPR to achieve satisfactory results as well as the ventilatory requirements during CPR are unclear. In a canine model of cardiac arrest, arterial pH, P_{CO_2}, and P_{O_2} demonstrated no significant change after 5 minutes of untreated ventricular fibrillation,[48] whereas arterial P_{O_2} decreased significantly in a swine model.[49] In a rat model, chest compression alone produced tidal volumes of 26% of baseline, and although arterial P_{CO_2} increased to 80 mm Hg after 9 minutes, the resuscitation rate was not impaired.[50] The animals were intubated in all of these studies. It is likely that ventilation induced by chest compression would be less in nonintubated models, but the effect this would have on blood gases is unknown.

Other studies have shown that ventilation plays an important role in resuscitation. An early study showed that well-oxygenated dogs had better carotid artery blood flow than did asphyxiated dogs. This was attributed to loss of peripheral vascular tone.[51] Yang and colleagues showed that spontaneous gasping during cardiac arrest in a swine model favored successful resuscitation and also showed that both the frequency and the duration of the gasps correlated with coronary perfusion pressure and predicted outcome.[52]

Three recent studies were specifically designed to test the effect of ventilation on outcome in swine models of CPR. One study compared a group receiving mechanical ventilation during CPR with a group receiving chest compression alone and with a group without chest compression or ventilation. The duration of untreated ventricular fibrillation was 30 seconds, followed by 12 minutes of CPR in the treatment groups. All animals were successfully defibrillated and entered a 2-hour intensive-care period. However, after 24 hours, only 2 of 8 animals that had had no CPR survived, whereas all 16 animals survived in the groups receiving chest compression, both with and without ventilation. Another study allocated 24 swine to groups with and without ventilation during 10 minutes of chest compression following 6 minutes of untreated ventricular fibrillation; 9 of 12 ventilated animals and only 1 of 12 nonventilated animals experienced a return of spontaneous circulation. The nonventilated animals died with significantly greater arterial and mixed venous hypoxemia and hypercarbia.[53] A follow-up study tested whether hypoxemia or hypercarbia independently affects survival of cardiac arrest. In a swine model of isolated arterial and mixed venous hypoxemia without hypercarbia in one group, and isolated hypercarbia without hypoxemia in another group, only 1 of the 10 animals in each group experienced the return of spontaneous circulation. There were important differences among the three studies, including the duration of untreated ventricular fibrillation, the use of 100% oxygen before cardiac arrest, and whether or not agonal respirations were prevented by administering a paralytic agent. Taken together, these studies provide some evidence that ventilation may possibly be withheld when chest compression is initiated promptly after cardiac arrest, but that ventilation is important for survival when chest compression is delayed.

Even fewer human studies of the role of ventilation during cardiac arrest are available. Because ventilation is such a well-accepted intervention, the ethical considerations involved in doing a controlled study by withholding ventilation in one group may be untenable. Nevertheless, there exists some indirect evidence pointing to the role of ventilation during resuscitation. For example, in Seattle, where ambulance response time is short, patients who had spontaneous agonal respiratory efforts immediately after cardiac arrest had higher rates of successful resuscitation.[54] Another study found that hypoxemia and hypercarbia were associated with the use of an esophageal obturator airway in the field and also with a lower resuscitation rate. Mixed venous oxygen saturation is associated with a prognosis for survival of hemorrhagic shock related to cardiac arrest, and mixed venous pH, P_{O_2}, and P_{CO_2} measured during cardiac arrest were significantly better in those with return of spontaneous circulation.[55] In the Netherlands, clinical CPR is given in the following order: chest compression, airway, breathing; ventilation is delayed and chest compression is initiated as soon as possible. Data

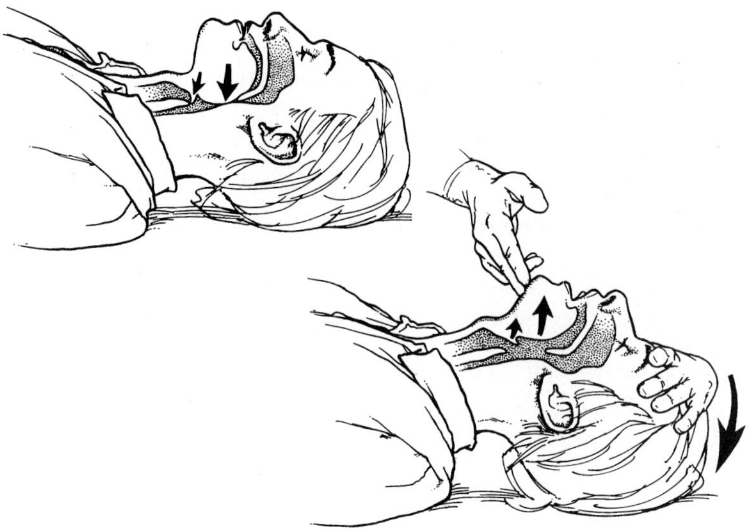

Figure 2–6. Opening the airway. Top: Airway obstruction produced by tongue and epiglottis. Bottom: Relief is provided by performing the head-tilt–chin-lift. (Reproduced with permission. *Advanced Cardiac Life Support,* 1997. © Copyright American Heart Association.)

from the Netherlands concerning survival after CPR show rates comparable to those reported in the United States.[56] Data concerning humans also suggest that prompt chest compression after cardiac arrest improves brain and heart perfusion and the success of defibrillation.

Thus, the role of ventilation during CPR is becoming more controversial. In the past it was thought that adequate ventilation was critical to delivering sufficient oxygenation to the tissues. Now it is being recognized that during the low-flow states of CPR, it is probable that much less than normal ventilation is needed. In addition, the time required to place an endotracheal tube may actually compromise the resuscitative efforts, if the patient was not initially hypoxic, as ischemia resulting from the lack of chest compressions may be more detrimental. If the cardiac arrest is due to hypoxia, however, securing a proper airway and adequate ventilation are critical (Figs. 2–6 and 2–7).

OUTCOMES

Overall survival rates average around 15% for cardiac arrests that occur in a hospital. For arrests that occur outside of the hospital, survival rates are generally lower. For arrests that occur in the setting of a procedure, survival rates can be much higher, as the cause is often reversible and there should be little delay in starting resuscitative measures. Arrests that occur in this setting can be caused by the patient's underlying disease or can be precipitated by an extrinsic event such as sudden occlusion of the airway, an adverse reaction to a medication, or an acute loss of vascular volume. Survival of cardiac arrest is related to the underlying cause as well as to the vigilance of the medical staff and the speed with which they recognize and appropriately treat the arrest. Rapidly reversible causes of arrest should be actively sought and definitively treated so as to produce the greatest number of survivors.

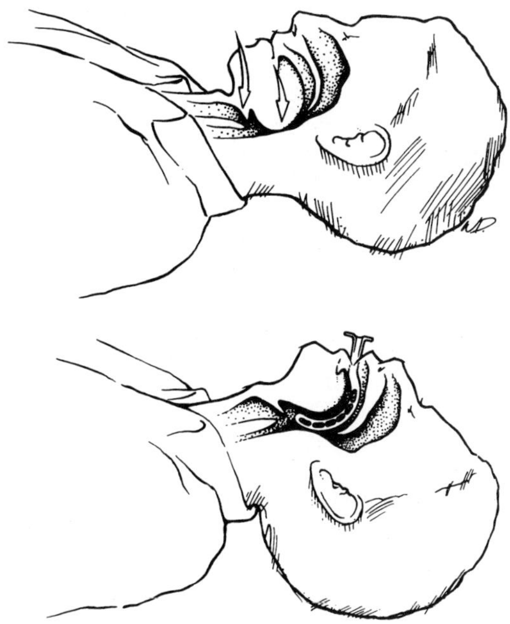

Figure 2–7. Correctly inserted oropharyngeal airway. Top: Before insertion; head position is incorrect. Bottom: After insertion; head is tilted and oropharyngeal airway is in place. (Reproduced with permission. *Advanced Cardiac Life Support,* 1997. © Copyright American Heart Association.)

REFERENCES

1. Guidelines for cardiopulmonary resuscitation and emergency cardiac care. Emergency Cardiac Care Committee and Subcommittees, American Heart Association, Part III: Adult advanced cardiac life support. JAMA 1992;268:2199–2241.
2. Gallagher J, Lombardi G, Gennis P. Effectiveness of bystander cardiopulmonary resuscitation and survival following out-of-hospital cardiac arrest. JAMA 1995;274:1922–1925.
3. Hoeyweghen R et al. Quality and efficacy of bystander CPR. Resuscitation 1993;26:47–52.
4. Cummins RO. From concept to standard of care? Ann Emerg Med 1989;18:1269–1275.
5. Atkins D, Kerber RE. Pediatric defibrillation: importance of paddle size in determining transthoracic impedance. Pediatrics 1988;82:914–918.
6. Atkins D, Kerber R. Pediatric defibrillation: current flow is improved by using "adult" paddle electrodes. Pediatrics 1994;94:90–93.
7. Bardy GH et al. Evaluation of electrode polarity on defibrillation efficacy. Am J Cardiol 1989;63:433–437.
8. Schuder JC et al. Is the effectiveness of cardiac ventricular defibrillation dependent upon polarity? Med Instrum 1987;21:262–265.
9. Lerman BB, Deale OC. Relation between transcardiac and transthoracic current during defibrillation in humans. Circ Res 1990;67:1420–1426.
10. Kerber RE et al. Self-adhesive pre–applied electrode pads for defibrillation and cardioversion: experimental and clinical studies. J Am Coll Cardiol 1984;3:815–820.
11. American National Standard Automatic External Defibrillators and Remote-control Defibrillarors. Arlington, VA, Association for the Advancement of Medical Instrumentation, 1993.
12. Martin DR et al. Initial countershock in the treatment of asystole. Resuscitation 1993;26:63–68.
13. Ewy GA et al. Ventricular fibrillation masquerading as ventricular standstill. Crit Care Med 1981;9:841–844.
14. Halperin HR et al. Vest inflation without simultaneous ventilation during cardiac arrest in dogs: improved survival from prolonged cardiopulmonary resuscitation. Circulation 1986;74:1407–1415.
15. Paradis NA, Martin GB, Rivers EP. Coronary perfusion pressure and the return of spontaneous circulation in human cardiopulmonary resuscitation. JAMA 1990; 263:1106–1113.
16. Eleff SM et al. Brain bioenergetics during cardiopulmonary resuscitation in dogs. Anesthesiology 1992;76:77–84.
17. Kowenhouven WB, Jude JR, Knickerbocker GG. Closed chest cardiac massage. JAMA 1960;173:1063.
18. Rudikoff MT, Maughan WL, Effron M, Freund P, Weisfeldt ML: Mechanisms of blood flow during cardiopulmonary resuscitation. Circulation 1980:61:345–352.
19. Halperin HR et al. A preliminary study of cardiopulmonary resuscitation by circumferential compression of the chest with use of a pneumatic vest. N Engl J Med 1993;329:762–768.
20. Cohen TJ et al. A comparison of active compression-decompression cardiopulmonary resuscitation with standard cardiopulmonary resuscitation for cardiac arrests occurring in the hospital. N Engl J Med 1993;329:1918–1921.
21. Sack JB, Kesselbrenner MB, Bregman D. Survival from in-hospital cardiac arrest with interposed abdominal counterpulsation during cardiopulmonary resuscitation [comments]. JAMA 1992;267:379–385.
22. Halperin HR, Weisfeldt ML. New approaches to CPR: four hands, a plunger, or a vest [editorial]. JAMA 1992;267:2940–2941.
23. Halperin HR et al. Determinants of blood flow to vital organs during cardiopulmonary resuscitation in dogs. Circulation 1986;73:539–550.
24. Taylor et al. Importance of prolonged compression during cardiopulmonary resuscitation in man. N Engl J Med 1977;296:1515–1517.
25. Halperin HR et al. Intrathoracic pressure fluctuations move blood during CPR: comparison of hemodynamic data with predictions from a mathematical model. Ann Biomed Eng 1987;15:385–403.
26. Babbs CF et al. Cardiac, thoracic, and abdominal pump mechanisms in cardiopulmonary resuscitation: studies in an electrical model of the circulation. Am J Emerg Med 1984;2:299–308.
27. Maier GW et al. The physiology of external cardiac massage: high-impulse cardiopulmonary resuscitation. Circulation 1984;70:86–101.
28. Ditchey RV, Slinker BK. Phenylephrine plus propranolol improves the balance between myocardial oxygen supply and demand during experimental cardiopulmonary resuscitation. Am Heart J 1994;127:324–330.
29. Lindner KH et al. Effects of active compression-decompression resuscitation on myocardial and cerebral blood flow in pigs. Circulation 1993;88:1254–1263.
30. von Planta I et al. Coronary perfusion pressure, end-tidal CO_2 and adrenergic agents in haemodynamic stable rats. Resuscitation 1993;25:203–217.
31. Berkowitz ID et al. Epinephrine dosage effects on cerebral and myocardial blood flow in an infant swine model of cardiopulmonary resuscitation. Anesthesiology 1991;75:1041–1050.
32. Halperin H, Guerci A. Vasoconstrictors during CPR: are they used optimally? Chest 1990;98:787–789.
33. Redding JS, Pearson JW. Evaluation of drugs for cardiac resuscitation. Anesthesiology 1963;24:203–207.
34. Yakaitis R, Otto C, Blitt C. Relative importance of alpha and beta adrenergic receptors during resuscitation. Crit Care Med 1979;7:293–296.
35. Berg RA et al. High-dose epinephrine results in greater early mortality after resuscitation from prolonged cardiac arrest in pigs: a prospective, randomized study. Crit Care Med 1994;22:282–290.
36. O'Neil BJ, Wilson RF. The controversies in cardiopulmonary resuscitation on high-dose epinephrine still continue [editorial]. Crit Care Med 1994;22:194–195.
37. Lipman J et al. High-dose adrenaline in adult in-hospital asystolic cardiopulmonary resuscitation: a double-blind randomised trial. Anaesth Intensive Care 1993;21:192–196.
38. Gonzalez ER, Ornato JP. The dose of epinephrine during cardiopulmonary resuscitation in humans: what should it be? [review]. DICP 1991;25:773–777.
39. Brown CG et al. The effect of high-dose phenylephrine versus epinephrine on regional cerebral blood flow during CPR. Ann Emerg Med 1987;16:743–748.
40. Gonzalez ER et al. Dose-dependent vasopressor response to epinephrine during CPR in human beings [comments]. Ann Emerg Med 1989;18:920–926.
41. Rayburn B et al. Cardiac output may not reflect levels of myocardial and cerebral flow during cardiopulmonary resuscitation [abstract]. Circulation 1988;78:II-239.
42. Falk JL, Rackow EC, Weil MH. End-tidal carbon dioxide concentration during cardiopulmonary resuscitation. N Engl J Med 1988;318:607–611.
43. Ditchey RV, Lindenfeld J. Potential adverse effects of

volume loading on perfusion of vital organs during closed-chest resuscitation. Circulation 1984;69:181–189.
44. Paradis NA et al. High atrial natriuretic peptide concentrations blunt the pressor response during cardiopulmonary resuscitation in humans. Crit Care Med 1994;22:213–218.
45. Safar P. Failure of manual respiration. J Appl Physiol 1959;14:84–88.
46. Safar P et al. Ventilation and circulation with closed-chest cardiac massage in man. JAMA 1961;176:574–576.
47. Safar P, Escarraga LA, Elam JO. A comparison of the mouth-to-mouth and mouth-to-airway methods of artificial respiration with the chest-pressure arm-lift methods. N Engl J Med 1958;258:671–677.
48. Meursing BTJ, Zimmerman ANE, van Heyst ANP. Experimental evidence in favor of a reversed sequence in cardiopulmonary resuscitation [abstract]. J Am Coll Cardiol 1983;1:610.
49. Tucker KJ et al. Changes in arterial and mixed venous blood gases during untreated ventricular fibrillation and cardiopulmonary resuscitation. Resuscitation 1994; 28:137–141.
50. Tang W et al. Myocardial function after CPR by precordial compression without mechanical ventilation. Chest 1991;100 (suppl):1325.
51. Pearson JW, Redding JS. Influence of peripheral vascular tone on cardiac resuscitation. Anesth Analg 1965;44:746–752.
52. Yang L et al. Spontaneous gasping increases the ability to resuscitate during experimental cardiopulmonary resuscitation. Crit Care Med 1994;22:879–883.
53. Idris AH et al. The effect of ventilation on resuscitation in an animal model of cardiac arrest. Circulation 1994;190:3063–3069.
54. Clark JJ et al. Incidence of agonal respirations in sudden cardiac arrest. Ann Emerg Med 1992;21:1464–1467.
55. Kazarian KK, del Guercio LRM. The use of mixed venous blood gas determinations in traumatic shock. Ann Emerg Med 1980;9:179–180.

CHAPTER **3**

Shock

Pamela A. Lipsett, MD

Circulatory shock is the single most common indication for admission to the intensive care unit (ICU). Shock is not a diagnosis but rather a physiologic state that is characterized by inadequate tissue oxygenation. A shock state can occur when the supply of oxygen is insufficient to meet metabolic demands or when the tissues are unable to use oxygen and other nutrients to meet these demands. Uncorrected, shock inevitably leads to the death of cells, tissues, organs, and the patient.

Although commonly regarded as inadequate blood pressure or hypoperfusion, shock stemming from all causes is best considered in terms of inadequate tissue oxygenation because that leads to a rational therapeutic approach—to deliver oxygen supply adequate to match the metabolic rate. Oxygen delivery (DO_2) is the rate of oxygen transport in arterial blood. It is defined as the product of cardiac output (Q) and the arterial oxygen content (CaO_2):

$$DO_2 = Q \times CaO_2$$

The arterial oxygen content is either bound to hemoglobin or dissolved in plasma. As seen in the equation

$$CaO_2 = (1.3 \times Hgb \times SaO_2)\ (0.003 \times PaO_2),$$

where Hgb is the hemoglobin, SaO_2 is the oxygen saturation, and PaO_2 is the arterial oxygen, the greatest changes in oxygen delivery occur with changes in cardiac output and hemoglobin, both of which are targets for directed therapy.

Oxygen uptake is the final step in the oxygen transport pathway. It represents the oxygen supply for tissue metabolism. The Fick equation defines oxygen uptake (VO_2) as the product of cardiac output and the arteriovenous difference in oxygen content ($CaO_2 - CvO_2$):

$$(VO_2 = Q \times (CaO_2 - CvO_2).$$

Because most tissue cannot store oxygen, the oxygen uptake from capillaries is considered to be the metabolic consumption of oxygen. When oxygen uptake is impaired, such as in sepsis, trauma, or burns, this relationship may not hold true.

The oxygen extraction ratio (O_2ER) is the fractional uptake of oxygen from the capillary bed. It is derived from the ratio of oxygen uptake to oxygen delivery:

$$O_2ER = VO_2/DO_2 \times 100$$

Normally, the rate of oxygen delivery exceeds the rate of uptake by a wide margin, which means that only a small amount of available oxygen is extracted from the capillary blood under normal conditions (22% to 32%). This allows tissue to adjust to decreases in blood flow by increasing oxygen extraction. This increase in oxygen extraction occurs in all vascular beds except the coronary circulation and the diaphragm. The inability of the coronary circulation to further increase its oxygen extraction partially explains why shock is a life-threatening condition.

Shock can be classified by clinical syndrome or cause or by considering the aspects of the circulation that have failed. No single manner of classifying shock is universally accepted; grasping the differences in hemodynamic presentation is critical. The conventional terms used to classify shock are hypovolemic, cardiogenic, neurogenic, and anaphylactic. However, these are probably better considered as syndromes—hypovolemic shock, cardiogenic shock, and vasogenic shock (Table 3–1). They are described in detail later.

The simplest way to understand shock and its assessment is to ask, Which part of the circulation has failed? The circulation can be divided into the pipes, the pump, and the perfusate.

Table 3–1. General Appearance of a Patient in Shock

Neurologic: Mental agitation, confusion, or obtundation
Respiratory: Tachypnea, increased minute ventilation
Skin: Diaphoresis, pallor, delayed capillary refill

Syndrome	Neck Veins	Pulmonary Exam
Hypovolemic	Flat	Tachypnea, shallow respirations
Cardiogenic	Distended	Tachypnea, shallow respirations
Vasogenic	Flat	Tachypnea, shallow respirations (wheezing in anaphylaxis, sepsis)

Pipe failure is equivalent to vasogenic shock and is characterized as failure to maintain adequate peripheral vascular tone and, therefore, failure to maintain adequate mean arterial blood pressure to sustain adequate oxygen delivery to the tissues. Patients with pump failure display either inadequate primary cardiac function or embarrassment of venous return such as that which occurs in a tension pneumothorax or in pericardial tamponade. One of the most common causes of circulatory failure in surgical patients is perfusate failure, which is hypovolemic shock resulting from hemorrhage or dehydration.

In general, these conditions can be distinguished easily by history and by careful clinical examination. A central venous line or even a Swan-Ganz catheter may be useful in guiding therapy, but these devices are rarely required to establish the presence of a shock state and begin correction of it. In the following sections, methods of recognizing various types of shock are followed by approaches to evaluation and management.

GENERAL CLINICAL APPEARANCE

Recognition and immediate treatment of shock are essential. The magnitude, depth, and duration of shock influence the outcome, as does the underlying cause of the shock state. Common to all shock states is the neuroendocrine response to inadequate oxygen delivery—an outpouring of the stress hormones, epinephrine, glucagon, cortisol, and growth hormone, all to aid in systemic stability. The most prominent of these are the catecholamines, which cause tachycardia and vasoconstriction, which may be seen as a narrowed pulse pressure, delayed capillary refill, and cool extremities. Therefore, patients who are cool to the touch and have even mild tachycardia and weak pulses should be assumed to be in circulatory shock until proven otherwise (Table 3–2).

Although blood flow to the central nervous system is often preserved until very late in the shock state, a patient with shock often presents with anxiety and apprehension that are sometimes confused with a drug ingestion or metabolic abnormality. A patient with mental obtundation and shock is demonstrating a profound degree of shock that requires immediate intervention.

Because in shock, oxygen delivery to local, regional, or global tissues is inadequate, the usual respiratory compensation for an increase in oxygen delivery is an increase in ventilatory rate. Usually, it is accompanied by somewhat shallow respiration, but the overall effect is an increase in minute ventilation.

HYPOVOLEMIC SHOCK

Presentation and Evaluation

Patients who present with hypovolemic shock are easily recognizable clinically. Aside from showing the general traits described above, a patient with hypovolemic shock may be diaphoretic and have cool extremities, a weak, thready pulse, and flat neck veins. Thus, quickly palpating an extremity pulse immediately conveys the

Table 3–2. Common Shock Syndromes

Syndrome	Cause
Hypovolemic	Hemorrhage
	Dehydration
Cardiogenic	Acute myocardial infarction
	Ischemia
	Valvular rupture
	Atrioventricular septal defect
	Arrhythmia
Vasogenic	Sepsis
	Neurogenic
	Anaphylaxis
	Pancreatitis
	Adrenal insufficiency
	Cirrhosis
	Arteriovenous fistula

temperature and perfusion of that extremity; looking for neck veins and listening to the lungs rapidly distinguishes the common shock syndromes (see Table 3–1).

The magnitude of the hypovolemia varies among patients; changes in vital signs are seen in proportion to the magnitude of the estimated blood volume lost. For example, in a 70-kg person, a 500-mL blood loss does not cause any alteration in hemodynamics and causes a minimal increase in heart rate and no change in blood pressure. This is the equivalent of donating a unit of blood and is well tolerated. In more significant blood loss, say 1,000 mL, the patient usually manifests changes in heart rate with a mild tachycardia (100), a narrowing of the pulse pressure, and an elevated diastolic pressure. Postural blood pressure, heart rate, or both are seen as is a mild decrease in urine output from the 0.5 mL/kg/h necessary to excrete a normal solute load.

Patients who lose more than 25% of their blood volume manifest changes in blood pressure. Tachycardia is then in the range of 120 to 140, depending on the magnitude of the volume loss. These patients require immediate restoration of blood volume and control of the underlying cause of the volume loss. Although measurement of central venous or pulmonary capillary wedge pressure and cardiac output is not necessary for a diagnosis of hypovolemic shock, these values can be predicted easily. Both central venous pressure and pulmonary capillary wedge pressure would be low, as would cardiac output. Because mean arterial blood pressure is often low, it follows that systemic vascular resistance is elevated, which is what would be expected, given the high catecholamine level (Table 3–3).

There are two common causes of hypovolemia in a surgical patient: hemorrhage and dehydration. The hypovolemia caused by dehydration is usually more gradual in onset and often can be diagnosed based on the patient's history of vomiting or diarrhea or on a serious mismatch in intake and output. In a patient with previously known hemoglobin levels, hemoconcentration is diagnostic of intravascular volume depletion. The effects of surgical procedures vary; some surgeries result in a large third-space fluid loss that demonstrates this physiology more acutely than fluid loss that results from vomiting.

In hemorrhagic states, the bleeding is either external and obvious, such as that which occurs with a carotid blow out, or it may be hidden internally, such as that which occurs with a ruptured aortic aneurysm or a mediastinal great vessel injury resulting from a central line mishap. If the bleeding is external, it should be immediately controlled by applying pressure directly to or just proximal to the site of bleeding. The use of tourniquets generally should be avoided.

Recognition of a hypovolemic patient is usually straightforward. One must be aware that patients who are being managed with agents that block the adrenergic system (atenolol, metoprolol, and so forth) may not manifest some of the classic findings of hypovolemic shock, namely tachycardia and elevation of the diastolic pressure. These patients may be at particular risk for injury caused by the shock state because of their diminished cardiac reserve, so knowing that these patients may have less of a response to volume loss may improve outcomes in this population.

CARDIOGENIC SHOCK

Presentation and Evaluation

Patients with cardiogenic shock have the same general characteristics as patients with hypovolemic shock. In addition, such patients present with distended neck veins, rales on chest auscultation, and cool extremities, which may also show signs of chronic congestive failure and peripheral edema (see Table 3–1). As is typical of patients in shock, the mean blood pressure is usually lower and the heart rate higher. Thus

Table 3–3. *Hemodynamic Picture: Shock Syndromes*

Syndrome	CVP	PCWP	CO	SVR
Hypovolemic	Low	Low	Low	High
Cardiogenic	High	High	Low	High
Vasogenic	Low/normal	Low/normal	High/normal	Low

CVP, central venous pressure; PCWP, pulmonary capillary wedge pressure; CO, cardiac output; SVR, systemic vascular resistance.

the pulmonary exam and the state of the neck veins are crucial in differentiating these patients from those with all other forms of shock. Patients in cardiogenic shock and with florid pulmonary edema generally do not benefit from any further intravascular volume expansion, whereas patients with the other forms of shock do benefit from fluid resuscitation. Jugular venous pressure and, usually, pulmonary capillary wedge pressure are substantially elevated (as is evidenced by distended neck veins), whereas cardiac output is low, and systemic vascular resistance is high (see Table 3–3). Thus, the major distinction between hypovolemic shock and cardiogenic shock is the status of the neck veins and the central venous pressure.

Cardiogenic shock can be intrinsic to the heart or extrinsic to the heart. Intrinsic cardiogenic shock results from primary cardiac failure, such as myocardial infarction, valvular rupture, acute atrioventricular septal defect, ischemia, or arrhythmia. The two most common circumstances in which a patient might develop intrinsic cardiogenic shock occur in the setting of perioperative care and in an elderly patient experiencing a cardiac event that precipitates a fall or an accident. The management of such a patient is aimed at minimizing myocardial oxygen consumption and eliminating ongoing ischemia, which are usually accomplished by normalizing the heart rate, thus allowing the coronary arteries time to fill during diastole, and by limiting myocardial work by optimizing preload and afterload.

Extrinsic cardiogenic failure can result from impaired venous return from the heart. Venous return is impaired in a pneumothorax, especially a tension pneumothorax, and also in pericardial tamponade. When a tension pneumothorax is present, the neck veins are distended; the trachea is shifted away from the side of the injury; breath sounds are absent or diminished (as heard in the axilla); and the side of the pneumothorax has a hyperresonant percussive sound. Based on these findings or on a high degree of clinical suspicion, a suspected tension pneumothorax should be treated with needle decompression of the affected hemithorax *prior* to obtaining a chest radiograph. As above, the hemodynamics are characterized by elevated central venous pressure and pulmonary wedge pressure, with low cardiac output and high systemic vascular resistance. Classically, the right and left heart pressures have been equalized in patients with cardiogenic failure and pericardial tamponade. Although patients with trauma are clearly at risk for tension pneumothorax and pericardial tamponade, either of these problems can present after an attempt at central line insertion. A tension pneumothorax can also result from barotrauma.

Pericardial tamponade is seen in patients with uremia and systemic inflammatory diseases, after a myocardial infarction and, increasingly, in patients afflicted with the human immunodeficiency virus. If possible, patients with suspected pericardial tamponade should undergo immediate echocardiography followed by pericardiocentesis.

VASOGENIC SHOCK

Presentation and Evaluation

Vasogenic shock may have a variety of clinical causes, but by far the most common is sepsis. Septic shock is the leading cause of death in the ICU, the 13th most common cause of death overall, and the most common type of shock encountered by internists. The primary problem in vasogenic shock is loss of tone in the arteries (low systemic vascular resistance). Usually, the cardiac output is elevated—thus the classic hyperdynamic and vasodilated state (see Table 3–3). This patient has the same general appearance as any other patient in shock, but often has warm extremities and flat neck veins (see Table 3–1). A patient may have a bounding distal pulse in spite of a low mean arterial blood pressure. This is the result of a characteristically low diastolic blood pressure and a widened pulse pressure. A patient may have wheezing as an early sign of endotoxemia and resulting acute pulmonary hypertension. Because of the associated tachypnea and hypotension, this is often confused with pulmonary embolus, but the classic hemodynamic findings differ.

Although cardiac output can vary dramatically in vasogenic shock, depending on the relative volume status, the volume status is usually low or low normal, the cardiac output normal or elevated, and the systemic vascular resistance low (see Table 3–3). Common causes of vasogenic shock are shown in Table 3–2. Previously considered separately as causes of shock, both neurogenic and anaphylactic shock are considered forms of vasogenic shock because of the primary defect in vascular tone that occurs in both of these conditions.

The pathogenesis of sepsis is very complex, and a number of studies have reported the likely sequence of events in the septic cascade. Sepsis progresses along a continuum from a localized nidus of infection, with local multiplication of the inciting organism, to the production or release of endotoxin (or other inflammatory cell-wall substances). The presence of endotoxin stimulates the production of both nonspecific and specific immune stimulants, such as the cytokines (tumor necrosis factor; TNF), the interleukins (IL), platelet activating factor (PAF), eicosanoids, complement components, kinins, and other molecular mediators that cause the systemic inflammatory response syndrome.

The sepsis cascade is classically triggered by the release of endotoxin into the circulation by gram-negative bacteria or by a comparable gram-positive or fungal cell wall substance. These substances then stimulate the release of mediators such as TNF, IL-1, IL-6, IL-8, PAF, and histamine from a variety of cells. There is activation of the coagulation, complement, and kinin cascades. Almost all of these substances directly or indirectly act on the vascular endothelium to cause vasodilatation or vasoconstriction, maldistribution of blood flow and, ultimately, endothelial damage with capillary leak syndrome. Failure of the microcirculation is the final common pathway in sepsis that results in or contributes to the development of the multiple organ dysfunction syndrome.

A patient should be suspected of having sepsis as the underlying cause of shock if the above hemodynamics are manifested, especially in the setting of previous episodes of mental confusion or glucose intolerance, which are early signs of infection in a postoperative patient.

A patient with neurogenic shock has low systemic vascular resistance and usually an adequate or high cardiac output. Most often such a patient has undergone neuraxial anesthesia or has suffered an acute neurologic or spinal injury. A patient with a lower spinal injury shows a hemodynamic profile similar to that of a septic patient, but without fever. A patient with a high spinal injury or block loses the cardiac accelerators and thus does not have tachycardia but displays the usual syndrome of low SVR, high cardiac output, and low (or normal) filling pressures.

Anaphylaxis is an immediate systemic hypersensitivity event that is produced by IgE-mediated release of chemicals from mast cells and basophils. The term "anaphylactoid reaction" designates a clinically similar event that is not mediated by antigen and IgE. Although the incidence of anaphylactic reactions is not known, it is estimated to be between 10 cases in 100,000 and 4 cases in 1,000,000. As new drugs and exposures occur, the incidence of anaphylaxis is likely to increase. Anaphylaxis must always be considered a possible cause in a patient with shock. Though some factors such as atopia predispose to anaphylaxis, this reaction can occur in any patient at any time. A rapid onset of 3 to 5 minutes is seen with exposure to intravenous antigens or latex. In hospitalized patients, agents that are especially likely to incite anaphylaxis are radiocontrast media, plasma expanders, anesthetics, aspirin, penicillin, and latex (Table 3–4).

The inflammatory, cytokine, complement, and kinin cascades are commonly activated in anaphylaxis. Histamine is perhaps the best-characterized and most important mediator of anaphylaxis. Histamine acts through both the H_1 and H_2 receptors to produce the clinical characteristics of anaphylaxis (Table 3–5). The three most life-threatening manifestations of anaphylaxis are airway edema, bronchospasm, and shock. The two events that lead to shock are vasodilatation and increased vascular permeability. This increase in vascular permeability, though generically like sepsis, can result in a dramatic shift of intravascular volume to extravascular fluid and resulting hypovolemia and shock. As much as 50% of intravascular volume can be lost in 10 minutes. The catecholamines and angiotensin I, which is converted to angiotensin II, are an attempt to cause vasoconstriction.

Table 3–4. *Agents that Cause Anaphylactic or Anaphylactoid Reactions*

Anaphylactic (IgE) Reactions
Food (peanuts, shellfish)
Drugs (antibiotics, insulin, colloid solutions)
Latex
Anaphylactoid Reactions
Direct release of mediators from mast cells
Drugs (especially morphine)
Environmental stimuli (cold, sunlight)
Exercise
Idiopathic sources
Disturbances in arachidonic acid metabolism
Aspirin
Nonsteroidal anti-inflammatory drugs
Administration of immune aggregates
Dextran and albumin
Intravenous gammaglobulin
Cytotoxins
Transfusion reactions
Miscellaneous and multimediator activity
Nonantigen/antibody-mediated complement
Radiocontrast material
Dialysis membranes
Protamine reactions (possibly)
Activation of complement system
Radiocontrast material
Dialysis membranes

Table 3–5. Mast Cell and Basophil Mediators in Anaphylaxis

Mediator	Event	Clinical Manifestations
Histamine	H_1 and H_2 receptors Rise in vascular permeability Contraction of smooth muscle Secretions from exocrine glands Irritation of sensory nerves	Flush, urticaria, angioedema, wheeze, hypotension, abdominal cramps, diarrhea
Lipo-oxygenase pathway (LTB4, LTC4, LTD4)	Chemotaxis Contraction of airway smooth muscles Rise in vascular permeability Secretions from goblet mucosal glands	Possible late phase Possible wheeze and hypotension
Cyclo-oxygenase pathway (PGD12, PGF2A, thromboxane A2)	Peripheral vasodilation Contraction of airway smooth muscles Coronary vasoconstriction Secretions from goblet and submucosal glands	Flush, hypotension, possible wheeze, myocardial ischemia

Because urticaria and angioedema are the most common signs of anaphylaxis, the absence of these findings mitigates against anaphylaxis as the cause of hypotension, especially if the patient does not have bronchospasm. If the mechanism of the shock episode remains in question, and the patient is seen promptly after the event, a serum tryptase level can be obtained. Serum tryptase levels peak 1.0 to 1.5 hours after the onset of anaphylaxis and can remain elevated for up to 5 hours. A serum histamine level is usually not helpful because it is elevated for only 1 hour after the event, but a 24-hour urine collection to determine levels of histamine and its metabolites can be useful.

PRIORITIES

Initial interventions are aimed at both diagnosis of and therapy for shock. The goal of therapy in all shock states is to ensure adequate delivery of oxygen to the peripheral tissue. As is true of any emergency, one must ensure that the ABCs (airway, breathing, circulation) are followed. Although it may not be immediately obvious, one must recognize that the airway may be compromised in a patient with anaphylaxis and neurogenic causes of shock. Ensuring the safety of a patient's airway is thus the first step. One must assess the overall neurologic status of the patient and the ability of the patient to protect his or her airway. Consideration must also be given to the overall condition of the patient. For example, a patient who has substantial hemorrhage from the neck and requires surgery will need airway control.

Providing oxygen is the single most important treatment to administer in a patient with shock. Oxygen should be immediately applied at a concentration of 100%. The only caution to observe in administering 100% oxygen is that a very few patients may have lost their CO_2 drive and are depending on hypoxic drive for ventilation. Ventilation is then ensured by bilateral auscultation of the chest, which is a critical step of the physical examination because it may identify a tension pneumothorax, a hemothorax, pulmonary edema, or wheezing consistent with anaphylaxis.

A tension pneumothorax is treated immediately upon suspicion of the diagnosis in a hypotensive patient with absent or diminished breath sounds and certainly in a patient with concurrent tracheal deviation and jugular venous distention. Treatment involves the use of a large-bore needle (angiocatheter), preferably a no. 14 or larger, in the midclavicular line and perpendicular to the skin in the second (or third) intercostal space, just over a rib. The presence of a tension pneumothorax is confirmed by the release of a large amount of air (hissing through the catheter) and clinical improvement of the patient. A chest tube should be placed irrespective of the identification of a sound, because lung injury would occur with the needle placement if a tension pneumothorax were not present. This is a small price to pay for a life-saving intervention by the few patients in whom the diagnosis is in error.

A bedside oxygen saturation monitor can provide immediate and ongoing information about the global saturation of the blood, and saturation should be monitored. Although

100% saturation is ideal, any saturation above 90% provides acceptable peripheral unloading of oxygen. Because the oxygen hemoglobin dissociation curve is sigmoidal in shape, a saturation of 90% is usually equal to a PaO_2 of more than 60 mm Hg. Recall that a patient receiving supplemental oxygen may not be adequately ventilated either primarily or as a compensation for another metabolic process. This is most notable in, for instance, a patient with a narcotic overdose who is ventilating inadequately. Oxygen saturation declines only at the very terminal stages of hypoventilation; with supplemental oxygen, saturation will be improved, but not ventilation. This can be seen by recalling the alveolar gas equation $\{PaO_2 = [(P_B - P_{H2O}) \times F_IO_2] - (PaCO_2/0.8)\}$. For example, a patient breathing room air with self-administering analgesia and too high a dose of narcotics can have supplemental oxygen doubled to 40% with a concomitant rise in the $PaCO_2$ to over 100 mm Hg before the saturation is affected. Therefore, an arterial blood gas is necessary when ventilation abnormalities or acidosis is suspected. If the clinical picture is severe, endotracheal intubation should be considered and the patient should be transferred immediately to an ICU.

Circulatory status is the next priority. Clinical assessment is performed as above. If hypotension is a reflection of hypovolemia, the patient has lost at least 25% of circulating blood volume, and this volume must be restored immediately. Two large-bore peripheral lines provide intravenous access adequate for most initial resuscitations. A large-bore catheter is preferred to a central venous catheter because of principles of flow and physics; flow is directly proportional to the length of the catheter and inversely proportional to the fourth power of the radius of the catheter. Once access is obtained, the hemoglobin level should be determined immediately and blood should be sent for typing.

In a patient in shock, the second major goal of therapy is to improve cardiac output. In virtually all shock states, except in a patient with florid pulmonary edema, the cardiac output can be improved immediately by a rapid increase in preload, that is, with volume infusion. Each patient in circulatory shock should receive a bolus of a balanced salt solution at a dose of 20 mL/kg. The choice of the balanced salt solution should be Ringer's lactate solution in most cases because it is iso-osmolar (Table 3–6) and has a pH closest to that of serum (though still acidic). Patients given large volumes of normal saline develop a hyperchloremic metabolic acidosis. However, normal saline is an acceptable alternative solution.

Table 3–6. *Resuscitation Fluids: Crystalloids*

Fluid	Osmolality	pH
Ringer's lactate solution	273	6.7
Normal saline (0.9%)	308	5.7
Saline 3%	1026	5.7

For the past three decades, an active debate has been going on about the value of crystalloid solutions over colloid solutions and vice versa. The fact that this debate has been ongoing for decades and has still failed to produce significant data that overwhelmingly supports a single position signifies that there is probably no major advantage to one solution over the other. Several meta-analyses have demonstrated no substantial benefit of colloid solutions over crystalloid solutions. In trauma, there is mildly convincing data that crystalloid solutions are preferable, with death as the primary outcome variable being examined. This finding has been attributed to the fact that colloidal solutions also leak across the capillary bed into the lung and may then provide an increase in interstitial oncotic pressure and prolong interstitial edema. These studies were done primarily with albumin as the colloidal solution. The common colloidal solutions are shown in Table 3–7. The most current cogent argument against colloidal solutions is the cost of these fluids and the remote possibility of an allergic reaction or infectious disease. Without evidence for a clear benefit of using colloidal solutions over using crystalloid solutions, the more cost-effective crystalloid solutions are recommended for most volume replacement.

The support of volume by using crystalloids

Table 3–7. *Resuscitation Fluids: Colloids**

Colloid	Osmolality	Colloid Oncotic Pressure
Albumin 5%	1500	20
Albumin 25%	300	70
Hetastarch (6%)	310	30
Dextran 40	308	40
Dextran 70	308	70

*Excluding fresh-frozen plasma, packed red cells, whole blood should also include assessment of the need for administration of blood or blood products. Transfusion of packed red cells is indicated to support oxygen delivery. The medical opinion on the exact level of hemoglobin at which a patient should be transfused has changed substantially over the past decade. Previously patients were transfused at a level of 10 g/dL. A recent study documented no ill effects when healthy patients were acutely exposed to a decline in hemoglobin to 5 g/dL. These patients were kept euvolemic. However, this finding cannot at this time be extrapolated to ill patients, and intravascular volume must be supplemented to euvolemia. Thus, assessment of the cardiac risk factors and assessment of ongoing blood loss should guide the trigger level for transfusion. In a patient with ongoing myocardial ischemia, myocardial oxygen delivery should be maximized, and most patients would benefit from a hemoglobin level higher than 10 g/dL. Transfusion of fresh-frozen plasma should be reserved for patients with a documented coagulopathy who have evidence of ongoing bleeding. These coagulopathies can occur in patients with underlying liver disease, in patients who have undergone massive transfusion, and in septic patients, for example. In patients who have had massive transfusions, thrombocytopenia is more likely to cause ongoing hemorrhage. A platelet count should be determined. Transfusion is usually necessary when there is persistent bleeding and the count is less than 50,000.

Hypertonic saline has been employed as an acute volume expander; initially, this solution was used for fluid administration in the field. Hypertonic saline is also used to treat elevated intracranial pressure. It is available in a variety of concentrations, but all solutions are substantially hyperosmolar and function by drawing fluid from the interstitium and cells to support the intravascular volume (see Table 3–6). Ideally, hypertonic saline should be administered by a central line because of its osmolality. It rapidly supports intravascular volume by increasing cardiac output and lowering systemic vascular resistance and is a good alternative for patients who require rapid intravascular volume expansion. Hypertonic saline can provide similar (or even greater) acute volume expansion when compared to colloid solution, and it has no allergic or infectious risk and is inexpensive. Extremely rapid shifts of sodium can be dangerous, and serum sodium should be monitored. When used for volume expansion (and not for elevations in intracranial pressure), serum sodium should not be maintained above 150 mEq/L. In patients with serious liver disease, caution should be employed in using hypertonic saline because of the incidence of central pontine myelinolysis associated with rapid serum sodium changes.

Once the ABCs have been addressed in a patient with shock from any cause, a patient who has any remaining signs or symptoms should be transferred to a setting in which more intensive nursing and physician care can be provided. At that point, searching for the underlying cause is paramount. Of course, if hemorrhage is the inciting cause of shock, bleeding sites are controlled immediately with digital pressure, followed by surgery when necessary.

As discussed previously, a patient may benefit from the placement of a central venous catheter or a Swan-Ganz catheter if left ventricular compliance is an issue. Although commonly employed as a monitoring device in patients in shock, the Swan-Ganz catheter has not actually been proven to impact outcome.

Once intravascular volume has been reestablished, any remaining deficits in cardiac output may have to be corrected with vasoactive agents. Agents such as α- and β-agonists may be used to supplement vascular tone and cardiac output. These agents are listed in Table 3–8. The use of these agents is directed by the cause of the shock state and by the patient's medical history, especially the cardiac function.

In a patient with sepsis, recognizing and identifying a potentially infectious pathogen and treating the infection appropriately is obviously of paramount importance. In a patient suffering from anaphylaxis, massive volume and the use of epinephrine are usually indicated when shock is present. If intravenous access is lacking, endotracheal or sublingual instillation of epinephrine can be given (0.3 to 0.5 mL of 1:1,000 aqueous solution). For intravenous use, a 1:10,000 solution can be used in increments of 0.1 to 0.2 mL, as required. Antihistamines may help to control cutaneous symptoms and may be helpful in the treatment of hypotension. The combined use of H_1 and H_2 antagonists is indicated. Therapy should therefore include diphenhydramine (25 to 50 mg intravenously) used together with ranitidine 1 mg/kg or cimetidine 4 mg/kg intravenously. The H_2 antagonist should be given somewhat slowly to avoid hypotension. Corticosteroids do not exert an immediate effect but their use is certainly warranted in biphasic or prolonged anaphylactic states. Intravenous routes of administration are suggested for severe cases, and either hydrocortisone (100 mg to 1 g) or methylprednisolone (80 to 125 mg) may

***Table 3–8.** Vasoactive Agents Commonly Used in the Treatment of Shock*

Agent	α Effect	β_1 Effect	β_2 Effect	Dopaminergic Effect
Phenylephrine	+ +	–	–	–
Dopamine	+ +→+ + +	+ +→+ + +	+→+ +	+ +
Norepinephrine	+ + +→+ + + +	+ + +→+ + + +	+→+ +	–
Epinephrine	+ + +→+ + + +	+ + +→+ + + +	+ + +→+ + + +	–
Dobutamine	–	+ +→+ + +	+ +→+ + + +	–

+→+ + + +, magnitude of effect of α and β receptor of commonly used vasoactive agents; + + + +, greatest magnitude.

be used. Aerosolized β-agonist nebulizers may have benefit much as they do in asthma. Occasionally, atropine is indicated for the treatment of bradycardia, and glucagon may be beneficial, as its action allows for positive inotropic and chronotropic effects on the heart that are independent of catecholamine receptors. This drug is especially useful in patients who have been receiving β-adrenergic blockers. Glucagon is given intravenously as a bolus dose of 1 to 5 mg followed by an infusion of 5 to 15 μg/min titrated according to the clinical response.

OUTCOMES

The outcome of an episode of shock depends substantially on the underlying medical condition of the patient and, most important, on the cause of the shock. For example, mortality after hemorrhagic shock secondary to a ruptured aortic aneurysm is about 50%, whereas hemorrhage secondary to a gunshot wound to the extremity, with vascular injury, in a young person is less than 10%. In a patient with cardiogenic shock, the long-term outcome is poor unless the underlying cardiac function can be improved. In a patient with reversible ischemic disease, reperfusion of the cardiac muscle may improve function.

For a patient with sepsis and shock, the mortality remains as high as 50%, with very little improvement over the past 25 years. The mortality resulting from sepsis today, however, is not acute within the first 24 to 72 hours, but occurs more than 14 days after the inciting event, when the patient may have developed multiple organ dysfunction syndrome. Much work is ongoing in modifying the inflammatory response in order to effect the outcome of sepsis. Virtually all clinical studies have shown limited efficacy at this time, and much work remains to define the ideal agent to administer to a septic patient. The outcome of anaphylactic shock depends on the recognition and immediate removal of the offending agent plus immediate volume and hemodynamic support, as required. The immediate therapy required and the time necessary to achieve this support in all forms of shock determine, in part, long-term survival. For a patient with spinal shock, providing respiratory support while maintaining cervical spine in-line position is life saving. The long-term outcome in this patient population is related to complications that develop secondary to ventilation and immobilization.

In summary, a patient in shock has inadequate delivery of oxygen to tissues. This state must be recognized and reversed immediately. In general, providing oxygen, and occasionally ventilatory support, volume, and vasoactive agents, can save lives. Ultimately, the identification and control of the inciting event determine the outcome.

SUGGESTED READING

American College of Chest Physicians/Society of Critical Care Consensus Conference. Definitions for sepsis and organ failure and guidelines for the innovative therapies in sepsis. Crit Care Med 1992;20:864–874.

Bone RC. Why sepsis trials fail. JAMA 1996;276:565–566.

Committee on Trauma. Manual: Advanced Trauma Life Support Program for Physicians. Chicago, American College of Surgeons, 1996.

Liberman P. Specific and idiopathic anaphylaxis: pathophysiology and treatment. In Bierman W et al., eds. Allergy and Asthma from Infancy to Adulthood, 3rd ed. WB Saunders, 1996, pp. 297–320.

Mollnes TE, Fosse E. The complement system in trauma-related and ischemic tissue damage: a brief review. Shock 1994;4:964–968.

Parillo JE. Pathogenic mechanisms of septic shock. N Engl J Med 1993;328:1471–1477.

Parillo JE. Septic shock in humans: advance in the understanding of pathogenesis, cardiovascular dysfunction and therapy. Ann Intern Med 1990;113:227–242.

Stone R. Search for sepsis drugs goes on despite past failures. Science 1994;264:365–367.

Szabo C, Thiemermann C. Invited opinion: role of nitric oxide in hemorrhagic, traumatic, and anaphylactic shock and thermal injury. Shock 1994;2:145–155.

Taylor RW, ed. Controversies in pulmonary artery catheterization. New Horizons 1997;5:173–296.

CHAPTER 4

Medical Emergencies

Todd Gress, MD, MPH,
and Alan Krasner, MD

Many life-threatening medical problems are treatable. Some emergencies, such as severe cutaneous drug reactions or anaphylaxis, have dramatic clinical presentations. Giant cell arteritis, on the other hand, is an urgent medical problem that requires diagnostic acumen because it often masquerades as other, more benign illnesses. Establishing the correct diagnosis often depends heavily on a careful history and physical exam, whereas other disorders are diagnosed on the basis of laboratory abnormalities, as is the case in acid-base disorders. Prompt diagnosis is essential so that effective therapy can be rendered. The following is an overview of diagnostic and therapeutic aspects of many medical emergencies encountered in hospitalized patients.

ALCOHOL WITHDRAWAL

Alcohol withdrawal is a potentially fatal syndrome that is often precipitated by hospitalization that causes abrupt cessation of alcohol intake. It is estimated that up to 20% of patients admitted to medical and surgical wards have alcohol dependence and are therefore susceptible to acute withdrawal.[1] Recognition and proper management of alcohol withdrawal is important so as to prevent withdrawal seizures, delirium tremens, exacerbation of preexisting medical problems, and mortality.

Alcohol withdrawal manifests as enhanced autonomic output which is demonstrated by an increase in pulse rate, respiratory rate, and temperature. A thorough history and physical exam should be performed to identify patients experiencing these symptoms and to reveal characteristics that may predict the development of withdrawal. Once it has been identified, the goal of treatment is to prevent the complications of withdrawal. It is important to remember that all patients should be screened for alcohol dependence because a significant proportion that develop withdrawal have unrecognized alcohol use.

Presentation

As pointed out by Lohr,[1] the description of alcohol withdrawal by Sir William Osler[2] in 1892 still applies today: "Delirium tremens (mania à potu) is really only an incident in the history of chronic alcoholism, and results from the long-continued action of the poison on the brain. . . . A spree in a temperate person, no matter how prolonged, is rarely if ever followed by delirium tremens; but in the case of an habitual drinker a temporary excess is apt to bring on an attack. It sometimes develops in consequence of the sudden withdrawal of the alcohol. . . . At the outset of the attack the patient is restless and depressed and sleeps badly. . . . The patient talks constantly and incoherently; he is incessantly in motion, and desires to go out and attend to some imaginary business. Hallucinations of sight and hearing develop. He sees objects in the room, such as rats, mice, or snakes, and fancies that they are crawling over his body. The terror inspired by these imaginary objects is great and has given the popular name 'horrors' to the disease. . . . There is much muscular tremor; the tongue is covered with a thick white fur, and when protruded is tremulous.

The pulse is soft, rapid, and readily compressed. There is usually fever, but the temperature rarely registers above 102° or 103°. . . . Insomnia is a constant feature. On the third or fourth day in favorable cases the restlessness abates, the patient sleeps, and improvement gradually sets in. The tremor persists for some days, and hallucinations gradually disappear, as the appetite returns."

The clinical picture is one of enhanced autonomic activity with increased pulse, respiratory rate, and temperature. A tremor of the hands is often present, along with generalized jitters or anxiety. Some patients develop nausea and gastrointestinal upset. These symptoms generally begin within 5 to 10 hours of cessation of alcohol intake, peak in intensity on day 2 or 3, and improve by day 4 or 5. Approximately 5% develop delirium tremens, a state defined by the presence of a clouded sensorium, sometimes accompanied by visual, tactile, and auditory hallucinations.[3] Seizures have been found in approximately 8% of patients with acute alcohol withdrawal; they occur most often between 6 and 48 hours after cessation of alcohol intake.[4]

Evaluation

Screening for alcohol dependence should begin with a thorough history and physical exam. The CAGE questionnaire[5] is a rapid and reliable tool for identifying alcohol dependence (Box 4–1). A single positive response suggests a problem with alcohol, and two or more positive responses correlate highly with severe alcohol abuse. Other medical illnesses such as infection that could worsen withdrawal should be sought as should those that may be exacerbated by withdrawal such as coronary artery disease. In a study involving consecutive patients admitted to an urban, university-affiliated hospital, those with concurrent medical illness were 5.1 times (95% confidence interval [95% CI] 2.1 to 12.6) more likely to develop delirium tremens.[6] History of previous alcohol withdrawal, seizures, or delirium tremens may also identify those likely to experience withdrawal and complications. Administration of the Clinical Institute Withdrawal Assessment for Alcohol, revised, scale (CIWA-Ar)[7] is a useful tool for determining the severity of alcohol withdrawal (Table 4–1). Total scores of 8 or higher identify patients who would benefit from pharmacologic management and close observation.[8] This scale is simple to use, but it is important not to confuse symptoms of coexisting medical illnesses with those of alcohol withdrawal when completing the questionnaire. The physical exam should concentrate on temperature, pulse rate, respiratory rate, and tremor. A baseline neurologic exam may be extremely valuable if the patient develops a change in mental status or has a seizure. A complete exam to identify coexisting medical conditions should be performed.

Laboratory analysis should include a complete blood count, chemistry panel, and serum magnesium level to search for alcohol-related illnesses, such as anemia, malnutrition, electrolyte disturbances, and hepatitis. An electrocardiogram should be considered in all patients with coronary artery disease, as the acute withdrawal may mask cardiac symptoms. Also, clinically relevant electrolyte abnormalities may be identified. Chest radiographs should be performed if clinically indicated.

Treatment Priorities

Attention to the fundamental elements of management is the cornerstone of successful treatment of alcohol withdrawal (Table 4–2). Dehydration is common, and adequate hydration with intravenous fluids should be provided. Nutritional support, including thiamine to prevent oculogyric crisis and Wernicke-Korsakoff syndrome, and a multivitamin, is also critical. Thia-

BOX 4–1

The CAGE Questionnaire

1. Do you feel you should *c*ut down on your alcohol consumption?
2. Have people *a*nnoyed you by criticizing your drinking?
3. Have you felt *g*uilty about your drinking?
4. Have you ever had a drink first thing in the morning to steady your nerves or get rid of a hangover (*e*ye opener)?

(Adapted from Ewing JA. Detecting alcoholism. The CAGE questionnaire. JAMA 1984; 252:1905–1907. Copyright 1984, American Medical Association.)

Table 4–1. *Clinical Institute Withdrawal Assessment Scale for Alcohol, Revised (CIWA-Ar)*

Nausea and Vomiting
Ask "Do you feel sick to your stomach? Have you vomited?"
Observation:
0—no nausea and no vomiting
1—mild nausea with no vomiting
2
3
4—intermittent nausea with dry heaves
5
6
7—constant nausea, frequent dry heaves and vomiting

Tremor
Arms extended and fingers spread apart
Observation:
0—no tremor
1—not visible, but can be felt fingertip to fingertip
2
3
4—moderate, with patient's arms extended
5
6
7—severe, even with arms not extended

Paroxysmal Sweats
Observation:
0—no sweat visible
1—barely perceptible sweating, palms moist
2
3
4—beads of sweat obvious on forehead
5
6
7—drenching sweats

Anxiety
Ask "Do you feel nervous?"
Observation:
0—no anxiety, at ease
1—mildly anxious
2
3
4—moderately anxious, or guarded, so anxiety is inferred
5
6
7—equivalent to acute panic states as seen in severe delirium or acute schizophrenic reactions

Agitation
Observation:
0—normal activity
1—somewhat more than normal activity
2
3
4—moderately fidgety and restless
5
6
7—paces back and forth during most of the interview, or constantly thrashes about

Tactile Disturbances
Ask "Have you any itching, pins-and-needles sensations, any burning, any numbness, or do you feel bugs crawling on or under your skin?
Observation:
0—none
1—very mild itching, pins and needles, burning or numbness
2—mild itching, pins and needles, burning or numbness
3—moderate itching, pins and needles, burning or numbness
4—moderately severe hallucinations
5—severe hallucinations
6—extremely severe hallucinations
7—continuous hallucinations

Auditory Disturbances
Ask "Are you more aware of sounds around you? Are they harsh? Do they frighten you? Are you hearing anything that is disturbing to you? Are you hearing things that you know aren't there?"
Observation:
0—not present
1—very mild harshness or ability to frighten
2—mild harshness or ability to frighten
3—moderate harshness or ability to frighten
4—moderately severe hallucinations
5—severe hallucinations
6—extremely severe hallucinations
7—continuous hallucinations

Visual Disturbances
Ask "Does the light appear to be too bright? Is its color different? Does it hurt your eyes? Are you seeing anything that is disturbing you? Are you seeing things that you know aren't there?"
Observation:
0—not present
1—very mild sensitivity
2—mild sensitivity
3—moderate sensitivity
4—moderately severe hallucinations
5—severe hallucinations
6—extremely severe hallucinations
7—continuous hallucinations

Headache, Fullness in Head
Ask "Does your head feel different? Does it feel like there is a band around your head?" Do not rate dizziness or lightheadedness. Otherwise, rate severity.
Observation:
0—not present
1—very mild
2—mild
3—moderate
4—moderately severe
5—severe
6—very severe
7—extremely severe

Orientation and Clouding of Sensorium
Ask "What day is this? Where are you? Who am I?"
Observation:
0—oriented and can do serial additions
1—cannot do serial additions or is uncertain about date
2—disoriented for date by no more than two calendar days
3—disoriented for date by more than two calendar days
4—disoriented for place and/or person

The total score is a simple sum of each item score (maximum score = 67)

(Adapted from Sullivan UT et al. Assessment of alcohol withdrawal: the revised Clinical Institute Withdrawal Assessment for Alcohol scale (CIWA-Ar). Br J Addict 1989;84:1353–1357.)

Table 4–2. *Initial Management of Alcohol Withdrawal*

Fluid and electrolytes	Intravenous hydration with crystalloids Replacement of electrolytes as indicated by laboratory values
Nutrition	Thiamine 100 mg IM/IV* on admission Thiamine 100 mg IM/IV*/oral daily for 1 week Oral multivitamin daily or intravenous with fluid replacement
Environment	Quiet as possible
Comorbid conditions	Identify on admission and watch carefully for exacerbations resulting from withdrawal

*See text regarding IV administration.

mine administration should occur prior to the administration of glucose-containing intravenous solutions, which may worsen thiamine deficiency. Thiamine should be given intramuscularly when there are no contraindications to intramuscular injection such as a coagulopathy. If a contraindication is present, thiamine can be given intravenously and has been demonstrated to be safe,[9] although there does exist a small risk of anaphylaxis. Magnesium should be administered if the patient is deficient in it, but there is no evidence that correction of hypomagnesemia improves withdrawal or its complications.[8]

Many patients require pharmacologic therapy to prevent the complications of withdrawal. The most effective pharmacologic agents for the treatment of alcohol withdrawal are the benzodiazepines. These agents reduce the unpleasant and comorbid symptoms of withdrawal and have been demonstrated in randomized, clinical trials to significantly reduce both seizures and delirium tremens.[8] The longer-acting benzodiazepines, chlordiazepoxide and diazepam, seem to contribute to a smoother withdrawal course with less breakthrough and rebound symptoms than the shorter-acting agents. However, oversedation, particularly in the elderly and those with liver disease, can be a problem with the longer-acting agents. Therefore, the shorter-acting lorazepam or oxazepam is preferred in these situations.[8]

Two methods of treatment using benzodiazepines have been studied—fixed-schedule and symptom-triggered (Table 4–3). In a randomized, controlled trial, both methods produced similar patient outcomes in the management of alcohol withdrawal; however, the symptom-triggered approach required less total medication administration and resulted in shorter treatment duration.[10] It is important to note that the symptom-triggered approach has been used only with the longer-acting agents and requires administration of the CIWA-Ar.[7] When used, the CIWA-Ar should be administered frequently (up to three times a day and after each medication administered for alcohol withdrawal). In the previously mentioned trial, 25 to 100 mg of chlordiazepoxide were given when the CIWA-Ar score was 8 or higher, which was assessed at baseline, every 8 hours, and 1 hour after chlordiazepoxide administration.[10] Both methods are outlined in Table 4–3, along with the dosage regimens of commonly used benzodiazepines.

Other agents that have been tried for alcohol withdrawal include β-blockers, clonidine, phenytoin, phenothiazines, and valproic acid. There are limited data on each, and none has been shown to be superior to the benzodiazepines in management of withdrawal. However, there are situations in which each may play an important role, such as using β-blockers to decrease blood pressure and heart rate in patients with coronary artery disease and clonidine in the management of concomitant heroin withdrawal. Cau-

Table 4–3. *Two Methods of Pharmacologic Management of Alcohol Withdrawal*

Fixed-schedule Dosing*
Chlordiazepoxide 50 mg every 6 h for 4 doses, then 25 mg every 6 h for 8 doses
Diazepam 10 mg every 6 h for 4 doses, then 5 mg every 6 hours for 8 doses
Lorazepam 2 mg every 6 h for 4 doses, then 1 mg every 6 hours for 8 doses
Provide additional medication as needed if symptoms are not controlled
Symptom-triggered Dosing
Monitor patient every 4 to 8 hours with the CIWA-Ar until the score is less than 8 to 10 for 24 h; use additional assessments as needed
Administer one of the following medications every hour when CIWA-Ar is higher than 8 to 10*:
Chlordiazepoxide 50 to 100 mg
Diazepam 10 to 20 mg
Lorazepam 2 to 4 mg
Repeat CIWA-Ar 1 hour after every dose to assess need for further medication

*Oxazepam may also be used, but no information about this medication was provided in this guideline.

(Adapted from Mayo-Smith MF. Pharmacological management of alcohol withdrawal: a meta-analysis and evidence-based practice guideline. American Society of Addiction Medicine Working Group on Pharmacological Management of Alcohol Withdrawal. JAMA 1997; 278:144–151. Copyright 1997, American Medical Association.)

tion should be exercised in the administration of phenothiazines, which may be useful for hallucinations that occur with delirium tremens but may precipitate seizures by lowering the seizure threshold.[8]

Alcohol withdrawal seizures are managed with supportive therapy, including oxygen and a safe environment to avoid self-induced physical injury. Other causes of seizure, such as hypoxia or hypoglycemia, should be excluded. In general, most alcohol withdrawal seizures are tonic-clonic and if focal, require a complete neurologic evaluation, including electroencephalography and brain imaging. Also, most recommend a complete evaluation in patients with new-onset seizure or a history of seizures without previous evaluation, regardless of alcohol use. A prospective study of computed tomography scans of the head in 250 patients with first alcohol-related, tonic-clonic seizures revealed intracranial lesions in 16 cases (6.2%).[4] Seizures can be treated with benzodiazepines, particularly if alcohol withdrawal is likely. Phenytoin is generally not necessary unless there is another cause for the seizure or if the patient develops recurrent seizures, including status epilepticus.

Treatment of delirium tremens is managed according to the same principles as those of alcohol withdrawal. However, patients may require more frequent dosing and intravenous administration of benzodiazepines. A dose of 10 mg of diazepam intravenously followed by 5 mg every 5 minutes to achieve a calm but awake state has been used with success,[11] but other benzodiazepines, including the short-acting agents, may be preferred. Regardless of which benzodiazepine is given, frequent assessment of the patient is imperative. Delirium tremens is the most severe form of withdrawal, and an intensive care setting for management is recommended. If phenothiazines are used for hallucinations, they should be instituted at a low dose and titrated to symptoms, as long as seizures do not occur. Delirium tremens generally persists for 3 to 5 days, regardless of treatment.[3]

Outcomes

Alcohol abuse is associated with an increased risk of postoperative complications and prolonged hospital stay. An increase in postoperative complications was found in a consecutive sample of patients undergoing elective hysterectomies who were consuming 60 g or more of ethanol daily (the equivalent of six 12-ounce portions of beer). The complication rate was 80% as opposed to 13% in the placebo group).[12] A similarly increased risk of postoperative complications was found in a prospective cohort of patients who consumed at least 60 g of ethanol daily and who underwent colorectal surgery; they were compared to patients who consumed less than 25 g of ethanol daily (67% versus 20%; $p < .05$). These patients also had longer hospital stays as compared to the control group (20 days versus 12 days; $p < .05$).[13]

Data concerning current mortality associated with the alcohol withdrawal syndrome are scarce. Patients with the highest risk of mortality resulting from alcohol withdrawal are those who develop delirium tremens. In the past, mortality rates due to this complication have ranged from 15% to 20%, but recent data suggest that mortality rates have decreased; they have been reported to be from 3% to 8%.[14, 15]

ACID-BASE DISORDERS

The body's ability to regulate serum pH can be critically challenged by many medical conditions. Identification and treatment of the underlying cause is the goal in the management of acid-base disorders, and a working knowledge of acid-base balance is necessary. There are four types of simple acid-base disorders—metabolic acidosis, metabolic alkalosis, respiratory acidosis, and respiratory alkalosis.

The pH of the body (the normal pH is 7.35 to 7.45) is carefully regulated by the renal and respiratory systems and intracellular buffering and can be calculated by using the Henderson-Hasselbach equation:

$$pH = 6.1 + \frac{[HCO_3^-]}{PaCO_2}$$

In acid-base disorders, a change in one system results in an expected compensatory response in the other in order to minimize the effect on pH. This compensatory response can be determined by the calculations presented in Table 4–4. The compensatory response usually does not completely correct the pH to normal; if it does, a mixed acid-base disorder is likely to be present. The body never overcorrects the pH when compensating for a simple acid-base disorder.

Presentation

Patients may present with a wide range of symptoms, depending upon the underlying

Table 4–4. *Calculation of Compensatory Responses in Simple Acid-Base Disorders*

Disorder	Compensation
Metabolic acidosis	$PaCO_2 = (1.5 \times [HCO_3-]) + 8$
Metabolic alkalosis	$PaCO_2$ will ↑ 0.75 mm Hg per mmol/L ↑ in $[HCO_3-]$
Respiratory alkalosis	
Acute	$[HCO_3-]$ will ↓ 2 mmol/L per 10 mm Hg ↓ in $PaCO_2$
Chronic	$[HCO_3-]$ will ↓ 4 mmol/L per 10 mm Hg ↓ in $PaCO_2$
Respiratory acidosis	
Acute	$[HCO_3-]$ will ↑ 1 mmol/L per 10 mm Hg ↑ in $PaCO_2$
Chronic	$[HCO_3-]$ will ↑ 4 mmol/L per 10 mm Hg ↑ in $PaCO_2$

(Adapted from Dubose TD. Acidosis and alkalosis. In Fauci AS et al., eds. Harrison's Principles of Internal Medicine, vol. 1. New York, McGraw-Hill, 1998, pp. 277–286.)

cause of the acid-base disorder, but there are no specific symptoms or signs associated with an acid-base disorder itself. Acidosis, if severe (pH < 7.2), may cause organ dysfunction and result in congestive heart failure, increased susceptibility to cardiac arrythmias, obtundation, and coma.[16] Metabolic acidosis causes an increase in the respiratory drive, so patients may be tachypneic. When it is severe, Kussmaul respirations, which are deep, regular, sighing respirations, are seen. Respiratory acidosis, on the other hand, typically occurs in a patient with a preexisting pulmonary disorder, such as chronic obstructive pulmonary disease, and such a patient often has symptoms of the disease. Any patient who is unconscious or sedated and has a suppressed respiratory drive may develop respiratory acidosis. Therefore, a patient with respiratory acidosis may be tachypneic, which causes impaired alveolar gas exchange, or hypopneic, which causes the accumulation of carbon dioxide.

Metabolic alkalosis may be caused by extracellular volume contraction, and signs of volume depletion, such as postural hypotension and tachycardia, may be evident. The compensatory change in ventilation may not be as obvious as that which occurs in metabolic acidosis. Respiratory alkalosis is associated with increased ventilation, and tachypnea is usually present.

Evaluation

The evaluation of an acid-base disorder is a two-step process. First, arterial blood gas and serum electrolyte levels should be obtained to correctly identify the primary disorder (or disorders, if a mixed acid-base disturbance is present). Then, secondary testing should be directed at identifying the underlying cause of the primary disorder.

The principal change in metabolic acidosis is a decrease in the serum bicarbonate, which lowers the pH. Compensatory tachypnea lowers the PCO_2 (partial pressure of carbon dioxide), helping somewhat to raise the pH. An increase in the anion gap (the normal gap is 12 ± 4 mEq/L) can help to narrow the differential diagnosis of the metabolic acidosis:

$$\text{Anion gap} = (Na^-) - (HCO^-_3 + Cl^-)$$

In addition, calculation of the serum osmolality can further narrow the diagnosis:

$$\text{Serum osmolality} = 2[Na^+] + \frac{[\text{Glucose}]}{18} + \frac{[\text{Urea}]}{2.8}$$

The difference between the measured and calculated serum osmolality should be no greater than 10 mOsm/kg, and if elevated in the presence of an anion gap metabolic acidosis, could indicate the addition of unmeasured metabolically active substances (ethanol, methanol, or ethylene glycol).

Among acid-base disturbances, metabolic acidosis with an elevated anion gap is most likely to have an underlying, life-threatening cause. Many times, the cause is obvious, such as when hyperglycemia is present in diabetic ketoacidosis. However, sometimes the cause may not be obvious, such as with salicylate ingestion, which causes an increased anion gap acidosis but may begin with a respiratory alkalosis (due to direct effects of salicylate on respiratory drive) or a mixed acidosis-alkalosis without any specific identifying clues. Therefore, in addition to the serum osmolality, a rapid laboratory evaluation, including a chemistry panel, a lactate level, and a search for possible ingestions (ethanol level, salicylate level, and volatile acid screen), should be performed. The causes of an anion gap, metabolic acidosis, can be remembered by using the mnemonic MUDPILES—(methanol ingestion, uremia, diabetic ketoacidosis, paraldehyde ingestion, iron or isoniazid ingestion, lactic acidosis, ethylene glycol ingestion or ethanol ingestion (ketoacidosis), and salicylate ingestion). Some causes of metabolic acidosis are listed in Table 4–5.

Metabolic alkalosis results in elevated serum bicarbonate and pH and a compensatory elevation in the PCO_2. It can be categorized as either chloride-responsive or chloride-nonresponsive metabolic alkalosis. In chloride-responsive alkalosis, dehydration is usually the underlying cause and can be rapidly reversed by the administration of normal saline to replenish fluid volume. Chloride-nonresponsive alkalosis is usually associated with mineralocorticoid excess as the underlying cause. This results in expansion of the extracellular fluid volume, so administration of normal saline will not correct the alkalosis. If the volume status is uncertain, measurement of the urine chloride can help to distinguish between the two types; a urine chloride level lower than 10 mEq/L (conservation by the kidney in a hypochloremic state) is found in chloride-responsive metabolic alkalosis. Some causes of metabolic alkalosis are listed in Table 4–5.

The primary change in respiratory acidosis is an increase in the P_{CO_2}. The kidneys respond by increasing the absorption and generation of bicarbonate. However, the measured bicarbonate concentration may be normal because the compensatory response by the renal system may take several hours to days to occur. On average, it takes 3 days to reach a 90% compensatory response.[17] A decrease in the P_{CO_2} is the primary change in respiratory alkalosis. Even though compensation by the renal system is often delayed, it eventually results in a decrease in the serum bicarbonate level. Some causes of respiratory acid-base disorders are listed in Table 4–6.

Changes caused by mixed disorders are more complicated, but in general, they should be suspected if the calculated compensatory response is not consistent with the measured values. For example, in a metabolic acidosis with a pH of 7.2 and a bicarbonate level of 10 mmol/L, an expected P_{CO_2} near $(1.5 \times 10) + 8 = 23$ mm Hg should occur. If the P_{CO_2} is 32 mm Hg, it means there is undercompensation, and a primary respiratory acidosis in addition to the primary metabolic acidosis should be suspected. Thus, by determining the primary disorder and calculating the compensatory response, mixed acid-base disorders can be defined. Estimation of the P_{CO_2} using this equation is valid only for the primary disorder, in this case, metabolic acidosis.

Table 4–5. *Common Causes of Metabolic Acidosis and Alkalosis*

Metabolic Acidosis	
High anion gap	Lactic acidosis Ketoacidosis: alcohol, diabetes, starvation Toxins: salicylates, methanol, ethylene glycol Renal failure
Normal anion gap	Gastrointestinal bicarbonate loss: diarrhea, small bowel drainage Renal acidosis, e.g., renal tubular acidosis Drug-induced hyperkalemia (with renal insufficiency) resulting from trimethoprim, nonsteroidal anti-inflammatory drugs, potassium-sparing diuretics
Metabolic Alkalosis	
Exogenous	Alkali administration
Chloride-responsive (extracellular volume contraction)	Vomiting, diuretics, posthypercapneic state
Chloride-unresponsive (extracellular volume expansion)	Renal artery stenosis, accelerated hypertension, Cushing's syndrome

(Adapted from Dubose TD. Acidosis and alkalosis. In Fauci AS et al., eds. Harrison's Principles of Internal Medicines, Vol. 1. New York, McGraw-Hill, pp. 277–286.)

Table 4–6. *Common Causes of Respiratory Acidosis and Alkalosis*

Respiratory Acidosis	
Central	Sedative medications, infection, stroke
Respiratory	Asthma, obstruction, emphysema, adult respiratory distress syndrome
Neuromuscular	Muscular dystrophy, kyphoscoliosis
Other	Obesity
Respiratory Alkalosis	Hypoxemia, pain, anxiety, hepatic failure

(Adapted from Dubose TD. Acidosis and alkalosis. In Fauci AS et al., eds. Harrison's Principles of Internal Medicine, vol. 1. New York, McGraw-Hill, 1998, pp 277–286.)

Treatment Priorities

Management of acid-base disorders, as emphasized earlier, is directed at the underlying cause. Many of the life-threatening acid-base disorders cause a high anion gap acidosis and require specific treatments. These include the infusion of ethanol for methanol ingestion, dialysis for salicylate ingestion, and the giving of insulin for diabetic ketoacidosis. Nonspecific treatment of metabolic acidosis is alkali therapy.

Severe metabolic acidosis with a pH below 7.2, may require treatment with sodium bicarbonate, particularly if there is evidence of organ dysfunction, such as heart failure or obtundation, or if the acidosis involves nonmetabolizable anions, which can accumulate in renal failure and toxic ingestions. Also, in all forms of severe acidosis, sodium bicarbonate may have to be administered to temporize the patient while the cause of the acidosis is determined or while waiting for definitive treatment to take effect. Sodium bicarbonate should be given as an infusion, with the goal of correcting the bicarbonate to approximately 10 mmol/L. The amount of bicarbonate needed can be estimated by multiplying 50% of the body weight by the number of mmol/L needed to raise the serum bicarbonate to 10 mmol/L.[16] This is a conservative estimate, and some patients may require more bicarbonate. For example, if the serum bicarbonate is 6 mmol/L in a 70-kg patient, then $0.50 \times 70 \times 4 = 140$ mmol of sodium bicarbonate that will be needed. Complications of administering the usual 1 N solution sodium bicarbonate therapy include hypernatremia and hyperosmolality, which can be avoided by creating an isotonic solution by mixing 3 ampules of sodium bicarbonate (50 mmol/L of sodium bicarbonate each) in 1 L of 5% dextrose in water. Other complications include volume overload and "overshoot" alkalosis (a rapid transition to alkalemia caused by exogenous administration of alkali and endogenous regeneration of bicarbonate), which occurs because of overcorrection of the bicarbonate level; it may be poorly tolerated by some patients.[16]

Metabolic alkalosis is most commonly caused by extracellular volume contraction and often responds to the infusion of normal saline, the so-called chloride-responsive alkalosis. If the volume status is uncertain and the alkalosis fails to respond to the infusion of saline, then a chloride-nonresponsive alkalosis may be the cause. If the volume status is unclear, a measurement of the urine chloride should be performed.

In respiratory acidosis, treatment may consist of inhaled β-agonists for the management of chronic obstructive pulmonary disease or antibiotics for an infection that is causing impairment of respiratory drive. Sedative drugs, particularly in patients with underlying pulmonary or neurologic disease, can depress respiratory drive and should be sought.

Respiratory alkalosis is caused by hyperventilation, so anything that increases respiration can be the underlying cause. Pain, anxiety, and infection are common causes, but caution must be exercised in assigning these causes without searching for more serious causes such as hypoxemia caused by an acute pulmonary embolus.

Outcomes

Outcomes of acid-base disorders are dependent upon the underlying causes of the disorder and, as mentioned previously, metabolic acidosis is more likely to have a life-threatening cause. Lactic acidosis, a common cause of metabolic acidosis in the hospitalized patient, carries a dismal prognosis. In a study of an ICU, only 17% of patients with lactic acidosis were discharged from the hospital.[18] On the other hand, diabetic ketoacidosis is an example of a reversible metabolic acidosis with a relatively good prognosis when treated adequately, and a prospective urban study found a mortality rate of less than 2%.[19]

HYPOKALEMIA

Hypokalemia, particularly when severe and acute in onset, is life threatening. Because potassium is the major intracellular cation and is responsible for maintaining the resting membrane potential, depletion of potassium can destabilize skeletal and heart muscle. The most severe effects, flaccid paralysis and cardiac arrest, can be prevented by proper repletion of this electrolyte.

A serum potassium of less than 3.5 mmol/L defines hypokalemia. Three main mechanisms that can lead to its development: decreased potassium intake, intracellular shift of potassium, and increased potassium loss. An understanding of these mechanisms can be used in the evaluation of the patient to determine the underlying cause of hypokalemia.

Presentation

Patients presenting with hypokalemia can be asymptomatic. Fatigue, myalgias, and muscular weakness are early symptoms that can progress to severe muscular weakness leading to hypoventilation and flaccid paralysis. Smooth muscle is much less affected than skeletal and cardiac muscle, but patients can develop paralytic ileus. Electrocardiographic changes are relatively nonspecific but when present could signal life-threatening hypokalemia. Electrocardiographic changes include T-wave flattening and inversion, prominent u waves, ST-segment depression, prolonged PR interval, decreased voltage, and a widened QRS complex. Without correction, patients may develop atrioventricular block, ventricular arrythmias, and cardiac arrest.

Evaluation

Once a diagnosis of hypokalemia has been established, a search for the cause should be undertaken (Table 4–7); it can often be obtained from the history. Use of diuretics, decreased intake, and gastrointestinal losses are common causes of hypokalemia. Shifts of potassium from the extracellular fluid compartments to the intracellular compartments occur in the presence of an alkalosis, but hypokalemia can also result in the development of an alkalosis. It is common for trauma patients to develop hypokalemia, which is thought to occur because of elevated levels of epinephrine and increased activity of the Na^+K^+ ATPase pump. α-Adrenergic antagonists and β-adrenergic agonists also increase Na^+K^+ ATPase pump activity, lowering potassium. Insulin decreases serum potassium by Na^+K^+ ATPase pump activity and by cellular uptake of potassium with glucose. A falsely low serum potassium level (pseudohypokalemia) can occur with leukemia because of white blood cell uptake of potassium.[20]

Table 4–7. *Causes of Hypokalemia*

Decreased intake
Redistribution into cells
- Metabolic alkalosis
- Insulin, β-adrenergic agonists, α-adrenergic antagonists
- Anabolic state
- Pseudohypokalemia
- Hypothermia
- Hypokalemic periodic paralysis
- Barium toxicity

Increased loss
- Nonrenal
  - Gastrointestinal (diarrhea)
  - Skin (sweat)
- Renal
  - Increased distal flow: diuretics, osmotic diuresis, salt-wasting nephropathies
  - Increased secretion of potassium
    - Mineralocorticoid excess: primary or secondary hyperaldosteronism, apparent mineralocorticoid excess (licorice, chewing tobacco), Cushing's syndrome, Bartter's syndrome
    - Distal delivery of nonreabsorbed anions: vomiting, nasogastric suction, type 2 renal tubular acidosis, diabetic ketoacidosis, glue-sniffing (toluene abuse), penicillin derivatives
    - Other: amphotericin B, Liddle's syndrome, hypomagnesemia

(Adapted from Brenner BM, Singer GG. Fluid and electrolyte disturbances. In Fauci AS et al., eds. Harrison's Principles of Internal Medicine, vol. 1. New York, McGraw-Hill, 1998, pp. 271–277.)

Treatment Priorities

The method used to correct hypokalemia is dependent upon the degree of hypokalemia present and on the underlying medical conditions. An asymptomatic patient with a serum potassium level between 3.0 and 3.5 mmol/L may be followed with serial laboratory assessment without replacement.[21] However, if there is a history of congestive heart failure and the patient is on digitalis, or if there is a history of ischemic heart disease, then such a potassium level should be corrected.

In most cases, oral replacement with potassium chloride is adequate. Oral potassium chloride may be given as a liquid (elixir), a powder, or a tablet. The elixir is the least costly, but many patients dislike the taste. The powder can be mixed with chilled water or orange juice and may be more palatable. Tablets usually contain less than half the amount of potassium in the elixir or powder, and the slow-release forms can cause intestinal ulceration and stenosis, although these problems are rare.[21]

If the potassium level is higher than 2.5 mmol/L and no electrocardiographic changes have occurred, 40 to 60 mEq/L of oral potassium should be given. The serum potassium level should then be measured every 4 hours and additional potassium given based on the results. In general, for each 10 mEq/L of potassium given, an increase of 0.1 mmol/L in the serum potassium occurs, but this is dependent on many variables and differs by patient, acid-base status, total body potassium deficit, and renal function.

For severe hypokalemia (serum potassium less than 2.5 mmol/L) or for any degree of hypokalemia with electrocardiographic changes, continuous electrocardiographic monitoring should be initiated. Potassium may be given orally, intravenously, or both. For those unable to take oral medications, potassium can be given at a rate of 10 mEq/h through a peripheral intravenous line. It is important to avoid dextrose-containing solutions that stimulate insulin secretion and can further lower serum potassium. For severe hypokalemia, particularly if concomitant oral supplemention cannot be given, potassium can be given at a rate of 20 mEq/h through a central intravenous line, which is preferable for higher concentrations of potassium because of direct toxicity to veins. Frequent monitoring of the serum potassium, at least every 4 hours, should be performed until the electrocardiographic changes have resolved and the serum potassium level is higher than 3.0 mmol/L. If the hypokalemia is refractory to potassium replacement, magnesium deficiency may be the underlying cause and should be repleted if low or if at the lower limits of the normal range.[21] Replacement of potassium in patients with impaired renal function should be undertaken with caution and with frequent monitoring of the serum potassium to avoid iatrogenic hyperkalemia.

HYPERKALEMIA

Hyperkalemia, a condition most commonly caused by acute or chronic renal failure, can lead to ventricular arrhythmias and death if prompt treatment is not instituted. Hyperkalemia causes few physical symptoms, but does cause fairly specific changes in the electrocardiogram (ECG). For these reasons, hyperkalemia is often identified on routine laboratory analysis or ECG.

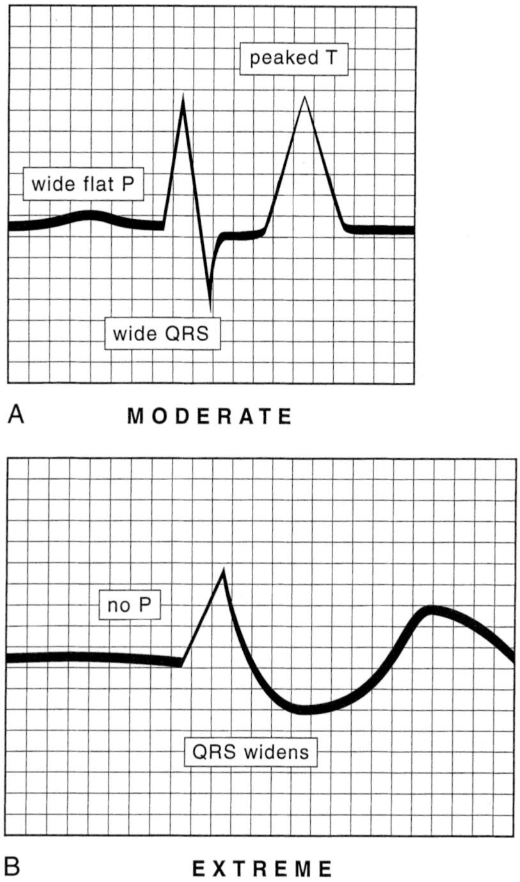

Figure 4–1. A: T waves are peaked and the QT interval is shortened. B: There is further widening of the QRS and flattening of the p waves.

Presentation

Patients with hyperkalemia may develop muscular weakness, which can progress to complete paralysis. The ECG reveals fairly specific changes. Early on, the T waves are peaked (Fig. 4–1A) and the QT interval is shortened. Then the PR interval lengthens and the QRS widens. Late findings include further widening of the QRS and flattening of the p waves (Fig. 4–1B).[22] Ultimately, a biphasic sine wave occurs, and at that point, ventricular standstill is imminent. This pattern and progression of electrocardiographic changes is highly variable among individuals and is more likely to develop when the increase in serum potassium has occurred acutely.

Evaluation

The most common cause of hyperkalemia is renal failure due to the inability of the kidney to excrete potassium. Hypoaldosteronism, hypoperfusion, and medications are other important causes of hyperkalemia. Patients may inadvertently receive exogenous potassium through salt substitutes, which should be looked for and discontinued. Pseudohyperkalemia, caused by a release of potassium from cells immediately prior to or following venipuncture, is an artificial elevation of potassium and can result from prolonged application of the tourniquet for venipuncture, hemolysis, leukocytosis, or thrombocytosis. Measurement of the plasma (not serum) potassium with proper venipuncture should be performed to rule out pseudohyperkalemia. Causes of hyperkalemia are listed in Table 4–8.

The initial evaluation of acute hyperkalemia should include a careful but urgent remeasurement of the plasma potassium to exclude pseudohyperkalemia. Medications should be reviewed as potential causes, particularly angiotensin-converting enzyme inhibitors and nonsteroidal anti-inflammatory drugs; if found to be present, these medications should be dis-

Table 4–8. *Causes of Hyperkalemia*

Renal failure
Decreased distal flow (decreased extracellular fluid volume)
Decreased potassium secretion
Impaired sodium reabsorption
Primary hypoaldosteronism
Secondary hypoaldosteronism: ACE inhibitors, NSAIDs
Resistance to aldosterone: tubulointerstitial disease, potassium-sparing diuretics
Enhanced chloride reabsorption
Gordon's syndrome
Cyclosporine

(Adapted from Brenner BM, Singer GG. Fluid and electrolyte disturbances. In Fauci AS et al., eds. Harrison's Principles of Internal Medicine, vol. 1. New York, McGraw-Hill, 1998, pp. 271–277.)

continued. The volume status, urine output, serum creatinine, and blood urea nitrogen should be assessed and an ECG should be performed. All of these steps should be taken as quickly as possible so that treatment is not delayed.

Treatment Priorities

Hyperkalemia, with symptoms of muscle weakness or electrocardiographic changes, requires immediate treatment. Initial measures are intended to stabilize a potentially fatal situation, provide time to remove the excess potassium and, ultimately, to identify and treat the underlying cause of the hyperkalemia. A dose of 10 mL of a 10% solution of calcium gluconate given intravenously over 2 to 3 minutes stabilizes cell membranes. This can be repeated if no change occurs in the ECG after 5 to 10 minutes. A dose of 10 units of regular insulin given simultaneously with 1 ampule of 50% dextrose intravenously increases cellular potassium uptake.[20] Nebulized albuterol can be used to cause an intracellular shift of potassium. Doses of 10 and 20 mg caused maximal decreases in serum potassium by 0.62 and 0.98 mmol/L, respectively, in a study of patients with chronic renal failure.[23] Onset of action was evident at 30 minutes and was sustained for 2 hours. Alkali therapy with sodium bicarbonate ($NaHCO_3$) also causes the shift of potassium into cells, but care must be taken in patients with renal failure or congestive heart failure who may be unable to handle the increased sodium load. If given, reassessment of volume status should be performed after administration of each ampule of bicarbonate.

Removal of potassium is the next step in acute correction of hyperkalemia. Loop or thiazide diuretics enhance potassium excretion if renal function is adequate. Cation-exchange resins act by exchanging sodium for potassium in the gastrointestinal tract and can be administered orally or rectally. The usual oral dose is 15 to 45 g of sodium polystyrene sulfonate mixed with 100 mL of sorbitol to avoid constipation. This usually lowers the serum potassium by 0.5 to 1.0 mmol/L within 1 to 2 hours and lasts up to 4 to 6 hours.[20] A dose of 50 g of sodium polystyrene sulfonate with 50 mL of 70% sorbitol in 150 mL of tap water can be administered as a retention enema in those unable to take oral medication, but in postoperative patients, the sorbitol should be omitted because of an increased risk of colonic necrosis.[20] Finally, for patients with life-threatening hyperkalemia who are unresponsive to these measures and for those with renal failure, dialysis may have to be performed.

ACUTE STROKE

Acute stroke occurred in 500,000 people in the United States in 1991; of those, 143,000 died.[24] It is now considered a medical emergency and should be managed as one. Advances in treatment have provided promising prospects not only for reducing infarct size but also for reversing the neurologic deficit by reestablishing blood flow through a once occluded cerebral vessel. Therefore, as in management of myocardial infarction, time is of the essence. Quick recognition of an acute stroke and rapid evaluation are the cornerstones of management. Consultation with a neurologist and transferring such patients to a unit specializing in the management of acute stroke may improve outcomes.[24]

Presentation

Patients with stroke can present in many different ways, depending upon which cerebral vessel is involved. A full discussion of vessel-dependent stroke syndromes is beyond the scope of this chapter; therefore, common stroke symptoms are presented here along with a table of common stroke patterns.

An alteration in consciousness may occur in a patient who is having stroke, but in general, loss of consciousness does not occur unless the stroke involves the brain stem or bilateral cerebral hemispheres or causes herniation of the

Table 4–9. *Common Patterns of Neurologic Abnormalities in Acute Ischemic Stroke*

Left (dominant) hemisphere	Aphasia, right hemiparesis, right-sided sensory loss, right visual field defect, poor right conjugate gaze, dysarthria, difficulty in reading, writing, and calculating
Right (nondominant) hemisphere	Neglect of the left visual space, left visual field defect, left hemiparesis, left-sided sensory loss, poor left conjugate gaze, extinction of left-sided stimuli, dysarthria, spatial disorientation
Brain stem/cerebellum/posterior hemisphere	Motor of sensory loss in all four limbs, crossed signs, limb or gait ataxia, dysarthria, dysconjugate gaze, nystagmus, amnesia, bilateral visual field defects
Small subcortical hemisphere or brain stem	
Pure motor stroke	Weakness of face and limbs on one side of the body without abnormalities of higher brain function, sensation, or vision
Pure sensory stroke	Decrease in sensation of face and limbs on one side of the body without abnormalities of higher brain function, motor function, or vision

(Adapted from Adams HP Jr et al. Guidelines for the management of patients with acute ischemic stroke: a statement for healthcare professionals from a special writing group of the Stroke Council, American Heart Association. Circulation 1994;90:1588–1601.)

brain stem. Varying degrees of aphasia may occur with or without dysarthria. Unilateral muscle weakness and sensory deficits are typically contralateral to the involved area. Changes in vision, such as loss of vision in one eye or visual field deficits, may occur. Ataxia and clumsiness may be noticeable when the patient walks or upon neurologic exam. Some common patterns of acute stroke are presented in Table 4–9.

Evaluation

A thorough history and physical exam should always be performed. The history may reveal a previous transient ischemic attack or stroke or previous diagnostic testing, such as carotid ultrasonography or cerebral angiography. The physical exam should focus on the cardiovascular and neurologic exam. Heart rhythm, carotid pulsations, and bruits may provide important clues to the cause of an acute stroke. Laboratory analysis, an electrocardiogram, a chest radiograph, and cerebral imaging should be included in the initial evaluation.[24]

The most important test to be performed is noncontrast computed tomography of the head. This should be done quickly to differentiate between hemorrhagic and ischemic stroke, as well as to rule out other possibilities such as a brain tumor or abscess. However, for suspected cerebellar or brain stem infarction, magnetic resonance imaging is more sensitive than computed tomography and may have to be performed.[24]

Laboratory studies should include a complete blood count, prothrombin time, partial thromboplastin time, and chemistry panel. Pulse oximetry and a fingerstick glucose test can be performed rapidly at the bedside to rule out hypoxia and hypoglycemia. Because of the strong association of heart disease and stroke, an ECG should be performed to assess for evidence of myocardial ischemia or infarction and arrythmias. Also, cardiac chamber enlargement may be identified on a chest radiograph.[24]

Treatment Priorities

Management of acute stroke should focus on the basics initially. The airway should be clear, adequate oxygenation should be maintained, and the blood pressure should be monitored frequently. The patient should be placed on continuous cardiac monitoring. Centers that specialize in acute stroke may be associated with improved outcomes.[24, 25] Therefore, transfer of the stable patient to a facility with excellence in stroke management may be appropriate.

Antihypertensive agents, in general, should be avoided, unless that patient has accelerated hypertension with a hemorrhagic infarction, aortic dissection, myocardial ischemia, or acute renal failure. However, if the mean arterial blood pressure is higher than 130 mm Hg, or the systolic blood pressure is higher than 220 mm Hg, treatment is indicated, according to recent guidelines.[24] Agents that provide good blood pressure control with minimal effect on cerebral blood pressure should be used. These include labetalol and enalaprilat if intravenous therapy is used, and captopril or nicardipine for oral therapy.[24] Low blood pressure is rare with acute stroke.

Table 4–10. *Complications of Acute Ischemic Stroke*

Neurologic
Cerebral edema
Hydrocephalus
Increased intracranial pressure
Seizures
Medical
Aspiration
Pneumonia
Myocardial infarction
Cardiac arrhythmias
Deep venous thrombosis/pulmonary embolism
Urinary tract infections
Decubitus ulcers
Contractures and stiff joints

(Adapted from Adams HP et al. Guidelines for the management of patients with acute ischemic stroke: a statement for healthcare professionals from a special writing group of the Stroke Council, American Heart Association. Circulation 1994;90;1588–1601.)

Treatment of acute stroke with anticoagulants and thrombolytics is still under investigation. There is no evidence that heparin improves outcome when administered in acute ischemic stroke, but it may be of benefit in cardioembolic stroke. Thrombolytics have been shown to improve outcome and neurologic recovery at the cost of increasing intracerebral hemorrhage.[26, 27] Consultation with a neurologist should be obtained to determine whether anticoagulants or thrombolytics are indicated and whether the risk-benefit ratio is favorable.

The most common complications of acute ischemic stroke are presented in Table 4–10. Consultation with a neurologist concerning any of the neurologic complications is appropriate. Seizures in stroke should be treated with anticonvulsants, but prophylactic administration of anticonvulsants is not recommended.[24] Pneumonia is common and should be suspect if hypoxia or fever develop. Prevention of deep vein thrombosis with subcutaneous heparin or low-molecular-weight heparin, or systematic compression devices if anticoagulants are contraindicated, should be attended to beginning at the initial evaluation.[24] Consultation with speech, occupational, and physical therapists is important in promoting functional recovery and may help to avoid problems with nutrition, decubitus ulcers, and contractures.

Outcomes

Population-based stroke registers have demonstrated a decline in stroke incidence and an even more pronounced decline in fatality rates. The rate of fatality at 1 month is about 20% to 30%.[28] A patient undergoing general surgery has up to a 3% risk of perioperative stroke.[29] A patient who suffers a stroke is at higher risk for recurrent stroke and myocardial infarction.

GIANT CELL ARTERITIS

Temporal (or giant cell) arteritis is a medical emergency. Without prompt glucocorticoid therapy, it can lead to severe visual loss or blindness. This disorder is characterized by focal areas of intense inflammation often containing characteristic multinucleated giant cells within the walls of elastin-containing arteries. Arteries affected by this disorder are typically limited to extracranial branches of the carotid artery.[30] These patients not uncommonly present with symptoms referable to the head, neck, and jaw regions.

Presentation

The diagnosis of temporal arteritis should be suspected based on the patient's history. Physical examination and blood testing help to support the clinical impression. The diagnosis is confirmed by temporal artery biopsy.

Temporal arteritis is generally a disease of the elderly. Onset of this disease before age 50 is extremely unusual. Women develop the condition more commonly than men, at a ratio of approximately 2:1.[30] The most common presenting symptom is headache, which affects 75% of patients and is classically bitemporal in distribution. The syndrome of polymyalgia rheumatica (PMR) accompanies temporal arteritis in at least 50% of patients. PMR is also a disease of the elderly that is characterized by pain and stiffness chiefly affecting the shoulders and pelvic girdle. Patients with PMR often describe difficulty in getting up from a reclining or seated position. Symptoms of PMR should raise suspicion of coexisting temporal arteritis.

Impaired vision occurs in 30% of patients with temporal arteritis. It may present with a variety of visual disturbances, including frank blindness. Urgent therapy (see later section) is mandated for patients with visual symptoms who are suspected of having temporal arteritis, even before supporting laboratory data are available.

Blood vessels supplying the muscles of mastication are frequently affected by the vasculitic process. One fourth of patients with temporal arteritis describe jaw claudication, which is pain in the masseter muscle that generally occurs during prolonged chewing. Fever may be the only clinical finding in some patients. Shaking chills, night sweats, weight loss, arthralgias, and malaise can occur as well, and such patients are often investigated for occult infection or malignancy.

Other symptoms of temporal arteritis may include throat pain, tongue pain, and scalp tenderness. The last problem is usually described as pain induced by combing the hair. Shoulder pain associated with polymyalgia rheumatica can also result in difficulty in combing the hair. Occasionally, larger elastic arteries outside the cranial distribution are involved, causing chronic cough, aortic regurgitation, or aortic aneurysm. Rarely, patients will present with posterior headaches due to occipital artery involvement.

Physical examination of patients with this disorder may be helpful. Patients are occasionally found to have palpable beading and tenderness of the temporal arteries. Less commonly, patients are found to have carotid bruits, aortic regurgitation, or frank synovitis.[30]

Evaluation

Certain routine blood tests support the diagnosis of temporal arteritis, although they are not diagnostic in and of themselves. The erythrocyte sedimentation rate is nearly always markedly elevated (often $>$ 100 mm/h by the Westergren method) in both temporal arteritis and polymyalgia rheumatica. Half of patients have normochromic, normocytic anemia, and one third of patients have elevated alkaline phosphatase. The diagnostic test that is the gold standard is temporal artery biopsy, which should be performed promptly when this diagnosis is suspected (Fig. 4–2A and B). Temporal artery involvement can be very localized, with intervening segments of artery histologically normal. Therefore, the surgeon should remove a 3- to 5-cm segment, and the pathologist may have to study several sections to demonstrate the arteritis.[30] In many cases, bilateral temporal

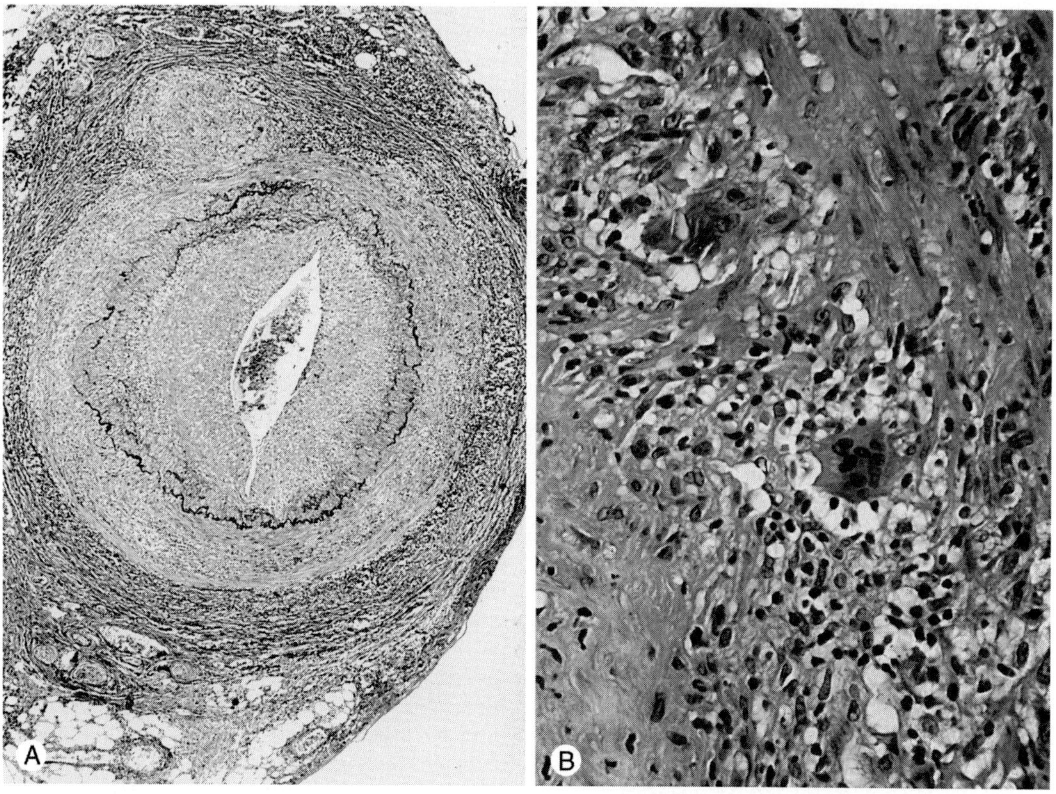

Figure 4–2. Histologic findings of giant cell arteritis. A: A cross-section of a temporal artery biopsy showing inflammation involving the entire thickness of the vessel wall. B: Higher-power magnification shows detail of the lymphocytic inflammation as well as multinucleated giant cells. (Photomicrographs courtesy of William Green, M.D.).

artery biopsies are performed to maximize sensitivity of the test. Sensitivities of 60% to 90% have been reported.[31–33] Giant cells are not always seen and are not necessary to establish this diagnosis. Although the biopsy is important, particularly with regard to justifying and guiding long-term therapy, empiric glucocorticoid therapy should not be delayed until after the procedure. Diagnostic histologic changes (particularly destruction of the elastic lamina) persist beyond the initiation of therapy, so most biopsies performed within 1 week of initiating therapy are usually reliable.[30, 33]

Treatment Priorities

The treatment for suspected or proven temporal arteritis is prednisone at a starting dose of 1 mg/kg/day (usually 40 to 80 mg/day). Other glucocorticoid preparations at equipotent doses can be used as well. Prompt institution of therapy is essential in order to prevent blindness, particularly in patients with early visual symptoms. A significant symptomatic response should be observed within days of initiating therapy. If a patient does not respond to therapy, the diagnosis should be called into question. In this situation, histologic information from an adequate temporal artery biopsy becomes essential. Laboratory tests, including the erythrocyte sedimentation rate, often normalize within 1 month of therapy. Prednisone is tapered very slowly, typically over a period of 6 to 24 months, as this disease is very prone to reactivation.[30] After a 6-month taper, approximately 50% of patients remain free of symptoms. If a patient relapses, resuming prednisone at a lower dosage (10 to 15 mg/day) is often adequate. A subpopulation of patients require treatment for 5 years or longer.[31]

Outcomes

Retrospective case studies suggest that the incidence of blindness is 20% or less. Once visual loss occurs in one eye, remaining vision can be lost within days. Prompt treatment, however, prevents total blindness in the vast majority of cases.[32]

ADVERSE DRUG REACTIONS

Adverse reactions to drugs are quite common and can lead to acutely life-threatening consequences. Up to 5% of all hospital admissions may be the result of adverse drug reactions.[34] Hospitalized patients are particularly at risk because of greater drug exposure, as they receive, on average, more than 10 different drugs. When fewer than 6 drugs are administered to an inpatient, the probability of an adverse reaction is 5%. Of patients receiving 15 or more drugs, more than 40% experience an adverse reaction.[35] It is estimated that 1 in every 1000 hospitalized patients has a serious dermatologic drug reaction.[36]

There are two categories of adverse drug reaction. Pharmacologic (type A) drug reactions are those that are predictable based on the pharmacology of the drug. They account for 80% of all drug reactions. A pharmacologic drug reaction is, by definition, dose-related; it resolves after discontinuation of the drug and recurs when the patient is rechallenged with the same substance. Rechallenge is not routinely recommended and should be considered only if the realistic benefits provided by the drug outweigh the risks. Idiosyncratic (type B) reactions cannot be predicted based on the known pharmacologic properties of the drug.[34]

The spectrum of potential adverse drug reactions is enormous and can affect every organ system. Dermatologic manifestations alone range from minor rash to the potentially fatal toxic epidermal necrolysis. Other drug reactions of urgent concern include anaphylaxis and angioedema.

Presentation

Toxic epidermal necrolysis (TEN) is an idiosyncratic drug reaction in adults. It is acute in onset and classically presents with poorly demarcated macules with purpuric centers concentrated around the face and upper trunk. These lesions spread rapidly and tend to coalesce into a confluent erythema. They then develop multiple flaccid bullae that rupture, sloughing large sheets of full-thickness necrotic epidermis, leaving behind denuded dermis. Most cases are associated with fever (>38°C) and extreme skin pain. TEN causes epidermal detachment of more than 30% of the body surface area. Lateral force applied to areas of normal-appearing skin next to intact bullae can cause the epidermis to separate from the dermis (Nikolsky's sign). Lesions that affect the oral, respiratory, intestinal, or urethral mucosa occur in 90% of patients. If this syndrome affects less than 10% of body surface area, it is referred to as the Stevens-Johnson syndrome and is associated with a more favorable prognosis. Patients who have the human immunodeficiency virus (HIV) are at significantly increased risk of drug-induced skin rashes, including TEN and Stevens-Johnson syndrome. The risk of cutaneous reactions to sulfonamides, in particular, is 10 to 1000 times higher among HIV-infected patients.[36]

Anaphylaxis is a clinically defined syndrome characterized by respiratory distress followed by hypotension (shock). It commonly involves the skin, producing urticaria, angioedema, and pruritis. Gastrointestinal symptoms are common as well and include diarrhea, nausea, vomiting, and abdominal cramping. It typically occurs seconds to minutes after the administration of a specific antigen to which a patient has previously been sensitized. Immunoglobulin E (IgE) antibodies mediate the release of histamine, prostaglandins, and other vasoactive agents that cause the syndrome. Anaphylaxis can result in death, most commonly by airway obstruction. Hypotensive collapse is the second most common cause of death. Respiratory arrest due to acute bronchospasm is generally preventable with prompt treatment. Shock may occur in the absence of respiratory symptoms.[37–39]

Anaphylactoid reactions are similar clinically to anaphylactic reactions but differ in that they are not mediated by IgE. Substances that precipitate anaphylactoid reactions are thought to cause direct release of vasoactive agents from mast cells or basophils. Hyperosmolar solutions such as intravenous contrast are common triggers of anaphylactoid reactions. Reactions occur in 5% to 10% of patients receiving intravenous contrast, and death occurs in 1 in 40,000 exposures.[39] Clinically, this syndrome is similar to anaphylaxis, although it is less likely to be associated with marked respiratory compromise or vascular collapse.

Angioedema appears as poorly demarcated areas of skin swelling, most commonly involving the lips, eyelids, and tongue. It tends to cause a burning discomfort unlike urticaria, which is usually associated with pruritis. Angioedema is characterized by edema in the deeper layers of skin, whereas urticaria affects superficial layers. When angioedema involves the airway, it is an emergency because it can lead to obstruction.

Evaluation

Evaluation of patients with adverse drug reactions begins with the identification and elimination of the offending agent. More than 95% of TEN in adults is caused by medication exposure. The most commonly implicated agents include carbamazepine, long-acting sulfadoxine and pyrimethamine, and trimethoprim-sulfamethoxazole. A list of 24 other agents and drug classes account for two thirds of cases of TEN or Stevens-Johnson syndrome. A skin biopsy should be performed in most cases to help rule out other disorders of desquamation, exfoliation, or blistering.[36]

A history of anaphylaxis in response to a particular agent is an absolute contraindication to rechallenge with the agent. Patients with a history of a mild systemic allergic reaction can have a severe reaction if rechallenged with the same agent.[39] Antibiotics (penicillins, cephalosporins, amphotericin B, nitrofurantoin), local anesthetics (procaine, lidocaine), bee venom, and foods are among the most common precipitants of anaphylactic reactions.[38] IgE-mediated systemic reaction to penicillin can be predicted by skin sensitivity testing. A patient with a history of penicillin allergy should be tested before receiving the drug. Anaphylaxis to penicillin has never been reported in a patient with a negative skin test. Three fourths of patients with a histories of penicillin sensitivity have negative skin tests and are therefore not at risk for anaphylaxis.[39] Two thirds of patients with histories of penicillin sensitivity and positive skin tests experience an allergic reaction if given the drug.[38]

Cephalosporins have in common with penicillin a β-lactam ring core structure. There is a 4- to 8-fold increase of risk of systemic reaction to first-generation cephalosporins in patients allergic to penicillin. Reaction rates to second- and third-generation cephalosporins are lower. Penicillin skin testing can help predict risk of anaphylaxis to cephalosporins. Isolated skin rashes in response to penicillin are not IgE-mediated and do not predict risk of anaphylaxis. It is generally safe to treat patients with a history of rash with second- or third-generation cephalosporins. Monobactams such as aztreonam do not cross-react with β-lactams; there is a 50% cross-reactivity with carbapenams such as imipenem.[39]

Many of the drugs that cause anaphylactic reactions can also result in isolated angioedema. Angioedema can also be caused by angiotensin-converting enzyme (ACE) inhibitors, nonsteroidal anti-inflammatory drugs, radiocontrast agents, and opiates through non-IgE mediated mechanisms.[36] The use of ACE inhibitors for the treatment of hypertension, congestive heart failure, and diabetic nephropathy has increased greatly over the past decade, and so too has the incidence of angioedema associated with ACE inhibitors. Angioedema occurs in 0.1% to 0.2% of patients within 3 weeks of starting ACE inhibitor therapy. It can resolve within hours of discontinuing the drug. The mechanism by which these drugs cause angioedema is unknown. ACE normally degrades bradykinin, so patients taking ACE inhibitors may be at risk for angioedema because of bradykinin accumulation.[40] Hemodialysis with high-flux membranes increases bradykinin production and so increases the risk of reaction to ACE inhibitors.[41]

Treatment Priorities

Treatment of severe drug reactions begins with discontinuing the causative agent. Patients with TEN should be transferred to an intensive care or burn unit. Aggressive fluid replacement is essential, as these patients are susceptible to massive fluid loss through denuded skin. Sepsis resulting from skin colonization is the most common cause of death in these patients. TEN is associated with a 30% mortality rate, whereas mortality for Stevens-Johnson syndrome is 5%. There are no proven ways to arrest the progression of TEN.[36]

Effective therapy for anaphylaxis, anaphylactoid reactions, and angioedema depends on prompt diagnosis. Airway integrity should be established, followed by urgent medical therapy. Proper airway management is determined by the nature of the respiratory embarrassment. Hypoxemia associated with severe bronchospasm not corrected by face mask oxygen supplementation is best managed with endotracheal intubation and assisted ventilation. Severe laryngeal edema may require emergent cricothyroidotomy or tracheotomy. Supplemental oxygen is indicated for most patients with respiratory symptoms.

The drug of choice for anaphylaxis is epinephrine; it is most effective when administered early. Epinephrine is usually given subcutaneously, 0.3 to 0.5 mg (0.3 to 0.5 mL of a 1:1000 solution) and can be given at 20-minute intervals. Epinephrine can also be given through an endotracheal tube (3 to 5 mL of a 1:10,000 solution). For hypotensive patients, 3 to 5 mL of a 1:10,000 solution can be given through a central line. A continuous epinephrine infusion titrated according to blood pressure may be needed for protracted anaphylaxis. Volume expansion with normal saline or Ringer's lactate solution is important in most hypotensive patients with acute hypovolemia due to capillary leakage or sudden drop in peripheral vascular resistance. A wide-open bolus of 500 to 1000 mL should be followed by a continuous infusion adjusted according to blood pressure and urine output. Vasopressive agents such as dopamine at 2 to 50 μg/kg/min are indicated for hypotension that does not respond to volume expansion and epinephrine. Bronchospasm should be treated with inhaled β-agonists such as albuterol 0.5 mL (2.5 mg). Previous exposure to β-blockers increases the risk of anaphylaxis and renders the reaction more resistant to treatment. Glucagon infusions can help to provide hemodynamic support in this setting.[39]

If the offending antigen is administered orally, induction of emesis with syrup of ipecac followed by activated charcoal in a cathartic can prevent continued absorption of the antigen. Both antihistamines and glucocorticoids are of little value in treating acute anaphylaxis, but both may be helpful in preventing recurrent reactions. Diphenhydramine 25 to 50 mg intravenously every 6 hours is the most commonly used antihistamine. Hydrocortisone 500 mg intravenously should be used initially in most cases and then tapered according to the patient's clinical status, although it does not relieve symptoms acutely.[39]

ILLICIT DRUG INTOXICATION

The use of cocaine, ethanol, and opioids can result in life-threatening intoxication syndromes. Medical complications resulting from drugs that are abused are a major burden on the health care system in this country. Cocaine use, for example, resulted in 30,900 emergency room visits in late 1992.[42] Of all deaths related to cocaine use, it is estimated that only one third are due to medical complications; the remainder are due to violent injuries.[43] Persistent opiate users have a 25% chance of dying within 20 years of active use from a variety of causes, including both medical complications and violence.[44] Ethanol dependence or abuse develops in 3% to 20% of the population.[3] Acute intoxications resulting from the use of these three drugs are often treatable, making prompt recognition essential.

Presentation

Cocaine is a stimulant, a local anesthetic, and a potent vasoconstrictor. Cocaine augments sympathetic nerve activity by inhibiting the reuptake of dopamine and norepinephrine. Its stimulant properties account for many of the symptoms and signs found in intoxicated patients. Mild stimulation can result in euphoria, agitation, emotional lability, and hallucinations. Physical findings include tachycardia, tachypnea, hyperpyrexia, nausea, vomiting, hypertension, mydriasis, muscle jerks, and diaphoretic, pale skin. Advanced cocaine intoxication can present with unresponsiveness, coma, and irregular or Cheyne-Stokes respiration and can end in respiratory arrest.[43]

The most common single complaint reported in one study of cocaine-related hospital visits was chest pain.[45] Only rarely was it caused by demonstrable cardiac ischemia. However, cocaine can result in a variety of life-threatening cardiovascular syndromes, including acute myocardial infarction, arrhythmias, and malignant hypertension in young people without other risks for cardiac disease. Cocaine use has a known association with either traumatic or nontraumatic rhabdomyolysis, a pathologic breakdown of muscle that can lead to renal failure. Potentially fatal central nervous system toxicity includes seizure activity and stroke induced by cerebral vasospasm. Smoking alkaloid cocaine (freebase) or the alkaloid prepared with sodium bicarbonate (crack) can result in a variety of pulmonary complications, including sudden pulmonary edema, pneumomediastinum, pulmonary hemorrhage, and hypersensitivity pneumonitis.[46] A patient with an especially fulminant course that is unresponsive to therapy may have swallowed packets of cocaine. Spillage of large amounts of cocaine in the intestinal tract can be fatal rapidly.

Cocaine withdrawal can be difficult to distinguish from major depression. A patient going through depression related to cocaine withdrawal is at significant risk for suicide.

Topical cocaine hydrochloride is commonly used as a local anesthetic in the mucous membranes of nasal, oral, and laryngeal cavities. The drug can be absorbed through mucous membranes but is generally broken down rapidly by plasma esterases. The plasma half-life is approximately 1 hour. Topical cocaine is available in 4% and 10% solutions. Typically, 5 mL of a 4% solution, or 200 mg, is the maximum dose used to anesthetize the nasal passageway. A lethal dose is approximately 1.2 g; however, idiosyncratic toxic reactions have been reported with doses as low as 20 mg. Symptoms of iatrogenic overdose can be identical to those experienced by recreational users and include restlessness, tachycardia, and hypertension.[47]

Opioids such as morphine or heroin can produce excessive sedation, hypoventilation, ileus, urinary retention, muscle flaccidity, and miosis when a patient has been overdosed. Less commonly, patients can develop hypotension, noncardiogenic pulmonary edema, bradycardia, coma, and respiratory arrest. Opioid withdrawal causes significant illness but is rarely life threatening. Withdrawal begins 8 to 12 hours after cessation of the drug and can last up to 5 days. It is characterized by nausea, vomiting, diarrhea, sweating, rhinorrhea, painful muscle cramping, mydriasis, piloerection, restlessness, and fever.[44]

Blood ethanol concentrations of more than 100 mg/dL generally meet the legal definition of intoxication. Patients at this level are often ataxic. As blood levels rise, patients become cognitively impaired and sedated. Lethal concentrations are highly variable but are generally within the range of 300 to 700 mg/dL. Death usually occurs as a result of respiratory depression that culminates in respiratory arrest.[48]

Evaluation

The history should include the types of drugs taken and the route of administration. Evidence of trauma and needle marks should also be sought. The physical examination of a hypertensive patient with cocaine intoxication should include inspection of the fundi for papilledema, which suggests malignant hypertension. Markedly hypertensive patients should also have a urinalysis, which can show cast formation or hematuria in the setting of acute hypertension-related renal damage. All such patients should have an ECG followed by continuous cardiac monitoring. Electrolytes, including serum creatinine and creatinine phosphokinase, should be measured. Freebase or crack smokers complaining of breathing difficulties or chest pain should undergo chest radiography to rule out pulmonary complications. Abdominal radiography is also indicated for individuals suspected of swallowing packets of cocaine ("body-packers").

Treatment Priorities

Treatment for all intoxicated patients begins with securing an adequate airway and supporting respirations and adequate circulation as necessary.

Many patients with cocaine-related syndromes do not require pharmacologic intervention; the figure was 24% in one series.[45] Because of cocaine's short half-life, severe toxicity rarely lasts for more than 2 hours. Agitated delirium, seizures, and hypertension not associated with acute end-organ damage are best treated with benzodiazepines such as 0.5 mg/kg of diazepam administered intravenously over 8 h.[42] Excessive muscular activity associated with agitation and seizures contribute to myocardial ischemia, hyperpyrexia, and myonecrosis, which can result in morbidity and mortality.[43] Extensive clinical experience and animal experimentation suggest that benzodiazepines should be the first-line drugs when pharmacologic intervention is warranted for cocaine toxicity. Patients felt to have cocaine-induced myocardial ischemia should be treated with oxygen and then aspirin to prevent thrombus formation, as long as there are no hemorrhagic contraindications. Nitroglycerin is also indicated, as it has been shown to reverse the coronary artery vasoconstriction induced by cocaine and because it relieves chest pain. If chest pain persists despite oxygen, benzodiazepines, aspirin, and nitrates, patients have been known to respond to α-receptor blockade using phentolamine at suggested beginning dose of 1 mg intravenously, which can reverse cocaine-induced vasoconstriction. Calcium channel blockers, especially verapamil, have also been used with success in this setting. If myocardial ischemia persists despite these measures, consideration should be given to thrombolytic therapy or angioplasty.[49] Although β-blockers are commonly used for patients with myocardial ischemia or infarction not related to cocaine use, they should not be used in a cocaine-intoxicated patient. β-Adrenergic stimulation helps to counterbalance the α-receptor–mediated vasoconstriction stimulated by cocaine. Blocking the β receptors can result in unopposed α stimulation and actually worsen cocaine-induced coronary vasoconstriction.[49, 50] Malignant ventricular arrhythmias such as ventricular tachycardia may be treated with lidocaine if several hours have elapsed since cocaine ingestion. However, lidocaine may not be safe if there is still circulating cocaine because the combination of drugs may lower arrhythmia and seizure thresholds. Sodium bicarbonate may be a safer choice for arrhythmia immediately following cocaine use.[49]

Mild to moderate hypertension related to cocaine use is best treated with benzodiazepines. If they are not adequate or if there is acute end-organ damage, the patient should be treated with intravenous phentolamine or sodium nitroprusside. Although β-blockers should be avoided, some authors have suggested the use of labetalol, which is a combined α- and β-blocker. However, the use of labetalol in a cocaine-intoxicated patient is controversial.[49]

Hyperthermia associated with cocaine use should be treated by controlling excessive muscular activity and seizures. Cooling blankets may also be helpful. A patient with rhabdomyolysis needs intravenous hydration to minimize myoglobin precipitation in the renal tubules.[43] A patient with packets of cocaine in the intestinal tract should be admitted for ICU monitoring; however, surgery often is not necessary; purgation induced by charcoal and mineral oil can be tried first.[48]

Opioid overdose is treated with naloxone hydrochloride, which is a specific opioid antagonist. It can reverse the sedation, hypoventilation, and hypotension associated with overdose. The beginning dose is 2 mg intravenously, although larger doses may be needed for overdoses of propoxyphene, diphenoxylate, or pentazocine. If there is no response to a cumulative dose of 10 mg of naloxone, the patient is unlikely to have simple opioid overdose. Naloxone has a 45-minute duration of action and is often given in a continuous intravenous infusion so the patient does not relapse after an intravenous bolus has worn off.[48] It can also be give intralingually[51] or via endotracheal tube when intravenous access is not possible. A patient who has overdosed on heroin should be observed for 24 hours. A patient who has overdosed on a longer-acting opioid such as methadone should be observed for 72 hours. Opiate withdrawal can be treated symptomatically. Nonopiate antidiarrheal agents and decongestants may be helpful. Clonidine, an α-2 adrenergic agonist that reduces catecholamine release from peripheral nerve endings is also effective in reducing hyperadrenergic symptoms of withdrawal. Recommended doses include 5 μg/kg or up to 0.3 mg 2 to 4 times per day. Some authors recommend a slow taper of opioid instead of acute discontinuation in addicted patients. Methadone is often used because of its ease of administration, as it is dosed once a day.[44]

A patient in a coma because of ethanol intoxication may require endotracheal intubation for airway protection. Gastric lavage should be performed in a comatose patient. Charcoal is not helpful because ethanol is rapidly absorbed. Hemodialysis can be used in life-threatening situations. Thiamine 100 mg intravenously followed by 50 mL of D-50-W should be given to a patient with severe alcohol intoxication.[48]

Outcomes

In a retrospective review of 233 cocaine-related visits to an urban emergency department, acute mortality was less than 1%. Only 9.9% of patients had to be admitted.[45] A patient who has suffered a cocaine-related myocardial infarction runs a high risk for recurrent ischemic chest pain or a second myocardial infarction. However, nonspecific chest pain is associated with a 1-year, 98% survival rate and a 1% risk of myocardial infarction.[49]

REFERENCES

1. Lohr RH. Treatment of alcohol withdrawal in hospitalized patients. Mayo Clin Proc 1995;70:777–782.
2. Osler W. The Principles and Practice of Medicine. New York, Appleton, 1892, pp. 1000–1005.
3. Schuckit MA. Alcohol and Alcoholism. In Fauci AS, Braunwald E, Isselbacher KJ et al., eds. Harrison's Principles of Internal Medicine, vol. 2. New York, McGraw-Hill, 1998, pp. 2503–2508.
4. Krasser C. The role of phenytoin in the management of alcohol withdrawal syndrome. Web/URL: <http://www.asam.org/publ/dilantin.htm> Last accessed 2/8/99:14.
5. Ewing JA. Detecting alcoholism. The CAGE questionnaire. JAMA 1984;252:1905–1907.
6. Ferguson JA et al. Risk factors for delirium tremens development. J Gen Intern Med 1996;11:410–414.
7. Sullivan JT et al. Assessment of alcohol withdrawal: the revised Clinical Institute Withdrawal Assessment for Alcohol scale (CIWA-Ar). Br J Addict 1989;84:1353–1357.
8. Mayo-Smith MF. Pharmacological management of alcohol withdrawal: a meta-analysis and evidence-based practice guideline. American Society of Addiction Medicine Working Group on Pharmacological Management of Alcohol Withdrawal. JAMA 1997;278:144–151.
9. Wrenn KD, Murphy F, Slovis CM. A toxicity study of parenteral thiamine hydrochloride. Ann Emerg Med 1989;18:867–870.
10. Saitz R et al. Individualized treatment for alcohol withdrawal: A randomized double-blind controlled trial. JAMA 1994;272:519–523.
11. Saitz R, O'Malley SS. Pharmacotherapies for alcohol abuse: withdrawal and treatment. Med Clin North Am 1997;81:881–907.
12. Filding C, Jensen LM, Tonnesen H. Influence of alcohol intake on postoperative morbitity after hysterectomy. Am J Obstet Gynecol 1992;166:667–670.
13. Tonnesen H et al. Postoperative morbidity among symptom-free alcohol misusers. Lancet 1992;340:334–347.
14. Dittmar G. Alcoholic delirium—a potentially life-threatening condition. Fortschr Med 1994;112:274–276.
15. Cushman PJ. Delirium tremens: update on an old disorder. Postgrad Med 1989;82:117–122.
16. Adrogue HJ, Madias NE. Management of life-threatening acid-base disorders. First of two parts [comments]. N Engl J Med 1998;338:26–34.
17. Dubose TD. Acidosis and alkalosis. In Fauci AS et al., eds. Harrison's Principles of Internal Medicine, vol. 1. New York, McGraw-Hill, 1998, pp. 277–286.
18. Stacpoole PW, Wright EC, Baumgartner TG et al. Natural history and course of acquired lactic acidosis in adults. DCA-Lactic Acidosis Study Group. Am J Med 1994;97:47–54.
19. Umpierrez GE et al. Hyperglycemic crises in urban blacks. Arch Intern Med 1997;157:669–675.
20. Brenner BM, Singer GG. Fluid and electrolyte disturbances. In Fauci AS et al., eds. Harrison's Principles of Internal Medicine, vol. 1. New York, McGraw-Hill, 1998, pp. 271–277.
21. Mandal AK. Hypokalemia and hyperkalemia. Med Clin North Am 1997;81:611–639.
22. Singer GG. Fluid and Electrolyte Management. In Carey CF, Lee HH, Woeltje KF, eds. The Washington Manual of Medical Therapeutics, Philadelphia, Lippincott-Raven, 1998, pp. 48–55.
23. Allon M, Dunlay R, Copkney C. Nebulized albuterol for acute hyperkalemia in patients on hemodialysis. Ann Intern Med 1989;110:426–429.
24. Adams HP Jr et al. Guidelines for the management of patients with acute ischemic stroke: a statement for healthcare professionals from a special writing group of the Stroke Council, American Heart Association Circulation 1994;90:1588–1601.
25. Langhorne P et al. Do stroke units save lives? [comments]. Lancet 1993;342:395–398.
26. Anonymous. Practice advisory: thrombolytic therapy for acute ischemic stroke—summary statement. Report of the Quality Standards Subcommittee of the American Academy of Neurology [comments]. Neurology 1996;47:835–839.
27. Hacke W et al. Intravenous thrombolysis with recombinant tissue plasminogen activator for acute hemispheric stroke. The European Cooperative Acute Stroke Study (ECASS) [comments]. JAMA 1995;274:1017–1025.
28. Numminen H et al. Declining incidence and mortality rates of stroke in Finland from 1972 to 1991. Results of three population-based stroke registers. Stroke 1996;27:1487–1491.
29. Landercasper J et al. Perioperative stroke risk in 173 consecutive patients with a past history of stroke. Arch Surg 1990;125:986–989.
30. Hellmann DB. Vasculitis. In Stobo JD et al., eds. The Principles and Practice of Medicine. Stamford: Appleton & Lange, 1996, pp. 215–221.
31. Nordborg E et al. Giant Cell Arteritis. Rheum Dis Clin North Am 1995;21:1013–1026.
32. Hunder GG. Giant cell arteritis and polymyalgia rheumatica. Med Clin North Am 1997;81:195–219.
33. Swannell AJ. Polymyalgia rheumatica and temporal arteritis: diagnosis and management. Br Med J 1997;314:1329–1332.
34. Pirmohamed M et al. Adverse drug reactions. Br Med J 1998;316:1295–1298.
35. Wood AJJ. Adverse reactions to drugs. In Fauci AS et al., eds. Harrison's Principles of Internal Medicine. New York, McGraw-Hill, 1998, pp. 422–430.
36. Roujeau JC, Stern RS. Severe adverse cutaneous reactions to drugs. New Engl J Med 1994;331:1272–1285.
37. Bochner BS, Lichtenstein LM. Anaphylaxis. N Engl J Med 1991;324:1785–1790.
38. Austen KF. Diseases of immediate type hypersensitivity. In Fauci AS et al., eds. Harrison's Principles of Internal Medicine. New York, McGraw-Hill, 1998, pp. 1860–1869.
39. Pittman A, Tillinghast J. Allergy and immunology. In Carey CF, Lee HH, Woeltje KF, eds. The Washington Manual of Medical Therapeutics. Philadelphia, Lippincott-Raven, 1998, pp. 213–226.
40. Israili ZH, Hall WD. Cough and angioneurotic edema

associated with angiotensin-converting enzyme inhibitor therapy. Ann Intern Med 1992;117:234–242.
41. Brunet P et al. Anaphylactoid reactions during hemodialysis and hemofiltration: role of associating AN69 membrane and angiotensin 1-converting enzyme inhibitors. Am J Kidney Dis 1992;19:444–447.
42. Mendelson JH, Mello NK. Cocaine and other commonly abused drugs. In Fauci AS et al., eds. Harrison's Principles of Internal Medicine, vol. 2. New York, McGraw-Hill, 1998, pp. 2512–2516.
43. Zafar H, Vaz A, Carlson RW. Acute complications of cocaine intoxication. Hosp Pract 1997;32:167–181.
44. Schuckit MA, Segal DS. Opioid drug abuse and dependence. In Fauci AS et al., eds. Harrison's Principles of Internal Medicine, vol. 2, 1998, pp. 2508–2512.
45. Brody SL, Slovis CM, Wrenn KD. Cocaine-related medical problems: consecutive series of 233 patients. Am J Med 1990;88:325–331.
46. Ettinger NA, Albin RJ. A Review of the respiratory effects of smoking cocaine. Am J Med 1989; 87:664–668.
47. Physician's Desk Reference. Montvale, Medical Economics, 1998, p. 3223.
48. Goodenberger D. Medical emergencies. In Carey CF, Lee HH, Woeltje KF, eds. The Washington Manual of Medical Therapeutics. Philadelphia, Lippincott-Raven, 1998, pp. 494–526.
49. Hollander JE. The management of cocaine-associated myocardial ischemia. N Engl J Med 1995;333:1267–1272.
50. Lange RA et al. Potentiation of cocaine-induced coronary vasoconstriction by beta-adrenergic blockade. Ann Intern Med 1990;112:897–903.
51. Maio RF, Gaukel B, Freeman B. Intralingual naloxone injection for narcotic-induced respiratory depression. Ann Emerg Med 1987;16:572–573.

CHAPTER 5

Endocrine Emergencies

Paul W. Ladenson, MD, and
Michael S. Boyne, MD

A number of endocrine and metabolic disorders, such as hypothyroidism, hyponatremia, and hypercalcemia, occur quite commonly in the general population, so their presence in patients with conditions requiring head and neck surgery can be expected. These diseases can have significant impacts on the cardiovascular function, nutritional state, neurologic status, and immune system of a surgical patient, potentially affecting a successful outcome. Therefore, it is necessary for a head and neck surgeon to be knowledgeable about the presentation and management of endocrine emergencies.

Condensed descriptions of the most common and severe endocrine and metabolic emergencies are presented in this chapter, which highlights measures for their prompt diagnosis and immediate management. The essential tests for biochemical confirmation of these endocrinopathies are detailed, but realistically, some of the endocrine emergencies require treatment before definitive laboratory results are available. Consequently, clinical acumen with a high index of suspicion for these disorders is required for early recognition of them, especially as many of their clinical manifestations are nonspecific and relatively common.

ADRENAL CRISIS

Adrenal crisis can occur in the setting of perioperative stress, particularly in a patient who has been taking exogenous glucocorticoid preparations and in a patient who is undergoing transsphenoidal pituitary surgery. Whether the patient suffers shock and death or is effectively treated depends, of course, on prompt diagnosis of the condition. Recognizing the possibility of acute adrenal insufficiency (adrenal crisis) in a patient with nonspecific symptoms and signs is the challenging part. Once this has been done, confirming the diagnosis and treatment is typically relatively straightforward.

Primary adrenal insufficiency can be caused by infectious, autoimmune, hemorrhagic, or tumor destruction of the adrenal cortex, with resulting glucocorticoid (cortisol) and mineralocorticoid (aldosterone) deficiencies. Hypothalamic and pituitary disorders cause secondary (or central) adrenal insufficiency with isolated glucocorticoid deficiency due to corticotropin releasing hormone (CRH) and corticotropin (ACTH) deprivation, respectively. The most common cause of adrenal insufficiency is long-term glucocorticoid therapy, which may cause prolonged suppression of the hypothalamic-pituitary-adrenal axis, even after therapy has been discontinued for several months.[1]

Presentation

Most of the symptoms of adrenal insufficiency are nonspecific: weakness, malaise, fatigue, anorexia, nausea, and vomiting are common initial symptoms, with weight loss if the condition has been subacute or chronic. The syndrome can then progress to fever, abdominal pain, intractable vomiting, delirium, hypotension, and vascular collapse that is resistant to catecholamines.

Signs of primary adrenal insufficiency may include hypotension, dehydration, and hyperpigmentation of the gingival and buccal mucosae and of the skin, especially the palmar creases, areolae, axillae, and old scars, and over extensor surfaces. Secondary adrenal insufficiency is associated with pallor and other signs of hypopituitarism such as hypogonadism, secondary hypothyroidism, diabetes insipidus, and growth failure.

The first clue that a patient with nonspecific symptoms or shock might have adrenal insufficiency may be abnormalities in routinely obtained laboratory tests, such as hyponatremia, hyperkalemia (typically only in primary adrenal insufficiency), azotemia, hypoglycemia, mild normocytic anemia, eosinophilia, or lymphocytosis.

Evaluation

It is crucial to consider adrenal insufficiency in patients with unexplained hypotension, vomiting, or abdominal, flank, or back pain, particularly in the settings noted above.[2] To confirm or exclude the diagnosis, serum and plasma samples should be obtained for measurement of cortisol and ACTH concentrations, respectively. This *must* be done before administration of glucocorticoid replacement therapy. A random cortisol level above 25 μg/dL excludes adrenal insufficiency, but lesser values in a critically ill patient—even values within the normal range for nonstressed individuals—do not rule out adrenal insufficiency.

In most circumstances, a 1-hour ACTH stimulation test should also be performed, in which the serum cortisol concentration is measured before as well as 30 and 60 minutes after the administration of 250 μg ACTH (cosyntropin). A peak serum cortisol concentration greater than 20 μg/dL is normal.[3] Because this test is predicated on the absence of an adrenal cortical response, it may yield falsely normal results in a patient with acute secondary adrenal insufficiency, for example, during the initial days or weeks after pituitary surgery, when the adrenal may not have yet atrophied as a result of ACTH deficiency.[4] Women taking estrogen preparations may also have falsely normal values due to an increase in cortisol-binding globulin.

The plasma ACTH concentration is helpful in distinguishing primary adrenal insufficiency, in which it is typically elevated, and secondary adrenal insufficiency, in which it is inappropriately normal or low. The CRH, metyrapone, and insulin tolerance tests for identification of secondary adrenal dysfunction are described by Grinspoon and Biller.[3]

Priorities

Parenteral glucocorticoid administration and fluid resuscitation are the cornerstones of management. Typical glucocorticoid regimens include 100 mg of hydrocortisone, intravenously, or 40 mg of methylprednisolone every 8 hours. In patients with primary adrenal failure, an additional 0.1 mg of fludrocortisone per day may be required to correct hyponatremia and hyperkalemia. Generous intravenous fluids should be administered, typically normal saline and 5% dextrose at a rate of 1 to 2 L/h. Any underlying precipitating factor such as systemic infection should be treated promptly.

Clinical improvement should begin within 4 to 6 hours and be clearly evident within 12 to 24 hours if adrenal insufficiency is solely responsible for the patient's symptoms. The glucocorticoid can be reduced to 50 mg every 6 hours when the clinical picture improves. The hyponatremia responds to normal saline and glucocorticoids and does not generally require the use of hypertonic saline. After the patient is stabilized, the cause of the adrenal insufficiency can be investigated. The ACTH level is invaluable in the evaluation, as high levels indicate primary disease, but other testing may be required.

Prevention

Adrenal crisis is preventable in patients being treated for previously diagnosed adrenal insufficiency, in those suspected of developing adrenal insufficiency after hypophysectomy, and in patients who have recently been treated with glucocorticoid medications.[5] A patient's maintenance glucocorticoid dose should be doubled in the setting of minor illness such as sinusitis or procedures such as bronchoscopy. A patient undergoing surgery under general anesthesia should receive 100 mg of hydrocortisone or 40 mg of methylprednisolone intravenously on-call to the operating room and 50 mg of hydrocortisone every 6 hours or 20 mg of methylprednisolone every 8 hours for the next 24 hours. In patients without complications, the dose can then be reduced by 50% for an additional 24 hours and then tapered to maintenance doses over the next 1 to 3 days. If any symptoms of adrenal insufficiency develop, the dose should be increased and a search should be initiated for the underlying stress that is responsible.

Outcome

Delayed diagnosis of an adrenal crisis can result in life-threatening shock with hypotension, cerebral hypoperfusion, coma, lactic acidosis, acute renal failure, and death. Proper recognition and treatment of the adrenal crisis typically results in prompt clinical recovery. However, it should be noted that supraphysiologic doses of glucocorticoid therapy may increase the risks of delayed wound healing, infection, hyperglycemia, and metabolic alkalosis.

DIABETES INSIPIDUS

Diabetes insipidus can occur in patients with tumors of the hypothalamic-pituitary region and in those with accidental or surgical trauma to the pituitary stalk. Diabetes insipidus is characterized by polyuria with urine that is inappropriately dilute in relation to serum osmolality and by associated thirst and polydipsia. Its causes are categorized as neurogenic or nephrogenic. Neurogenic diabetes insipidus results from intracranial disorders that cause an absolute or relative deficiency of vasopressin (antidiuretic hormone, ADH), such as hypothalamic tumors or sarcoidosis; from stalk injury due to trauma or tumors, particularly craniopharyngiomas; and from pituitary tumors or surgery. Nephrogenic diabetes insipidus occurs when there is renal insensitivity to an appropriate circulating ADH concentration. Acquired nephrogenic diabetes insipidus can be caused by hypercalcemia, hypokalemia, chronic renal disease, and certain drugs, such as lithium and demeclocycline.

Presentation

The symptoms of diabetes insipidus are passage of large volumes of urine, between 2.5 and 20.0 liters per day, both day and night, and excessive thirst and polydipsia, with a preference for cold water. If the patient is unable to access water because of coma, mechanical ventilation, or physical or chemical restraints, for example, or if the thirst mechanism is impaired or there is inadequate fluid replacement in a hospitalized patient, then life-threatening dehydration and hypernatremia can occur. They can present as lethargy, confusion, weakness, and seizures and progress to obtundation, coma, and death.

The underlying disease causing diabetes insipidus may contribute to or dominate the clinical picture. A patient with neurogenic diabetes insipidus may also have other elements of hypopituitarism, including hypothyroidism and adrenal insufficiency. These deficiencies may partially mask the signs of diabetes insipidus by impairing water excretion by the kidneys; the diabetes insipidus may become fully evident only when these components of hypopituitarism are treated.

After pituitary surgery, a patient may have a triphasic course of water imbalance.[6] There can be initial transient diabetes insipidus, occurring from 12 to 36 hours after surgery, due to paralysis of ADH release. This can be followed, between 24 and 72 hours after surgery, by the syndrome of inappropriate of ADH caused by unregulated ADH release from the hypothalamus. Finally, a patient may develop permanent diabetes insipidus.

Evaluation

Each patient should be evaluated clinically to determine the severity of the dehydration and to find clues that identify the underlying disorder that is responsible for the diabetes insipidus. Laboratory testing should include serum electrolytes, glucose, calcium, and osmolarity with simultaneous determination of urine osmolarity or specific gravity. It is essential that the volumes of fluid administered or consumed and of urine excreted be recorded accurately.

The diagnosis of diabetes insipidus can be made if the 24-hour urine volume is more than 30 mL/kg, with a urine osmolality of less than 300 mOsm/kg H_2O or a urine specific gravity of less than 1.010.[7] If there is associated hypernatremia with a serum sodium concentration greater than 145 mEq/L and plasma osmolality greater than 295 mOsm/kg H_2O, the diagnosis is secure. In a patient with an incomplete form of diabetes insipidus and in one who is not dehydrated, a water deprivation test can be performed to determine the ADH and the renal responses to volume depletion and hyperosmolarity.[8] Details of the test protocol are available elsewhere.[8,9] Consideration should also be given to evaluating anterior pituitary and renal functions in the appropriate clinical settings.

Priorities

The aim in managing a patient with diabetes insipidus is to correct fluid and electrolyte imbalances. This requires careful serial monitoring of "ins and outs" and serum electrolytes. Isosmotic volume depletion should be corrected with intravenous normal saline. The free-water deficit can be calculated by using the following equation:

$$\text{Free-water deficit} = 0.6 \times \text{weight in kg} \times (\text{Na} - 1)/140$$

One half of the estimated water deficit should be administered over the first 24 hours as hyposmotic fluids (0.45% saline or dextrose); the balance should be given over the next 48 hours. This approach lessens the risk of cerebral edema.

In general, a patient with neurogenic diabetes insipidus who is excreting more than 4 liters of urine per day can be given arginine vasopressin to decrease fluid requirements. In an acute setting, arginine vasopressin can be given parenterally; the usual initial dose is 2 to 5 IU subcutaneously, intramuscularly or intravenously. Its duration of action is only 3 to 6 hours. Consequently, fluid balance, serum sodium, and urine osmolarity must be monitored and repeat doses given when hypotonic urine reemerges. Alternatively, arginine vasopressin can also be given as an intravenous infusion starting at 2.5 IU/h and then titrated to maintain a urine output of 0.5 to 1.0 mL/kg/h.[10] Vasopressin can cause myocardial ischemia, which can be treated with topical nitrates to reverse the vasospasm.

The preferred therapy for chronic diabetes insipidus is 1-deamino-8-D-arginine-vasopressin (DDAVP), which has a longer duration of action (6 to 24 hours). The starting dose is 5 to 10 μg intranasally at bedtime, with titration of dose and frequency of administration being determined according to urine volume and serum sodium concentration. In general, the serum sodium level should be maintained in the high-normal range to avoid water intoxication and hyponatremia.

A patient with nephrogenic diabetes insipidus does not respond to vasopressin; that is the pathogenesis of the problem. Reversible causes, such as hypercalemia or lithium toxicity, should be corrected. Treatment with a thiazide diuretic, usually 50 to 100 mg/day of hydrochlorothiazide plus sodium restriction, can increase renal tubular water reabsorption.[11] Alternatively, 1.5 to 3.0 mg/kg of indomethacin has similar efficacy. The best responses may be achieved with a combination of thiazide, indomethacin, and vasopressin therapies.

Outcome

Delayed or inadequate treatment of diabetes insipidus can result in neurologic sequelae. Patients can develop neuromuscular irritability, chorea, seizures, obtundation, and coma. Mortality is high in the young and the elderly. Appropriate treatment of hypernatremia caused by diabetes insipidus brings about complete resolution of all symptoms and signs. However, survivors may have irreversible focal neurologic deficits due to venous sinus thrombosis or cerebral hemorrhage.

THE SYNDROME OF INAPPROPRIATE ANTIDIURETIC HORMONE SECRETION AND OTHER HYPONATREMIC EMERGENCIES

Hyponatremia and associated hypo-osmolality, which have been reported to occur in 3% to 15% of hospitalized patients, can produce significant morbidity. Fundamentally, hyponatremia can be caused by excessive sodium loss from, or excessive water retention in, extracellular fluid.[12] Head and neck patients most commonly develop hyponatremia in two situations: first, when limited fluid intake and resulting volume depletion have been treated with hypotonic fluids, and second, when there is inappropriate antidiuretic hormone secretion, either perioperatively or as a paraneoplastic syndrome.

When the plasma osmolality falls below 275 mOsm/kg, typically equivalent to a serum sodium concentration of 135 mEq/L, secretion of ADH normally ceases.[13] When it does not, the syndrome of inappropriate ADH secretion (SIADH) develops. Initially, there is retention of free water that causes volume expansion. The activation of baroreceptors then induces urinary sodium loss and water excretion. SIADH is, therefore, classically characterized by (1) hyponatremia and hypo-osmolality; (2) an inappropriately high urinary osmolality, usually more than 100 mOsm/kg; (3) absence of hypovolemia and edema-forming states; (4) normal renal, adrenal, and thyroid functions.

A number of neoplasms cause SIADH through ectopic ADH production, including squamous cell carcinomas of the head and neck. Virtually any intracranial disorder (such as infection, hemorrhage, infarction, tumor, and seizure) can cause SIADH by enhancing hypothalamic ADH secretion. Through unclear mechanisms, any intrathoracic disorder (such as pneumonia, abscess, asthma, and pneumothorax) can also cause SIADH. Several drugs that potentiate the effect of ADH or stimulate its release (such as chlorpropamide, vinca alkaloids, phenothiazines, oxytocin, clofibrate, narcotics, and carbamazepine) can cause SIADH. General anesthesia, surgery,[14] and positive pressure ventilation can also produce SIADH.

Presentation

The clinical manifestations of hypo-osmolality are related to its severity and to the rapidity of its onset. As plasma osmolality falls, an influx of water into central nervous system neurons results in cerebral edema. The serum sodium rapidly falls below 125 mEq/L, and the patient then typically complains of malaise and nausea. Headache, confusion, and stupor can develop when the sodium level falls further, to 115 to 120 mEq/L. If there is a continued decline to below 115 mEq/L, seizures, coma and, eventually, death can occur. If the fall in sodium concentration is very gradual, however, the patient may remain asymptomatic. At any given level of hyponatremia, women, particularly premenopausal women, are more susceptible to the development of neurologic consequences than are men.[15]

Evaluation

When significant hyponatremia is documented, a plasma osmolality should be determined to rule out pseudohyponatremia, such as that which can be caused by severe hypertriglyceridemia. In the absence of direct plasma osmolality determination, it may be estimated by using the following formula:

$$\text{Plasma osmolality} = 2(\text{Na}) + \text{glucose}/18 + \text{BUN}/2.8$$

Normal osmolality is approximately 290 mOsm/kg H_2O.

In patients with documented hypo-osmolality and no clinical evidence of hypovolemia or edema, the urine osmolality and sodium concentration are helpful in making a further differential diagnosis. A urine osmolality of less than 100 mOsm/kg suggests primary polydipsia or a reset osmostat. A urine osmolality of more than 100 mOsm/kg indicates impairment of free-water excretion. The urine sodium concentration is then useful in identifying the cause. Urine sodium levels lower than 20 mEq/L indicate effective volume depletion such as that which occurs in cardiac failure, advanced nephrosis, and cirrhosis. Serum sodium levels higher than 40 mEq/L are typically seen in SIADH, salt-losing nephritis, adrenal insufficiency, diuretic use, and hypothyroidism.

Priorities

The intensity of treatment for hyponatremia depends on its severity, the rate at which it has developed, and whether the patient is symptomatic. On the one hand, an asymptomatic patient with moderate hyponatremia (serum sodium 120 to 130 mEq/L) that has developed over weeks (e.g., due to diuretic therapy) can be quite slowly corrected with conservative interventions such as fluid restriction. On the other hand, a symptomatic patient with severe hyponatremia (e.g., serum sodium 100 to 115 mEq/L) that has developed rapidly (e.g., due to anesthesia and hypotonic intravenous fluids) must be aggressively treated to avoid irreversible injury to the central nervous system.

A volume-depleted patient should receive normal saline to correct the deficits. A patient with edema usually responds to fluid restriction, cardiac afterload–reducing agents, and, if needed, dialysis. A patient with SIADH can usually be treated with water restriction, a high-salt/high-protein diet, and loop diuretics, if necessary. For sustained SIADH, 300 to 600 mg of demeclocycline twice daily can be employed to induce partial nephrogenic diabetes insipidus. Alternatively, 600 to 1800 mg of lithium carbonate per day can also be used but is less effective and is more likely to cause toxicity.

Emergency treatment for a more severely affected patient includes fluid restriction, discontinuation of contributing drugs, treatment of the underlying condition, and administration of hypertonic 3% saline at a rate of less than 0.5 mEq/hour or 12 mEq/L/day.[16] Faster rates of correction can lead to central pontine myelinosis, a syndrome of dysarthria, spastic quadriplegia, obtundation, seizures, and death.[17] After attaining a plasma sodium of 125 to 130 mEq/L, water restriction and correction of the underlying cause can be used to restore a fully normal serum sodium concentration. A woman's total body sodium deficit can be roughly estimated by using the following formula:

Sodium deficit = total body water (TBW) × sodium deficit/L, i.e., equals 0.5 × lean body weight (kg) × (desired Na^+ concentration − plasma Na^+)

In men, TBW is approximately 60% of lean weight, so the factor in the formula becomes 0.6.

Outcomes

A patient with prolonged, severe hyponatremia can suffer metabolic encephalopathy, including lethargy, coma, respiratory arrest, and a persistent vegetative state or death. A premenopausal woman has a 25-fold greater risk of experiencing these complications than a man.[18] A patient who has had a prior cerebral infarct may have irreversible focal neurologic deficits.

In the treatment of hyponatremia, fewer of the poor outcomes are the result of late diagnosis than of excessively rapid correction of the hyponatremia, which causes the syndrome of central pontine myelinosis (CPM). A patient with CPM develops mutism, pseudobulbar palsy, quadriplegia, and a locked-in syndrome several days after reversal of hyponatremia. Demyelinating lesions can be confirmed by computed tomography or magnetic resonance imaging, but radiographic signs may take as long as 4 weeks to develop. There is no effective treatment for CPM.

HYPOCALCEMIA

Hypocalcemia is a relatively common occurrence in patients undergoing head and neck surgery. Its significance can range from a mild asymptomatic biochemical abnormality to a life-threatening condition. Approximately 50% of circulating calcium is in the free ionized form that is physiologically important for neuromuscular functions; the remainder is bound to plasma proteins, mainly albumin, and inorganic anions. The ionized calcium concentration is homeostatically regulated by parathyroid hormone (PTH) and vitamin D. PTH levels rise rapidly in response to hypocalcemia, resulting in increased bone resorbtion and renal calcium reabsorbtion in the distal tubule. PTH also stimulates renal production of 1,25-dihydroxyvitamin D [$1,25(OH)_2D$], which promotes the absorption of calcium and phosphate from the gastrointestinal tract. The maximal effects of $1,25(OH)_2D$ require 24 to 48 hours to take place, unlike the effects of PTH, which occur in minutes. Clinically significant hypocalcemia occurs, therefore, when there is an absolute or partial failure of the PTH homeostatic mechanisms.

The most common cause of hypocalcemia is hypoalbuminemia, which lowers total calcium concentration while the ionized calcium concentration remains normal. The total calcium concentration can be approximately corrected for a low serum albumin level by the following formula:

Corrected calcium (mg/dL) = measured serum calcium (mg/dL) + 0.8[4.0 − serum albumin (g/dL)].

Common causes of a true decrease in the ionized calcium concentration include hypoparathyroidism, hypomagnesemia, renal failure, and abnormalities of vitamin D metabolism. Postsurgical hypoparathyroidism after parathyroid, thyroid, or other neck surgeries can be the result of resection of or trauma to the parathyroid glands or their vascular supply. Transient hypoparathyroidism is also commonly seen following removal of a parathyroid adenoma previously causing primary hyperparathyroidism.[19] In this setting, the normal parathyroid glands are suppressed and after removal of the adenoma, the serum PTH levels become undetectable within hours. The serum calcium falls to a nadir at 20 hours, with recovery of PTH and calcium levels within 48 hours in most cases. This scenario can also be complicated by the avid deposition of calcium in bone, referred to as the "hungry bone syndrome." The incidence of the syndrome is directly related to the patient's age, the preoperative levels of the calcium, alkaline phosphatase, PTH, and blood urea, and the volume of the parathyroid adenoma.[20]

Other causes of hypoparathyroidism include congenital absence of the glands, congenital resistance to PTH action, and injury to the glands caused by autoimmunity, infiltration by metastatic tumor or hemochromatosis, or neck irradiation. Of course, hypoparathyroidism must be distinguished from other causes of hypocalcemia. These include vitamin D deficiency due to malabsorption, dietary deficiency, lack of sunlight, renal failure, liver disease, or anticonvulsant therapy; hyperphosphatemia; pancreatitis; multiple transfusions with citrated blood; and drugs, such as bisphosphonates, mithramycin, cisplatin, doxorubicin, ketoconazole, and pentamidine. Critically ill patients in intensive care units commonly have multifactorial hypocalcemia resulting from decreased serum protein binding, respiratory alkalosis, hypomagnesemia, or suppressed PTH secretion.[21]

Presentation

Patients with mild to moderate hypocalcemia may experience numbness and paresthesias of the fingers, toes, and circumoral area; fasciculations; and muscle cramps of the hands, lower limbs, and back. Increased neuromuscular irritability can be demonstrated by eliciting Chvostek's (Weiss's) and Trousseau's signs. The former is elicited by gently tapping over the main trunk of the facial nerve just anterior to the ear. In a positive test, there is visible twitching of the ipsilateral angle of the mouth. Approximately 8% to 10% of normal subjects have a positive test, but patients with severe hypocalcemia may also have twitching of the alae nasi and other facial muscles. Trousseau's sign is the production of carpopedal spasm in response to inflation of a sphygmomanometer cuff to 20 mm Hg above systolic blood pressure for 3 to 5 minutes.

Tetany and focal or generalized seizures can occur in patients with more profound hypocalcemia or underlying seizure disorders. Irritability, personality disturbances, psychosis, and other organic brain syndromes have been described. Cardiac effects include prolongation of the QT interval, decreased myocardial contractility and, rarely, hypotension and congestive heart failure.[22] Other manifestations of hypocalcemia include laryngospasm, bronchospasm, dysphagia, abdominal pain, and biliary colic.

Evaluation

If only the total serum calcium is obtained, the serum albumin should be determined and the serum calcium corrected for hypoalbuminemia. An ionized calcium should also be obtained in most cases, particularly in critically ill patients who often also have abnormalities of serum proteins. In a symptomatic patient, emergency treatment may have to be administered before the cause of the hypocalcemia is determined.

The serum magnesium should also be determined. Hypomagnesemia of less than 1.0 mg/dL can contribute to hypocalcemia by impairing PTH secretion and inducing target tissue PTH resistance.[23] If hypomagnesemia is ruled out, an intact PTH level should be determined next. This differentiates hypoparathyroidism from other causes of hypocalcemia associated with appropriate secondary hyperparathyroidism. Among the causes of secondary hyperparathyroidism, a high serum phosphate level is seen in renal failure, rhabdomyolysis, tumor lysis syndrome, and pseudohypoparathyroidism. A low serum phosphate suggests vitamin D deficiency or resistance or the hungry bone syndrome.

Priorities

Patients with moderate to severe clinical manifestations of hypocalcemia, such as painful muscle cramps, carpopedal spasm, tetany, seizures, cardiac arrhythmias, or hypotension, should receive intravenous calcium. Between 100 and 200 mg of elemental calcium should be infused; this will typically raise the ionized calcium level by 0.5 to 1.5 mM/L.[24] Calcium gluconate (containing 90 mg of elemental calcium per 10-mL ampule) should generally be used because it does not cause venous irritation. The alternative is calcium chloride (272 mg of elemental calcium per 10-mL ampule). Initially, one or two ampules of calcium gluconate should be diluted in 100 mL of 5% dextrose solution and infused over 5 to 10 minutes. The effects of this single pulse disappear within several hours, so a continuous intravenous infusion of calcium gluconate should then be started by adding 10 ampules to 1 L 5% dextrose and infusing this solution at 50 mL/h (45 mg of elemental calcium per hour). Some protocols recommend rates of 0.3 to 0.5 mg/kg/h for moderate hypocalcemia and 1.0 to 1.5 mg/kg/h for severe cases. Regardless, serial calcium measurements should be obtained every 2 to 4 hours, and the rate of infusion should be titrated to maintain low normal calcium concentrations. If the hypocalcemia is likely to persist, oral calcium supplements (approximately 2 g of elemental calcium) should be started along with 0.5 to 1.0 μg/day of $1,25(OH)_2D$ (calcitriol).

Asymptomatic or mild cases of hypocalcemia need only oral calcium supplementation, for example, 1 to 2 g of elemental calcium as calcium carbonate (40% elemental calcium) or calcium citrate (21% elemental calcium), and careful observation. Because calcium carbonate is best absorbed in an acidic environment, tablets should be taken after meals and may not be well absorbed in patients with gastric achlorhydria. It is generally best to administer calcium citrate or calcium glubionate (115 mg calcium/5 mL syrup) to patients with achlorhydria such as pernicious anemia, after gastric pull-up, after vagotomy, or with jejunostomy feeding tubes. Patients with refractory hypocalcemia and hypomagnesemia should receive magnesium supplementation in addition to their calcium therapy. Patients with severe magnesium deficiency can receive 2 g of magnesium sulfate intravenously over 2 hours; patients with mild or chronic deficiency can be treated with 400 to 800 mg/day of oral magnesium oxide.

Outcomes

Severe untreated hypocalcemia causes tetany, seizures, laryngospasm, respiratory failure, and congestive heart failure. Chronic hypocalcemia can result in calcifications of the basal ganglia and cerebellum, which can sometimes be associated with parkinsonian symptoms, choreoathetosis, or tremor of the hands, and ataxia can develop in these individuals. Prompt and appropriate therapy of hypocalcemia eliminates all acute and chronic sequelae.

HYPERCALCEMIA

Severe hypercalcemia commonly occurs in two settings: severe hyperparathyroidism and hypercalcemia of a malignancy in head and neck patients. This metabolic syndrome may escape detection. Its symptoms and signs of hypercalcemia are nonspecific. In some cases, the severity of hypercalcemia may not be apparent due to hypoalbuminemia and a misleadingly mild degree of serum total calcium elevation. In these cases, it is important to correct for the altered serum albumin concentration (see later) or monitor the ionized calcium level.

Although the differential diagnosis of hypercalcemia includes many other conditions, most patients with severe hypercalcemia have either hyperparathyroidism or hypercalcemia of malignancy. These two conditions are distinguished by the concomitant serum parathyroid hormone concentrations. Hyperparathyroidism is most commonly caused by a single adenoma, less often by four-gland hyperplasia, and rarely by parathyroid carcinoma.[25] Malignancy-related hypercalcemia can be caused by several mechanisms.[26] Lymphomas, myeloma, and breast carcinoma produce local osteolysis by means of the paracrine effects of the cytokines that activate osteoclasts. Humoral mediation of hypercalcemia such as can be seen in squamous cell carcinomas is caused by production of the PTH-related peptide (PTHrP). Rarely, certain tumors can convert excessive amounts of 1-hydroxyvitamin D to 1,25-dihydroxyvitamin D; even more rarely, they can secrete true PTH.

Other causes of hypercalcemia are sarcoidosis and other granulomatous diseases that produce 1,25-dihydoxyvitamin D, vitamin D intoxication, endocrinopathies (thyrotoxicosis, adrenal insufficiency, acromegaly, pheochromocytoma, and VIPoma), thiazides, vitamin A intoxication, aluminum intoxication, milk-alkali syndrome, immobilization, and renal failure.[27]

Presentation

The severity of the clinical syndrome generally correlates with the magnitude of hypercalcemia. Neurologic effects can range from apathy, depression, and drowsiness to psychosis, ataxia, stupor, and coma. Neuromuscular manifestations of hypercalcemia can include weakness, proximal myopathy, and hypertonia. A short QT interval is commonly seen, and bradycardia can occur in severe cases. Hypercalcemia can induce renal insensitivity to vasopressin, causing polyuria, polydipsia, and volume depletion, which can then exacerbate hypercalcemia. Other renal effects can include hyperchloremic acidosis, nephrocalcinosis, and chronic renal failure. Gastrointestinal complaints of anorexia, nausea, vomiting, and constipation are common. Abdominal pain can be seen, but classic reports of its association with peptic ulcer disease are now questioned. Metastatic calcium deposition can cause band keratopathy and pancreatitis.

Evaluation

The history and physical examination should be directed toward identifying the cause of the hypercalcemia. If the serum albumin is abnormal, an ionized calcium level should be obtained or, alternatively, the total calcium can be corrected by using the following formula:

Corrected serum calcium $=$ measured serum calcium $+ 0.8 \times (4.0 -$ serum albumin).

The serum intact PTH concentration should be measured as the first step in determining the cause of hypercalcemia. An elevated or inappropriately normal serum PTH level is indicative of hyperparathyroidism in all but the very rare cases of ectopic secretion of true PTH. On the other hand, a low PTH level implies a parathyroid-independent process, usually malignancy. The serum level of thyroid-stimulating hormone (TSH) should be obtained to rule out hyperthyroidism. An elevated PTHrP confirms humoral hypercalcemia of malignancy, whereas an increased 1,25$(OH)_2$ vitamin D concentration indicates a granulomatous process or lymphoma.

Priorities

In severe hypercalcemia, repletion of extracellular fluid volume is almost always the essential first step.[28] After dehydration has been confirmed clinically, and as it is confirmed by measurement of the serum urea nitrogen level and other routine chemical parameters, a normal saline infusion should be started at 200 to 400 mL/h. In addition to diluting the circulating calcium pool, the increased renal perfusion and glomerular filtration increase calcium excretion. The serum calcium typically falls by 2 to 4 mg/dL in the first 24 hours. The patient's volume status should be carefully monitored by frequent physical examinations, measurement of urinary volumes and, if necessary, central venous pressure measurements. Overly aggressive infusion rates can lead to pulmonary edema, hypokalemia, hypomagnesemia, and hypophosphatemia. A loop diuretic can be added if there is volume overload or simply to augment renal losses of calcium once the patient is rehydrated.

Specific therapy can then be given to ensure chronic control of the hypercalcemia. The majority of the agents inhibit bone resorption. Bisphosphonates such as pamidronate block osteoclastic function and are generally considered the first-line drugs. Pamidronate is given as an intravenous infusion of 60 to 90 mg over 4 to 6 hours. The onset of its action is usually seen after 24 to 48 hours, the nadir of serum calcium occurring 3 to 6 days later, and the duration of action lasting 1 to 8 weeks. Patients with hypercalcemia of malignancy may need repeated administrations every 2 to 4 weeks.[29] Of these patients, 15% experience a transient fever and myalgias and an increase in serum creatinine concentration.

Salmon calcitonin can also be used, but it is not as potent as pamidronate, tachyphylaxis occurs after a few days, and it is expensive. Calcitonin can be used as an antiresorptive agent while awaiting the onset of the effect of pamidronate. The usual dose is 4 to 8 IU/kg subcutaneously every 12 hours. Patients should undergo skin testing for hypersensitivity before its use.

There is also a role for mithramycin (now plicamycin), which is given in doses of up to 25 μg/kg intravenously over 8 hours. The serum calcium concentration falls within 24 to 36 hours, and its effects last 5 to 8 days. Its use is, however, limited by the side effects of thrombocytopenia, hepatic toxicity, and renal insufficiency. Consequently, it is recommended for patients who fail pamidronate therapy.

Glucocorticoids such as prednisone, 40 to 60 mg/day, can be tried if the cause of hypercalcemia is myeloma, granulomatous processes, lymphoma, or vitamin D intoxication. Other medications such as gallium nitrate, nonsteroidal anti-inflammatory agents, etidronate, and oral phosphates are rarely used. The treatment for primary hyperparathyroidism is surgical resection.

Outcomes

The natural history of untreated severe hypercalcemia is progressive obtundation, coma, dehydration, renal and respiratory failure, and death. When patients receive appropriate treatment, all symptoms can be reversed and complications avoided. The prognosis of the patient is then dependent on the underlying condition. Hypercalcemia of malignancies is usually a poor prognostic sign that heralds advanced disease, especially if it is mediated by PTHrP.[30] Even then, however, control of the hypercalcemia may result in improved quality of life and may prolong survival.

HYPOGLYCEMIA

Hypoglycemia is the most common metabolic emergency encountered. Whipple first described the triad of criteria that define hypoglycemia: (1) symptoms of aberrant behavior, confusion, altered level of consciousness, or seizure; (2) a simultaneous plasma glucose concentration less than 40 mg/dL; and (3) the resolution of symptoms with the administration of glucose.[30a] All three criteria should be met to establish the diagnosis with certainty. The temporal pattern of the hypoglycemia helps to distinguish the cause. Fasting hypoglycemic disorders can be potentially lethal and often reflect the presence of serious underlying disorders, whereas postprandial (or reactive) states are usually less serious and are modifiable by diet. The most common cause of hypoglycemia in a surgical patient is medication, usually due to insulin or sulfonylurea therapy.[31] Other causes of fasting hypoglycemia are distinctly less common; they include severe malnutrition, insulinoma, extrapancreatic malignancies, adrenal insufficiency, severe hepatic diseases, chronic renal failure, inborn errors of carbohydrate metabolism, alcohol, and factitious causes. Postprandial hypoglycemia is seen after gastric surgery, in disordered gastrointestinal motility syndromes, in early type 2 diabetes mellitus, with ethanol, in reaction to other substrates (e.g., fructose, leucine, galactose), and as an idiopathic disorder.

Presentation

Symptoms of hypoglycemia can be categorized as adrenergic and neuroglycopenic. Adrenergic symptoms include sweating, anxiety, tremor, and palpitations and are caused by the activation of the sympathetic nervous system. They generally precede neuroglycopenic symptoms. The effects of hypoglycemia on the central nervous system include confusion, headache, blurred vision, incoherent speech, ataxia, inappropriate behavior, drowsiness, coma, convulsions, and death.

Evaluation

Clinical suspicion of hypoglycemia should prompt immediate acquisition of a blood sample for determination of the plasma or whole blood glucose concentration. It is important that the blood sample be obtained before administration of therapy whenever possible. If the cause of the hypoglycemia is not evident, a plasma aliquot can be stored for later measurement of the insulin and C peptide levels.

Priorities

If the patient is conscious and able to swallow, glucose-containing foods such as juice or candy can be given. If the patient is unconscious, 25 to 50 g of glucose should be given as an intravenous push with 50% dextrose. This dose should be repeated if the patient does not begin to recover within 3 to 5 minutes.[32] If there is no recovery in 10 to 15 minutes, other diagnostic possibilities should be considered. When intravenous glucose is not available or intravenous access is impossible, 1 mg of glucagon can be given intramuscularly or intravenously. In cases of hypoglycemia induced by alcohol or malnutrition, 100 mg of thiamine should also be given to prevent Wernicke's syndrome from developing. Once the patient recovers, an infusion of 5% dextrose should be started until hourly blood sugars reveal consistent normoglycemia and the patient is feeding orally. If the hypoglycemia is due to sulphonylureas, recurrent hypoglycemia can occur for hours or days, depending on the agent's duration of action; for example, chlorpropamide lasts for 50 to 60 hours and glyburide for 12 to 24 hours. When the resuscitation has been accomplished, the precipitating cause of the hypoglycemia can be investigated if it is not clinically obvious.[33]

Outcome

Permanent focal neurologic injury has been reported to occur in 3% of patients with prolonged or recurrent hypoglycemia. In one series, the mortality rate directly attributable to hypoglycemia was less than 1%.[34] All of these complications and the morbidity of hypoglycemia can be avoided if hypoglycemia is promptly recognized and treated.

PHEOCHROMOCYTOMA AND HYPERTENSIVE CRISIS

Pheochromocytoma and related neuroendocrine tumors of the sympathetic nervous system are rare catecholamine-producing neoplasms that can be encountered in two settings. First, pheochromocytoma may occur in multiple endocrine neoplasia (MEN), type II, along with hyperparathyroidism and medullary thyroid carcinoma, for which neck surgery may be indicated. Second, chemodectomas are related tumors of the carotid body and cervical sympathetic chain, which can present as a cervical mass requiring biopsy or excision.

Presentation

In patients with unrecognized and untreated pheochromocytoma, anesthesia and surgery can precipitate an adrenergic crisis, including the development of potentially life-threatening hypertension and tachyarrhythmias along with atrial and ventricular fibrillation.[35] Other cardiovascular complications can include pulmonary edema, myocarditis, myocardial infarction, dissecting aortic aneurysm, hypovolemic shock, seizure, and cerebrovascular accident due to infarction or hemorrhage. Conscious patients may experience headache, anxiety, chest pain, and vomiting. Metabolic complications can include postoperative hypoglycemia and lactic acidosis, even in the absence of shock.

Evaluation

Preoperative evaluation of a patient with hyperparathyroidism should include at least clinical consideration of the possibility of pheochromocytoma. A personal history of severe or labile hypertension, paroxysmal symptoms, previous thyroid carcinoma, or adrenal tumor should prompt further review of the patient's past records to discern whether a catecholamine-secreting tumor is a possibility.

For a patient in whom there is only a moderate index of suspicion, a 24-hour urine collection for metanephrines is an appropriate preoperative screening procedure.[36] For an individual at higher risk—one with convincing paroxysmal symptoms or a personal or family history of MEN-II features—additional analyses of urinary fractionated catecholamines and plasma catecholamines may be appropriate to exclude the diagnosis with even greater certainty. In general, imaging the adrenals is not a sufficiently specific procedure to be warranted until there is a biochemical diagnosis, as up to 3% of individuals have nonfunctioning adrenal adenomas.

A previously undiagnosed patient with a syndrome that suggests hypertensive crisis with cardiovascular complications may require cardiac enzymes, chest radiographs, telemetry, echocardiograms, and computerized tomography of the chest if aortic dissection is considered a possibility.

Priorities

A patient suffering a hypertensive crisis caused by known or suspected pheochromocytoma or another underlying disorder such as renal artery stenosis is usually managed in an intensive care setting and with an arterial line to monitor the blood pressure. Hypertension can be controlled with 5 to 10 mg of intravenous phentolamine mesylate as a slow push after a test dose of 0.5 mg; the dose is repeated in a few minutes if necessary.[37] Alternatively, 0.5 to 10.0 μg/kg/min of intravenous sodium nitroprusside to a maximum dose of 800 μg/min can be used. The maximum dose should not be exceeded, as the risk of thiocyanate and cyanide toxicity increases. Intravenous labetalol (a combined α- β-receptor blocker) as an infusion of 0.5 to 2.0 mg/min or as 20- to 80-mg boluses up to a total of 300 mg has also been used successfully. A patient with tachycardia or tachyarrhythmias may need β-blockers for rate control. The selective β_1 blocking agent esmolol hydrochloride is ideally suited for this purpose, as it has a very short duration of action, with a plasma half-life of 8 minutes. Esmolol can be administered as a 500-μg/kg loading dose of over 1 minute, followed by an infusion of 50 μg/kg/min for 4 minutes. The esmolol loading dose is repeated if no therapeutic effect is seen within 5 minutes, and the maintenance infusion is then increased to 100 μg/kg/min. These titrations are repeated until the heart rate and arterial blood pressure approach normal. It is advisable to reduce the mean arterial pressure by 25% or to reduce the diastolic blood pressure to 100 to 110 mm Hg. The maintenance infusion is continued until a longer-acting therapy is instituted.

Hypotensive crises, which can occur with predominantly epinephrine-secreting tumors or with excessive antihypertensive therapy, may require fluid replacement with both saline and colloidal solutions. Patients should be monitored for hypoglycemia perioperatively and treated appropriately (see the previous section on hypoglycemia). Lactic acidosis can be treated with large-volume infusions of saline and bicarbonate.

Prevention

The best approach to dealing with perioperative hypertension and other complications related to pheochromocytoma is to avoid them by means of preoperative diagnosis, as noted above. In families with suspected MEN-IIa, the presence of RET proto-oncogene mutations can also be used to identify individuals at high risk.

In a patient with pheochromocytoma, surgical resection of the adrenal tumor after appropriate preoperative preparation becomes the highest priority; other surgery and angiographic procedures should be deferred. Typically, phenoxybenzamine is used, initially 10 to 20 mg two to four times a day and then in a gradually increasing dose until blood pressure is controlled and the patient has a postural blood pressure drop of 10 to 20 mm Hg in diastolic pressure). Prazosin, 1 mg four times a day to a maximum of 20 mg/day, can also be used. Labetalol, 100 mg four times a day to a maximum of 1600 mg/day, has also been employed. A patient is at a low risk for an adrenergic crisis perioperatively if (1) the blood pressure is less than 160/90 mm Hg for 48 hours; (2) orthostatic hypotension does not exceed 45 mm Hg; (3) there have been no ST-segment or T-wave changes for 2 weeks; and (4) there is less than one premature ventricular contraction every 5 minutes.

Outcome

A patient with a hypertensive crisis caused by pheochromocytoma may experience grave consequences, including acute myocardial infarction, congestive heart failure, cerebrovascular accident, hypertensive encephalopathy, postoperative hypotensive shock, and severe lactic acidosis. The risk of these events can be lessened by prompt diagnosis and treatment. Overenthusiastic treatment can cause hypotension and the consequences of shock.

MYXEDEMA COMA

Myxedema and complicated myxedema are the final stages of severe, long-standing hypothyroidism. The head and neck surgeon may encounter this entity as an incidental perioperative crisis. The syndrome is seen most frequently in the elderly and during the winter season. The diagnosis should be considered in all patients with unexplained coma or obtundation, especially if hypothermia is present. Although uncommon, myxedema coma has a high mortality rate, even when promptly recognized and treated effectively. Obtundation is typically precipitated by the stress of sepsis, surgery, myocardial infarction, cerebrovascular accident, gastrointestinal hemorrhage, trauma, cold exposure, or pharmacologic agents.[38] In hospitalized patients, the administration of sedative and narcotic agents is often responsible.

Presentation

There may be an antecedent history of hypothyroidism, and a thyroidectomy scar or goiter may be evident. Hypothermia is common. The patient generally has edematous facies with periorbital puffiness; dry, rough skin and coarse, scant hair; and nonpitting edema of the hands and ankles. Macroglossia may be present. Neurologic abnormalities can range from somnolence and mild confusion to delirium, seizures, obtundation, and coma.

Bradycardia, hypotension, distant heart sounds, findings consistent with pleural effusion, and delayed deep-tendon reflex responses can be seen. Severe hypothyroidism can diminish ventilatory responses to hypoxia and hypercapnea and result in alveolar hypoventilation and carbon dioxide narcosis.[39]

If a precipitating factor is present, such as sepsis or a cerebrovascular accident, it may dominate the clinical picture.

Evaluation

Whenever clinically suspected, serum TSH and free thyroxine (T_4) levels should be obtained, although initial management should not be delayed until these results have returned. A random serum cortisol concentration should also be requested before starting glucocorticoid therapy, as coexisting adrenal insufficiency can occur in a hypopituitary patient and in a patient with combined autoimmune thyroiditis and adrenal failure (Schmidt's syndrome). A complete blood count, routine serum chemistry analyses, an arterial blood gas determination, appropriate blood and other cultures, a chest radiograph, and an electrocardiogram should also be obtained.

Management

Patients should be managed in an intensive care setting. Optimal general medical care, including cardiopulmonary support and detection and treatment of underlying infection or cardiovascular events, may be more important in determining survival than the thyroid hormone replacement regimen.[40] Hypothermia is best treated with passive rewarming such as blankets, rather than with rapid active warming, which induces peripheral vasodilation that may worsen hypotension. Hypotension, if present, is initially treated with gradual volume expansion with normal saline, and myocardial infarction should be considered. Unremitting hypotension may justify dopamine administration. Hypoxia and hypercapnea may necessitate tracheal intubation and mechanical ventilation. Sedative drugs should to be avoided because of their impaired metabolic clearance and their potential to further weaken respiratory drive. Sepsis is present in one third of patients but may not be heralded by fever because of the presence of hypothermia. Infection should be routinely sought by appropriate clinical and laboratory examinations, including cultures of blood, urine, and cerebrospinal fluid. Myocardial infarction should be excluded by electrocardiography and, when indicated, serum cardiac enzyme determinations. Mild to moderate hyponatremia (a serum sodium concentration greater than 125 mEq/L), can be corrected with restriction of fluids to 1.0 to 1.5 L/day. More severe hyponatremia should be treated with cautious administration of normal or hypertonic saline until the serum sodium concentration is greater than 120 mEq/L.

In settings in which complicated myxedema is strongly suspected, thyroid hormone therapy should be started before thyroid function test results return. Two regimens have been advocated, although no comparative trial has demonstrated which might be superior. Thyroxine (T_4; Synthroid) therapy can be initiated with a

500-μg intravenous loading dose followed by 1.5 to 2.0 μg/kg/day intravenously. Thyroxine treatment has the theoretical advantage of a controlled onset of action with extrathyroidal T_4-to-T_3 conversion at a rate that is appropriate for the patient's overall state of illness. Triiodothyronine (T_3; Triostat), 25 to 50 μg every 8 hours intravenously may be faster-acting in the restoration of myocardial contractility, ventilatory drive, and renal free water excretion. It should be reemphasized that the clinical outcome is probably more dependent on meticulous attention to general medical management than to which thyroid hormone regimen is selected.

Glucocorticoids should generally be given for two reasons. First, adrenal insufficiency can occur in a hypothyroid patient with underlying hypopituitarism or combined autoimmune glandular failure (Schmidt's syndrome). Second, profound hypothyroidism itself can impair the responsiveness of the hypothalamic-pituitary-adrenal axis. Glucocorticoid therapy may be given as 100 mg of intravenous hydrocortisone every 8 hours until the results of the initial plasma cortisol test are known.

The patient's response to therapy will be seen as a gradual resolution of hypothermia, usually commencing within 24 hours. Bradycardia, hypotension, and hyponatremia may begin to improve within the first day. Coma and ventilatory failure typically take longer to respond. Once the patient is able to take oral medication, 1.5 to 2.0 μg/kg/day of thyroxine is the treatment of choice.

Outcome

In earlier reported series, myxedema coma was associated with a mortality rate of 60% to 70%. More recently, with improved intensive, supportive care, mechanical ventilation, and the use of parenteral thyroid hormone replacement, the mortality rate has fallen to 15% to 20%.[41] Poor prognostic factors include advanced age, a pulse rate of less than 44 beats per minute, infection, coincidental myocardial infarction, persistent hypothermia, severe hypotension, and a core body temperature of less than 93°F.[42]

COMPLICATED THYROTOXICOSIS

Thyrotoxicosis (thyroid crisis) complicated by severe cardiovascular, neurologic, gastrointestinal, or infectious manifestations is uncommon but is associated with a high mortality (10% to 75%).[43] Classical thyroid crisis is characterized by severe thyrotoxicosis with fever, delirium, and heart failure, often with manifestations in other organ systems. The syndrome is often precipitated when a previously hyperthyroid patient suffers a superimposed infectious, cardiovascular, metabolic, surgical, or other traumatic insult. Other conditions that can act directly on the thyroid gland to provoke thyroid hormone release include thyroid surgery, withdrawal of thionamide therapy, radioiodine treatment, iodine administration, and vigorous palpation of the thyroid gland.

Presentation

Patients typically have accentuated symptoms of thyrotoxicosis. They may also have other characteristics of Graves' disease, such as goiter and orbitopathy. A thyroidal bruit or thrill may be present. Hyperpyrexia, with a body temperature higher than 102°F, may be present. Mental status changes in the sensorium can include severe agitation, hyperkinesis, delirium, and psychosis. In some cases, there has been progression to obtundation and coma.

Cardiovascular manifestations include tachycardia and tachypnea. Congestive heart failure with atrial fibrillation is among the classic features of fully developed thyroid crisis, but other tachyarrhythmias, such as sinus tachycardia and atrial premature beats, and myocardial ischemia can also occur. Gastrointestinal complaints include diarrhea, nausea, vomiting, and abdominal pain. Mild hepatic dysfunction is commonly present, and severe hepatic necrosis may occur, but rarely. Consequently, jaundice is a poor prognostic factor. Other clinical features can include malnutrition and hypoglycemia.

Complicated thyrotoxicosis is most often seen in patients with underlying cardiovascular disease, in postpartum women, and in noncompliant patients with disturbed psychology and social circumstances and poor access to health care.[44]

Evaluation

Clinical diagnosis is dependent on recognizing that a febrile, agitated patient with heart failure may have thyrotoxicosis as the fundamental precipitant. A goiter and, in a patient with Graves' disease, ophthalmopathy can be the decisive clinical clues. Thyroid function tests confirm the presence of an elevated free T_4 concentration in association with a suppressed serum TSH level[45]; but treatment typically has to be instituted before thyroid function tests results have returned from the laboratory. Other common laboratory abnormalities include leucocytosis, normocytic anemia, hyperbilirubinemia, elevated serum transaminase concentrations, and azotemia. There may also be hypercalcemia and elevated alkaline phosphatase secondary to increased bone resorption.

If the precipitating factor is not readily apparent, underlying infection must be excluded. Consequently, blood, urine, sputum, and cerebrospinal fluid may have to be collected for culture. Initiation of broad-spectrum antibiotics is often appropriate until sepsis is excluded.

Priorities

A patient with thyrotoxic crisis is best managed in an intensive care setting. Extracellular volume depletion secondary to fever and diarrhea should be corrected. In a patient with heart failure, hemodynamic monitoring is essential to avoid excessive hydration. Hypotension may require vasopressor agents. Dextrose with saline may be useful to restore depleted hepatic glycogen stores. Fever should be corrected with antipyretics and, in severe cases, with external cooling blankets and other measures. Acetaminophen rather than aspirin is used as an antipyretic, as aspirin displaces T_4 from binding sites and theoretically could worsen the clinical condition.[46]

Congestive heart failure and tachyarrhythmias often require urgent treatment. In addition to oxygen and measures to reverse hyperpyrexia, very rapid ventricular response rates in a patient with atrial fibrillation should be reduced to the range of 90 to 120 beats per minute with β-adrenergic blocking agents. In patients with significant left ventricular failure, this should be done with pulmonary capillary wedge pressure monitoring and a short-acting β-adrenergic blocking agent such as esmolol.[47] Although a patient may benefit from diuresis, it should be undertaken cautiously, in view of the expanded intravascular spaces of a vasodilated, thyrotoxic patient. Similarly, vasodilator agents should be used with caution in a patient with thyrotoxic heart failure. In a patient with atrial fibrillation and heart failure, anticoagulation should usually be instituted unless it is contraindicated.

Although glucocorticoid therapy has long been advocated for a patient in thyroid storm, the rationale for it is not well established. Glucocorticoids do decrease extrathyroidal conversion of T_4 to T_3. Similarly, vitamin supplements have traditionally been recommended. Justification for their use is lacking, but they may be harmlessly administered.

Treatments that are specifically directed against thyroid gland hyperactivity include inhibition of further thyroid hormone synthesis, inhibition of thyroid hormone release, inhibition of peripheral conversion of T_4 to T_3, β-adrenergic blockade of target tissue thyroid hormone actions, and removal of excess circulating thyroid hormone. Thionamides, propylthiouracil (PTU; 200 to 250 mg every 4 to 6 hours, orally), or methimazole (30 to 40 mg every 6 to 8 hours, orally or rectally), should be started immediately to decrease further thyroid hormone biosynthesis. PTU has the theoretical advantage of decreasing peripheral conversion of T_4 to T_3. After thionamide administration for 1 to 2 hours to prevent exacerbation of the thyrotoxicosis, thyroid hormone release from the gland can be blocked by with iodine as ipodate (a 3-g loading dose followed by 1 g/day, orally), Lugol's iodine solution (0.5 mL every 6 hours, orally), saturated solution of potassium iodide (10 drops twice a day, orally) or sodium iodide (0.5 to 1.0 g every 12 hours, as an intravenous infusion. This combined therapy usually brings about a rapid decrease in free T_4 levels, with achievement of a biochemically euthyroid state within 4 to 7 days. In severe cases, excess circulating hormone can be removed with dialysis, plasmapheresis,[48] charcoal plasma perfusion,[49] or cholestyramine.

Outcome

Poor prognostic signs for a patient with complicated thyrotoxicosis include jaundice, hypotensive shock, congestive heart failure, and severe pyrexia. The patient's outcome is also dependent on the nature of the medical illness that typically precipitates this syndrome. Prompt diagnosis, a comprehensive treatment plan addressing every aspect of thyroid hormone production and peripheral action, and meticulous attention to the management of complicating cardiopulmonary and infectious complications are essential.

GOITROUS OBSTRUCTION

Goitrous enlargement of the thyroid gland can displace and obstruct the trachea, esophagus, and venous structures in the neck. The vast majority of such cases are caused by nontoxic multinodular goiter. Symptoms are generally attributable to extraluminal compression of the trachea or esophagus. Thyroid malignancies can also cause extraluminal or intraluminal obstruction, particularly when poorly differentiated. In these cases, hemoptysis and vocal cord paralysis are the predominant signs. Goiters extending beneath the thoracic inlet, which occur in 1 of 5,000 persons, descend along fascial planes into the mediastinum, maintaining their anatomic and vascular connections to the cervical thyroid. Less than 1% are truly intrathoracic, arising congenitally in the mediastinum and deriving their blood supply from intrathoracic vessels.

Presentation

The presentation of obstructing goiters varies depending on their location. Cervical goiters, which compress the trachea or esophagus, can cause exertional or positional dyspnea, stridor, dysphagia, nonproductive cough, and wheezing. The cervical sympathetic nervous system chain, the recurrent laryngeal nerves, and the superior vena cava can also be involved, causing a Horner's syndrome, vocal cord paralysis, and a superior vena caval syndrome, respectively. However, these are unusual presentations for nonmalignant goiters. When dyspnea and stridor develop suddenly, they are usually caused by spontaneous hemorrhage into the gland, which causes a rapid increase in the volume of the gland.

Retrosternal goiters cause compression of the trachea, esophagus, and superior vena cava at the level of the thoracic inlet.[50] Tracheal compression, with or without respiratory compromise, is three times more common than esophageal compression. Rarely, the superior vena cava may be obstructed, with resulting edema of the face and upper limbs, facial plethora, hoarseness, dizziness, dyspnea, and elevation of the jugular venous pulse. Patients with retrosternal goiters are usually euthyroid but can have autonomously functioning nodules that cause hyperthyroidism.

Physical examination typically reveals a clinically euthyroid patient and a cervical goiter with its inferior margin extending beneath the sternum. Occasionally, no cervical component can be appreciated when intrathoracic goiters are connected to the gland by only a thin bridge of fibrous tissue. Symptomatic dyspnea and facial plethora may occur when a patient raises his or her arms over the head (Pemberton's sign) as the result of obstructing the already narrowed thoracic inlet.[51]

Evaluation

Computed tomography or magnetic resonance imaging of the neck and chest is the best way to define the extent of the goitrous mass and the degree of tracheal compression. Computed tomography scans should be performed without iodinated radiocontrast agents to avoid iodine-induced thyrotoxicosis. Pulmonary function flow-volume loops can be valuable to define the pathophysiologic significance of airway narrowing, whether obstruction is intrathoracic or extrathoracic.[52] Cervical goiters can cause extrathoracic obstruction, diminishing primarily inspiratory airflow and flattening the inspiratory phase of the loop. A peak inspiratory flow of less than 1.5 L/sec may be an indication for surgical intervention. Radionuclide thyroid scans are useful principally to confirm that a superior mediastinal mass is thyroid tissue. If dysphagia is present, a barium swallow study may confirm whether esophageal compression is likely to be responsible. Fine-needle aspiration biopsies should be performed when malignancy is suspected and before virtually all surgical procedures. Finally, the serum TSH concentration should be measured to ensure that the patient is euthyroid.

Management

Surgical resection is the preferred treatment for acutely obstructing goiters. Intrathoracic goiters are usually resectable with a standard cervical collar incision, but in difficult cases, sternotomy may be required. Large posterior goiters more often require this approach. Sternotomy may also be required in emergency surgeries for airway obstruction and for recurrent intrathoracic goiters. True mediastinal goiters separate from the cervical thyroid gland may also require sternotomy to deal with their mediastinal vascular supply. Hemorrhage is of concern during thyroidectomy, and morcellation should also be avoided.

For patients who have nonacute, mild compressive symptoms and who are not surgical candidates or who refuse to consider surgery, radioiodine therapy is an alternative. In one series,[53] patients received single intravenous doses of I^{131} at 100 μCi per estimated gram of thyroid tissue, followed by daily administration of thyroxine to maintain the serum TSH concentration at less than 1.5 mU/L. After 1 year, the mean reduction in goiter volume was 40%. The narrowest diameter of the tracheal lumen was increased by 36%. Symptoms of dyspnea and inspiratory stridor improved in 66% of patients. However, these benefits of radioiodine treatment may take 12 to 24 months to occur, and patients must be carefully monitored for the possible development of thyrotoxicosis due to radiation thyroiditis.

Outcome

Thyroidectomy for obstructive symptoms usually results in significant clinical improvement. Peak and midinspiratory flow rates can increase by 100% postoperatively. Patients may have tracheomalacia from long-standing goiters. (Tracheomalacia is discussed in Chapter 9, Airway Emergencies.) Injury to the recurrent laryngeal nerve and surgical hypoparathyroidism remain potential surgical complications. Up to 20% of patients may have recurrence of retrosternal goiters after successful surgery.

SUPPURATIVE THYROIDITIS

The thyroid gland is rarely infected as the result of spread from contiguous structures or hematogenously from a distant focus. Children with acute suppurative thyroiditis usually show a left pyriform sinus or a fistula as the route of infection. Infectious material can also spread via fascial planes from the retropharyngeal space (as in tonsillitis or pharyngitis) or from the lateral pharyngeal space (as in otitis, mastoiditis, tonsillitis, or parotiditis.[54] Direct infection of the thyroid gland after subtotal thyroidectomy also occurs rarely.

Acute suppurative thyroiditis, in one series, was caused by pyogenic bacteria in 68% of 224 cases, mycobacteria in 9%, parasites in 5%, syphilis in 3%, and fungi in 15%.[55] Individuals with preexisting thyroid disease (e.g., adenoma, nodular and simple goiters, carcinoma, and thyroiditis) are predisposed to infection of the gland and account for more than one half of cases. Consequently, women are more often affected than men. The most commonly responsible bacterial organisms are *Staphylococcus aureus*, *Streptococcus pyogenes*, *Streptococcus pneumoniae*, and genera of the Enterobacteriaceae family. Anaerobes including *Bacteroides* species may occasionally be involved. Thyroidal tuberculosis is typically associated with miliary dissemination and follows an indolent course with few symptoms. Fungal thyroiditis is generally attributable to *Aspergillus* species in immunocompromised patients, although there have also been reported cases of *Coccidiodes immitis*, *Histoplasma capsulatum*, and *Candida albicans* infections of the thyroid gland.

Presentation

Patients with acute thyroiditis present with a brief history of fever, malaise, and swelling and severe pain of the thyroid. Dysphonia and dysphagia may be prominent complaints. On examination, there is typically erythema, warmth, tenderness, and swelling of the thyroid gland with cervical adenopathy. The absence of pain and erythema suggests a tuberculous or syphilitic cause. Fluctuance of the gland implies abscess development. There may also be evidence of contiguous or distant foci of infection elsewhere.

Leukocytosis is normally present. Serum thyroid function tests are usually normal, unless there was preexisting thyroid dysfunction. Sonography or computed tomography imaging can demonstrate the presence of thyroid enlargement and fluid collection.

Management

Fine-needle aspiration, with or without ultrasonic guidance, should be performed and the aspirated material submitted for Gram stain and culture. Blood cultures should also be obtained. Treatment includes appropriate antibiotics and local heat. If no organisms are seen in the initial smear, broad spectrum antibiotics should cover staphylococci until culture results are available. An abscess should be surgically drained. The absence of a clinical response to appropriate antibiotics should prompt surgical exploration. After recovery, a barium swallow or computed tomography scanning is indicated in children to rule out a pyriform sinus or fistula.

Outcome

The prognosis after infection of the thyroid gland is generally good, with few complications, although permanent vocal cord paralysis may occur. Thyroid function usually remains normal, although there can be transient hypothyroidism or, rarely, permanent thyroid gland failure.

REFERENCES

1. Oelkers W. Adrenal insufficiency. N Engl J Med 1996;335:1206–1212.
2. Werbel SS, Ober KP. Acute adrenal insufficiency. Endocrinol Metab Clin North Am 1993;22:303–328.
3. Grinspoon SK, Billet BM. Laboratory assessment of adrenal insufficiency. J Clin Endocrinol Metab 1994;79:923–931.
4. Streeten DHP, Anderson GH Jr, Bonaventura MM. The potential serious consequences from misinterpreting normal responses to the rapid adrenocorticotropin test. J Clin Endocrinol Metab 1996;81:285–290.
5. Salem M, Tainsh RE, Bromberg J, et al. Perioperative glucocorticoid coverage: a reassessment 42 years after emergence of a problem. Ann Surg 1994;219:416–425.
6. Blevins LS, Wand GS. Diabetes insipidus. Crit Care Med 1992;20:69–79.
7. Robertson GL. Differential diagnosis of polyuria. Ann Rev Med 1988;39:425–442.
8. Ober KP. Diabetes insipidus. Crit Care Clinics 1991;7:109–125.
9. Bichet DG. Diabetes insipidus and vasopressin. In Moore WT, Eastman R, eds., Diagnostic Endocrinology, 2nd ed. St. Louis, Mosby, 1996, pp. 157–175.
10. Levitt MA, Fleischer AS, Meislin HW. Acute posttraumatic diabetes insipidus: treatment with continuous intravenous vasopressin. J Trauma 1984;24;532–535.
11. Lewis DJM, Thomas JP. Treatment of nephrogenic diabetes insipidus. N Engl J Med 1986;315:1292–1293.
12. Mans OH, Carroll HJ. Disorders of sodium metabolism: hypernatremia and hyponatremia. Crit Care Med 1992;20;94–103.
13. Rose BD. Hypoosmolal states: hyponatremia. In Clinical Physiology of Acid-Base and Electrolyte Disorders, 4th ed. New York, McGraw-Hill, 1994, pp. 651–694.
14. Steele A, Gowrishankar M, Abrahamson S, et al. Postoperative hyponatremia despite near-isotonic saline infusion: a phenomenon of desalination. Ann Intern Med 1997;126:20–25.
15. Ayus JC, Wheeler IM, Arieff AI. Postoperative hyponatremic encephalopathy in menstruant women. Ann Intern Med 1992;117:891–897.
16. Mulloy AL, Caruana RJ. Hyponatremic emergencies. Med Clin North Am 1995;79:155–168.
17. Laureno R, Karp BI. Myelinolysis after correction of hyponatremia. Ann Intern Med 1997;126:57–62.
18. Fraser CL, Arieff AI. Epidemiology, pathophysiology and management of hyponatremic encephalopathy. Am J Med 1997;102:67–77.
19. Falk SA, Birken EA, Baran DT. Temporary postthyroidectomy hypocalcemia. Arch Otolaryngol Head Neck Surg 1988;114:168–174.
20. Brasier AR, Nussbaum SR. Hungry bone syndrome: clinical and biochemical predictors of its occurrence after parathyroid surgery. Am J Med 1988;84:654–660.
21. Zaloga GP, Chernow B, Cook D, et al. Assessment of calcium homeostasis in the critically ill surgical patient: the diagnostic pitfalls of the McLean Hastings nomogram. Ann Surg 1985;202:587–594.
22. Guise TA, Mundy GR. Evaluation of hypocalcemia in children and adults. J Clin Endocrinol Metab 1995;80:1473–1478.
23. Zaloga GP. Hypocalcemic crisis. Crit Care Clin 1991;7:191–200.
24. Reber PM, Heath H. Hypocalcemic emergencies. Med Clin North Am 1995;79:93–106.
25. Al Zahrani A, Levine ML. Primary hyperparathyroidism. Lancet 1997;349:1233–1238.
26. Mundy GR, Guise TA. Hypercalcemia of malignancy. Am J Med 1997;103:134–145.
27. Shane E. Hypercalcemia: pathogenesis, clinical manifestations, differential diagnosis and management. In Favus MJ, ed. Primer on the Metabolic Bone Diseases and Disorders of Mineral Metabolism, 3rd ed. Philadelphia, JB Lippincott, 1996, pp. 177–181.
28. Bilezikian JP. Management of acute hypercalcemia. N Engl J Med 1992;326:1196–1203.
29. Wimalawansa SJ. Optimal frequency of administration of pamidronate in patients with hypercalcemia of malignancy. Clin Endocrinol 1994;41:591–595.
30. Pecherstorfer M, Schilling Y, Blind E, et al. Parathyroid hormone–related protein and life expectancy in hypercalcemic cancer patients. J Clin Endocrinol Metab 1994;78:1268–1270.

30a. Whipple AD. The surgical therapy of hyperinsulinism. J Int Chir 1938;3:257–276.

31. Jennings AM, Wilson RM, Ward JD. Symptomatic hypoglycemia in NIDDM patients treated with oral hypoglycemic agents. Diabetes Care 1989;12:203–208.
32. Comi RJ. Approach to acute hypoglycemia. Endocrinol Metab Clin North Am 1993;22:247–262.
33. Service FJ. Hypoglycemia. Endocrinol Metab Clin North Am 1997;26:937–955.
34. Malouf R, Brust JCM. Hypoglycemia: causes, neurological manifestations and outcome. Ann Neurol 1985;17:421–430.
35. Bravo EL, Gifford RW. Pheochromocytoma. Endocrinol Metab Clin North Am 1993;22:329–341.
36. Bravo EL. Evolving concepts in the pathophysiology, diagnosis, and treatment of pheochromocytoma. Endocrine Rev 1994;15:356–368.
37. Calhoun DA, Oparil S. Treatment of hypertensive crisis. N Engl J Med 1990;323:177–183.
38. Nicoloff JT, LoPresti JS. Myxedema coma: a form of decompensated hypothyroidism. Endocrinol Metab North Am 1993;22:279–290.
39. Ladenson PW, Goldenheim PD, Ridgeway EC. Prediction of reversal of blunted respiratory responsiveness in patients with hypothyroidism. Am J Med 1988;84:877–883.
40. Myers L, Hays J. Myxedema coma. Crit Care Clin 1991;7:43–56.
41. Jordan JM. Myxedema coma: the prognosis is improving. Endocrinologist 1993;3:149–153.
42. Hylander B, Rosenqvist U. Treatment of myxedema coma: factors associated with a fatal outcome. Acta Endocrinol 1985;180:65–71.
43. Wartofsky L. Thyrotoxic storm. In Braverman LE, Utiger RD, eds. Werner and Ingbar's The Thyroid, 7th ed. Philadelphia, JB Lippincott, 1995, pp. 701–707.
44. Sherman SI, Simonson L, Ladenson PW. Clinical and socioeconomic predispositions to complicated thyrotoxicosis: a predictable and preventable syndrome. Am J Med 1996;101:192–198.
45. Brooks MH, Waldstein SS. Free thyroxine concentrations in thyroid storm. Ann Intern Med 1980;93:694–697.
46. Burch HB, Wartofsky L. Life-threatening thyrotoxicosis: thyroid storm. Endocrinol Metab North Am 1993;22:263–277.
47. Brunette DD, Rothong C. Emergency department treatment of thyrotoxic crisis with esmolol. Am J Emerg Med 1991;9:232–234.

48. Tajiri J, Katsuya H, Kiyokaya T, et al. Successful treatment of thyrotoxic crisis with plasma exchange. Crit Care Med 1984;12:536–537.
49. Candrina R, DiStefano O, Spandrio S, et al. Treatment of thyrotoxic storm by charcoal plasmaperfusion. J Endocrinol Invest 1989;12:133–134.
50. Madjar S, Weissberg D. Retrosternal goiter. Chest 1995;108:78–82.
51. Blum M, Biller BJ, Bergman DA. The thyroid cork: obstruction of the thoracic inlet due to retroclavicular goiter. JAMA 1974;227:189–191.
52. Karbowitz SR, Edelman LB, Nath S, et al. Spectrum of advanced upper airway obstruction due to goiters. Chest 1985;87:18–21.
53. Huysmans D, Hermus A, Corstens F, et al. Large compressive goiters treated with radioiodine: Ann Intern Med 1994;12:757–762.
54. Basgoz N, Swartz MN. In Braverman LE, Utiger RD, eds. Werner and Ingbar's The Thyroid, 7th ed. Philadelphia, JB Lippincott, 1995, pp. 1049–1056.
55. Berger SA, et al. Infectious diseases of the thyroid gland. Rev Infect Dis 1983;5:108–122.

CHAPTER **6**

Hematologic Emergencies

Alyson D. Buckner, MD
William R. Bell, MD

ANEMIA

Erythropoiesis is the process by which red blood cell (RBC) precursors in the bone marrow mature and are released into the circulating blood pool. In normal individuals, erythrocyte production and destruction (effected by the spleen) are nearly equivalent. Thus, a dynamic equilibrium is achieved such that the erythron is of stable size, configuration, and number. A decrease in RBC production, an increase in destruction, and extracorporeal blood loss result in a reduction of the erythrocyte mass. Anemia is defined as a reduction in the collective volume of red blood cells (the hematocrit) below 41% in adult males and below 36% in adult females.

Profound anemia, especially if it occurs rapidly, is an emergency commonly encountered in surgical patients. Acute blood loss, intraoperatively, postoperatively, or in the setting of trauma, accounts for a large subset of patients that suffer from significant anemia. Additionally, there are a number of common congenital and acquired disorders affecting the erythron that result in a chronic anemic state, with or without superimposed periods of more acute reductions in hemoglobin. It is imperative to recognize and treat these in the perioperative period, as any further declines in hemoglobin levels from the baseline may disrupt the tenuous, compensated state achieved physiologically in a patient with one of these disorders (Fig. 6–1).

Classic examples of congenital RBC disorders characterized by chronic anemia are the

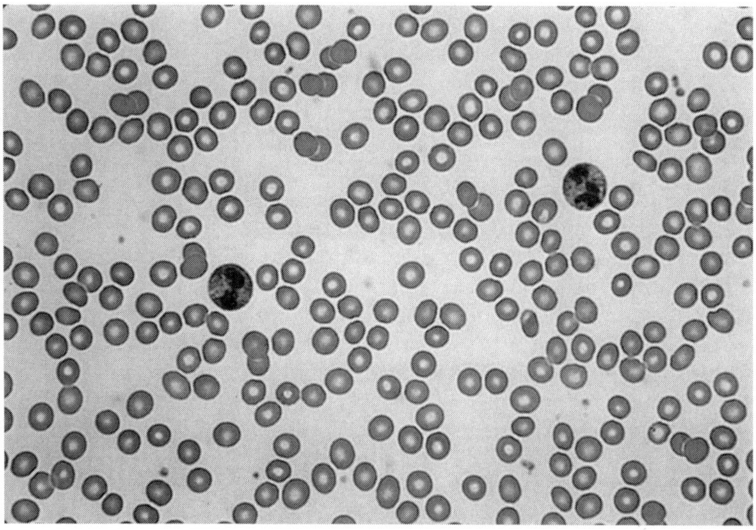

Figure 6–1. Normal peripheral blood smear.

hemoglobinopathies. Sickle cell disease (SSD) and sickle cell trait are hemoglobinopathies resulting from the production of dysfunctional hemoglobin molecules; in SSD, all hemoglobin produced is defective, and in sickle cell trait, less than one half of the hemoglobin produced is defective. The abnormal hemoglobin tends to form a thick gel within the erythrocyte under conditions of decreased oxygen tension. Continued polymerization of the sickle hemoglobin is reflected in the conversion of the biconcave RBCs into rigid, viscous erythrocytes with a characteristic sickled shape. The deleterious consequences of this include decreased ability of the deformed RBCs to traverse the microvasculature effectively, which produces local tissue hypoxia and necrosis, and premature destruction of erythrocytes by the reticuloendothelial system, with resultant anemia. The sickle globin gene is most prevalent in the populations of equatorial Africa and their descendants, but there are substantial numbers of affected individuals of Middle Eastern, Indian, and Mediterranean heritage. SSD affects approximately 75,000 to 85,000 African Americans in the United States (about 0.25%), and sickle cell trait occurs in 8% to 10% of this population.[1]

The thalassemia syndromes constitute the most prevalent of all known genetic diseases.[2] They are characterized by a disturbance in hemoglobin production whereby a reduced rate of synthesis of one or more of the globin chains leads to imbalances in the relative proportions of the various globin chains within the erythrocyte. The chains present in excess are highly unstable and insoluble. They precipitate and ultimately become deposited on the RBC membranes, with subsequent increased hemolysis and diminished RBC survival. This, in turn, leads to a state of ineffective erythropoiesis and chronic anemia. Thalassemia syndromes occur widely in people indigenous to the Mediterranean basin, the Middle East, Africa, and Southeast Asia.[3]

In addition to the congenital anemias, there are a number of acquired anemic states that are commonly encountered in surgical patients. Chronic excessive alcohol ingestion, a common habit among many head and neck surgery patients, is often associated with an anemia of mild to moderate severity. The cause of the anemia is multifactorial and includes profound nutritional deficiencies (iron and folate),[4] chronic gastrointestinal bleeding, and direct toxic effects of alcohol on erythropoiesis.[5]

It is also recognized that many infectious and noninfectious disorders are accompanied by an anemia of moderate severity, with hemoglobin concentrations in the range of 7 to 11 g/dL. This anemia of chronic disease is often associated with tuberculosis, subacute bacterial endocarditis, AIDS, rheumatoid arthritis, and metastatic carcinoma.[6] It is characterized by a moderately reduced RBC life span, disturbed iron metabolism, and impaired compensatory erythropoietic response.

Anemia is one of the most characteristic manifestations of chronic renal failure, with the degree of anemia being proportional to the degree of azotemia present.[7] The life span of RBCs in patients with chronic renal disease is foreshortened because of red cell fragility and hemolysis.[8] Compounding this problematic state of increased erythrocyte destruction is the failure of the marrow to show the appropriate compensatory erythroid hyperplasia.[9] Marrow suppression in renal failure is a consequence of deficient erythropoietin production by the kidneys.

Presentation

Patients presenting with severe, acute anemia most often have a recent history of surgery, trauma with hemorrhage, or massive gastrointestinal bleeding. An acute, severe decrease in intravascular volume causes tachycardia and postural hypotension, followed by impairment of cardiac output, vasoconstriction, and shock if progressive volume loss continues. Major hemodynamic compromise may be seen with acute loss of 30% to 40% of blood volume. The loss of circulating RBCs with ongoing hemorrhage decreases oxygen-carrying capacity, increases tissue hypoxia, and further exacerbates the shock state. Pallor of the skin, conjunctivae, and mucous membranes are typical of profoundly anemic patients.

The chronic anemia seen in congenital hemoglobinopathies may be mild or severe, with patients in variable states of precarious compensation. Many patients with SSD or sickle trait have been previously diagnosed with these maladies and come to surgical attention for treatment of unrelated problems, although some patients with milder forms of the disease might have eluded prior recognition. It is essential to determine the degree of anemia present preoperatively, as a low hemoglobin level implies decreased reserve and thus decreased tolerance of any further exacerbation of anemia. Patients with SSD also tend to develop jaundice and hepatomegaly, renal dysfunction and failure, splenomegaly and functional asplenia, and disorder of bone growth secondary to repeated episodes of bone infarction. Susceptibility to infection is increased.[1] Painful vaso-occlusive crises may be induced in the postoperative period as a result of the hypoxemia and venous stasis that accompany general anesthesia.[10]

Patients with any of the thalassemias are anemic to various degrees. Children with thalassemia display bossing of the skull, prominence of the maxilla, and trabeculation of the long bones and phalanges on plain radiographs due to expansion of the marrow spaces. Iron overload and its attendant consequences (from chronic transfusion) are the major complications recognized in adolescence and adulthood.[11]

Evaluation

Severe anemia is suspected when there is a history of significant bleeding or trauma. Measurement of hematocrit value immediately after profound bleeding may not show a commensurate decrement in RBC mass. The hematocrit value tends to fall gradually over a period of 24 to 48 hours after sudden hemorrhage, such that the magnitude of the blood loss may not be fully appreciated initially. Clinical signs and symptoms are important in order to determine the degree of anemia and the ability of the patient to compensate for the disturbance in homeostasis.

Sickle cell disease, sickle cell trait, and the thalassemias may be recognized by anemia in the clinical context of a patient with the aforementioned ethnicities or a positive family history. Hemoglobin values range from 2 to 11 g/dL, with somewhat higher (even normal) levels in patients with sickle cell trait. The anemia in SSD and sickle trait is normochromic and normocytic, whereas it is hypochromic and microcytic in thalassemia. Peripheral blood smears display irregular, sickled red cell forms in the former disease states, and anisocytosis with occasional target cell formation in the latter. Hemoglobin electrophoresis confirms the diagnosis of SSD and sickle trait; diagnosis of thalassemia involves direct quantification of the various globin chains and chain lengths (Fig. 6–2).[2]

Marked anemia may be an incidental finding in a patient undergoing preoperative assessment, and it frequently reflects underlying systemic illness. Unexplained anemia, therefore, warrants investigation. A thorough history, focusing on any potential occult sources of blood loss, should be obtained. Initial laboratory evaluation for anemia without an obvious source includes guaiac tests on serial stool samples, a complete blood count, and microscopic examination of a peripheral blood smear.

Assessment of RBC size and pigmentation is the cornerstone of accurate diagnosis of the cause of the anemia. Microcytosis and hypochromia are characteristic of iron deficiency anemia, thalassemia, and anemia of chronic diseases (including inflammatory, renal, and malignant diseases). Further evidence of iron deficiency includes a decrease in serum iron concentration, total iron binding capacity, and serum ferritin. Iron deficiency is confirmed by the absence of stainable iron on examination of

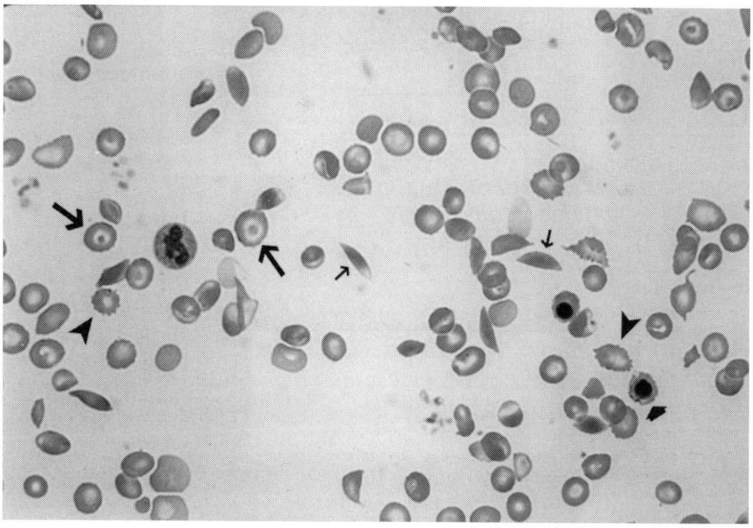

Figure 6–2. Sickle cell anemia. Arrowheads, burr cells; long arrows, target cells; small arrows, sickled cells; single fat arrow, nucleated red blood cell.

aspirated bone marrow.[12] Macrocytic erythrocytes are associated with deficiencies of folic acid or B_{12}, resulting in megaloblastic anemia. Hypersegmentation of polymorphonuclear leukocytes is also commonly observed in the setting of megaloblastic anemia.[13]

Priorities

Acute hemorrhage is managed by control of the bleeding source, restoration of intravascular volume, and replenishment of RBC stores. Hemostasis may be achieved by direct pressure if the source of bleeding is visible, but may require surgical intervention. Correction of decreased intravascular volume is accomplished with rapid infusion of warmed crystalloid (isotonic normal saline or Ringer's lactate solution) or colloid (Hespan). Transfusion of packed RBCs is necessary in circumstances of severe hemorrhage and will provide some expansion of the intravascular volume as well as replenishment of oxygen-carrying capacity. Associated coagulopathy must be controlled since it can contribute to ongoing bleeding. In the instance of hemorrhage in a patient unwilling to accept transfusion of blood and blood products such as a Jehovah's witness, this strategy must be amended. Control of bleeding is essential for optimal treatment. In addition, limitation of cellular metabolism and oxygen requirements by means of sedation, intubation, mechanical ventilation, and paralysis may be necessary.

Aggressive supplementation of endogenous iron stores with intramuscular or intravenous iron dextran is advisable. The total dose of iron dextran sufficient for replenishment of RBC mass may be calculated on the basis of the patient's weight and hemoglobin level (Box 6–1).

BOX 6–1

Calculation of Iron Dextran Dose Based on Patient Weight and Hemoglobin Deficit

$D_{Fe(g)} = (D_h/100) \times W_{kg} \times 65 \times 0.0034$
$D_{Fe(mg)} = D_h \times W_{kg} \times 2.2$
$D_{Fe(mg)} = D_h \times W_{lb}$

D_{Fe}, total hemoglobin iron (Fe) deficit
D_h, whole blood hemoglobin deficit, g/dL
W_{kg}, patient weight in kilograms
W_{lb}, patient weight in pounds
Total blood volume, 65 mL/kg
Iron (Fe) content of hemoglobin, .34%

Caution must be observed with administration, as this iron preparation may be associated with serious side effects, including arthralgias, fever, nausea, hypotension, thrombophlebitis, indelible discoloration at the injection site (intramuscular), and anaphylaxis.[14, 15] Erythropoietin may be administered to accelerate maturation and release of RBC forms from the marrow. Dosages range from 50 to 150 units/kg, with injections typically given every other day for 1 to 2 weeks.[16] Erythropoietin therapy may be rejected by some Jehovah's witnesses because the preparation commercially available contains human albumin.

Modest anemia without hemodynamic compromise is optimally treated with an oral iron supplement such as ferrous sulfate. Therapy is initiated at 325 mg twice daily and should continue for at least 8 months in menstruating females and 6 months in adult males and nonmenstruating females.

Optimal perioperative treatment of SSD frequently involves transfusion of packed RBCs to decrease the relative proportion of abnormal hemoglobin (and therefore the rate of sickling) and improve the anemia. Sickle hemoglobin should be reduced to less than 40% of the total hemoglobin value before any surgical procedure.[2] Measures to prevent hypoxia and intravascular volume depletion should be undertaken, as they also contribute significantly to sickling and sludging of blood in the microvasculature. The thalassemias are managed with chronic transfusion of packed RBCs, administration of iron chelators, and splenectomy in patients with massive splenomegaly.[17]

Outcomes

Acute hemorrhage with severe anemia is responsive to the supportive measures outlined above. Transfusion of blood products is not a benign course of action and, if possible, should be avoided. There are risks of transmission of infectious diseases, transfusion reaction, and fluid and iron overload inherent in transfusion.

The prognosis and outcome for patients with SSD are variable. Multiple episodes of painful vaso-occlusive crises throughout life are observed; pulmonary infarction, renal failure, and cerebrovascular accidents are later sequelae. Survival of patients through middle age is now common with aggressive health maintenance.

The chronic need for transfusion, as is the case with the thalassemias, may result in profound and irreversible iron overload. Deposition of iron in the heart, liver, and endocrine glands leads to organ failure. Siderosis is the leading cause of death in all types of thalassemia syndromes.[18]

TRANSFUSION REACTIONS

A transfusion reaction may be defined as any untoward event or physiologic consequence that occurs as a result of receiving blood or blood products. It is estimated that between 0.5% and 3.0% of all transfusions are associated with some type of adverse effect, although serious, life-threatening effects are much more rare. Each year in the United States, approximately 14 million units of blood products are transfused to 3.2 million patients, resulting in 120,000 immediate adverse reactions.[19] This does not include infectious sequelae or the more nebulous immunomodulation (i.e., immunosuppression) that may accompany transfusion (Table 6–1).

Transfusion reactions may be very broadly divided into hemolytic and nonhemolytic. The hemolytic variety occurs once for every 6,000 to 25,000 units of RBCs transfused.[20, 21] These reactions are the direct effect of intravascular RBC destruction by immune mechanisms. Preexisting anti-RBC antibodies (isohemagglutinins) in the recipient bind to transfused RBCs, activate the complement system, and lyse the target cells. Hemolysis is not necessarily limited to the donor cells; activated complement may adhere to native RBCs as well, such that substantial amounts of the recipient's own RBCs are lysed too. Involved antibodies are almost invariably those directed against antigens of the ABO group and are naturally occurring in transfusion-naive patients. They are most often associated with clerical error and transfusion of ABO-incompatible blood into a patient (Table 6–2 and Fig. 6–3).[22]

Table 6–1. *Estimated Risks of Transfusion per Unit**

Minor allergic reactions	1 in 100
Bacteremia†	1 in 2500
Viral hepatitis	1 in 5000
Hemolytic transfusion reaction	1 in 6000
HIV infection	1 in 420,000
Acute lung injury	1 in 500,000
Anaphylaxis	1 in 500,000
Septicemia‡	1 in 500,000
Fatal hemolytic reaction	1 in 600,000
Immunosuppression	?

Data from Klein HG. Allogeneic transfusion risks in the surgical patient. Am J Surg 1995;170(suppl 6A):21–26.
*Statistics are for the United States in 1995.
†Platelets.
‡Platelet-associated.

Table 6–2. *Blood Type Frequencies in Caucasian Population*

Blood Type	% in Population	Antigen or RBC	Antibody in Serum
A	44.5	A	Anti-B
B	8.5	B	Anti-A
O	43.5	O	Anti-A, anti-B
AB	3.5	A, B	None
Rh+	85	D	None
Rh−	15	−	Anti-D (only if immunized)

Febrile reactions are the most common nonhemolytic reactions, with a rate of occurrence of 1% with RBC transfusions and up to 20% with platelet transfusions.[23] These reactions are the result of the recipient's producing antibodies to passenger leukocytes from the donor (commonly antibodies to donor human leukocyte antigens present on granulocytes, lymphocytes, and platelets) and cytokines (especially the endogenous pyrogens interleukin-1 and -2 and tumor necrosis factor) synthesized by donor leukocytes during storage.

Allergic complications of transfusion also occur and range from minor urticarial reactions to bronchospasm and, rarely, even fulminant anaphylaxis with subsequent shock and death. These reactions occur when recipient antibodies and donor plasma proteins combine to form immune complexes that activate the complement system. These anaphylatoxins then trigger the degranulation of mediators from mast cells and basophils in the recipient. They are most often seen in the context of plasma infusion and

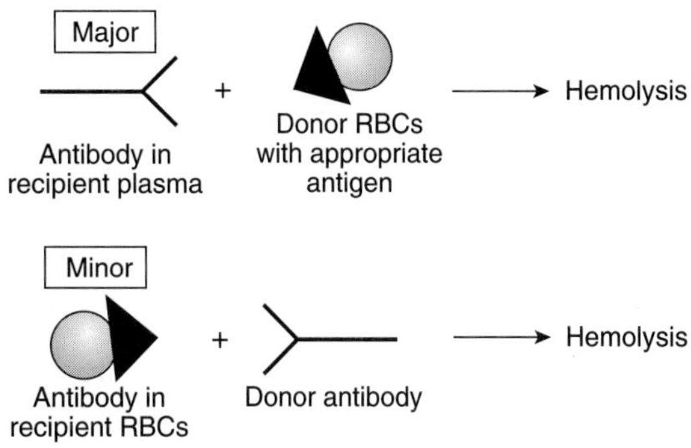

Figure 6–3. Hemolytic transfusion reactions and incompatabilities.

high-volume plasma exchange.[24] A patient who is deficient in immunoglobulin A (IgA) is at particular risk for anaphylactic reaction to a blood product, as many of these individuals have preformed anti-IgA antibodies that will react with the IgA present in donor plasma.[25]

Bacterial contamination of blood products, although not a transfusion reaction in the pure sense, should be considered, as it is in the differential diagnosis of a serious transfusion reaction that manifests with profound hemodynamic compromise. Fulminant bacterial sepsis is seen once for every 2.5 million units of blood products transfused, and bacteremia is associated with one of every 4000 units of platelets transfused.[26] The cryophilic organisms *Streptococcus lactus*, *Enterobacter agglomerans*, and *Yersinia enterocolitica* are most often responsible for the contamination and are thought to be direct contaminants from the donor venipuncture sites.[27, 28] Units of blood products that are older are at greatest risk of having clinically significant numbers of bacteria, which are capable of multiplying during storage. This is more common with units of platelets than with other blood components because of the need to store them at room temperature (Table 6–3).[26]

Presentation

Acute hemolytic transfusion reactions are typified by the onset of fever (virtually 100%), chills, nausea, flushing, dyspnea, flank pain, vague feelings of uneasiness, and progressive hypotension soon after infusion of 5 to 20 mL of blood product. Diagnosis in sedated, anesthetized, or neurologically impaired patients who are unable to report subjective symptoms is problematic. The only initial symptom may be fever or hemorrhage.[29] Disseminated intravascular coagulation (DIC) and renal failure are expected sequelae in this situation. In febrile, nonhemolytic transfusion reactions, a temperature rise of 3° to 5°C during transfusion without other precipitating factors is diagnostic. Some patients also experience constitutional symptoms, such as nausea, vomiting, and headache. Manifestations of allergic reactions are protean and differ in clinical severity. Urticarial reactions are mild and are characterized by hives and pruritus. Progression to more serious symptoms of nausea, vomiting, dyspnea, and bronchospasm may occur. Anaphylaxis is the most rare of the allergic complications and is recognized shortly after initiation of transfusion by transient hypertension, followed by profound hypotension, flushing, chills, laryngeal edema, and sometimes anuria.[30]

Evaluation

Evaluation of a patient exhibiting signs or symptoms of a transfusion reaction is centered on ascertaining whether the reaction is severe (hemolytic, anaphylactic, or septic) or whether it is of lesser clinical significance (febrile or minor allergic). If hemodynamic or respiratory compromise is evident on clinical evaluation of the patient, the diagnosis of a severe transfusion reaction should be entertained. The evaluation for a severe transfusion reaction involving red cells is designed to rule out an acute hemolytic reaction. First, witnessed review of the donor unit and recipient identification numbers should be quickly accomplished, as most cases of acute hemolytic reactions can be traced to clerical error and infusion of ABO mismatched blood.[22] Samples of blood from the donor unit and the recipient should be obtained and sent to the blood bank for immediate retyping and crossmatching. A direct antiglobulin (Coombs') test should also be performed. Because intravascular hemolysis releases free hemoglobin into the plasma, hemoglobinemia and hemoglobinuria will be present in an acute hemolytic reaction. A direct smear of the recipient's peripheral blood

Table 6–3. *Storage Conditions and Properties of Selected Blood Products*

Blood Product	Storage Temperature	Number of Cells or Activity	Volume of Infusion	Maximum Storage Life
Packed RBCs	1° to 6°C	Hematocrit = 70%–80%	200–250 mL	35 days
Whole blood		Hematocrit = 40%		
Platelets	20° to 24°C	≥ 5.5 × 10^{10} cells	50–60 mL	5 days
Fresh-frozen plasma	−18 to −20°C	—	200–250 mL	1 year
Coagulation factor concentrates	2° to 6°C	Variable	10–25 mL	Years
Cryoprecipitate	−20°C	Variable	10–15 mL	1 year

should also be examined for evidence of visible hemolysis. If hemolysis is intravascular, shistocytes are usually seen on a peripheral blood film.

Anaphylactic reactions to blood products may present with the same clinical manifestations as acute hemolytic reactions, so distinguishing the two is initially problematic. The laboratory evaluation outlined above will be negative in a severe allergic reaction; no evidence of intravascular hemolysis will be present. Once an acute hemolytic reaction is ruled out, the possibility of an allergic reaction must be investigated. The recipient's blood may be tested for plasma IgA level and the presence of anti-IgA antibodies, as most anaphylactic reactions occur in the context of a recipient with IgA deficiency and high-titer anti-IgA antibodies.[31]

If there is high clinical suspicion of bacterial contamination as the cause of hemodynamic collapse in a patient undergoing transfusion of a blood product, and the initial laboratory investigation for an acute hemolytic reaction is negative, culture of the remaining untransfused blood product and the patient's blood is the most helpful and appropriate test to perform. A Gram's stain should be performed as well. Heightened clinical suspicion of bacterial contamination is warranted if the blood product in question has had a prolonged storage time—platelets that are 4 to 5 days old or RBCs that are 25 to 35 days old.[29]

Minor transfusion reactions of limited clinical significance (febrile reactions, urticaria, and pruritus) usually do not warrant initiation of any specific laboratory investigation. An exception to this involves the patient who is sedated, anesthetized, or neurologically impaired such that a rise in temperature may be the only clue to an acute hemolytic reaction. A lower threshold for complete evaluation should be present in these clinical situations.

Priorities

Upon recognition of a potentially severe reaction, whether due to acute intravascular hemolysis, anaphylaxis, or bacterial contamination, transfusion should be discontinued immediately. Hemodynamic collapse in any of these situations should be addressed with intravenous crystalloid or colloid infusion, pressor support may be necessary to maintain blood pressure, and transfer of the patient to an intensive care setting.

If an acute hemolytic reaction is diagnosed, additional therapy is required to prevent renal damage from the released hemoglobin. Diuretics (furosemide and "renal dose" dopamine infusion at 3 to 10 μg/kg/min) are helpful to maintain brisk urinary output. Alkalinization of the urine with intravenous bicarbonate may also be useful for clearance of nephrotoxic free hemoglobin.[32]

Management of a true anaphylactic reaction consists of administration of epinephrine, antihistamines (diphenhydramine and H_2 blocker), and corticosteroids. To minimize further exposure to plasma proteins, patients who have had severe allergic reactions should receive only washed cell products in any future transfusion.[29] These patients should not be given plasma unless it is absolutely necessary, because it is impossible to ascertain the presence of the responsible antigen.

Treatment for sepsis in the setting of bacterial blood contamination is supportive. Antibiotics such as the antipseudomonal penicillins (piperacillin and tazobactam) and third-generation cephalosporins (ceftriaxone) are efficacious against the most commonly isolated bacteria (*Streptococcus lactus*, *Enterobacter agglomerans*, and *Yersinia enterocolitica*) and should be instituted before the results of the cultures are available.[28, 33]

In the setting of a more minor transfusion reaction, interruption of the blood product infusion is not always necessary. Febrile reactions are common and self-limited. Continuation of the transfusion is acceptable if review of the clinical situation indicates that a more serious transfusion reaction is unlikely. Symptomatic treatment with antipyretics is usually effective. Depletion of donor leukocytes can be accomplished by the use of leukocyte-reduction filters for future transfusions. Urticaria and pruritic reactions may also be treated symptomatically without interruption of the transfusion.[34] Diphenhydramine is the therapy of choice, and patients may be pretreated with it for prevention. Progression of allergic symptoms may occur, and discontinuation of the infusion is essential under such circumstances.

Outcomes

The vast majority of transfusion reactions are self-limited in nature and rarely produce long-term sequelae. Acute hemolytic transfusion reactions and progressive anaphylactic reactions to blood products occur much less frequently than do the minor transfusion reactions, but

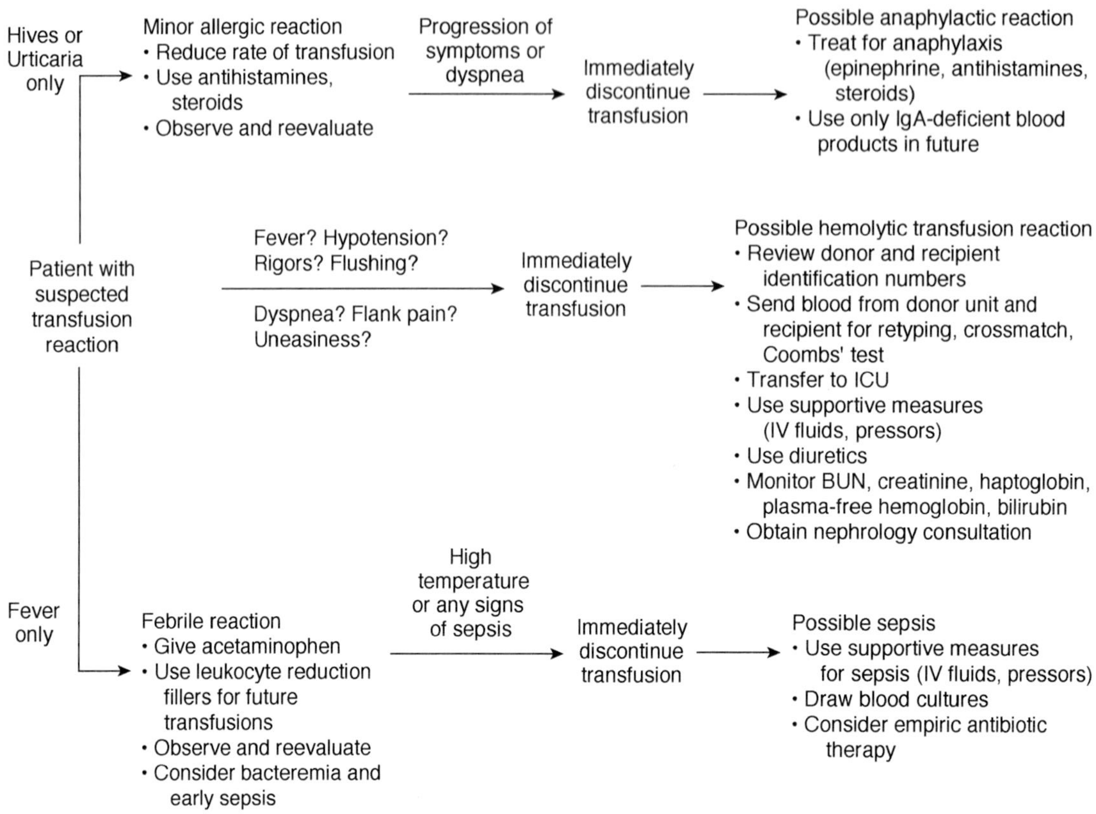

Figure 6–4. Algorithm for clinical evaluation and management of suspected transfusion reaction.

they are more likely to produce significant morbidity, including permanent renal dysfunction, and mortality (Fig. 6–4).

DISSEMINATED INTRAVASCULAR COAGULATION

A cogent and lucid definition of DIC, a life-threatening hemostatic disorder, has been put forth by Bick: "DIC is a systemic thrombohemorrhagic disorder in association with defined clinical situations and laboratory evidence of procoagulant and fibrinolytic activation, inhibitor consumption, and evidence of organ damage or failure."[35] DIC is not an independent entity, but rather a pathologic syndrome recognized in the setting of a systemic and usually severe disease process. In essence, it is the normal sequence of coagulation gone awry, with diffuse microvascular thrombosis and systemic fibrinolysis occurring simultaneously. The sequelae of unchecked activation of these two arms of the coagulation pathway include hemorrhage and small vessel thrombosis, and may even progress to large vessel thrombosis. Bleeding may be massive and recalcitrant to therapeutic measures. The associated thrombosis produces ischemia and end-organ damage in the cardiac, pulmonary, renal, hepatic, and central nervous systems.[36]

The pathophysiology of DIC is complex, as there are multiple initiators, activated coagulation factors, and effectors involved. A triggering event such as the release of endotoxin from bacterial cell walls, the presence of tumor tissue thromboplastin antigens in patients with malignancy, massive transfusion, or intravascular hemolysis activates the tissue-plasminogen-platelet system via the extrinsic pathway of coagulation, mediated by tissue thromboplastin. Alternatively, the intrinsic pathway of coagulation may be activated by many of the same inciting factors. Thrombin and plasmin are generated, and they circulate systemically. Circulating thrombin cleaves fibrinogen, producing fibrin. Fibrin polymerizes within the vascular compartment, producing thrombosis in capillary beds and in larger vessels. Ischemia and anoxic damage to organs ensue. Platelets become trapped in the evolving, diffuse clots and are destroyed, thereby producing thrombocytopenia. Plasmin in the circulation degrades soluble fibrin, fibrin, and fibrinogen (generating the fibrinogen-fibrin degradation products), along with activation of factors V, VII, IX, and XI. Clotting factors are destroyed out of proportion to production. Plasmin also activates the complement system, resulting in complement-induced lysis of RBCs and platelets, leading to more profound anemia and thrombocytopenia. Activation of the kinin system also occurs, with a resultant increase in vascular permeability, hypotension, and shock (Fig. 6–5).[35]

Table 6–4. *Disease States Associated with Disseminated Intravascular Coagulation*

Obstetric conditions
Amniotic fluid embolism
Placental abruption
Retained fetus
Eclampsia
Abortion
Intravascular hemolysis
Hemolytic transfusion reactions
Massive transfusion
Septicemia
Gram-negative (endotoxin release)
Gram-positive (mucopolysaccharide release)
Viremia
Metastatic cancer and leukemias
Trauma
Multiorgan system trauma
Burns
Extensive crush injuries with tissue necrosis
Acute liver disease
Prosthetic devices
LeVeen and Denver shunts
Intra-aortic balloon pumps

Presentation

Patients with the clinical syndrome of DIC are acutely ill with an underlying disease process (Table 6–4). DIC is not a primary disease entity, so there are no clinical findings specifically diagnostic for it. Prominent in the constellation of systemic signs are fever, hypotension, acidosis, proteinuria, hypoxia, and hemorrhage. Some or all of these signs may be present in a patient before the onset of DIC.

Physical examination indicators of DIC include petechiae and purpura, wound bleeding postoperatively, oozing from venipuncture and intra-arterial line sites, and deep-tissue bleeding resulting in hematoma formation. In addition, bleeding in the gastrointestinal and genitourinary systems may be evident. Just as impressive, although not as clinically obvious initially, is the thrombosis that is produced throughout the vasculature. Acute renal failure is common; it results from a combination of microvascular thrombosis in the capillary beds of the kidney (at the level of the glomeruli) and the reduced renal blood flow that accompanies hypotension. General cortical and brain-stem dysfunction are attributable to widespread thrombosis in the brain. Focal neurologic defects, impaired con-

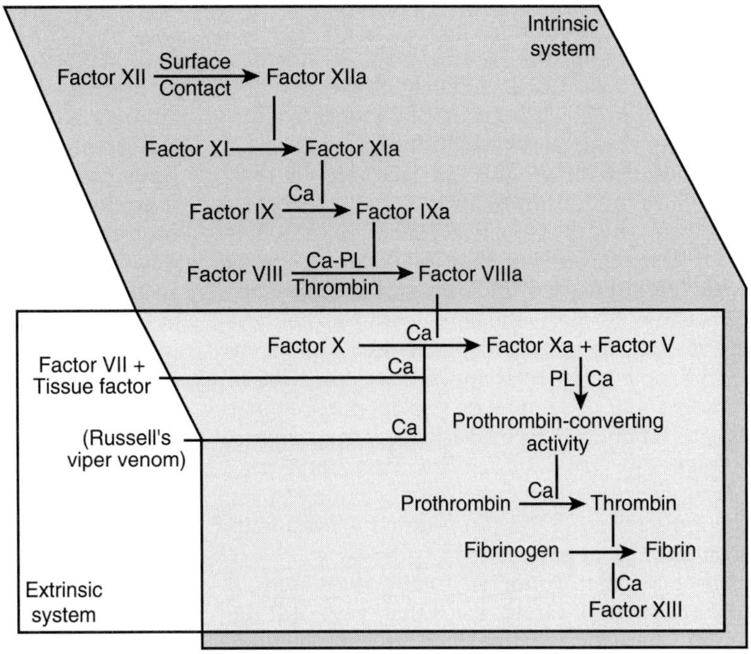

Figure 6–5. Coagulation cascade.

sciousness, seizures, and coma may all occur in the setting of DIC. Thrombosis and hemorrhage in the lungs inhibit oxygenation and ventilation, producing hypoxia, acidosis, and respiratory failure.[35]

Evaluation

Laboratory evaluation is essential in DIC, as there are neither pathognomonic clinical signs nor symptoms. Likewise, there is no single test to confirm or completely rule out the diagnosis. A body of evidence must be generated to support the diagnosis in the appropriate clinical setting. Laboratory evidence of procoagulant activation, fibrinolytic activation, inhibitor consumption, and end-organ damage should be sought.

Global tests of coagulation are only minimally useful in confirming the diagnosis. The prothrombin time (PT) should be prolonged in the setting of DIC, but for multiple reasons beyond the scope of this text, it may be normal or shortened in up to 50% of patients. Likewise, the activated partial thromboplastin time (aPTT) should also be increased in DIC, but it is actually prolonged in only 50% to 60% of patients. The thrombin time (TT) is expected to be prolonged as well, but may be normal or shortened due to the same confounding factors that affect the PT and aPTT. A bonus test of the thrombin (or reptilase) time may be performed, whereby the resultant clot is observed for dissolution. If the clot does not dissolve within 10 minutes, a clinically significant amount of plasmin is unlikely to be present. Lysis of the clot indicates that there is a clinically significant level of fibrinolysis present.[37] Measurement of coagulation factor levels provides little useful information.

Fibrin and fibrinogen degradation products (FDPs) are elevated in 85% to 100% of patients with DIC. They are indicative of the presence of plasmin, as this is the endogenous proteolytic agent that acts to degrade fibrin and fibrinogen. Antithrombin III levels are decreased in 89% of cases of DIC.[38] A newer test is the D-dimer assay. D-Dimer is formed when plasmin digests soluble and cross-linked fibrin (but not fibrinogen). It is considered the most reliable test for the presence of DIC, as D-dimer elevation is seen in 93% of patients.[39]

The platelet count is usually decreased in DIC, although rarely the value may still be within the normal range. Thrombocytopenia is at times profound, with counts down to 2000 to 3000/mm^3.

***Table 6–5.** Laboratory Diagnosis of Disseminated Intravascular Coagulation*

Test	Percentage of Patients with Abnormal Values
D-dimers	93%
Antithrombin III	89%
Fibrinopeptide A	88%
Fibrin(ogen) degradation products	75%
Platelet count	90%–100%
Thrombin time	100%
Fibrinogen level	Variably decreasing
Prothrombin and thromboplastin times	Often normal

Examination of the peripheral blood smear may reveal evidence of RBC fragmentation (schistocytes, helmet cells, and burr cells) and thrombocytopenia (Table 6–5).[35]

Priorities

The essential first step in the control and elimination of DIC is aggressive treatment of the underlying disease process, which serves as the nidus for ongoing DIC. Broad-coverage antibiotic therapy and generous restoration of intravascular volume are appropriate initial interventions for sepsis. Chemotherapy and surgery may be necessary for an oncology patient with fulminant DIC. Victims of thermal injuries and patients with tissue necrosis as the triggering event may be improved by surgical debridement.

Specific therapies aimed at treating the concomitant thrombosis and hemorrhage make up the second principle of relieving DIC. Thrombosis has the greatest impact on morbidity and mortality in patients with DIC, so impeding ongoing intravascular clotting is imperative. The stimulus for secondary fibrinolysis is also reduced by this intervention. Heparin therapy is somewhat controversial, and the decision to institute anticoagulation must be based on the individual patient's characteristics, such as the inciting cause of the DIC and its response to therapy, the hemodynamic status, the sites and severity of hemorrhage, and the sites and severity of thrombosis. It may be reasonable to use heparin in situations in which the patient continues to bleed or clot significantly 4 to 6 hours after initiation of therapeutic interventions for the underlying illness. Unfractionated and low-molecular-weight heparins are available and both have shown efficacy in limited clinical studies. Unfractionated heparin may be used for subcutaneous low-dose injections or for larger-dose intravenous infusions. There is no evidence that intravenous heparin is less effective than low-dose subcutaneous heparin. Low-molecular-weight heparin may be associated with fewer bleeding complications and has less effect upon platelet function.[40] Heparin therapy is clearly contraindicated in any circumstance of central nervous system insult or fulminant liver failure. DIC has been treated successfully in small numbers of patients with antithrombin III concentrates.[41]

Persistent hemorrhage after treatment of the primary disease process and addition of heparin suggests significant depletion of clotting factors. These components may be safely replaced if the underlying disease process is controlled, but preparations should be devoid of fibrinogen. Supplementation of fibrinogen in the face of fulminant DIC where plasmin is in excess will produce additional FDPs that further impair hemostasis and is not recommended. Fresh-frozen plasma should therefore be used with caution. Transfusion of washed, packed RBCs and platelet concentrates is indicated to ameliorate the anemia and thrombocytopenia once specific treatment of the inciting disease has been instituted.[35]

Outcomes

Survival rates of approximately 75% to 95% have been reported for DIC when aggressive, individualized treatment is used for fulminant DIC; the exception is intractable, progressive neoplastic disease.

OTHER COAGULOPATHIES

In addition to DIC, there are a number of other coagulopathies, both congenital and acquired, that may be present in surgical patients and require immediate attention perioperatively to prevent or control hemorrhage.

The most commonly encountered causes of congenital coagulopathies are the congenital factor deficiencies, including factor VIII deficiency (hemophilia A), factor IX deficiency (hemophilia B or Christmas disease), and von Willebrand's factor deficiency (von Willebrand's disease, or vWD). Together, these three entities account for approximately 95% of all known congenital factor-deficiency disorders.[42] Both types of hemophilia are inherited as X-linked recessive disorders and occur, therefore, almost exclusively in males. Female carriers of factor IX deficiency may be symptomatic and experience significant hemorrhage. As a result of important advancements in the recognition and treatment of these diseases, the relative proportion of adults with these disorders is rising.

The acquired clotting abnormalities are a more heterogeneous group. Hepatic insufficiency or fulminant liver failure, vitamin K deficiency, and azotemia/uremia are common causes of coagulopathy in critically ill patients. It is estimated that 15% of patients in intensive care units develop clinical or laboratory evidence of hepatic insufficiency, with prolongation of the PT and aPTT as a prominent manifestation. Clotting factor synthesis (not only the vitamin K–dependent factors II, VII, IX, and X, but also factor V) is depressed in these patients. In vitamin K deficiency, the hemostatic defect results directly from the inability of factors II, VII, IX, and X to undergo gamma-carboxylation in the hepatocytes, a biochemical reaction for which vitamin K serves as a cofactor. Patients who are malnourished, unable to absorb nutrition effectively enterally, or on broad-spectrum antibiotics are particularly susceptible to vitamin K deficiency. Coagulopathy in the uremic patient is multifactorial and is associated with intrinsic platelet dysfunction secondary to the effects of urea.[43]

Acquired inhibitors to coagulation factors (circulating anticoagulants) are seen, although rarely, in association with neoplastic disease, including squamous cell carcinoma of the head and neck.[44]

Iatrogenic coagulopathies are acquired disturbances of blood clotting that are caused by prior or ongoing medical interventions. Massive transfusion syndrome results from large-volume transfusion of packed RBCs in a short time without replenishment of coagulation factors or platelets with fresh-frozen plasma and platelet concentrates. In this setting, production of coagulation proteins is reduced and circulating concentrations fall to very low levels, resulting in bleeding. This occurs most commonly in the setting of severe hemorrhage and profound trauma.[43] Therapeutic anticoagulation is often desired, as is the case with the administration of anticoagulant (heparin and warfarin) and antiplatelet (aspirin) drugs. This is an increasingly prevalent problem because of the aging of the population and the proportionately larger number of patients with heart disease, cerebrovascular disease, and thromboembolic events for which these drugs are the mainstays of treatment.[45]

Presentation

Congenital disorders of blood coagulation are most commonly recognized during infancy, childhood, or adolescence by pediatricians and family practitioners, although this is not absolute. Those severely afflicted with hemophilia display spontaneous hemarthroses, intramuscular hematomas, and bleeding diatheses associated with minor trauma. Rare hemophiliac patients may develop pharyngeal and retropharyngeal hematomas, usually in the setting of a mild viral pharyngitis.[46] Patients with mild disease (factor activities exceeding 5% of normal) and those with vWD may experience excessive bleeding only in the setting of dire trauma, surgery, or invasive procedures. Mucocutaneous bleeding is the most common symptom in patients with vWD. Epistaxis occurs in 60% of these patients.[47] Eliciting a thorough and accurate personal and family history preoperatively is crucial to the discovery of undiagnosed hemostatic disorders. A tendency toward easy bruising, prolonged bleeding following dental or minor surgical procedures, and menorrhagia (in women) or a family history of any of these or the aforementioned problems may portend a congenital coagulopathy and therefore merit thorough investigation prior to surgery. In some instances a patient's personal history and family history are negative in this regard, and a congenital coagulopathy may not be appreciated until the postoperative period when prolonged and excessive bleeding become apparent.

Clinical suspicion and diagnosis of the acquired coagulopathies, especially in a critically ill patient, are based on the recognition of excessive bleeding and abnormalities in the PT and aPTT in the appropriate context. A history of malnutrition, alcoholism, preexisting liver or kidney disease, and prolonged broad-spectrum antibiotic use may be present.[43]

Iatrogenic coagulopathies are usually apparent from the patient's history or PT and aPTT values. Coagulopathy caused by massive transfusion is evident from the clinical context and is expected when bleeding, prolonged PT and aPTT, and thrombocytopenia occur in a patient who has received more than 5 to 10 units of packed RBCs within a short time. Children are at risk when their transfusion requirements approach one blood volume—approximately 250 to 750 mL for neonates and infants and 1 to 3 L for older children.[48] A history of anticoagulant or antiplatelet drug use should be elicited from a patient preoperatively. Warfarin and heparin prolongs the PT and the aPTT. Patients taking aspirin for cardiovascular or cerebrovascular disease may omit this piece of information if they are unaware that aspirin is an ingredient in over-the-counter medications they have ingested recently or because they do not recognize that nonprescription use of aspirin is of any potential consequence. Detailed questioning concerning aspirin is exceedingly important. If a positive history is obtained, surgery should be, if possible, delayed for 14 or more days. Patients should be firmly informed that they must absolutely discontinue aspirin and any aspirin-containing compounds 14 to 21 days before surgical intervention.

Evaluation

The congenital coagulopathies are to be suspected when a pertinent history is obtained and when serious or unexplained episodes of bleeding occur. A patient with severe hemophilia A, hemophilia B, or vWD has a prolonged aPTT and bleeding time. The PT is characteristically normal in both hemophilias. A mixing test, combining the hemophilic plasma with normal plasma and then repeating the aPTT, shows a normal value for the aPTT. Assays for the specific deficient factors may also be carried out to confirm decreased activity and the hemophilic state. For the diagnosis of vWD, an assay of the level of von Willebrand's factor and ristocetin cofactor (which quantitates the ability of plasma von Willebrand's factor to agglutinate platelets) must be performed.[42]

Elevated liver enzymes and rising creatinine, in addition to prolongation of the PT, are frequently seen in the setting of liver and kidney disease when they are the causes of acquired coagulopathies. To identify vitamin K deficiency as the cause of coagulopathy, measurement of factors II, VII, IX, and X must be performed. This is confirmed when the PT normalizes after vitamin K administration. A circulating anticoagulant is present if a prolonged PT or aPTT is not corrected by mixing normal plasma with patient plasma. Isolation of the offending inhibitor is possible by the employment of known specific factor-deficient plasma.[49]

The degree of coagulopathy produced by the administration of anticoagulant drugs is assessed by the commensurate magnitude of elevation of the PT (warfarin) and aPTT (heparin). Platelet dysfunction in the setting of aspirin therapy can be assessed by obtaining a bleeding time, but this test may be unreliable as an indicator of surgical bleeding in general and for that associated with aspirin ingestion in particular. Most patients on chronic aspirin therapy have a prolongation of bleeding time above their own baseline, but their values on aspirin may still fall within the upper limit of the normal range.[50] Ticlopidine, another antiplatelet drug, produces effects on bleeding time similar to those of aspirin. This agent may also depress the white blood cell count and has an association with thrombotic thrombocytopenic purpura.[51]

Priorities

Once a diagnosis of a congenital coagulopathy has been made, it is imperative to involve the hematologist in the perioperative management of the patient. Hemophilia is treated with supplemental factor VIII or IX. Milder forms of hemophilia A and vWD are amenable to treatment with intranasal DDAVP, which acts to release factor VIII and von Willebrand's factor from intracellular stores. Cryoprecipitate infusion remains the first-line treatment for severe vWD.[46, 47]

Hematologic consultation is also important in the clinical setting of acquired coagulopathies so as to optimize treatment. Intrinsic liver disease and hepatic insufficiency may be treated with transfusion of fresh-frozen plasma perioperatively to replenish coagulation factors. Supplemental vitamin K is also therapeutic for cases of suspected vitamin K deficiency. Uremic patients who have bleeding diatheses may benefit from the administration of intranasal DDAVP, as this agent increases the release of clotting factors from intracellular locations and thereby augments the circulating levels of these factors.[43]

The coagulopathy associated with massive transfusion of packed RBCs is predictable and preventable. Prophylaxis may be achieved by transfusion of fresh-frozen plasma and platelets for every 5 to 10 units of packed RBCs infused, or for every total blood volume equivalent.

Perioperative warfarin and aspirin therapy is managed in consultation with the prescribing physician. A hematologist should be consulted in complex situations. In general, warfarin can be discontinued 3 to 7 days prior to elective surgical procedures, depending on the dose being employed and on the underlying condition being treated, and it may be reinstituted when all bleeding has ceased after surgery; in this way, potentially massive surgical and postoperative hemorrhage is avoided.[52] In patients who are at high risk of thromboembolic complications when warfarin is discontinued (e.g., patients with prosthetic heart valves, patients with very strong tendencies to develop thromboses, and patients in hypercoagulable states), it is advisable to stop the warfarin and simultaneously institute heparin therapy before surgery. Removal of the heparin is performed 4 to 6 hours before surgery, with resumption of both heparin and warfarin postoperatively when all bleeding has ceased. Discontinuation of heparin is appropriate only after therapeutic warfarin levels have been achieved. Some patients at lower risk for complications (e.g., those under treatment for deep venous thrombosis (DVT) or prevention of stroke with atrial fibrillation) can be safely advised to stop warfarin 3 days prior to surgery and resume the normal dose 1 day after surgery, when no active bleeding is present. Emergency surgery may be necessary in the face of full anticoagulation. Patients on warfarin may need fresh-frozen plasma and vitamin K to reduce the chance of intraoperative and postoperative bleeding, and protamine sulfate can be used reverse the effects of heparin. Patients taking aspirin and other nonsteroidal anti-inflammatory drugs may be advised to discontinue their use of aspirin 2 weeks before surgery and of NSAIDs 2 to 3 days before surgery. There is conflicting evidence as to whether aspirin actually increases clinically significant bleeding in the setting of surgical intervention.[50, 53] If the antiplatelet effects of aspirin are deemed to be contributory to the presence of bleeding diathesis, therapy with DDAVP may be instituted, as there is some evidence to suggest that it is beneficial in this circumstance.[54]

Outcomes

Successful treatment of the congenital coagulopathies with factor supplements and/or DDAVP is well established. Meticulous attention to surgical hemostasis and optimization of the supplementation regimen are crucial. Poor wound healing and infections of wound hematomas are common in postsurgical patients with congenital coagulopathies when factor supplementation is not utilized. Acquired coagulopathies are manageable with the appropriate interventions.

Bleeding diatheses caused by anticoagulant medications are avoidable with the proper preoperative instructions for discontinuation of the anticoagulant medicine. Patients on aspirin and antiplatelet therapies have been shown to have increased operative blood loss, especially those undergoing cardiac surgery, but this conclusion is controversial. There may be a certain subset of aspirin hyperresponders who are at particular risk of intraoperative and postoperative bleeding. It is wise to have all patients stop taking aspirin 10 to 14 days prior to surgery. If inordinate bleeding does occur, there is evidence that treatment with DDAVP during the postoperative period is highly effective in controlling this problem.

DEEP VENOUS THROMBOSIS AND PULMONARY EMBOLISM

DVT with pulmonary emboli (PE) is among the most dreaded complications of the postoperative period. Venous thrombi form, usually within the veins of the lower extremities, as a consequence of changes in the coagulation mechanisms of the blood, damage to the endothelial linings of the vessels, and venous stasis. All of these conditions tend to occur in postoperative patients. Part or all of the formed clot may eventually be dislodged from its place of origin and travel via the vena cava and right heart to the pulmonary vasculature.

It is estimated that 260,000 patients are diagnosed with venous thromboembolism each year in the United States. The actual frequency of this disease is probably three times this number, as most experts agree that venous thromboembolic events are grossly underrecognized and underreported. Pulmonary embolism as a sequela of DVT accounts for the deaths of 50,000 to 100,000 patients per year, or 5% to 10% of all deaths occurring in hospitals.[55] Risk factors predisposing to venous thromboembolic events include major surgery, orthopedic procedures (especially lower extremity arthroplasty), hip and long bone fractures, obesity, increasing age, malignancy, multiple trauma, pregnancy, oral contraceptive use, congenital deficiencies of coagulation factor inhibitors, and a history of a previous thromboembolic event. The frequency of DVT and PE after head and neck surgery is lower than that seen after major general and orthopedic procedures, and is most often associated with oncologic procedures and maxillofacial trauma.[56]

Presentation

Deep venous thrombosis affecting the lower extremities is characterized by edema, erythema, and pain. Palpable venous cords or pain on passive flexion of the foot (Homans' sign) may be present as well, although their absence does not rule out the diagnosis. Postoperative day 5 is the most common time for recognition and diagnosis of DVT. Resultant pulmonary emboli may be clinically occult or massive and fatal. Clinical signs of PE include dyspnea, tachypnea, pleuritic chest pain, increased oxygen requirement, low-grade fever, increased pulmonic component of the second heart sound (P_2), tachycardia or atrial fibrillation, diaphoresis, and a sense of impending doom.

Evaluation

The presence of any of the signs and symptoms listed above, especially when found in combination in a postsurgical patient, warrants immediate clinical evaluation to rule out PE. Acute respiratory decompensation requires review of an urgently obtained plain chest radiograph and electrocardiogram and arterial blood gas studies. Atelectasis and parenchymal opacities are commonly found on chest radiographs of patients with confirmed PE. Signs of right heart strain may be manifested on a 12-lead electrocardiogram as an S wave in lead I, a Q wave in lead III, and a prominent T wave, also in lead III. New-onset atrial fibrillation or tachycardia may be evident as well. A large A–a gradient, as calculated from PO_2 and inspired oxygen values, is also characteristic of PE (Box 6-2).

Doppler ultrasound of the lower and upper

BOX 6-2

Calculation of Alveolar–Arterial Oxygen Gradient

$PA\text{–}aO_2 = PAO_2 - PaO_2$
$PAO_2 = PIO_2 - (PaCO_2/RQ)$
$PIO_2 = FIO_2\ (P_{atm} - P_{H2O})$

$PA\text{–}aO_2$, alveolar–arterial oxygen gradient
PAO_2, partial pressure of oxygen in alveolar air
PaO_2, partial pressure of oxygen in arterial blood
PIO_2, partial pressure of oxygen in inspired air
$PaCO_2$, partial pressure of CO_2 in arterial blood
RQ, respiratory quotient, usually 0.8
FIO_2, fraction of inspired oxygen (21% for room air)
P_{atm}, atmospheric pressure (760 mm Hg at sea level)
P_{H2O}, vapor pressure of H_2O (47 mm Hg)

extremities is the most widely available and well-established noninvasive technique for the diagnosis of DVT. Its advantages include cost-effectiveness and portability, as it may be performed at the bedside in critically ill patients. A recent large study compiling the results of multiple investigations found the sensitivity of ultrasound to be 95%, with a specificity of 98%.[57] Invasive contrast venography remains the gold standard of tests, but is less frequently employed now because of the excellent record of ultrasound in the diagnosis of DVT.

A lung scan to determine the ventilation-perfusion ratio ($\dot{V}/\dot{Q}$ scan) is the best initial test to evaluate for the potential presence of a PE. A normal $\dot{V}/\dot{Q}$ scan (6 to 8 views) excludes the possibility of clinically significant PE. If the $\dot{V}/\dot{Q}$ scan indicates an intermediate probability in the setting of convincing clinical data, it is reasonable to institute therapy. If the $\dot{V}/\dot{Q}$ scan is abnormal and there are confounding clinical problems such as congestive heart failure, chronic lung disease, or asthma, then pulmonary angiography is indicated to confirm the diagnosis.[58] Other clinical situations in which absolute confirmation of PE by angiography is important include cases in which there is a history of bleeding or untoward reactions to anticoagulants and cases in which surgical embolectomy or placement of a vena cava filter is contemplated.

Priorities

Once the diagnosis of DVT has been established, therapy with thrombolytic agents or intravenous heparin should be instituted immediately. Treatment with heparin should continue for 4 to 7 days, after which time warfarin may be started. Prolongation of the aPTT to 1.5 to 2.5 times control is desirable.[59] There is mounting evidence that low-molecular-weight heparin provides comparable or superior efficacy and safety, and it has the added advantages of once- or twice-daily subcutaneous dosing, superior bioavailability, and not requiring laboratory monitoring.[60] Ideally, warfarin is given such that a prothrombin time–international normalized ratio (PT-INR) of 2.5 to 3.5 is maintained on PT testing. Warfarin is continued for 3 to 6 months in a patient with a first episode of proximal DVT or PE. Treatment for 6 to 12 months is indicated for a patient with recurrent DVT or with an ongoing risk factor for DVT, such as a hypercoagulable state.[59]

Thrombolysis is indicated in those situations in which significant hemodynamic compromise is present and is unrelenting despite anticoagulant therapy. Thrombolysis is also indicated to reduce the morbidity associated with the postphlebitic syndrome. Streptokinase or urokinase is administered intravenously or via pulmonary arterial catheter as a bolus dose, followed by continuous infusion for up to 72 hours.[61] Surgical embolectomy may be necessary in rare cases of hemodynamic collapse.

Effective prevention of DVT and PE is achieved in most cases with the use of lower and/or upper extremity sequential compression devices during surgery and with continuation of their use postoperatively until regular ambulation is achieved. Low-dose subcutaneous heparin is likewise effective for prophylaxis. There is much evidence to suggest that combination therapy with these two modalities is even more effective than the use of either alone.[62]

Outcomes

DVT with PE is associated with high mortality rates, as described above. Failure of adequate anticoagulation to prevent subsequent episodes of DVT and PE is not uncommon. In these patients, investigation for the presence of a hypercoagulable state (occult malignancy, lupus anticoagulant, coagulation factor inhibitor deficiencies, and so forth) is indicated. Interruption of the vena cava with filter devices is extremely rarely indicated, but may be the only therapeutic option to control this disease when anticoagulation fails or when recurrent thrombosis exists concomitantly with hemorrhage.

Other significant morbidity from this disease includes the postphlebitic syndrome, which is characterized by pain, chronic edema, and cutaneous ulceration of the affected extremity. The true frequency of this complication is unknown because of the paucity of data and the lack of a uniform definition, but it has been estimated that half of all patients with recurrent thrombophlebitis are found, on long-term follow-up, to be affected.[60]

Chronic thromboembolic pulmonary hypertension represents an alternative natural history and outcome of pulmonary emboli: the pathogenesis of this situation is that organized, recanalized clot significantly narrows major pulmonary arteries. This sequela occurs in a minority of patients who survive an embolic event but has severe manifestations, including persistently increased right ventricular afterload, pulmonary hypertension, and right ventricular failure.[63]

REFERENCES

1. Beutler E. The sickle cell diseases and related disorders. In Beutler E et al., eds. Williams' Hematology, 5th ed. New York, McGraw-Hill, 1995.
2. Sharon, BI. Transfusion therapy in congenital hemolytic anemias. Hematol Oncol Clin North Am 1994;8:1053–1086.
3. Weatherall DJ, Clegg JB. The Thalassemia Syndromes, 3rd ed. Oxford, Blackwell, 1981.
4. Lindenbaum J. Folate and vitamin B_{12} deficiencies in alcoholism. Semin Hematol 1980;17:119–129.
5. McCurdy PR, Pierce LE, Roth CE. Abnormal bone marrow morphology in acute alcoholism. N Engl J Med 1962;266:505–507.
6. Erslev AJ. Anemia of chronic disease. In Beutler E et al., eds. Williams' Hematology, 5th ed. New York, McGraw-Hill, 1995.
7. Radtke HW, Claussner A, Erbes PM. Serum erythropoietin concentration in chronic renal failure: relationship to degree of anemia and excretory function. Blood 1979;54:877–884.
8. Caro J, Erslev AJ. Anemia of chronic renal failure. In Beutler E et al., eds. Williams' Hematology, 5th ed. New York, McGraw-Hill, 1995.
9. Cotes M et al. Characterization of the anemia of chronic renal disease and the mode of its correction by r-HuEPO. Q J Med 1989;70:113–137.
10. Homi J et al. General anesthesia in sickle cell disease. Br J Med 1979;1:1599–1601.
11. Rebulla P, Modell B. Transfusion requirements and effects in patients with thalassemia major. Lancet 1991;337:277–280.
12. Beutler E, Robson MJ, Buttenwiesser E. A comparison of the plasma iron, iron-binding capacity, sternal marrow iron, and other methods in the clinical evaluation of iron stores. Ann Intern Med 1958;48:60–82.
13. Sullivan L. Differential diagnosis and management of the patient with megaloblastic anemia. Am J Med 1970;48:609–617.
14. Auerbach M et al. Clinical use of the total dose of intravenous infusion of iron dextran. J Lab Clin Med 1988;111:566–570.
15. Amitai A, Acker M. Adverse effects of intramuscular iron injection. Acta Haematol 1982;68:341–342.
16. Flaharty KK et al. Pharmacokinetics and erythropoietic response to human recombinant erythropoietin in healthy men. Clin Pharmacol Ther 1990;47:557–564.
17. Fosburg MT, Nathan DG. Treatment of Cooley's anemia. Blood 1990;76:435–444.
18. Zurlo MG et al. Survival and causes of death in thalassaemia major. Lancet 1989;2:27–30.
19. Wallace EL et al. Collection and transfusion of blood and blood components in the United States, 1989. Transfusion 1993;33:139–144.
20. Klein HG. Allogeneic transfusion risks in the surgical patient. Am J Surg 1995;170(suppl 6A):21–26.
21. Dodd RY. Adverse consequences of blood transfusion: quantitative risk estimates. In Nance ST, ed. Blood Supply: Risks, Perceptions, and Prospects for the Future. Bethesda, MD, American Association of Blood Banks, 1994.
22. Honig CL, Bove JR. Transfusion-associated fatalities: review of Bureau of Biologies reports, 1976–1978. Transfusion 1980;20:653–661.
23. Chambers LA et al. Febrile reactions after platelet transfusion: the effect of single versus multiple donors. Transfusion 1990;30:219–221.
24. Isbister JP. Adverse reactions to plasma and plasma components. Anesth Intens Care 1993;21:31–38.
25. Pineda A, Taswell HF. Transfusion reactions associated with anti-IgA antibodies: report of four cases and review of the literature. Transfusion 1985;15:10–15.
26. Koll BS, Brown AE. Infections associated with blood product transfusions in patients with cancer. Infect Med 1993;10:12–18.
27. Blajchman MA. Bacterial contamination of blood products and the value of pretransfusion testing. Immun Invest 1995;24:163–170.
28. Nicolls MD. Transfusion: morbidity and mortality. Anesthes Intens Care 1993;21:15–19.
29. Sloop GD, Friedberg RC. Complications of blood transfusions. Postgrad Med 1995;98:159–172.
30. Dabrow MB, Wilkins JC. Hematologic emergencies. Postgrad Med 1993;93:183–190.
31. McBride JA, O'Hoski P. Immediate and delayed adverse reactions to transfusions. In Brian MC, Carbone PP, eds. Current Therapy in Hematology-Oncology, 4th ed. Philadelphia, BC Decker, 1992, p. 136.
32. Ewald GA, McKenzie CK. The Washington Manual of Medical Therapeutics, 28th ed. Boston, Little, Brown, 1995.
33. Gilbert DN, Moellering RC Jr, Sande MA. The Sanford Guide to Antimicrobial Therapy, 28th ed. Vienna, Antimicrobial Therapy, 1998.
34. Chambers LA et al. Febrile reactions after platelet transfusions: the effect of single versus multiple donors. Transfusion 1990;30:219–221.
35. Bick RL. Disseminated intravascular coagulation: objective criteria for diagnosis and management. Med Clin North Am 1994;78:511–543.
36. Baglin T. Disseminated intravascular coagulation: diagnosis and treatment. Br Med J 1996;312:683–687.
37. Wheeler A, Rubenstein EB. Current management of disseminated intravascular coagulation. Oncology 1994;8:69–73.
38. Bick RL, Kunkel LA. Disseminated intravascular coagulation syndrome. Int J Hematol 1992;55:1–26.
39. Bick RL, Baker W. Diagnostic efficacy of the D-dimer assay in DIC and related disorders. Blood 1986;68:329.
40. Holmer F et al. Heparin and its low-molecular-weight derivatives: anticoagulant and anti-thrombotic properties. Haemostasis 1986;16S:1–7.
41. Emerson TE et al. Efficacy of ATIII supplementation in animal models of fulminant *E. coli* endotoxemia or bacteremia. Am J Med 1989;87S:27–33.
42. Lusher JM. Transfusion therapy in congenital coagulopathies. Hematol Oncol Clin North Am 1994;8:1167–1177.
43. Parker RI. Etiology and treatment of acquired coagulopathies in the critically ill adult and child. Crit Care Clin 1997;13:591–609.
44. Shastri KA et al. Acquired factor VIII inhibitor with squamous cell carcinoma of the epiglottis. Arch Otolaryngol Head Neck Surg 1990;116:350–353.
45. Humphries JE. Transfusion therapy in acquired coagulopathies. Hematol Oncol Clin North Am 1994;8:1181–1201.
46. Roberts HR, Hoffman M. Hemophilia and related conditions—inherited deficiencies of prothrombin (factor II), factor V, and factors VII to XII. In Beutler E et al., eds. Williams' Hematology, 5th ed. New York, McGraw-Hill, 1995.
47. Aledort LM. Treatment of von Willebrand's disease. Mayo Clin Proc 1991;66:841–846.
48. Lim RC et al. Platelet response and coagulation changes following massive blood replacement. J Trauma 1973;18:577–583.
49. Staudinger T, Locker GJ, Frass M. Management of

acquired coagulation disorders in emergency and intensive-care medicine. Semin Thromb Hemos 1996;22:93–104.

50. DeCaterina R et al. Bleeding time and bleeding: an analysis of the relationship of the bleeding time test with parameters of surgical bleeding. Blood 1994;84:3363–3370.
51. Love BB, Biller J, Gert M. Adverse hematological effects of ticlopidine: prevention, recognition, and management. Drug Safety 1998;19:89–98.
52. Goldsmith SM, Leshin B, Owen J. Management of patients taking anticoagulants and platelet inhibitors prior to dermatologic surgery. J Dermatol Surg Oncol 1993;9:578–581.
53. Ferraris VA et al. Preoperative aspirin ingestion increases operative blood loss after coronary artery bypass grafting. Ann Thorac Surg 1995;59:1036–1037.
54. Kan PCA. Use of DDAVP in controlling aspirin-induced coagulopathy after cardiac surgery. Heart Lung 1994;23:333–336.
55. Daven JE, Alpen JS. Natural history of pulmonary embolism. Prog Cardiovasc Dis 1995;17:259–270.
56. Lowry JC. Thromboembolic disease and thromboprophylaxis in oral and maxillofacial surgery: experience and practice. Br J Oral Maxillofac Surg 1995;33:101–106.
57. Cronan JJ. Venous thromboembolic disease: the role of ultrasound. Radiology 1993;186:619–630.
58. Worsley DF, Alavi A. Comprehensive analysis of the PIOPED (Prospective Investigation of Pulmonary Embolism Diagnosis) study. J Nucl Med 1995;36:2380–2387.
59. Wood AJJ. Management of venous thromboembolism. N Engl J Med 1996;335:1816–1828.
60. Tapson VF, Hull RD. Management of venous thromboembolic disease: the impact of low-molecular-weight heparin. Clin Chest Med 1995;16:281–284.
61. Goldhaber SZ. Thrombolytic therapy in venous thromboembolism: clinical trials and current indications. Clin Chest Med 1995;16:307–328.
62. Kalodiki EP et al. DVT prophylaxis with low-molecular-weight heparin and elastic compression in patients having total hip replacement: a randomized controlled trial. Intern Angiol 1996;15:162–168.
63. Fedullo PF et al. Chronic thromboembolic pulmonary hypertension. Clin Chest Med 1995;16:353–374.

CHAPTER 7

Thermal Emergencies

Lesley Wong, MD

The initial emergency management of thermal injuries focuses primarily on resuscitation of the cardiovascular system and on airway protection and oxygenation. The burn wound itself is addressed only secondarily. This chapter outlines the initial emergency evaluation and management of a burn patient, the diagnosis and treatment of smoke inhalation, and the early management of a burn wound, and then discusses related injuries, electrical injury, and frostbite.

Thermal injury to the skin and mucosa can occur by way of flame, contact with heat, scalding, or chemical exposure. The majority of serious burn injuries are treated in specialized burn centers where the overall mortality rate has declined to 4%. Coinciding with this decline in mortality has also been a decline in the incidence of large surface area burn injuries. More than 80% of injuries now involve less than 20% of the total body surface area (TBSA). Many burns involving smaller percentages of the body surface area are cared for in general hospitals where nonspecialists must treat them and so must be aware of key points in emergency management.

PRESENTATION AND EVALUATION

The emergency department evaluation for thermal injuries begins, as with any trauma patient, by using an ABCDEF algorithm (airway, breathing, circulation, cervical spine stabilization, disability/neurologic deficit, exposure/examination, fluid resuscitation).[1] High-flow oxygen (100%) is begun immediately. Early establishment of an airway by endotracheal intubation is indicated for impending or existing upper airway obstruction (see the later section on inhalation injuries), and for patients with altered mental status or loss of consciousness due to carbon monoxide poisoning, other asphyxiants, intoxication, or other associated trauma. Breathing is assessed by observation of adequate chest wall expansion and chest auscultation. Circumferential full-thickness chest wall burns can restrict adequate chest wall expansion, and if ventilation is impaired, escharotomies are needed to release the constricting eschar. Associated lung pathology such as pneumothorax is also evaluated at this time. Blood pressure and peripheral pulses are assessed to evaluate circulation, and large-bore peripheral intravenous lines are inserted to begin fluid resuscitation. Cervical spine stabilization is carried out in the appropriate clinical circumstances. The level of alertness and response to verbal and painful stimuli are documented. These can be affected by associated injury, hypoxia, substance abuse, and preexisting conditions.

A secondary full body survey is then undertaken to localize associated injuries. Preinjury medical history, medications, allergies, and tetanus immunization status are determined. An estimate of the percentage of TBSA burned determines the need for triage to a specialized burn center (based on American Burn Association criteria, Box 7–1) and serves as the basis for fluid resuscitation calculations. A Lund and Browder chart assigns a percentage of TBSA to each anatomic area; it varies according to the patient's age (Fig. 7–1). For example, an infant's head makes up almost twice as much of the percentage of TBSA as does an adult's head. Only second- and third-degree burns, burns in-

BOX 7–1

Burn Center Referral Criteria (American Burn Association)

- Second- and third-degree burns of more than 10% BSA in patients under 10 years or over 50 years old
- Second- and third-degree burns of more than 20% BSA in patients in other age groups
- Second- and third-degree burns with serious threat of functional or cosmetic impairment that involve face, hands, feet, genitalia, perineum, and major joints
- Third-degree burns greater than 5% BSA in any age group
- Significant electrical burn injuries, including lightning injury
- Chemical injuries with serious threat of functional or cosmetic impairment
- Inhalation injury with burn injury
- Circumferential burns of an extremity or chest
- Burn injury in patients with significant preexisting medical disorders
- Any burn patient with concomitant trauma in which the burn injury poses the greatest risk of morbidity or mortality

BSA, body surface area.

volving some or all of the dermis, are included in the calculations. First-degree burns involving only the epidermis do not have physiologic consequences and therefore do not contribute to fluid loss.

Determination of peripheral pulses and capillary refill is important in determining the need for escharotomies. Skin injured by full-thickness burns loses its ability to stretch because of damage to elastin fibers; thus, it cannot expand with underlying swelling of the soft tissue. This results in circumferential compression of underlying neurovascular structures. An escharotomy is a full-thickness incision along the midlateral axis of an extremity, through the eschar into the subcutaneous tissues; it is similar in concept to bivalving a tight cast.

As part of the initial resuscitative interventions, peripheral access is secured, and a Foley catheter and nasogastric tube are inserted. Central venous lines are placed in patients with burns of more than 30%, in elderly patients, in patients with associated medical conditions, and in patients with severe smoke inhalation. Central access through burned skin is sometimes necessary when large surface areas are involved. Initially, the burn wound is clean, but a high incidence of sepsis occurs if sites in burned skin continue to be used.

Initial laboratory values are obtained— hematocrit, electrolytes, urinalysis, toxin screen, electrocardiogram, chest radiographs, and carboxyhemoglobin and arterial blood gas, if indicated. Initial chest x-rays are often clear and initial arterial oxygenation is often relatively normal, even in the presence of smoke inhalation. Tetanus prophylaxis is given if tetanus immunization is not current or if the status is unknown. Analgesics are administered as needed, preferably intravenously to avoid unpredictable absorption.

FLUID RESUSCITATION

Fluid resuscitation is symptomatic treatment of the hypovolemic shock that results from a systemic capillary leak not limited to the area of the burn injury. Little can be done to treat the underlying cause of the shock, so resuscitation is essentially treatment of symptoms. Experimental protocols for the use of antioxidants, growth hormone, and prostaglandin inhibitors may eventually be useful against inflammatory mediators released by macrophages, platelets, and activated neutrophils.[2] The edema formation occurs most rapidly during the first 8 hours after the injury and then tapers at approximately 12 to 24 hours postinjury. This time course is the rationale behind many of the formulas consisting of sodium-containing fluids. The Parkland formula is the most commonly used (Box 7–2), but practitioners should not adhere rigidly to a single formula. Instead, patients should be given what is needed to maintain urine output and vital signs and normalize electrolytes. A target urine output of 0.5 mL/kg/h in adults and 1.0 mL/kg/h in children and

BOX 7–2

Parkland Formula for Fluid Resuscitation

Lactated Ringer's solution: 4 mL/kg/% burn	½ given over the first 8 hours, ½ given over the next 16 hours
then	
Colloid: 0.5 mL/kg/% burn	Given over the second 24 hours
plus	
D-5-W 2000 mL	

Date of Admission: ______________________ Weight: ______________________

AREA	PERCENT OF BURN					SEVERITY OF BURN		TOTAL PERCENT
	0-1 Year	1-4 Years	5-9 Years	10-15 Years	ADULT	2°	3°	
Head	19	17	13	10	7			
Neck	2	2	2	2	2			
Ant. Trunk	13	17	13	13	13			
Post. Trunk	13	13	13	13	13			
R. Buttock	2½	2½	2½	2½	2½			
L. Buttock	2½	2½	2½	2½	2½			
Genitalia	1	1	1	1	1			
R.U. Arm	4	4	4	4	4			
L.U. Arm	4	4	4	4	4			
R.L. Arm	3	3	3	3	3			
L.L. Arm	3	3	3	3	3			
R. Hand	2½	2½	2½	2½	2½			
L. Hand	2½	2½	2½	2½	2½			
R. Thigh	5½	6½	8½	8½	9½			
L. Thigh	5½	6½	8½	8½	9½			
R. Leg	5	5	5½	6	7			
L. Leg	5	5	5½	6	7			
R. Foot	3½	3½	3½	3½	3½			
L. Foot	3½	3½	3½	3½	3½			
				Total				

Code: Blue areas indicate 2°
Red areas indicate 3°

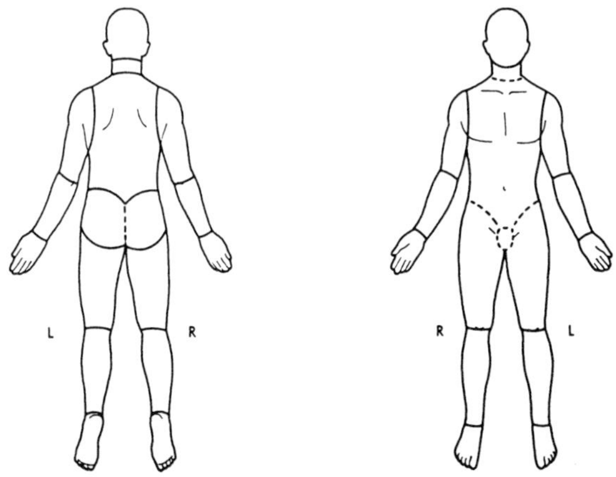

Figure 7–1. Lund and Browder chart to calculate percent total body surface area burned. (Adapted from the Baltimore Regional Burn Center admission burn evaluation sheet.)

maintenance of a mean arterial pressure of 65 to 70 mm Hg indicates adequate organ perfusion. Ringer's lactate solution is the basis for most formulas with a sodium concentration of 130 mEq/L and a physiologic pH of 6.5. The calculated volume required for the first 24 hours postinjury (4 mL/kg/% TBSA burned) is based on the loss of sodium from the extracellular space that is estimated to be 0.5 to 0.6 mEq sodium/kg/% TBSA burned.

Hypertonic or modified hypertonic solutions are potentially beneficial in reducing the volume required to deliver the same amount of sodium, but closer monitoring of serum electrolytes is required, and a clear benefit has not been established in all clinical studies reported.[3–5]

The administration of colloid-containing solutions, used for their oncotic properties, is begun during the second 24 hours postinjury. At some point in the first 12 to 24 hours postinjury, the return of normal capillary permeability enables more of the administered volume to remain within the intravascular space. The benefit to patient outcome of administering colloid, however, has not been clearly proven. Adverse effects have been documented, including increased fluid accumulation in the lungs, which is associated with increased clinical pulmonary complications, and a decreased glomerular filtration rate despite increases in the plasma volume.[6] Nevertheless, colloid is still commonly used as a primary fluid in the second 24 hours

BOX 7-3

Classic Clinical Indicators for Smoke Inhalation

History: Closed-space injury
- Altered mental status
- Known inhaled toxins

Physical Examination: Facial burns
- Singed facial hair
- Hoarseness
- Wheezing, stridor
- Carbonaceous sputum

in addition to the administration of free water and glucose-containing fluids. Also at 24 hours postinjury, enteral alimentation is attempted, as this has beneficial effects on the immune system.[7]

INHALATION INJURY

As incomplete products of combustion are inhaled, an oxidant-mediated chemical injury occurs to the mucosa of the airways and, ultimately, to the alveoli. Also, direct respiratory injury can occur with facial exposure to direct flame, inhalation of hot steam, or aspiration of hot liquids. Exposure to toxic gases such as oxides of nitrogen or phosgene is associated with delayed onset of pulmonary edema. Mortality is increased by as much as 20 times in the presence of inhalation injury for the same percentage of surface burned.[8]

Factors that are likely to indicate the presence of inhalation injury include closed space fires in which the patient was asleep or unconscious in a burning building, extensive facial burns, altered levels of consciousness, singed facial hairs, and carbonaceous sputum (Box 7–3).[9] The classic physical findings of facial burns and singed facial hairs have a positive predictive value of only 40% to 70%, but it becomes higher if burns of the central face and lips are considered. This physical finding correlates with prolonged exposure to flames. Fiberoptic laryngoscopy demonstrates edema and erythema (Fig. 7–2). Serial nasopharyngoscopy provides concrete documentation of the presence of inhalation injury and helps to determine the need for intubation. Changes in the pharynx alone do not portend serious injury, but findings of laryngeal edema, including epiglottic edema, interarytenoid edema, and true vocal cord edema constitute indications for intubation. Impaired vocal cord abduction can occur as a result of inhalation injury and cause physiologic upper airway obstruction even with only minor swell-

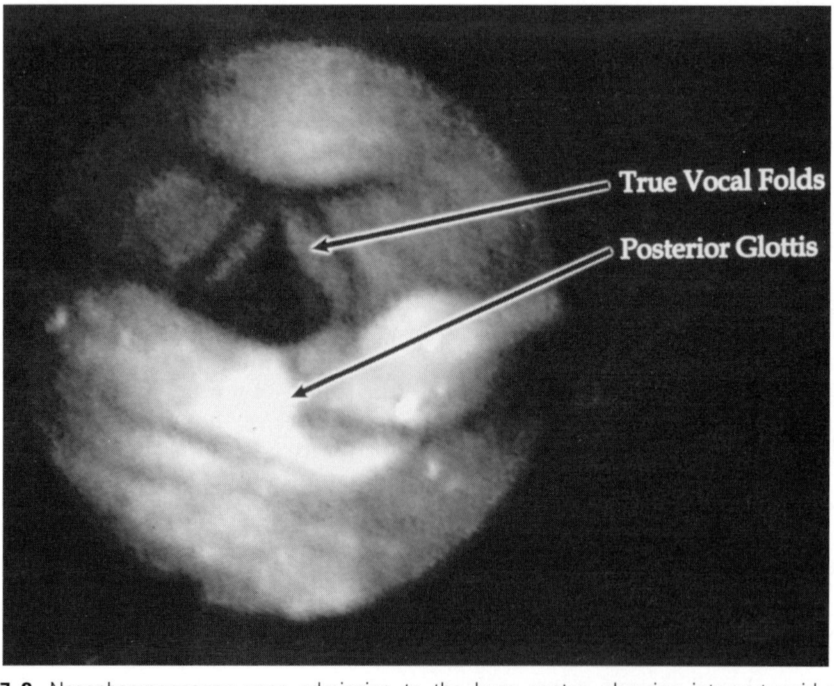

Figure 7–2. Nasopharyngoscopy upon admission to the burn center, showing interarytenoid swelling. (Courtesy of T. Muehlberger, M.D.)

ing. Laryngeal findings do not necessarily correlate with the degree of lower airway parenchymal injury. Subglottic injury can be more pronounced than more proximal airway injury because of chemical irritants in eddies of airflow below the vocal cords.

Spirometric flow-volume curves correlate well with nasopharyngoscopy but require a cooperative patient without oral burns.[10] A decrease in both inspiratory and expiratory flow rates is seen with a "sawtooth" pattern (Fig. 7–3). It has a high negative predictive value in that a patient with a normal test result is not likely to have significant obstruction. Bronchoscopy and xenon-133 ventilation-perfusion lung scans evaluate lower airway burns but do not correlate with the severity of the injury and may be difficult to perform in an emergency setting.

Additional testing is unnecessary in a patient with massive burns in whom intubation is indicated for massive volume resuscitation and administration of sedating analgesics. A patient with minor or absent cutaneous burns and a suspicious clinical history and examination, but with normal arterial blood gas and a normal chest radiograph, requires more sensitive testing. Arterial blood gas, carboxyhemoglobin, and chest radiographs identify established respiratory abnormalities early in the clinical course and should be followed by direct visualization of the airway because they are nonspecific and may be normal in the presence of pharyngeal edema. If these tests are normal and there is still some question of inhalation injury, further testing that has high negative predictive value (normal results more likely to indicate no injury), based on institutional availability, is performed—flow-volume curves, lower endoscopy/bronchoscopy, and radionuclide scans (Fig. 7–4).

Injury to the upper airway manifests as laryngeal edema. A patient presenting with hoarseness, cough, or stridor requires emergent intubation. Any signs of respiratory distress such as use of accessory muscles, dyspnea, or paradoxic chest excursion, or loss of conscious-

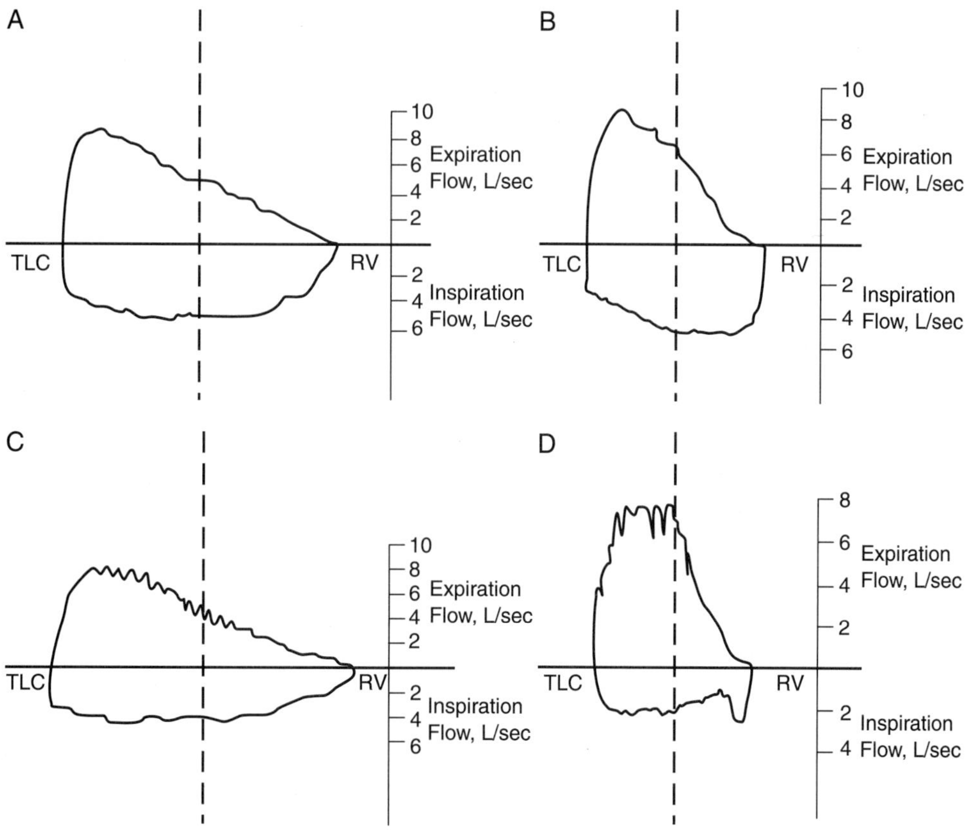

Figure 7–3. Flow volume curve patterns seen in victims of smoke inhalation. A: Normal. B, C, and D: Variable extrathoracic airway obstruction. C and D: Sawtoothing. RV, residual volume; TLC, total lung capacity. (From Haponik EF, Munster AM, Wise RA, et al. Upper airway function in burn patients: correlation of flow volume curves and nasopharyngoscopy. Am Rev Respir Dis 1984;129:251.)

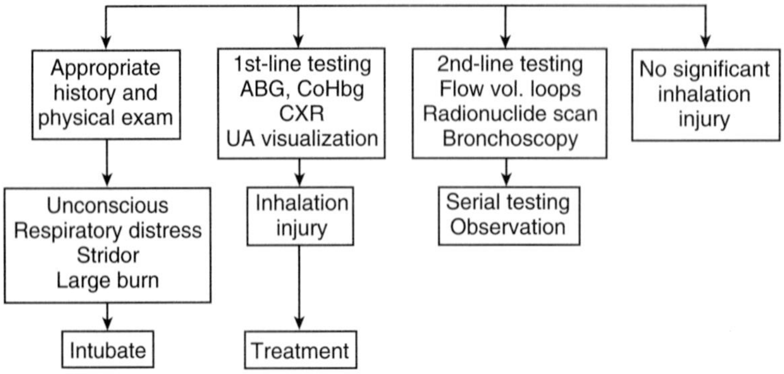

Figure 7–4. Smoke inhalation diagnostic algorithm.

ness (which is predictive of the need for prolonged intubation) should prompt urgent intubation. Edema can progress rapidly (Fig. 7–5), peaking at 24 hours postinjury. The degree of edema is also associated with burns covering a larger surface area and with increased fluid requirements. Lower airway injury may not be evident for 12 to 24 hours postinjury. Initial chest radiographs and arterial blood gases are normal and it is only when mucosal sloughing and secretions accumulate that atelectasis and airway obstruction produce clinical findings. Intubation should be carried out before landmarks become distorted. Thick secretions require an endotracheal tube of at least 7.5 mm in internal diameter for pulmonary toilet.

Carbon monoxide poisoning can be associated with airway injury or can be present as an isolated injury. A product of oxygen combustion, carbon monoxide displaces the oxyhemoglobin curve to the left, impairing oxygen delivery, and binds with greater affinity to hemoglobin (Fig. 7–6). Ultimately, mitochondrial function and adenosine triphosphate (ATP) production are affected. Symptoms correlate with carboxyhemoglobin levels and eventually culminate in coma and cardiac arrest as a result of ischemia as oxygen is displaced from hemoglobin. The arterial oxygen tension remains normal, reflecting oxygen dissolved in plasma, whereas the measured oxygen saturation of hemoglobin decreases. Administering 100% oxygen decreases the half-life of carboxyhemoglobin to 45 minutes from 250 minutes on room air.

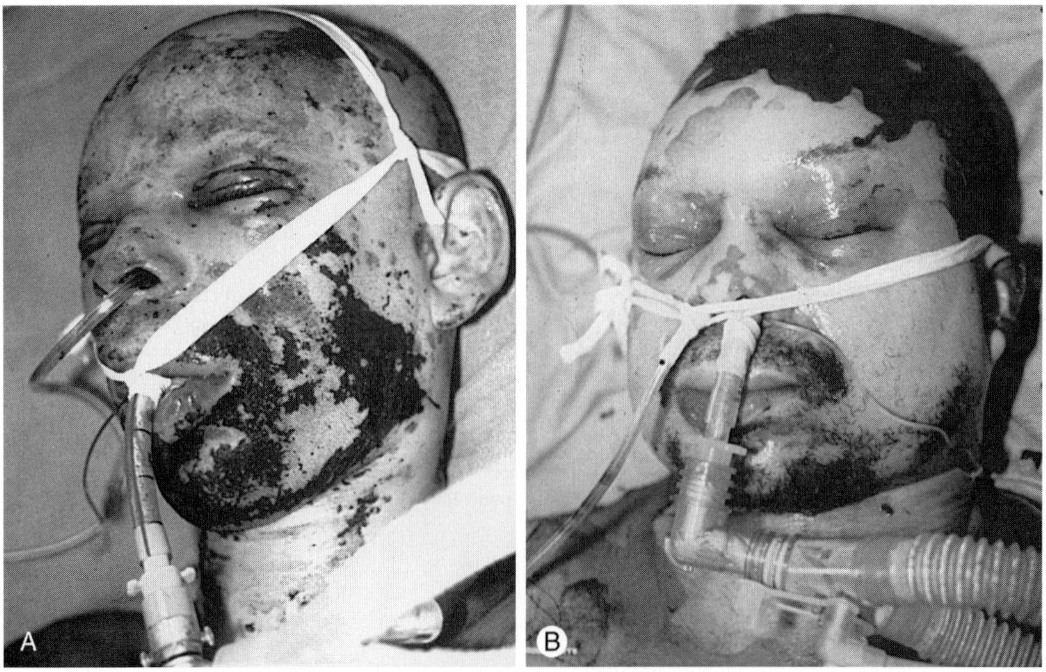

Figure 7–5. A: Diffuse facial burns on admission. B: The same patient 24 hours later.

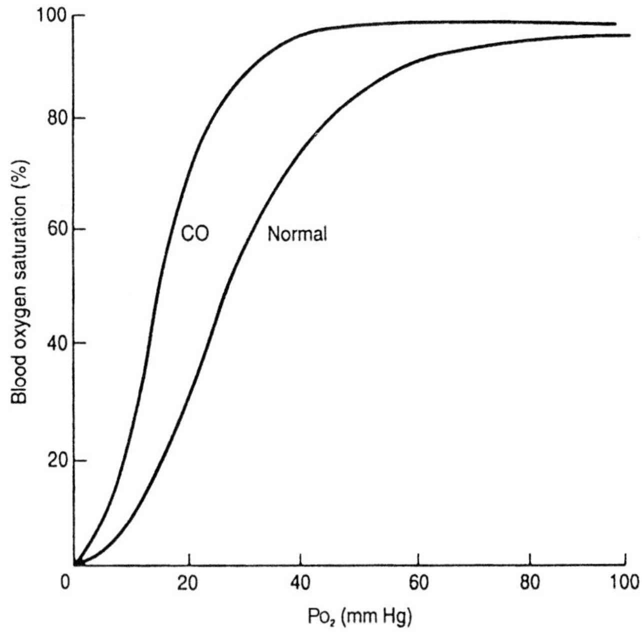

Figure 7–6. Oxygen-hemoglobin dissociation curve in the presence of carbon monoxide (CO). (From Strongin J et al. Pulmonary disorders in the burn patient. In Martyn JAJ, ed. Acute Management of the Burned Patient. Philadelphia, WB Saunders, 1990.)

Cyanide toxicity resulting from inhaled hydrocyanide is another aspect of inhalation injury. Cyanide binds to the cellular cytochrome system and inhibits cellular metabolism and ATP production. Persistent metabolic acidosis despite adequate volume resuscitation and cardiac output correlates with elevated cyanide levels.[11] Treatment consists of sodium nitrite and sodium thiosulfate to convert cyanide to excretable sodium thiocyanate. In France, hydroxocobalamin is administered as an antidote to all patients with loss of consciousness, severe mental confusion, or elevated plasma lactate levels, at the scene or on arrival at the treating facility.[12] This treatment is controversial, as the correlation between cyanide levels, clinical findings, and mortality is not clear.

Lower airway injury is treated with bronchodilators, positive end-expiratory pressure (PEEP) ventilation, and aggressive pulmonary toilet to clear secretions. Later in the hospital course, pneumonia and adult respiratory distress syndrome contribute to pulmonary pathology. In intubated patients, barotrauma is common secondary to stiff airways and noncompliant chest walls. Early escharotomies of chest burns are indicated for rising peak airway pressures. Permissive hypercapnia, high-frequency jet ventilation, or pressure-controlled inverse ratio ventilation have also been of benefit in some studies.[13]

Tracheostomy is generally performed when prolonged intubation is anticipated. Early tracheostomy may result in both short-term and long-term complications in 30% of patients. Higher infection rates, tracheomalacia, and tracheal stenosis are seen when tracheostomy is performed acutely.[14] Tracheal intubation, either nasally or via tracheostomy, in the setting of inhalation injury can result in ulcerative tracheobronchitis. Tracheobronchial infection is caused by mechanical trauma from the tube and the flora of the surrounding burn wound, which gains direct access to the tracheobronchial tree in the setting of absent natural airway defenses. Long-term complications include complex strictures of the larynx and trachea requiring prolonged tracheal stenting and resection or stenting of subglottic stenoses.[15]

Prophylactic antibiotics do not result in long-term improvement in outcome.[16] Systemic steroids are potentially detrimental, but aerosolized steroids can be helpful in bronchospasm refractory to β-adrenergic inhalers.

BURN WOUND MANAGEMENT

Definitive treatment of the burn wound—excision and skin-grafting—is delayed until systemic stability has been restored. Immediate intervention consists of eliminating or neutralizing the source by removing all clothing and irrigating copiously for 1 hour in the case of chemical injury. Cooling appears to produce some benefit by decreasing the progression of tissue damage, but it may be complicated by hypothermia and is therefore not routinely employed. During initial resuscitation, airway management, and triage to a burn care center, the burn wound is best kept covered with a sterile sheet and body temperature kept within a normal range.

Once the patient has arrived at the definitive treatment location, topical antimicrobial therapy should be initiated. Three agents are used in common practice: silver sulfadiazine cream with a broad spectrum and little toxicity; mafenide acetate cream with better eschar penetration, but some pain on application and inhibition of carbonic anhydrase when used over large surface areas; and 0.5% silver nitrate solution, which can leach electrolytes from the wound and causes staining of the wound.

For partial-thickness wounds, the goal of treatment is to prevent desiccation and infection of the dermis until epithelialization can occur. For smaller wounds, antimicrobial therapy is not necessary, and synthetic dressings can be placed on the wounds and allowed to adhere while epithelialization occurs under the dressing. Silver-impregnated dressing are also undergoing clinical evaluations and may allow healing with less pain during dressing changes. Enzymatic agents have also been shown to achieve healing in partial-thickness wounds.

Bacitracin ointment can be used for facial burns if they are superficial. Ophthalmic preparations are used near the eyes to avoid chemical conjunctivitis. Crusting should be gently cleaned with mild soap and water. For deeper facial burns, silver sulfadiazine should be used, necessitating gauze bandages. Early excision and grafting with unmeshed sheet grafts may prevent future development of hypertrophic scarring. Various anatomic regions of the head and neck have special considerations.[17]

Neck injuries require early excision and grafting and aggressive splinting, as the development of burn scar contractures has an impact on the ability to intubate during later procedures that require general anesthesia (Fig. 7–7).

Eye burns require consultation with an ophthalmologist as soon as they are apparent. Copious irrigation of the eye with a balanced salt solution is indicated. Fluorescein examination with a Wood's light will reveal corneal defects. The majority of these injuries heal rapidly by reepithelialization with frequent application of ophthalmic antibiotic ointment. Lid injury may result in corneal exposure, desiccation, and resulting infection, which can lead to globe rupture (Fig. 7–8). Compulsive lid and corneal lubrication and possible early lid release and tarsorrhaphy are indicated to prevent these sequelae.

Burns to the auricle are managed initially with topical antibiotics. Mafenide, which has the ability to penetrate eschar, is often used, with the goal of preventing auricular chondritis. The poorly vascularized auricular cartilage, if infected, requires debridement, leading to permanent ear deformity. Avoidance of pressure on the helical rim protects against cartilage exposure (Fig. 7–9).

Full-thickness nasal burns often lead to exposure of cartilage. Viability may be preserved by temporary coverage with allograft skin until a flap coverage procedure can be performed. The incidence of deformity is high.

A newly reported mechanism of facial burn-

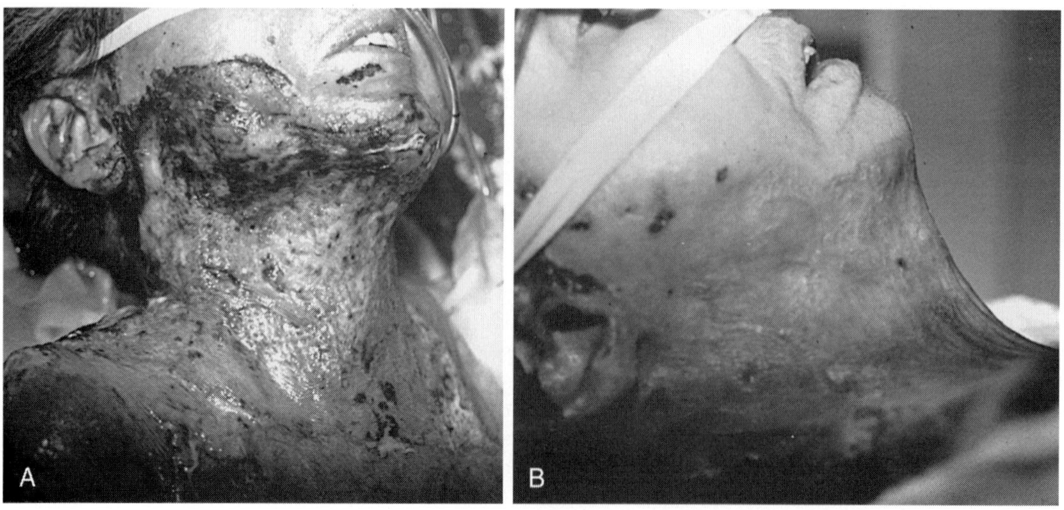

Figure 7–7. A: Extensive neck burn following debridement. B: Resulting scar contracture.

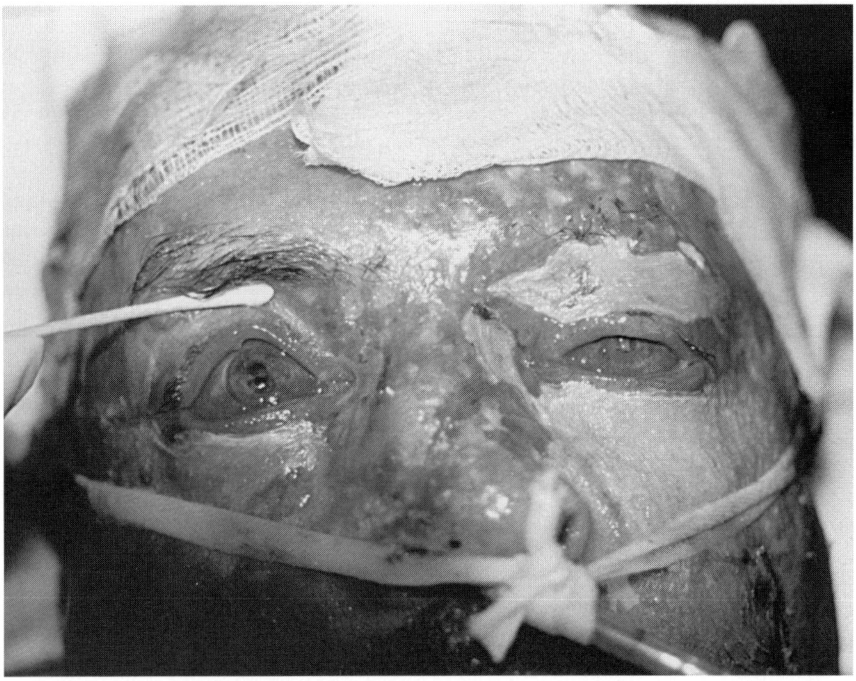

Figure 7–8. Bilateral lid burns and exposure keratitis.

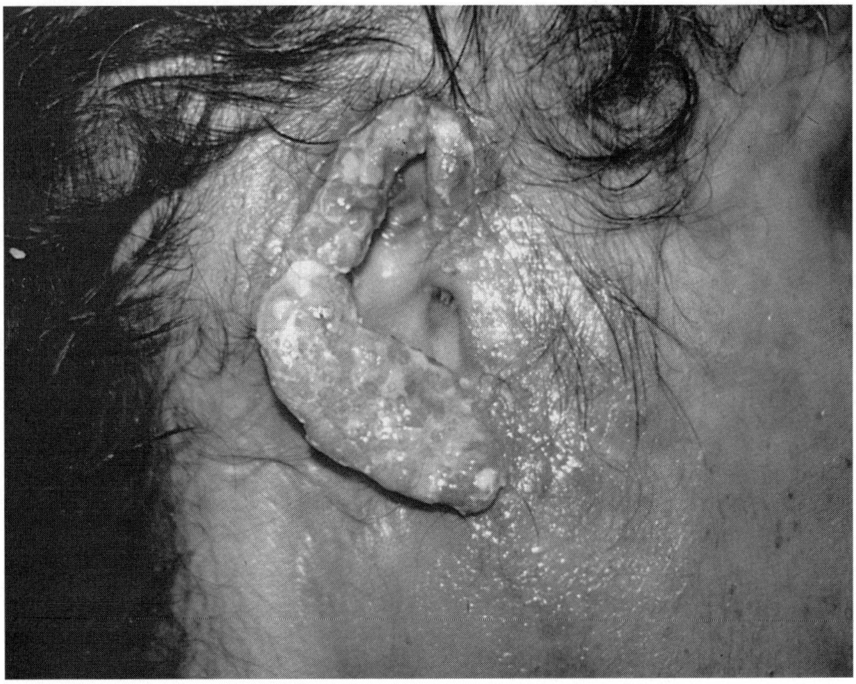

Figure 7–9. Burn to helical rim with cartilage exposure.

ing is automobile airbag deployment.[18] Facial contusions, abrasions, and fractures occur from direct contact or friction. Thermal burns can be caused by the high-temperature gases that are released in a series of exothermic chemical reactions that occur during inflation of the airbag, and chemical burns can be caused by an alkali (sodium hydroxide) or other particulates that are produced within the generated gaseous plume. These then come into contact with the driver or passenger during airbag deflation when the gases are vented.

ELECTRICAL INJURY

Approximately 5% of burns are caused by electrical injury; the mortality rate is 3% to 15%. High-voltage electrical injury causes tissue damage by direct electrical injury of cell membranes that causes cell lysis or by direct heat injury that results from the conversion of electricity as it meets tissue resistance. The smaller the diameter of the body part, the more intense is the heat that is generated. This heat is capable of charring hands, feet, and extremities. Bone, the tissue with the greatest resistance, is capable of generating more heat than skin is able to generate, which results in injuries that include extensive muscle damage but relatively little damage to overlying skin. Electric current travels along the vessels with the least resistance, resulting in damage that causes delayed vessel thrombosis and progressive ischemia. Thromboxane, a vasoconstricting arachidonic acid metabolite, is released from injured cells and contributes to progressive vasoconstriction and necrosis.[19]

Fluid resuscitation after electrical injury does not follow specific formulas, as fluid requirements are higher than the involved body surface area would suggest. Muscle damage and myoglobinuria put a patient at risk for renal tubular obstruction. Alkalinizing the urine helps to prevent pigment deposition in the kidney tubules. Unlike thermal burns, electrical burns can cause compartment syndrome, which develops because of muscle swelling and requires urgent fasciotomy. Symptoms of nerve compression or nerve deficit (tingling, pain, decreased sensation) require carpal or tarsal tunnel release.

The history of the accident takes on great importance in the situation of cardiac arrest or associated musculoskeletal trauma. Perforation of abdominal viscera, neurologic injury, such as physiologic spinal cord transection, aphasia, seizure, and pneumothorax are among possible associated injuries. Cardiac arrhythmias range from cardiac arrest at the scene to ventricular and atrial arrhythmias. Electric current passing though the heart can cause ventricular fibrillation. Other common changes in heart rate include sinus tachycardia and nonspecific ST-T wave changes.

The management of wounds caused by electrical burns is different from that of wounds cause by flames. Early fasciotomy and nerve decompression are followed by serial debridement as the wound demarcates. Functional viable structures such as tendon and nerves can be protected by allograft skin until definitive free-tissue transfer or flap coverage can be planned (Fig. 7–10). Mafenide is the topical agent of choice because of its high degree of penetration into eschar.

Oral Commissure Burns

The most common electrical burn in children occurs at the corner of the mouth when a chewed electric cord frays and produces an electrical short. Bleeding from the labial artery at 1 to 3 weeks following the injury occurs in up to one fourth of patients as the local necrotic tissue begins to slough. Initial treatment of the burn wound and debridement of necrotic tissue are conservative to avoid overresection of viable tissue.

After the wound has healed and during the ensuing period of scar maturation, prolonged splinting with orthodontic appliances for up to 6 to 8 months is often recommended to minimize contracture. This is difficult in young children and requires the cooperation of both the patient and the family. Delayed commissure reconstruction, with scar excision and lateral advancement of the orbicularis oris muscles from the upper and lower lips, vascularized by the labial arteries, allows functional restoration of the modiolus labii. The vermilion border is reconstructed, and oral mucosal flaps are advanced to cover the muscle flaps. This method results in less recurrent contracture than simple mucosal or vermilion advancement flaps.[20]

COLD INJURY

Cold injury to tissue is termed "frostbite" and is included with thermal injuries because both are injuries to the skin. The initial injury subsequently triggers mediator responses that result in progressive damage. Frostbite comprises extra- and intracellular ice formation, cell dehy-

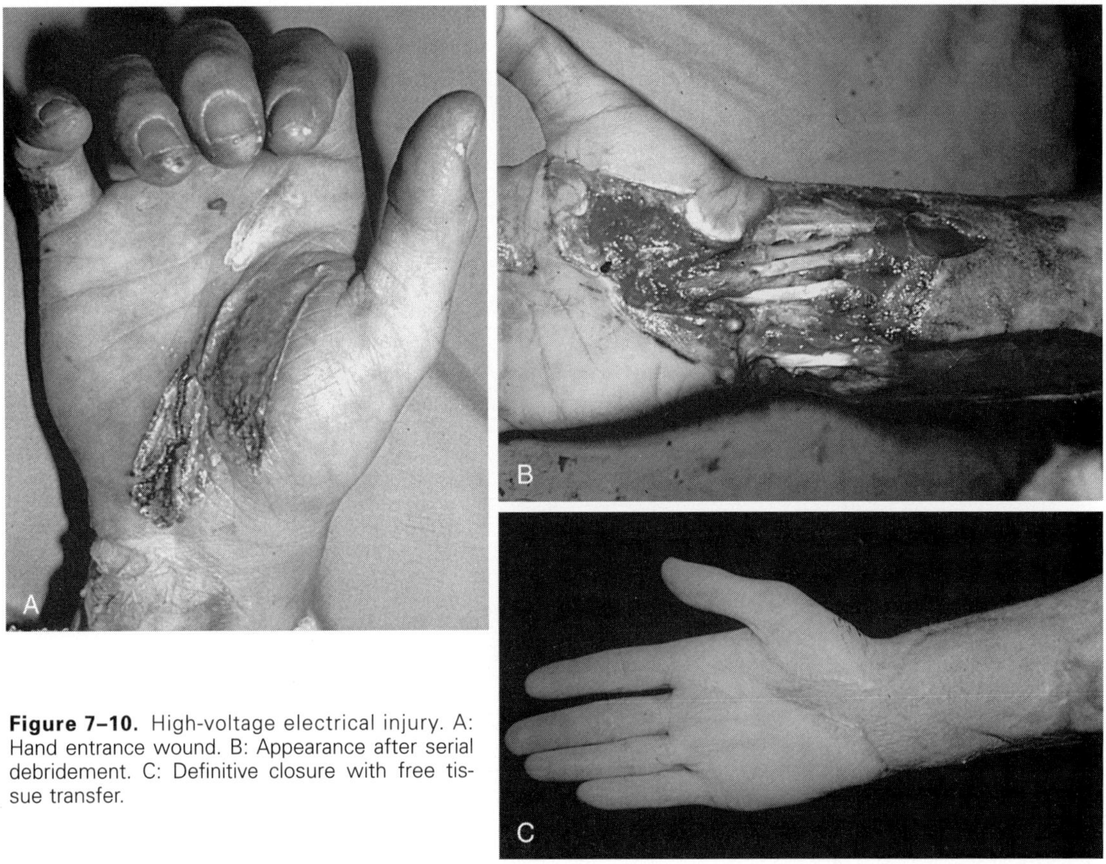

Figure 7–10. High-voltage electrical injury. A: Hand entrance wound. B: Appearance after serial debridement. C: Definitive closure with free tissue transfer.

dration, and shrinkage. The skin also undergoes intense vasoconstriction in order to preserve the body's core temperature, which then adds to the local injury. As tissue temperature falls, a plasma leak is followed by ice crystal formation, cellular dehydration, vascular stasis and, finally, thrombosis leading to ischemia and gangrene. The vasoconstrictor thromboxane has been found in frostbite blisters as well as in burn blisters and in electrically injured tissue. In all these types of injuries, microvascular thrombosis contributes to increased tissue damage. On initial presentation, the tissue is yellow-white or mottled. Tissue injury spans a spectrum, the severity of injury depending on temperature and length of exposure as well as on the wind-chill factor and moisture. Superficial injury presents with clear blistering and a blanching, pink-red wound base. These tissues are sensitive and edematous and heal by reepithelialization. Deep injury involves full-thickness skin damage and damage to tendon, muscle, and bone. Blisters are violaceous or hemorrhagic, and the wound base is blue-gray and insensate, eventually becoming dry and mummified. Clear blisters are debrided upon presentation; hemorrhagic blisters often are aspirated but left so as to prevent desiccation. Topical antimicrobial agents such as silver sulfadiazine are also employed.

During initial transport of the frostbite patient, care is taken to avoid a thaw/refreezing cycle. Rapid rewarming is facilitated in circulating warm water (40° to 42°C or 104° to 108°F). Higher temperatures may cause further tissue damage. Rewarming relieves direct injury by ice crystals in the tissue but does not relieve the progressive mediator-induced injury. Topical prostaglandin inhibitors such as aloe vera may be of benefit. Systemic ibuprofen can be given to inhibit the eicosanoid cascade.[21] Tetanus prophylaxis and analgesics are also administered.

Hyperemia, edema, and the formation of vesicles and bullae occur between 6 and 24 hours after rewarming. Progression to dry, blackened tissue with demarcation continues up to 45 days postinjury.

Adjunctive measures such as prophylactic antibiotics, heparin, and low-molecular-weight dextran have not proven to be of benefit for frostbite. The fibrinolytic agent urokinase, used to prevent fibrin deposition on injured epithelium, has anecdotal benefit. Research efforts currently focus on prostaglandin inhibitors and free-radical scavengers.

OUTCOMES

The early treatment of thermal, electrical, and cold injury and smoke inhalation has an impact on the outcome in terms of survival and long-term function. Prompt, aggressive resuscitation has improved survival in intensive care units and has diminished the incidence of organ failure, especially renal failure. Three major risk factors that increase the chance of death after burn injury have been identified: age above 60, a burn size greater than 40% TBSA, and inhalation injury.[22] The overall mortality rate in this series was 4%, but the addition of just a single risk factor increases the mortality rate from 3%, with one factor present, to 33% with two factors present, to 90% with all three factors present. This analysis emphasizes the importance of smoke inhalation as a prognostic factor for survival. Late septic complications, both pulmonary and systemic, still remain a challenge for survivors of the resuscitation phase.

As the mortality rate after burns approaches a minimal level, an emphasis on prevention will take on greater importance in future attempts to improve survival. The physical sequelae of skin injury, especially the skin of the head and neck, affect a survivor's interaction with society. Despite advances in skin coverage, such as artificial skin, cultured skin, and skin substitutes, the ability to control hypertrophic scarring remains a challenge for the future.

REFERENCES

1. National Burn Institute. Advanced Burn Life Support Course. Lincoln, NE, National Burn Institute, 1994.
2. Knox J et al. Increased survival after major thermal injury: the effect of growth hormone therapy in adults. J Trauma 1995;39:526–530.
3. Monafo WW, Halverson JD, Schechtman K. The role of concentrated sodium solutions in the resuscitation of patients with severe burns. Surgery 1984;95:129–134.
4. Gunn ML et al. Prospective, randomized trial of hypertonic sodium lactate versus lactated Ringer's solution for burn shock resuscitation. J Trauma 1989;29:1261–1267.
5. Huang PP et al. Hypertonic sodium resuscitation is associated with renal failure and death. Ann Surg 1995; 221:543–557.
6. Gore DC, Dalton JM, Gehr TW. Colloid infusions reduce glomerular filtration in resuscitated burn victims. J Trauma 1996;40:356–360.
7. McDonald WS, Sharp CW, Deitch EA. Immediate enteral feeding in burn patients is safe and effective. Ann Surg 1991;213:177–183.
8. Shirani KZ, Pruitt BA, Mason AD. The influence of inhalation injury and pneumonia on burn mortality. Ann Surg 1987;205:82–87.
9. Pruitt BA et al. Evaluation and management of patients with inhalation injury. J Trauma 1990;30(suppl 12):S63–S69.
10. Haponik EF et al. Acute upper airway injury in burn patients: serial changes of flow-volume curves and nasopharyngoscopy. Am Rev Respir Dis 1987;135:360–366.
11. Baud FJ et al. Elevated blood cyanide concentrations in victims of smoke inhalation. N Engl J Med 1991; 325:1761–1766.
12. Hantson P, Butera R, Clemessy JL. Clinical and paraclinical observations in victims of smoke inhalation without burns. Chest 1997;111:671–675.
13. Rue LW et al. Improved survival of burned patients with inhalation injury. Arch Surg 1993;128:772–780.
14. Moylan JA et al. Tracheostomy in thermally injured patients: a review of five years' experience. Ann Surg 1972;38:119–123.
15. Gaissert HA, Lofgren RH, Grillo HC. Upper airway compromise after inhalation injury: complex strictures of the larynx and trachea and their management. Ann Surg 1993;218:672–678.
16. Sears SD. Pulmonary infections in the burn patient and their management. In Haponik EF, Munster AM, eds. Respiratory Injury: Smoke Inhalation and Burns. New York, McGraw-Hill, 1990.
17. Ahrenholz DH, Clayton MC, Solem LD. Burns and wound management. Otolaryngol Clin North Am 1995; 28:1039–1055.
18. Hallock GG. Mechanisms of burn injury secondary to airbag deployment. Ann Plast Surg 1997;39:111–113.
19. Robson MC, Murphy RC, Heggars JP. A new explanation for the progressive tissue loss in electrical injuries. Plast Reconstr Surg 1984;73:431–437.
20. Pensler JM, Rosenthal A. Reconstruction of the oral commissure after an electrical burn. J Burn Care Rehab 1990;11:50–53.
21. McCauley RL et al. Frostbite: methods to minimize tissue loss. Postgrad Med 1990;88:67.
22. Ryan CM et al. Objective estimates of the probability of death from burn injuries. N Engl J Med 1998; 338:362–366.

CHAPTER 8

Anesthetic Emergencies

Tamora Carter Bynoe, MD
Lee A. Fleisher, MD

Numerous emergencies are related to the administration of anesthesia. These situations can develop on induction, intraoperatively, or postoperatively. During induction, an unrecognized or unanticipated difficult airway can result in an airway emergency, which is discussed in Chapter 10. A number of other situations require extensive preoperative evaluation, change in intraoperative management, or cancellation of the case. This chapter reviews these emergency situations and their impact on perioperative care.

MALIGNANT HYPERTHERMIA

Malignant hyperthermia (MH) is a syndrome characterized by a hypermetabolic response following exposure to certain general anesthetic agents. MH is a genetic disease with autosomal dominant transmission and variable penetrance. It has a reported incidence of 1 in 14,000 children and 1 in 50,000 adults.[1]

MH was first described as a clinical syndrome in the 1960s after the identification of a patient with a strong family history of perioperative mortality. The pathophysiology of MH was better defined after the discovery of the porcine animal model. A particular inbred line of pigs were known to have high mortality rates under stressful conditions such as fighting and during transport for slaughter. This phenomenon was coined "porcine stress syndrome" (PSS). PSS was found to be a disorder of skeletal muscle, and when susceptible pigs were exposed to succinylcholine and volatile anesthetics they experienced acidosis, rigidity, and hyperthermia. MH in humans and PSS have virtually identical clinical and laboratory findings.

The hypermetabolism of MH is the result of abnormal and excessive release of intracellular calcium from the sarcoplasmic reticulum of susceptible muscle cells. The released calcium binds to troponin, permitting the interaction of actin and myosin filaments and leading to muscle contraction. Because of the overwhelming calcium release, the contraction is intense and prolonged. This causes a chain of reactions that result in the hydrolysis of adenosine triphosphate and in carbon dioxide and lactate production, oxygen consumption, and skeletal muscle cell destruction with release of intracellular potassium, calcium, creatinine kinase, and myoglobin.

An abnormality in the ryanodine receptor protein is believed to be responsible for the derangement of skeletal muscle in PSS. Ryanodine is the calcium-release channel of the sarcoplasmic reticulum. PSS results from a single-point mutation found in all susceptible breeds of swine. In humans, there is marked heterogeneity involving more than one mutation. The presence of the abnormal ryanodine protein reduces the activation threshold for the release of calcium from the sarcoplasmic reticulum. Volatile anesthetics depolarize susceptible muscle sufficiently to reduce transmembrane voltage to the activation threshold, thus causing release of sarcoplasmic calcium and subsequent contraction.

Presentation and Evaluation

The clinical onset of MH is variable but can be triggered by all volatile anesthetics and succinylcholine. Even the newer volatile anesthetics (desflurane, sevoflurane) are capable of triggering MH. Nondepolarizing neuromuscular blocking agents and intravenous anesthetics do not cause MH. Previous uneventful anesthetic exposures do not guarantee that a patient is not MH-susceptible. The onset of symptoms may occur minutes to hours after exposure.

The hallmark of the MH syndrome is hypermetabolic activity. Early signs include tachycardia, hypertension, and tachypnea. These signs can be misinterpreted as light anesthesia and improperly treated by increasing the concentration of the volatile anesthetic. Increasing end-tidal carbon dioxide caused by the patient's rising metabolism is also an early sign. Cardiac dysrhythmias are frequently noted on continuous electrocardiogram monitoring. Hyperthermia is a late sign of MH and can be quite dramatic, with temperatures as high as 46°C having been reported. Generalized rigidity may be noted but is a variable finding. Laboratory findings include hypercarbia, metabolic acidosis, hyperkalemia, hypercalcemia, and myoglobinuria. Masseter spasm (jaw muscle rigidity) after the administration of succinylcholine has been considered a precursor to MH and should alert the anesthesiologist to the possibility of an impending MH event.

Priorities

One controversy surrounding MH is the degree of masseter spasm that warrants aborting a surgical procedure. Spasm of the jaw muscle occurs in varying degrees in normal individuals. If increased muscle tone prevents mouth opening, the risk of MH rises greatly, and elective surgery should be aborted. Masseter spasm of lesser degree is more controversial. Patients who exhibit a lesser degree of trismus after the administration of succinylcholine should be monitored very closely. Arterial blood gases should be evaluated for metabolic acidosis, and vital signs should be carefully monitored for any signs of hypermetabolism. If blood gases are normal and there are stable vital signs, some anesthesiologists believe that surgery can proceed safely. Nontriggering drugs (barbiturates, benzodiazepine, propofol, etomidate, ketamine, etc.) should be used for the maintenance of anesthesia.

In 1979 dantrolene became available as a treatment for MH. Dantrolene blocks the release of calcium from the sarcoplasmic reticulum. It is a life-saving and integral part of the management of MH. When MH is suspected in an anesthetized patient and other causes of tachycardia, hypertension, and fever have been ruled out, treatment of MH should be promptly implemented.

The first step in treating MH is to discontinue use of the triggering agent and begin hyperventilating the patient with 100% oxygen. Elective surgery should be halted or expedited so that the patient can be stabilized. Help should be obtained from other anesthesia providers or operating room personnel to dissolve the dantrolene from its powdered form into solution. Danotrolene 2.5 mg/kg should be administered every 5 minutes to a total dose of 10 mg/kg, if needed. Blood should be sent to the laboratory for arterial blood gas and electrolyte analysis. Urine output should also be promoted and evaluated for the presence of myoglobinuria. Because of the profound metabolic acidosis that can develop during a fulminant MH episode, treatment with sodium bicarbonate is necessary. If the patient is hyperthermic, measures should be taken to cool the patient, such as administering cold intravenous solutions, applying ice packs to the groin and axilla, or using cooling blankets. Once stabilized, the patient should be monitored in an intensive care unit (Box 8–1).

A patient with a personal or family history of MH can safely be anesthetized for elective surgical procedures. Regional anesthesia is a safe alternative for appropriate cases, or general anesthesia can be administered with a "clean" anesthesia machine. A clean anesthesia machine can be prepared by removing vaporizers, using

BOX 8–1

Treatment of Malignant Hyperthermia

1. Discontinue use of triggering agent and hyperventilate patient with 100% oxygen.
2. Inform surgeon that the surgical procedure must be expedited or aborted.
3. Call for help.
4. Administer dantrolene 2.5 mg/kg IV. Repeat dantrolene every 5 to 10 minutes using end-tidal carbon dioxide and temperature as therapeutic guides.
5. Monitor and treat acidosis using sodium bicarbonate based on arterial blood gas analysis.
6. Actively cool patient using cold IV solutions and ice packs to the axilla and groin.
7. Monitor and maintain urine output.
8. Transfer to an intensive care unit.

a new disposable circle system, and replacing the fresh gas outlet. Oxygen at 10 L/min is flushed through the anesthesia machine for at least 10 to 20 minutes.[2, 3] There are many safe drugs available for the induction and maintenance of anesthesia. Intravenous induction agents (barbiturates, benzodiazepines, etomidate, ketamine, propofol), narcotics, nondepolarizing neuromuscular blocking agents (atracurium, mivacurium, rocuronium, vecuronium, pancuronium), local anesthetics, anticholinergics, and anticholinesterase used to reverse paralysis can all be used safely in patients susceptible to MH.

Outcomes

The long-term sequelae can vary according to the medical course of the MH episode. In fulminant cases, neurologic injury may be permanent, presumably due to impaired cerebral blood flow and oxygenation. Once it was associated with high mortality, but prompt recognition and proper treatment have reduced mortality caused by MH to less than 10%.[4]

Patients suspected of having an episode of MH should be sent for the halothane-caffeine contracture test. This test, which requires a muscle biopsy, has 100% sensitivity and is the gold standard for the diagnosis of MH. Currently, there are only 11 centers in the United States and 24 centers in Europe that perform this test.

DENTAL TRAUMA

Dental trauma is the most commonly reported complication of general anesthesia, with an incidence of 1 in 1,000 intubations. In a multicenter retrospective study, 75% of dental injuries occurred during intubation, 9% occurred at the time of extubation, and 9% occurred in the recovery room (presumably in patients emerging from anesthesia who were inadvertently grinding their teeth or biting on a hard oral airway). Of the dental injuries, 50% were reported to occur in situations in which intubation was either emergent or difficult. The most commonly injured tooth is the left upper central incisor (51%), followed by the left lateral incisor (19%) and right central incisor (16%). The types of injuries include the loosening, dislodgment, fracturing, or avulsing of teeth and damage to dental prostheses. Teeth that are diseased, have been recently restored, or are loose are at highest risk of being dislodged or broken during general anesthesia.[5]

Each patient's dentition should be evaluated and documented preoperatively. Dentures should be identified and removed prior to the induction of anesthesia. During the discussion of the risks of general anesthesia, patients should be made aware of the small risk of dental injury. Patients, including children (who begin to lose primary teeth), with severely decayed or very loose teeth should be informed of the possibility that the tooth will be removed by the anesthesiologist prior to intubation. In some cases, it may be appropriate for dental treatment to be performed prior to elective surgery.[6]

Damage can be minimized if patients with characteristics associated with difficult intubations are identified. Those factors known to make intubation difficult include protruding maxillary incisors, decreased cervical extension, retrognathia, and limited jaw excursion. In such cases, regional anesthesia or oral or nasal fiberoptic intubations may be preferable to direct laryngoscopy. Significant dental trauma may occur during direct laryngoscopy, especially if improper technique is employed. Care should always be taken to avoid applying pressure to the central incisors during intubation. However, protection of the airway should not be sacrificed for fear of dental injury. The use of tooth protectors has been advocated by dentists to reduce the risk of dental injury. Avoiding hard oral airways as bite blocks should be considered. Rolled gauze placed over the molars and premolars is an alternative to the inflexible oral airway as a bite block.

Presentation and Evaluation

When inadvertent fracture or dislodgment of a tooth occurs, attempts should be made to locate all of the pieces, including those that may have been aspirated or swallowed. Locating whole or partial teeth may require radiographs of the head, chest, or abdomen. Bronchoscopy may be required to retrieve the damaged tooth, as aspiration of a tooth may lead to pulmonary complications, including lung abscess.

Priorities

Once the tooth is located, it should be held by the crown to avoid contact with the root. It should be rinsed with saline only. If it is possible, the tooth can be placed in its anatomic position, even though the risk of repeated avulsion during the course of the anesthetic period still exists. Alternatively, the tooth can be kept in saline-soaked gauze, and consultation with a dental service made as soon as possible for further management.

Outcomes

See Chapter 16 for further details on the management of avulsed teeth. The injury should be documented in the patient's medical chart, and the patient should be informed of the injury. Each institution has a risk-management protocol regarding compensating the patient for dental injuries.

ASPIRATION

Aspiration of gastric contents and resultant aspiration pneumonitis is an ever-present risk for any patient undergoing anesthesia. Concern about this event was first raised in 1848 after 15-year-old Hannah Greener died from aspiration while under chloroform. Almost a century later an obstetrician, Curtis Mendelsohn, published an article that highly influenced the current anesthetic practice regarding aspiration pneumonia.

Mendelsohn had performed experiments in which he instilled acidic solution into the tracheobronchial trees of rabbits and noted the severe damage that occurred in the lungs. Solutions of neutral pH caused minimal damage even if large volumes were used.[7] Many studies have been published subsequently regarding the pathophysiology of aspiration pneumonitis (Mendelsohn's syndrome). The threshold for developing Mendelsohn's syndrome is a gastric pH of 2.5 and a gastric volume of 0.4 mL/kg. The presence of particulate matter in the aspirate leads to severe lung injury regardless of the pH of the material. Thus, the most severe lung injury is caused by aspiration of highly acidic and particulate matter.

Aspiration during the perioperative period is a rare occurrence. In a large retrospective study (n = 215,488) the reported incidence was 1 in 3,216.[8] Risk factors that were identified included emergency surgery (1 in 895) and comorbid disease. Only 37% of patients who aspirated developed symptoms, and they became apparent within 2 hours of the event. The overall mortality rate secondary to aspiration was reported to be 1 in 71,829. No risk factors for aspiration were found in 57% of patients. An earlier study (n = 185,358) showed a high risk for aspiration in the pediatric and elderly age groups.[9] The rate of incidence in patients age 0 through 9 years was three times that of patients in the 20 through 49 age group. The overall mortality was 1 in 46,340. Risk factors were not present in 18% of aspiration cases, though difficulty in intubation was described in 67% of those cases.

Factors that predispose patients to aspiration under anesthesia are shown in Box 8–2. The anesthesiologist should consider preemptive measures to prevent aspiration in at-risk patients or to reduce its severity if it occurs.

Premedication of patients at risk includes histamine (H_2) blocking agents and nonparticulate antacids that increase the pH of gastric contents. Metoclopramide, which stimulates gastric emptying and increases lower esophageal sphincter tone, may also provide prophylaxis for aspiration.[10]

Observing appropriate fasting times prior to elective surgery to allow for adequate gastric emptying has been a mainstay of surgery. Recently, there has been controversy over the current guidelines for fasting. Studies have shown that the gastric volume and gastric pH of patients presenting for elective surgery who have fasted for 6 to 8 hours and those who have been allowed to consumed clear liquids 2 hours prior to surgery do not differ substantially. Guidelines differ at individual institutions; at the Johns Hopkins Hospital most anesthesiologists would delay elective surgery for 6 to 8 hours after a patient has eaten solid food. Surgery may be delayed 2 to 4 hours after consumption of clear liquids.

Aspiration is mostly likely to occur during induction of general anesthesia. A rapid-sequence technique is desirable for patients at risk because it allows the shortest period of time

BOX 8–2

Aspiration Risk Factors

- Bowel obstruction
- Gastrointestinal motility disorders
- Pregnancy
- Morbid obesity
- Diabetes mellitus
- Hiatal hernia
- Recent ingestion of food
- Depressed level of consciousness
- Esophageal disease

between the induction of anesthesia and the securing of the airway with a cuffed endotracheal tube. This technique involves denitrogenation by breathing 100% oxygen via mask for 5 minutes or by taking four vital capacity breaths. Cricoid pressure is applied as an induction dose of an intravenous anesthetic is administered, followed by a rapid-onset neuromuscular blocking agent. No attempt to ventilate the patient is made prior to intubation to prevent insufflation of the stomach with gas. Once proper placement of the endotracheal tube is confirmed, cricoid pressure is released. Success of the rapid-sequence induction assumes that the anesthesiologist has examined the airway preoperatively and feels confident that intubation will not present a problem. If the ease of intubation is questioned, then an awake intubation may be necessary.

Emergence from anesthesia is another time when aspiration is more likely to occur. A patient at risk for aspiration should not be extubated until fully conscious, alert, and able to follow commands. If vomiting occurs after extubation, the patient will be able to protect his or her airway and not regurgitate material into the lungs.

Presentation and Evaluation

Unless regurgitation of gastric contents is witnessed, the diagnosis of aspiration may be difficult. The clinical manifestations of aspiration are quite variable, ranging from asymptomatic minor aspiration to tachypnea, wheezing, hypoxemia, and acute airway obstruction with more significant aspiration. Chest x-rays may be normal in up to 10% of cases and may not reveal any abnormalities for several hours after the incident. Patients with early and extensive radiographic changes tend to have more unstable hospital courses.

Priorities

Treatment of massive pulmonary aspiration is largely supportive. Bronchoscopy and lavage is reserved for patients who have aspirated material that is causing significant airway obstruction. There is some concern that pulmonary lavage may wash aspirated material to more distal areas of the tracheobronchial tree. Mechanical ventilation is appropriate for patients with depressed levels of consciousness or increased FIO_2 or positive end-expiratory phase requirements for maintenance of an adequate PaO_2. There is no role for the routine use of corticosteroids or prophylactic antibiotics. Antibiotics are reserved for patients who have high likelihood of a pulmonary infection or patients who have aspirated obviously contaminated material.

Outcomes

Mortality after aspiration is approximately 5%.[8, 9] Morbidity after a severe aspiration episode may include reactive airway disease, lung abscess formation, or multiorgan failure resulting from prolonged hypoxemia. The elderly and patients with comorbid diseases are at greater risk for poor outcomes.

ANAPHYLAXIS

Anaphylaxis is a potentially life-threatening allergic reaction that may involve the cardiovascular, respiratory, and dermatologic systems. This exaggerated immunologic response is a type I immediate-hypersensitivity reaction resulting from the interaction of an antigen with preexisting antigen-specific immunoglobulin E (IgE) antibodies located on the surfaces of tissue mast cells and basophils. The initial exposure to the foreign molecule stimulates IgE antibody production. Reexposure to the antigen or a chemically similar molecule causes the binding of the antigenantibody complex and the release of the vasoactive mediators stored in the cytoplasmic granules. These mediators (histamine, arachidonic acid, leukotrienes, kinins, eosinophilic chemotactic factor, and prostaglandins) cause increased capillary permeability, bronchoconstriction, vasodilation, coronary vasoconstriction, and myocardial depression. These effects produce the clinical manifestations of the anaphylactic reaction (see Chapter 3 for more details).[11]

Life-threatening anaphylaxis under general anesthesia occurs 1 in 5,000 to 1 in 15,000 instances of anesthesia.[12] Because of the multiple medications used in the delivery of anesthesia, it may be difficult to determine which was the offending agent that induced the anaphylactic reaction. Moscicki and colleagues performed skin tests on 27 patients who had survived anaphylactic reactions in the operating room, and found that 44% had a history of atopy, compared to the incidence of atopy in the general population of 15% to 20%.[12] Of the 13 patients who had positive skin tests, the most common offending agents were neuromuscular blocking agents (46%) followed by thiobarbiturates (38%) and penicillin derivatives (15%). Patients who had developed more than one sign of anaphylaxis were more likely to have positive skin tests. In 1993, a group of French investigators looked at 813 anaphylactic reactions that occurred intraoperatively.[13] Neuromuscular blocking agents accounted for 70.3% of the allergic reactions, followed by latex (12.6%) and colloid volume expanders (4.6%). Antibiotics accounted for only 2.6% of the anaphylactic reactions.

Recently, latex allergy has gained more interest as a potent allergen in severe life-threatening anaphylaxis. Latex is a natural product found in the milky sap of the rubber tree, *Hevea brasiliensis.* Although it has been widely used in the medical field for over a century, the first allergic reaction to latex was not described until 1979. Numerous cases of IgE-mediated latex allergies have been reported since then. People at risk for severe latex allergy are those who have repeated exposure to rubber products. Children with congenital genitourinary defects or myelomeningocele are chronically exposed to latex products such as urinary catheters and gloves.[14, 15] Other high-risk groups include patients with occupational exposure to rubber products, health care workers, orthopedic patients, and patients who have spinal cord injuries that require frequent urinary instrumentation. People with latex sensitivity may describe symptoms of watery eyes or rash when in contact with balloons or household gloves. Patients with allergies to chestnuts, bananas, kiwi, or avocados are also at risk for latex allergy because of antigenic similarities.

Sensitization to latex may occur because of systemic absorption of antigenic material through microscopic mucosal tears that are the result of repeated catheterization. Patients who have severe latex sensitization may develop symptoms of anaphylaxis from the aerosolized latex particles that originate from gloves. Because of the seriousness and growing prevalence of latex allergy, many hospital centers are creating a latex-free environment for their patients and employees.

In the operating room, many latex products are used in the delivery of anesthesia, including gloves, blood pressure cuffs, tourniquets, rebreathing bags, syringes, medication vials, cloth adhesive tape, intravenous bag ports, and other items.[15] Latex-free substitutes are available for some of the necessary equipment needed to safely anesthetize a patient. When a patient who is known to have a latex allergy or who is at high risk for latex allergy presents for surgery, the team should take special precautions to prevent or minimize the risk of an anaphylactic event. Some institutions advocate prophylactic use of steroids and H_1 and H_2 histamine receptor antagonists 1 hour prior to surgery. However, anaphylactic events have occurred despite the pretreatment. At Johns Hopkins Hospital, effort is made to schedule elective surgery on latex-allergic patients early in the day because there should be fewer aerosolized latex particles in the environment. There is a special latex-free cart that contains equipment such as gloves, tourniquets, and rebreathing bags. Patients are not routinely pretreated with steroids and histamine receptor antagonists.

Presentation and Evaluation

The symptoms of anaphylaxis can vary from predominantly respiratory complications to cardiovascular collapse. In the awake patient, early symptoms may include hoarseness or the sensation of a lump in the throat caused by laryngeal edema. Progression to total airway obstruction may be imminent. Complaints of chest tightness, shortness of breath, coughing, or wheezing are indicative of lower respiratory tract involvement. Patients may have a sense of impending doom or complain of feeling lightheaded. Clinically, hypotension and arrhythmias may be seen. Gastrointestinal complaints such as nausea, vomiting, cramps, and bloody diarrhea are also common in the awake patient. Cutaneous signs and symptoms include erythema, pruritus, and angioedema.

In an anesthetized patient, the most common presenting clinical sign of anaphylaxis is acute cardiovascular collapse. Early cutaneous signs may not be evident because the patient is hidden under drapes. Other causes of sudden hypotension should be excluded such as myocardial ischemia or infarction, aspiration, or pulmonary embolus. The concomitant development of bronchospasm, hypoxemia, generalized edema, and arrhythmia may aid in the diagnosis of an allergic reaction.

Priorities

When the diagnosis of anaphylaxis is made intraoperatively, the anesthesiologist must initiate treatment promptly. First, the offending agent should be identified and removed. As mentioned earlier, this may prove challenging because of the number of drugs that have been used. Allergies to thiobarbiturates and muscle relaxants usually present within 10 to 20 minutes of injection, whereas latex allergic reactions usually occur well after induction of anesthesia. All patients should be ventilated with 100% oxygen. In a patient not yet intubated, secure the airway with an endotracheal tube because of the risk of rapidly progressing laryngeal edema. Rapid volume resuscitation, preferably with intravenous crystalloid, should begin immediately. Epinephrine restores membrane permeability, decreases the release of vasoactive mediators, and relaxes bronchial smooth muscle and is the first-line agent in the treatment of anaphylaxis. Boluses of 0.1 to 0.2 μg/kg of epinephrine should be administered to maintain adequate blood pressure, and epinephrine infusion may be necessary. Once the patient has been hemodynamically stabilized, the administration of diphenhydramine and histamine H_2 antagonists should be considered. If bronchospasm is persistent, aminophylline (5 to 6 mg/kg over 20 min) can be infused. Steroids prevent a late-phase reaction but do not demonstrate any immediate effects. The patient's acid-base status should be monitored and treatment (sodium bicarbonate) instituted if necessary. If the patient has been stabilized and does not require aggressive resuscitation (epinephrine infusion), the decision to proceed with or abort surgery should be made in a careful discussion between the anesthesiologist and surgeon. The patient should be monitored for at least 24 hours in an intensive care setting.

Outcomes

The mortality rate for anaphylactic reactions under general anesthesia is between 4% and 6%.[12] After recovery from the anaphylactic event, the patient should be sent for skin testing to determine the agent responsible. The patient should obtain a Medic Alert bracelet that notes the name of the offending drug as well as the reaction of anaphylaxis.

INTRAOPERATIVE HYPOXEMIA

There are many causes of hypoxemia that may confront the anesthesiologist in the operating room (Box 8–3). Prompt recognition and intervention are necessary to prevent catastrophic events.

BOX 8-3

Causes of Intraoperative Hypoxemia

Endotracheal tube malposition
Laryngospasm
Pneumothorax
Bronchospasm
Aspiration
Pulmonary edema
Pulmonary embolism
$\dot{V}/\dot{Q}$ mismatch

Endotracheal Tube Malposition

After intubation has been achieved, the proper position of the endotracheal tube must be confirmed.[16] Esophageal placement of the endotracheal tube (ETT) is a risk of intubation. A review of closed claims cases involving anesthesia reveals that most intraoperative cardiac arrests are related to difficulty in airway management, with unrecognized esophageal intubations playing a major role. ETT disconnects and inadvertent extubations are also dangers that should be looked for during surgery.

PRESENTATION AND EVALUATION

Many techniques can be employed by anesthesia providers to detect ETT malposition. Direct visualization of the vocal cords with a laryngoscope as the ETT passes through them is the simplest technique that is employed. In cases in which intubation is difficult, full view of the glottis may not be achieved or movement of the head may change the final position of a correctly placed tube. Extension of the head may cause inadvertent extubation, whereas flexion of the head may cause endobronchial intubation. This is a major concern in pediatric patients because of the shorter tracheal length.

The presence of bilateral breath sounds is usually indicative of proper ETT placement. However, there are numerous case reports in which breath sounds were auscultated with the ETT located in the esophagus. Positive-pressure ventilation of the esophagus can produce coarse sounds that can be auscultated through the chest wall. Obese patients and patients with obstructive lung disease may have decreased breath sounds that are difficult to hear, or severe bronchospasm may reduce ventilation. The rise of the chest wall associated with positive-pressure ventilation may also be obscured in these patients.

The fiberoptic bronchoscope has been exceedingly helpful in the practice of anesthesiology. It can be useful for intubation when direct laryngoscopy is difficult or impossible. With the fiberoptic bronchoscope, direct visualization of the glottis and tracheal rings offers assurance that the ETT has been properly placed. This technique, however, requires experience and enough time to properly anesthetize the patient's upper airway with topical anesthesia or with nerve blocks. The flexible endoscopic equipment is expensive and fragile.

Capnometry, the measurement of carbon dioxide concentration, has become the most reliable method of detecting improper ETT placement. In the presence of intact pulmonary circulation, carbon dioxide can be measured from gas exiting the endotracheal tube as the patient is ventilated. Mass spectrometry can produce a continuous carbon dioxide waveform that can be visualized. Initially, carbon dioxide may be detected by the capnometer if the endotracheal tube has been placed in the esophagus, but the carbon dioxide levels are low and quickly disappear with continuing ventilation. The use of continuous carbon dioxide monitoring intraoperatively also detects mishaps such as disconnection and kinking of the ETT and inadvertent extubations.

PRIORITIES

Unrecognized ETT malposition may be revealed by declining oxygen saturation, as measured by continuous pulse oximetry. A systematic approach should be taken to identify the cause of the hypoxemia. Auscultation of the chest wall will determine whether the breath sounds are present and equal. The absence of breath sounds suggests esophageal intubation, ETT disconnect, a kink in the ETT, a turned-off ventilator, or inadvertent extubation. Unequal breath sounds may be due to endobronchial intubation or pneumothorax.

The anesthesia machines in the United States are equipped with a ventilator disconnect alarm that is activated when there is a decrease in the breathing circuit pressure of an intubated patient. Often in otolaryngologic surgery, the patient's head is rotated away from the anesthesiologist's direct line of vision which makes identifying ETT disconnects and extubations difficult. The anesthesia machine's alarm plays an important role in alerting the anesthesiologist to that possibility.

If the disconnect alarm sounds, the anesthesiologist should immediately investigate the endotracheal tube. This may involve interrupting surgery to go under the surgical drapes and visualize the ETT. If the ETT has come out, the patient must be immediately reintubated. Surgery around the airway can distort the anatomy and make reintubation difficult. It may be necessary to obtain a surgical airway.

OUTCOMES

If ETT malposition is identified early, and appropriate intervention is employed, morbidity is low. If the malposition is not identified or if correcting the problem is difficult and prolonged, the patient is at risk for hypoxia, which can lead to neurologic injury, cardiac arrest and, ultimately, the death of the patient.

Laryngospasm

Laryngospasm is the sudden involuntary contraction of laryngeal muscles which causes adduction of the vocal cords and, thus, airway obstruction. If not recognized in a timely fashion, the airway obstruction will lead to hypoxemia followed by brain injury or death. It is usually prompted when the glottis of an anesthetized patient is exposed to noxious stimulation, commonly during emergence from anesthesia. The stimulation of the glottis by secretions or instrumentation, such as a suction catheter or an oral airway, can initiate reflexive closure of the vocal cords.

Children have a high incidence of laryngospasm during induction and emergence. Patients in the recovery phase of an upper respiratory infection are prone to laryngospasm and hypoxemia.[17]

PRESENTATION AND EVALUATION

Laryngospasm should be considered in any patient with airway obstruction not relieved by maneuvers such as neck extension, jaw thrust, or placement of a nasal or oral airway.

PRIORITIES

Treatment consists of clearing secretions from the pharynx, supplying positive airway pressure (15 to 20 cm H_2O) with mask and 100% oxygen. Manual displacement of the jaw anteriorly stretches the hyoepiglottic ligament, the epiglottis, and the aryepiglottic folds, thereby opening the forced closure of the glottis. If the laryngospasm is not relieved, administering a small dose of succinylcholine may be necessary to prevent progression to hypoxia.

OUTCOMES

Morbidity and mortality are low if laryngospasm is recognized in a timely fashion and proper treatment is initiated.

Postobstructive Pulmonary Edema

The development of pulmonary edema following relief of airway obstruction is a risk of laryngospasm and other obstructive conditions. Postobstructive pulmonary edema was first described in 1977. It has been well documented in children who have been intubated because of airway obstruction while suffering from croup or epiglottis. There have been a number of reports of adult patients who developed pulmonary edema after relief of laryngospasm.[18, 19]

The proposed mechanisms are controversial. The most commonly held theory is that significant negative intrathoracic pressure develops as the patient attempts to breathe against a closed glottis. This pressure is transmitted to the pulmonary interstitial tissues, and that increases the hydrostatic pressure gradient, causing the transudation of fluid out of the pulmonary circulation. Increased venous return caused by the negative intrathoracic pressure increases pulmonary blood volume and pulmonary arterial pressure. These changes contribute to further hydrostatic transudation of fluid. Hypoxia leading to pulmonary capillary damage and increased membrane permeability has also been implicated as a cause of fluid in the lungs. Increased sympathetic tone results from hypoxemia and hypercarbia and leads to the release of catecholamines. This situation is associated with a decline in ventricular function, systemic vasoconstriction, and the shunting of blood into the pulmonary circulation, which further augments pulmonary blood volume and pulmonary arterial pressure.

PRESENTATION AND EVALUATION

Once the airway obstruction has been relieved by mask or by intubation, patients develop pink frothy sputum and hypoxemia, and chest radiography reveals abnormalities consistent with pulmonary edema.

PRIORITIES

The treatment of postobstructive pulmonary edema is largely empiric. Supplemental oxygen should be supplied to maintain adequate oxygenation. In severe cases, intubation and mechanical ventilation may be required. The addition of a positive end-expiratory phase may be necessary. The usefulness of diuretics is unclear in the treatment of this type of pulmonary edema, but diuretics such as furosemide are commonly administered. There is no role for steroids in the treatment of postobstructive pulmonary edema.

OUTCOMES

Regardless of the type of treatment given, the time course of postobstructive pulmonary edema is quite rapid. Resolution generally occurs within 24 hours.

VENOUS AIR EMBOLISM

Venous air embolism (VAE) is caused by the entrainment of air into the venous circulation when the level of the surgical site is higher than the right atrium. The greater the gradient between the surgical site and the right atrium, the greater the risk of air entrainment. A gradient as little as 5 cm H_2O is sufficient for the entry of air into open veins. VAE occurs more frequently than is clinically significant; however, the entrainment of a significant volume of air (7.5 mL/kg in dogs) can lead to cardiovascular collapse and death.

In neurosurgery performed in the sitting position, the incidence of VAE is as high as 10% to 80%.[20] Urologic and orthopedic surgeries also produce significant incidence of VAE. The increasing use of laparoscopy has led to a number of reported cases of VAE.[21] The abdomen is insufflated with carbon dioxide at 12 to 15 mm Hg, which is higher than venous pressure and can enable the passage of gas into the circulatory system if there are any open veins.

Presentation and Evaluation

Cardiovascular collapse is caused when a significant volume of air has accumulated in the right ventricular outflow tract, causing obstruction of blood flow to the lungs. The clinical signs and symptoms are based on the rate and volume at which the air enters the circulatory system. Right-to-left shunting of air through a patent foramen ovale may cause paradoxical embolization of air into cerebral or coronary arteries with devastating results.

An abrupt drop in end-tidal carbon dioxide caused by the increase in pulmonary dead space and a decrease in the oxygen saturation are early signs of clinically significant VAE. Electrocardiography may reveal brady- or tachyarrhythmias. If a pulmonary artery catheter is present, increases in pulmonary artery pressures would be noted. Precordial Doppler ultrasound placed over the right heart is able to detect the presence of 0.25 mL of air in the venous system. The classic "mill-wheel" murmur heard by precordial or esophageal stethoscope is a late sign that is present after cardiovascular collapse has occurred. Transesophageal echocardiography, which can detect as little as .02 mL/kg of air, is the most sensitive method of detecting air in the right heart. This method of detection is expensive and requires an anesthesiologist trained in its use.

Priorities

When a patient presents for surgery in which VAE represents a significant risk such as posterior fossa surgery in the sitting position, steps can be taken prior to surgery to minimize the risk of VAE. The patient should be kept well hydrated to maintain elevated right atrial pressure, thus reducing the gradient between the surgical site and the right atrium. Precordial Doppler ultrasound should be placed along the right sternal border to detect the presence of air. A multiorificed right atrial catheter should be positioned so that the tip of the catheter is 2 cm below the superior vena cava-atrial junction so that air can be aspirated from the right atrium.

If VAE is suspected, nitrous oxide should be discontinued and the patient placed on 100% oxygen. Nitrous oxide will diffuse into the air bubbles in the right heart and increase the size of the embolus. The surgeon should flood the field with normal saline to prevent further entry of air. If possible, the patient should be positioned so that the surgical site is lower than the right atrium. Placing the patient in the left lateral decubitus position may be necessary to relieve air lock in the right heart. If the surgical site is the face or head, gentle compression of the bilateral jugular veins may prevent further entrainment of air into the right heart. The anesthesiologist should attempt to aspirate air from the right atrial catheter. Pharmacologic support should be started in patients who remain hemodynamically compromised despite appropriate intervention.

Outcomes

Perioperative mortality from VAE is less than 1%.

CARDIOVASCULAR COMPLICATIONS

Cardiovascular dysfunction represents an urgent or emergent situation that could lead to cardiovascular collapse or death. In the past 2 decades, a great deal of effort to identify patients at risk for cardiovascular complications has surrounded noncardiac surgery. Two recent guidelines from the American Heart Association, American College of Cardiology, and the American College of Physicians have identified clinical risk stratification and appropriate use of diagnostic testing.[22, 23] Traditionally, an anesthesiologist has required a full understanding of a patient's cardiovascular status before proceeding with noncardiac surgery, yet in the current climate of cost-containment, a full evaluation is frequently abbreviated. Additionally, cardiovascular disease can progress during the perioperative period and precise identification of the patient at greatest risk is difficult or impossible.

Perioperative cardiovascular dysfunction can be broadly divided into two categories, ischemic and nonischemic. Myocardial ischemia can lead to myocardial infarction, left ventricular dysfunction, and eventual death.[24] A patient may also have a history of nonischemic cardiomyopathy and may be at high risk for developing left ventricular dysfunction and acute pulmonary edema, which rarely progress to irreversible cardiovascular changes. This section will focus on the more worrisome ischemic dysfunction.

Presentation and Evaluation

Identification of a patient at great risk for developing perioperative myocardial ischemia depends upon an accurate clinical and exercise history as well as on factors specific to the surgical procedure. In a recent analysis of patients in the Coronary Artery Surgery Study who subsequently underwent noncardiac surgery, head and neck surgery was associated with an intermediate risk of cardiovascular complications, similar to the risk level of patients undergoing abdominal or thoracic procedures.[25] A patient with overt angina pectoris has ongoing myocardial ischemia. The severity of the coronary artery disease is determined by the stability of symptoms and by exercise tolerance. A patient with progressive symptoms or angina at rest (unstable angina) is at a prohibitively high risk for perioperative cardiovascular morbidity and should undergo only emergency procedures.[26] A patient who develops angina at high workloads (Table 8–1) is at risk for perioperative ischemia but the probability of overt dysfunction is rare. In contrast, a patient who develops signs of angina at low work loads and has clinical signs of left ventricular dysfunction such as dyspnea or orthopnea has a prior probability of developing perioperative ischemia and frequently develops left ventricular dysfunction. A patient in this category may benefit from more invasive monitoring, as intraoperative hypertension may be the result of either hypovolemia or left ventricular dysfunction.

The standard method of diagnosing intraoperative myocardial ischemia is the electrocardiogram. An ST segment shift from baseline is associated with myocardial ischemia. With the advent of computerized ST segment trending, most monitors began to display the extent of the ST segment shift, updated approximately every 20 to 30 seconds. Numerous studies have documented that this form of analysis greatly improves the observer's ability to detect perioperative myocardial ischemia and has high sensitivity compared to other modalities.[27] It is important to realize that not all episodes of significant ST segment depression represent true myocardial ischemia, as electrolytes, position, and pharmacologic agents can affect the electrocardiogram.

If true myocardial ischemia is detected, it is important to treat the episode so as to potentially prevent overt myocardial necrosis, infarction, or death. Perioperative myocardial ischemia has been shown to be the strongest predictor of perioperative cardiac morbidity, and postoperative myocardial ischemia is more important than preoperative or intraoperative episodes.[24] Additionally, several investigators have shown that the duration of ST segment depression correlates with the probability of cardiac morbidity.[28, 29] Although new trials have evaluated the beneficial effects of early treatment of perioperative ischemia, most clinicians believe that such action decreases the probability or the extent of myocardial necrosis.

Table 8–1. *Estimated Energy Requirements for Various Activities*

1 MET
Can you
Take care of yourself?
Eat, dress, or use a toilet?
Walk indoors around the house?
Walk a block or two on level ground at 2 to 3 mph or 3.2 to 4.8 km/h?
Do light work around the house like dusting or washing dishes?
4 METs
Can you
Climb a flight of stairs or walk up a hill?
Walk on level ground at 4 mph or 6.4 km/h?
Run a short distance
Do heavy work around the house like scrubbing floors or lifting or moving furniture?
Participate in moderate recreational activities like golf, bowling, dancing, doubles tennis, or throwing a baseball or football?
>10 METs
Can you
Participate in strenuous sports like swimming, singles tennis, football, basketball, or skiing?

MET, metabolic equivalent.
(Adapted from the Duke Activity Status Index and American Heart Association Exercise Standards. Reproduced with permission from AHA/ACA Guidelines.)

Priorities

Treatment of perioperative ischemia is determined by its cause. Numerous studies have documented the importance of tachycardia in the development of myocardial ischemia.[30] Tachycardia may be related to inadequate anesthesia or analgesia or to exaggerated sympathetic response, particularly in a patient with a history of hypertension. Therefore, treatment can consist of deepening the anesthetized state, administering narcotics, or administering beta blockade. Electrocardiographic evidence of myocardial ischemia can also occur in the absence of any hemodynamic changes; coronary vasomotor changes resulting in decreased coronary blood flow can lead to myocardial ischemia. Administration of nitroglycerin frequently results in the resolution of such ischemia.

Myocardial ischemia is of greatest concern when it is associated with hypotension. Hypotension, particularly in the presence of tachycardia, can lead to myocardial ischemia. Additionally, myocardial ischemia can lead to left ventricular dysfunction and further hypotension. This represents a true emergency, as the situation can quickly deteriorate into cardiogenic shock. If time permits, additional monitoring may be required to direct therapy. Therapy consists of blood pressure support with phenylephrine or norepinephrine. Low cardiac output states may require inotropic support with agents such as dopamine, dobutamine, or epinephrine. Relief of myocardial ischemia may require coadministration of nitroglycerin once the blood pressure is normalized, particularly if cardiac output and blood pressure are low while the pulmonary capillary wedge pressure is high. If treatment does not improve hemodynamics, an intra-aortic balloon pump should be considered for support of the circulation. The need to insert such a device occurs rarely but may provide the only means of adequate support. In any case, surgery should be aborted or quickly completed in order to facilitate stabilization of the patient.

Cardiovascular collapse may occur as a result of an acute thrombosis or a myocardial infarction in evolution. In such a circumstance, the goals must be to support the circulation and limit infarct size. Some investigators have advocated acute coronary angiography and angioplasty, if these techniques are available, in order to salvage the myocardium. Such aggressive treatment could result in increased surgical bleeding. Minimizing potential surgical stress is important to decreasing potential cardiovascular complications.

Myocardial ischemia and ventricular dysfunction can lead to congestive heart failure, but low cardiac output states related to aggressive fluid administration and the myocardium-depressing effects of anesthetic agents can also lead to pulmonary edema. Signs of acute pulmonary edema include decreased oxygen saturation and pink frothy liquid in the endotracheal tube. Treatment is determined by cause. Overhydration can be acutely corrected by the administration of nitroglycerin or of a diuretic, which should improve the situation over a longer period of time. Myocardial depression may require the administration of an inotrope, and dobutamine frequently improves the situation. Although it is prudent to complete the surgical procedure quickly, these circumstances rarely result in the same level of emergency as acute ischemia.

Outcomes

Supply-and-demand mismatches can lead to myocardial ischemia. Prolonged myocardial ischemia (more than 30 minutes or accumulative duration of more than 2 hours in 24 hours) has been associated with an increased incidence of perioperative myocardial infarction. Patients who sustain a perioperative myocardial infarction have a high 30-day mortality rate and decreased long-term survival compared to similar high-risk patients without perioperative complications.[31] There are currently no published studies demonstrating that early treatment with anti-ischemic agents would decrease the incidence of cardiac morbidity, but such an approach has been advocated and is currently being tested. Future research will determine if prophylactic or acute treatment of myocardial ischemia is the optimal and most cost-effective approach.

REFERENCES

1. Sessler DI. Malignant hyperthermia. Acta Anaesthesiol Scand 1996;109(suppl):25–30.
2. Beebe JJ, Sessler DI. Preparation of anesthesia machines for patients susceptible to malignant hyperthermia. Anesthesiology 1988;69:395–400.
3. McGraw TT, Keon TP. Malignant hyperthermia and the clean machine. Can J Anaesth 1989;36:530–532.
4. Carr AS et al. Incidence of malignant hyperthermia reactions in 2,214 patients undergoing muscle biopsy. Can J Anaesth 42:281–286.
5. Lockhart PB et al. Dental complications during and after tracheal intubation. J Am Dent Assoc 1986; 112:480–483.
6. Chadwick RG, Lindsay SM. Dental injuries during general anesthesia. Br Dent J 1996;180:255–258.
7. Mendelsohn CL. The aspiration of stomach contents into the lungs during obstetric anesthesia. Am J Obstet Gynecol 1946;52:191–205.
8. Warner MA, Warner ME, Weber JG. Clinical significance of pulmonary aspiration during the perioperative period. Anesthesiology 1993;78:56–62.
9. Olsson GL, Hallen B, Hambraeus-Jonzon K. Aspiration during anaesthesia: a computer-aided study of 185,358 anaesthetics. Acta Anaesthesiol Scand 1986;30:84–92.
10. Ellmauer S. Prophylaxis and therapy of the acid aspiration syndrome. Anaesthetist 1987;36:599–607.
11. Levy JH. Allergic reactions during anesthesia. J Clin Anes 1988;1:39–46.
12. Moscicki RA et al. Anaphylaxis during induction of general anesthesia: subsequent evaluation and management. J Allergy Clin Immunol 1990;86:325–332.
13. Laxenaire M. Drugs and other agents involved in anaphylactic shock during anaesthesia. A French multicenter epidemiological inquiry. Ann Fr Anesth Reanim 1993;12:91–96.
14. Gol M et al. Intraoperative anaphylaxis: an association with latex sensitivity. J Allergy Clin Immunol 1991;87:662–666.
15. Pollard RJ, Layon AJ. Latex allergy in the operating room: case report and brief review of the literature. J Clin Anes 1996;8:161–167.
16. Birmingham PK, Cheney FW, Ward RJ. Esophageal intubation: a review of detection techniques. Anesth Analg 1986;65:886–891.
17. Tait AR, Knight PR. Intraoperative respiratory compli-

cations in patients with upper respiratory infections. Can J Anaesth 1987;34:300–303.
18. Herrick IA, Mahendra B, Penny FJ. Postobstructive pulmonary edema following anesthesia. J Clin Anesth 1990;2:116–120.
19. Holmes JR, Hensinger RN, Wojtys EW. Postoperative pulmonary edema in young athletic adults. Am J Sports Med 1991;19:365–371.
20. Palmon S et al. Venous air embolism: a review. J Clin Anesth 1997;9:251–257.
21. Cottin V, Delafosse B, Viale JP. Gas embolism during laparoscopy. Surg Endosc 1996;10:166–169.
22. Eagle K et al. Guidelines for perioperative cardiovascular evaluation of the noncardiac surgery: a report of the American Heart Association/American College of Cardiology Task Force on Assessment of Diagnostic and Therapeutic Cardiovascular Procedures. Circulation 1996;93:1278–1317.
23. American College of Physicians. Guidelines for assessing and managing the perioperative risk from coronary artery disease associated with major noncardiac surgery. Ann Intern Med 1997;127:313–328.
24. Mangano DT et al. Association of perioperative myocardial ischemia with cardiac morbidity and mortality in men undergoing surgery. N Engl J Med 1990; 323:1781–1788.
25. Eagle KA et al. Cardiac risk of noncardiac surgery: influence of coronary disease and type of surgery in 3368 operations, CASS Investigators and University of Michigan Heart Care Program, Coronary Artery Surgery Study. Circulation 1997;96:1882–1887.
26. Shah KB et al. Angina and other risk factors in patients with cardiac diseases undergoing noncardiac operations. Anesth Analg 1990;70:240–247.
27. Eisenberg MJ et al. Monitoring for myocardial ischemia during noncardiac surgery: a technology assessment of transesophageal echocardiography and 12-lead electrocardiography, the Study of Perioperative Ischemia Research Group. JAMA 1992;268:210–216.
28. Fleisher LA, Nelson AH, Rosenbaum SH. Postoperative myocardial ischemia: etiology of cardiac morbidity or manifestation of underlying disease. J Clin Anesth 1995;7:97–102.
29. Landesberg G et al. Importance of long-duration postoperative ST-segment depression in cardiac morbidity after vascular surgery. Lancet 1993;341:715–719.
30. Slogoff S, Keats AS. Does perioperative myocardial ischemia lead to postoperative myocardial infarction? Anesthesiology 1985;62:107–114.
31. Mangano DT et al. Long-term cardiac prognosis following noncardiac surgery, the Study of Perioperative Ischemia Research Group. JAMA 1992;268:233–239.

CHAPTER 9

Airway Emergencies

David W. Eisele, MD

Acute upper airway obstruction is a life-threatening emergency that requires immediate intervention. Ensurance of an adequate airway is the primary priority in patient resuscitation. All physicians should be capable of basic emergency airway control.

Airway obstruction can be the result of a variety of disorders, including trauma, neoplasm, infection, inflammatory process, neurologic dysfunction, presence of a foreign body, hemorrhage, and anatomic conditions. A thorough understanding of the causes of airway obstruction is necessary in order to properly manage airway emergencies. This chapter discusses the evaluation and management of acute upper airway obstruction in general as well as specific techniques for airway control. In addition, management principles related to specific causes of acute upper airway obstruction in adults are covered. Pediatric airway emergencies are discussed in Chapter 21.

ACUTE UPPER AIRWAY OBSTRUCTION

Acute upper airway obstruction can result from a variety of disorders. Affected sites can include the oral cavity, oropharynx, hypopharynx, larynx, and trachea (Table 9–1). Compromise of the airway can occur at any of these levels as a result of various causes, including swelling, collapse, scarring, a foreign body, hemorrhage, neoplasm, or neurologic dysfunction.

Emergency airway management principles include the determination of the site and degree of obstruction, airway control by forced ventilation, intubation, or surgical bypass of the obstructed site with a cricothyroidotomy or tracheotomy, and treatment of the precipitating cause of obstruction.

Presentation

Patients with acute upper airway compromise may exhibit varying degrees of dyspnea or may be unresponsive if complete airway obstruction has occurred. Symptoms of upper airway obstruction can be relatively nonspecific or may relate to the underlying pathologic process causing the obstruction. In addition, symptoms of upper airway obstruction can be variable. In most patients, dyspnea is the primary complaint. Anxiety coupled with distress and a sense of impending doom may accompany this symptom. Dyspnea may not be present until significant airway compromise occurs. Depending on the cause of the obstruction, patients may complain of such associated symptoms as pain, dysphagia, odynophagia, hoarseness, otalgia, hemoptysis, cough, or fever.

Signs of upper airway obstruction include cessation of breathing, in the setting of complete obstruction, or stridor if a partial obstruction is present. Stridor is noisy respiration and is usually high-pitched and harsh. Stridor can occur during inspiration, expiration, or both phases of breathing. The pattern of stridor relative to the respiratory cycle can help to localize the site of obstruction. Inspiratory stridor is associated with obstruction at or above the glottis. Expiratory stridor is related to obstruction of a major bronchus. Biphasic stridor usually relates to subglottic or tracheal obstruction. Stridor may be present at rest or may be evoked

***Table 9–1.** Causes of Adult Upper Airway Obstruction*

Trauma	**Foreign Body**
Maxillofacial	Food
Oral cavity	Vomitus
Pharyngeal	Dentures/teeth
Laryngotracheal	Blood clot
Penetrating neck	Miscellaneous ingested objects
Blunt neck	
Infection	**Inflammatory**
Ludwig's angina	Caustic ingestion
Peritonsillar abscess	Radiation therapy
Retropharyngeal abscess	Thermal
Deep neck space infection	Anaphylaxis
Supraglottitis	Angioedema
Tetanus	Granuloma
Respiratory papillomatosis	Granulation tissue
	Neurologic
	Coma
	Vocal cord paralysis
Neoplasm Intrinsic	**Miscellaneous**
Oral cavity	Tracheomalacia
Pharynx	Lingual thyroid enlargement
Larynx	Tracheostomal stenosis
Trachea	Functional laryngeal dyskinesia
Neoplasm Extrinsic	
Thyroid	
Esophagus	
Lymphoma	

during deep, rapid breathing. A patient with upper airway obstruction usually demonstrates an inspiratory phase that is longer than the expiratory phase; the normal inspiratory phase is less than two thirds as long as the expiratory phase.

Chest retractions or use of accessory muscles for breathing may be noted. These signs indicate the need for increased effort to inspire. Patients may become fatigued because of this effort and may display restlessness or agitation. Clearly, sedation is contraindicated for these symptoms. Tachypnea and tachycardia commonly occur with airway obstruction. A respiratory rate of more than 20 breaths per minute is considered elevated. Increased respirations compensate for reduced tidal volumes.

Voice or speech alterations may be noted. Hoarseness can occur because of vocal cord abnormalities or dysfunction. A muffled voice can be caused by supraglottic and pharyngeal masses. Complete aphonia may occur with severe laryngeal injuries. The patient may be unable to swallow his or her own secretions and may expectorate saliva or bloody secretions. This difficulty may be related to pain or to dysfunction of the swallowing mechanism as well as to mechanical obstruction. Blood and blood-tinged secretions are signs of mucosal injury. Subcutaneous emphysema may be present and indicates disruption of the aerodigestive tract.

Additional signs may or may not be present, depending on the cause of the airway obstruction. There may be obvious blunt or penetrating injuries of the head and neck. Neck swelling resulting from infection, hemorrhage, or neoplasm may be present. Skin discoloration caused by subcutaneous bleeding, infection, or other agents may be noted. Deformities of the maxillofacial region may be present because of fractures.

Evaluation

For a patient with a compromised airway, an immediate, thorough assessment of the degree of airway obstruction is required. A general overall primary survey of the patient and determination of the precipitating event causing the airway obstruction is also necessary. Impending or complete airway obstruction mandates that an emergency airway be secured by mouth-to-mouth resuscitation, mask ventilation, endotracheal intubation, or surgical intervention (cricothyroidotomy or tracheotomy). Clinical judgment must determine the urgency with which the airway is controlled in the case of a compromised but stable airway. (Emergency airway procedures are described in detail in subsequent sections of this chapter.)

The potential for associated cervical spine injury should be recognized in all trauma patients, and care should be exercised to protect the patient from neurologic injury during airway management. Emergency airway control in a patient with a cervical spine injury is discussed later.

HISTORY

A patient should be questioned about the onset, duration, and progression of dyspnea. Any history of injury, trauma, caustic or foreign body ingestion, or prior intubation or tracheotomy should be elicited. The presence of associated symptoms should be determined, too, specifically, stridor, pain, loss of consciousness, dysphagia, odynophagia, otalgia, bleeding, hoarseness, or fever. If the patient is unresponsive or unable to communicate, a history should be obtained from family members, friends, or witnesses. A history of prior medical problems or airway events such as angioedema should be obtained.

PHYSICAL EXAMINATION

A complete head and neck examination should be performed if the airway is stable and immediate airway intervention is not necessary. Particular attention should be directed to the oral cavity, oropharynx, larynx, and hypopharynx. The integrity of the dentition should be determined in trauma patients. Mirror or fiberoptic laryngoscopy should be performed.

The source and degree of active hemorrhage should be determined if possible. The inferior limit of the airway obstruction should be determined, as airway control below that level is necessary.[1] The chest should be examined visually and by auscultation. Breath-sound intensity and distribution should be determined. Associated chest injuries and pneumothorax should be considered in trauma patients. Bronchial obstruction as a result of foreign bodies such as fractured teeth or blood clots may occur.

Vital signs—respiratory rate, heart rate, blood pressure, and temperature—should be determined. Arterial blood gases should be obtained, but patients with evolving upper airway obstruction may have minimal decreases in PaO_2 and mild increases in $PaCO_2$ compared to baseline values. Pulse oximetry is also useful for the evaluation of the degree of hypoxemia. Pulse oximetry measures arterial oxygen saturation. Below an arterial oxygen saturation level of 90%, the PaO_2 can be estimated by subtracting 30 from the arterial oxygen saturation value.

The severity of the obstruction and the decision to perform airway intervention should be based on clinical factors, not laboratory results. In particular, the physician should not be lulled into a false sense of security regarding the patient's airway status if normal blood gas values are noted.

IMAGING STUDIES

Imaging studies can be helpful in identifying the site of obstruction and the extent of disease in some patients. They may be particularly helpful in assessing the subglottic larynx and trachea, which are difficult to visualize by indirect laryngoscopy.

The cervical spine should be examined radiographically in a trauma patient. This is extremely important in order to rule out injury to the cervical spine, should spine manipulation be necessary in the patient's management. Chest radiographs should also be obtained in a trauma patient, in a patient with an abnormal chest examination, and in a patient with a history of foreign body ingestion.

Lateral and posteroanterior soft tissue radiographs of the head and neck may be helpful in evaluating the pharynx, larynx, and trachea. Some foreign bodies are radiopaque and can be localized by performing imaging studies. A narrowing or displacement of the air column may be observed. It should be emphasized that the degree of airway obstruction in general is not determined by imaging studies but, rather, is determined clinically.

Transportation of the patient from a controlled environment, such as the emergency room, intensive care unit, or operating room, to an imaging suite can be hazardous if the airway obstruction worsens. Position changes such as the supine positioning of a patient for a computed tomography (CT) scan may further compromise the airway. Therefore, any patient with a compromised airway who is transported should be accompanied by a physician equipped with the necessary airway equipment who can secure the patient's airway should intervention be necessary.

CT scanning may be helpful to evaluate maxillofacial injuries, infections, and neoplasms. The information provided by a CT scan may give the physician additional information regarding compromise of the airway and may aid in directing therapeutic intervention for these conditions. In general, magnetic resonance imaging is not used for the evaluation of acute upper airway obstruction.

Arteriography may be indicated in cases of penetrating facial and neck trauma (penetrating neck trauma is discussed in Chapter 12).

FLOW-VOLUME LOOPS

Flow-volume loops are respiratory function tests that may provide additional information regarding the severity, location (extrathoracic or intrathoracic), and nature (fixed or variable) of the obstruction.[2–4] In this study, the patient achieves a single, maximal effort, respiratory cycle (inspiration and expiration). Airflow is plotted against volume for both inspiration and expiration, creating a graph in the shape of a loop (Fig. 9–1). The study is effort-dependent and thus requires a cooperative patient as well as special equipment and examiner expertise.

Airway obstruction results in diminished airflow. The effect of airway lesions on flow-vol-

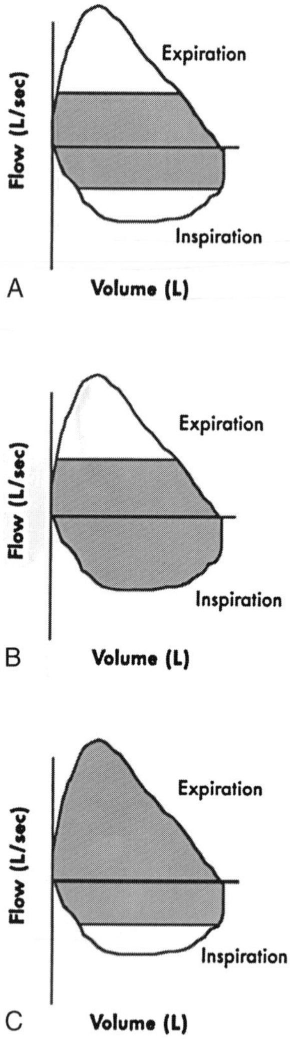

Figure 9–1. Flow-volume loops in upper airway obstruction. A normal flow-volume loop is shown by the solid lines. The shaded area represents the flow limitation for each type of upper airway obstruction. A: Fixed obstruction. B: Variable intrathoracic obstruction. C: Variable extrathoracic obstruction. (From Lynch JP, Quint LE. Tracheobronchial and esophageal manifestations of systemic diseases. In Cummings CW et al., eds. Otolaryngology: Head and Neck Surgery, 3rd ed. St. Louis, Mosby–Year Book, 1998, p. 2344.)

ume loops varies according to whether the obstruction is stiff (fixed) or pliable (variable). A fixed obstruction such as tracheal stenosis causes similar limitations in airflow during both inspiration and expiration (Fig. 9–1A). In contrast, variable obstructions, because they are subject to transmural pressure gradients, affect inspiration and expiration differently, depending on their location relative to the thorax. Variable intrathoracic lesions preferentially diminish expiratory airflow (Fig. 9–1B), whereas variable extrathoracic obstructions compromise primarily inspiratory airflow (Fig. 9–1C). The Bernoulli effect may contribute to further flow compromise in cases of flaccid airway lesions.

In normal individuals, the inspiratory and expiratory flow rates at mid–vital capacity ($\dot{V}I_{50}$ and $\dot{V}E_{50}$) are nearly equal.[5] In variable extrathoracic obstruction, the ratio of $\dot{V}E_{50}$ to $\dot{V}I_{50}$ ($\dot{V}E_{50}/\dot{V}I_{50}$) is greater than 1.15. In contrast, in variable intrathoracic obstruction, the $\dot{V}E_{50}/\dot{V}I_{50}$ ratio is usually less than 0.90.[5] For a fixed obstruction, $\dot{V}E_{50}$ and $\dot{V}I_{50}$ are generally equal.

In general, we use the airflow at midinspiration ($\dot{V}I_{50}$) to gauge the degree of inspiratory airflow impairment. Most patients do well at rest with a $\dot{V}I_{50}$ airflow of more than 1.5 L/sec. Flow-volume loops can be repeated serially in order to objectively monitor the clinical course or the result of therapeutic intervention.[4]

ENDOSCOPY

Direct inspection by direct laryngoscopy, tracheoscopy, bronchoscopy, and esophagoscopy is indicated if major injury to the oropharynx, hypopharynx, larynx, trachea, or esophagus is suspected.[1] In general, flexible bronchoscopes and esophagoscopes are preferred to rigid endoscopes because of the ease of insertion, visual quality, and diminished risk of esophageal perforation. Rigid bronchoscopes and esophagoscopes are indicated for the retrieval of foreign bodies in the bronchus or esophagus. In penetrating neck injuries, endoscopy should be performed prior to neck exploration, if possible, to assess the neuromuscular integrity of the pharynx and larynx and to incorporate this information into the surgical plan.[1]

Priorities

AIRWAY MANAGEMENT

A number of options for managing the airway are available for use in a patient with upper airway obstruction. The decision to use a particular approach depends upon numerous factors, including the degree, cause, location, and evolution of the obstruction, as well as factors unique to the patient. Proper judgment is necessary to differentiate a patient who can be carefully observed and managed medically from a patient who requires immediate or expeditious interventional airway control. The following sections discuss the various options for airway management.

LOCATION TO BE USED FOR AIRWAY MANAGEMENT

If immediate airway control is necessary, it should be performed emergently without transfering the patient to another location. Some situations arise, however, in which the patient's airway is stable enough to allow safe transport to a more controlled environment such as an operating room. The decision to transport a patient requires sound clinical judgment and careful weighing of the benefits of moving the patient against the risks of doing so. The stability of the patient and the location of the destination are factors that must be considered. If a decision is made to transfer the patient to another location, the patient must be accompanied by personnel capable of airway intervention who have airway management equipment, should intervention be necessary en route.

MEDICAL MANAGEMENT

Careful observation with medical management is a reasonable plan for selected patients with mild or moderate, stable upper airway obstruction. This plan requires patient management in an intensive care unit with close observation by health care professionals who are able to monitor the airway status and detect changes in the degree of airway impairment. Intubation equipment, a tracheotomy set, and a physician capable of airway management must be readily available. Should the airway deteriorate, interventional control by intubation or creation of a surgical airway is necessary.

Vital signs and pulse oximetry should be monitored and a baseline arterial blood gas reading obtained. The patient's respiratory and mental status should be carefully watched and symptoms intermittently assessed.

A patient who has a bacterial infection should receive appropriate intravenous antibiotics. Infectious emergencies of the neck are covered in Chapter 19. Inflammatory processes require medications appropriate for the condition. Adjuncts to observational airway management include oxygen administration, racemic epinephrine, corticosteroids, heliox, and continuous positive airway pressure (CPAP). These adjuncts are discussed in the following sections.

Supplemental oxygen delivered by humidified face mask is helpful in maintaining blood oxygenation (Fig. 9–2). Humidity in the respiratory circuit moistens the airway mucosa and thins secretions. Supplemental oxygen may depress the respiratory drive in some patients with

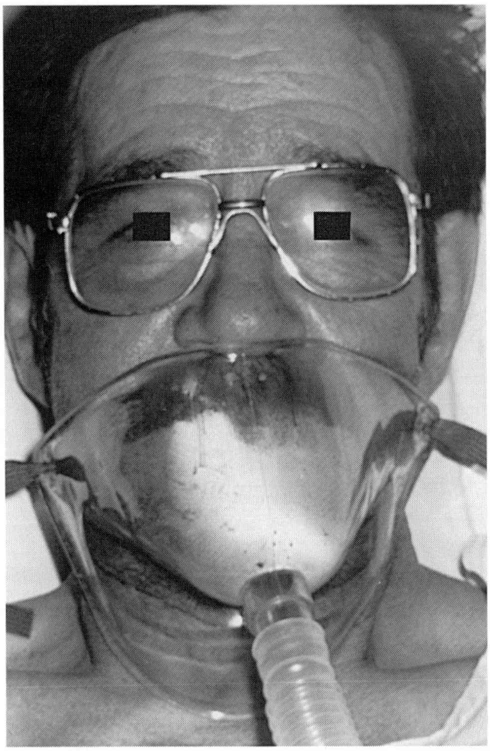

Figure 9–2. A humidified face mask for oxygen administration.

chronic lung disease, and for this reason, arterial blood gases should be followed to monitor for hypercapnia.

Racemic epinephrine can be delivered by nebulizer and may reduce upper airway edema; however, it has a relatively short duration of effect. Intravenous corticosteroids such as dexamethasone 1.0 to 1.5 mg/kg or methylprednisolone 5 to 7 mg/kg may also be beneficial in reducing edema and preventing further swelling.[6] Dexamethasone can be given every 8 hours for several days without the need to perform a steroid taper.

Heliox, a mixture of helium and oxygen, benefits some patients with moderate airway obstruction by improving ventilation.[7–9] Heliox, which is given in a mixture of 70% to 80% helium and 30% to 20% oxygen, has less density than either air or oxygen. Because of Graham's law, this lower density provides improved airflow. The work of breathing is decreased because of decreased airway resistance to flow. Clinical effectiveness is normally apparent in several minutes.[9] Mixtures of heliox containing less than 60% helium are too dense to be clinically valuable, so patients who require an FIO_2 of more than 40% are not candidates for heliox. Administration of heliox may decrease fatigue in patients with partial airway obstruction who are struggling to breathe. Heliox is also useful for patients who have reversible airway obstructions that are expected to be transient and for temporizing before a definite means of airway control, such as a tracheotomy, is performed. CPAP delivered by face mask may be beneficial for patients with airway obstruction due to loss of tone of the upper airway musculature such as that which occurs after general anesthesia and periodic upper airway obstruction such as that which occurs in obstructive sleep apnea. A face mask that achieves a seal around the nose and mouth and is secured in place with straps allows positive pressure to be delivered by bag or ventilator. The positive pressure prevents upper airway collapse during inspiration.

THE UNCONSCIOUS PATIENT

When faced with a patient who appears to be unconscious, the rescuer should attempt to awaken the victim in order to confirm the unconscious state. If the patient is unresponsive, resuscitation should commence and help should be requested. The steps of cardiopulmonary resuscitation, the ABCs (airway, breathing, circulation), should follow an initial assessment.

The first priority in resuscitation is the airway. It should be opened by neck extension (Fig. 9–3) if there is no suspected cervical injury, and the mandible should be displaced forward (the jaw-thrust maneuver) (Fig. 9–4). These positional maneuvers help to alleviate obstruction caused by tongue prolapse and hypotonia of the pharyngeal musculature, which can occur in an unconscious patient. An oropharyngeal airway (Fig. 9–5A) or a nasopharyngeal airway (Fig. 9–5B), if available, can be placed to open the pharyngeal airway.

The next priority is breathing (ventilation). Signs of adequate respirations should be assessed by inspection and auscultation. If breathing is not adequate, assisted ventilation should be initiated using a mouth-to-mouth, mouth-to-mask or bag-to-mask technique.[10] If resuscitation equipment is available, a bag-valve hand resuscitator is preferred for ventilation because supplemental oxygen can be administered (Fig. 9–6). If ventilation is impaired, the presence of an obstructed airway must be considered. A supine Heimlich maneuver should be performed and the pharynx swept with an index finger to clear away any dislodged foreign body. If

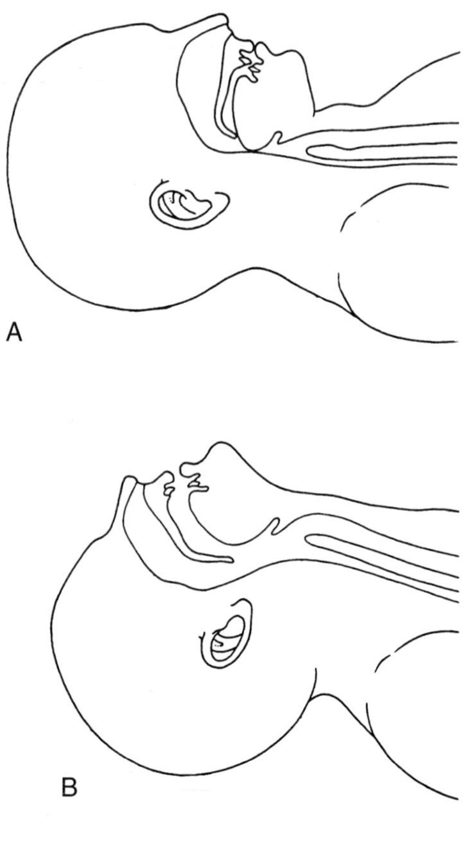

Figure 9–3. A: Obstructed airway. B: Neck extension to open airway.

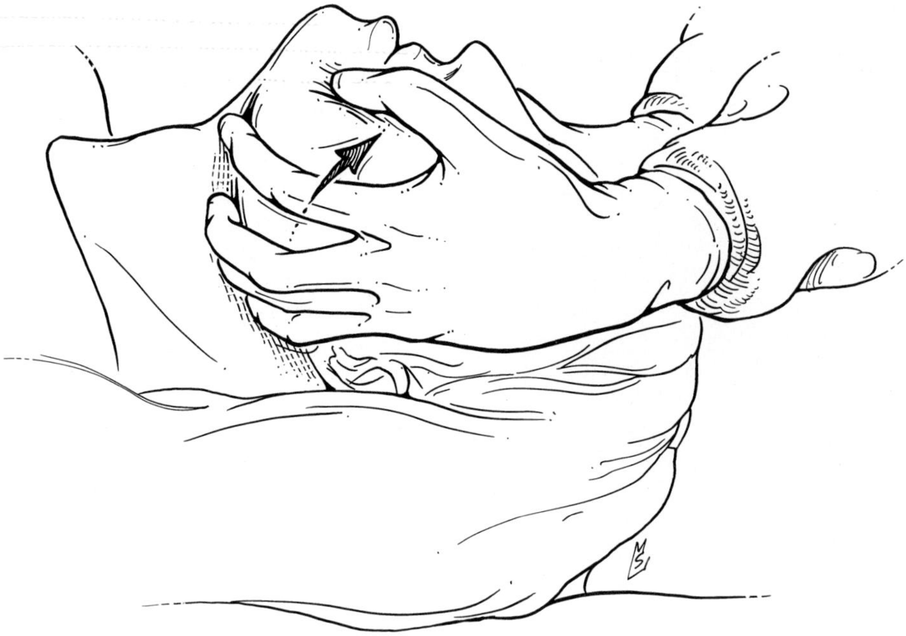

Figure 9–4. The jaw-thrust maneuver.

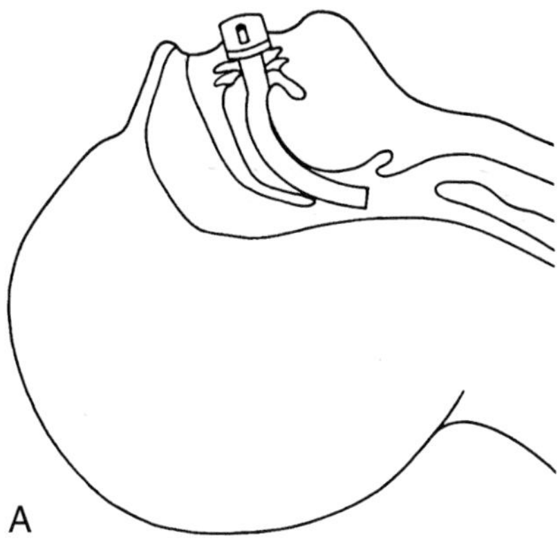

A

Figure 9–5. A: Oropharyngeal airway. B: Nasopharyngeal airway.

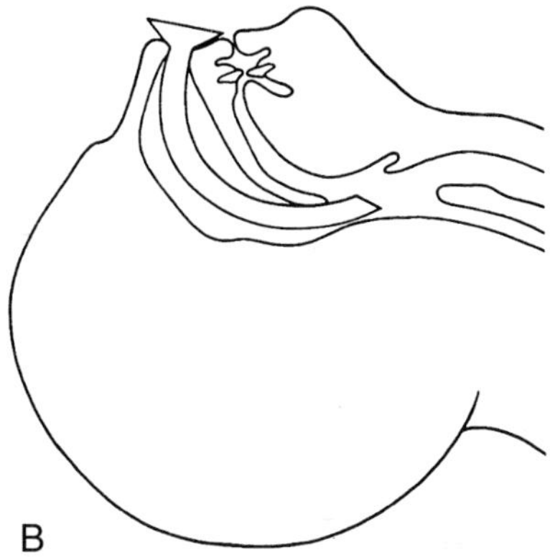

B

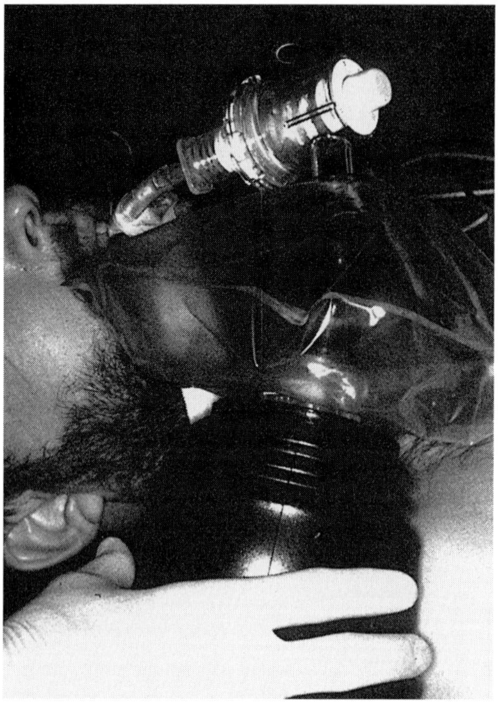

Figure 9–6. Ventilation with a hand resuscitator.

ventilation is still unsuccessful, intubation should be attempted when intubation equipment is available. Lack of intubation equipment or inability to intubate the patient requires that a cricothyroidotomy or tracheotomy be performed to secure the airway.

Circulation should be assessed by palpating the carotid pulse. The absence of a pulse is an indication to begin closed chest compression. Chest compressions should be given at a rate of 80 to 100 per minute. For every five compressions, an assisted breath is delivered. Cardiopulmonary resuscitation is covered in Chapter 2.

THE HEIMLICH MANEUVER

In conscious patients with witnessed or suspected foreign body obstruction of the upper airway, the Heimlich maneuver should be performed.[11, 12] Patients commonly display a universal choke sign, with the hands grasping the throat (Fig. 9–7). Foreign body airway obstruction can occur while eating; this is referred to as the "café coronary."[13] Factors that contribute to this problem include alcohol ingestion, dentures, incomplete chewing of food, and talking while eating.[13]

The Heimlich maneuver consists of forceful subdiaphragmatic thrusts and is performed by standing behind the victim, placing a fist below the xiphoid process, holding the fist with the other hand, and forcefully compressing the abdomen with superiorly directed thrusts (Fig. 9–8). The thrusts should continue until the foreign body has been dislodged or the victim loses consciousness. The Heimlich maneuver can also be performed in the supine position if the patient is unconscious. The pharynx then should be swept with an index finger in order to clear a dislodged foreign body. Next, ventilation or intubation should be attempted. If these interventions fail to secure the airway, a cricothyroidotomy or tracheotomy should be performed.

FACE-MASK VENTILATION

Mask ventilation is the primary airway intervention for an unconscious patient who requires airway control and ventilation when mask ventilation equipment is available. A form-fitting mask, a self-inflating bag-valve hand ventilator (Ambu bag), and an oxygen source are the necessary equipment. The mask (Fig. 9–9) is placed

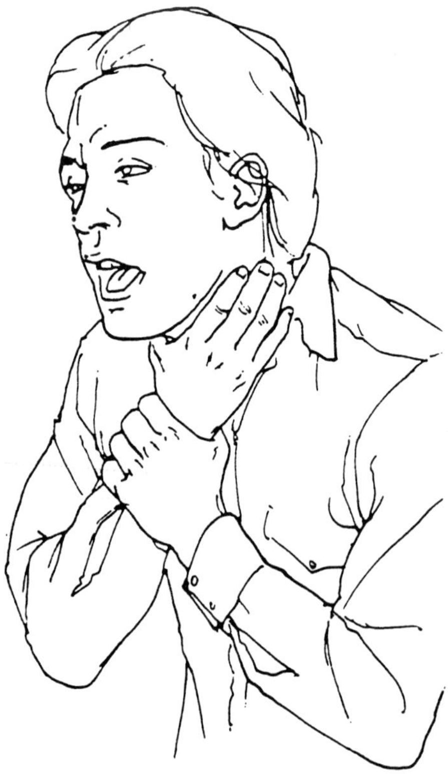

Figure 9–7. Universal choke sign. (From Emergency Cardiac Care Committee and Subcommittees, American Heart Association. Guidelines for cardiopulmonary resuscitation and emergency cardiac care, II: adult basic life support. JAMA 1992; 268:2192. Copyright 1992, American Medical Association.)

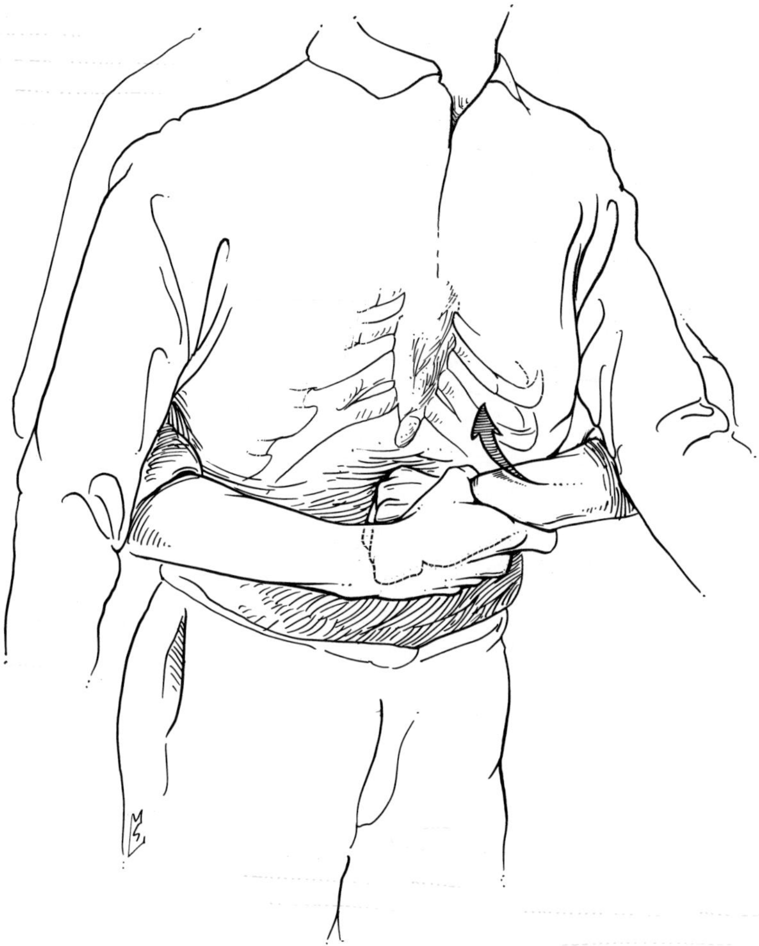

Figure 9–8. The Heimlich maneuver. The rescuer stands behind the victim and grasps the fist with the other hand, placing both hands just below the rib cage. The fist is pressed into the abdomen with a quick upward thrust.

over the nose and mouth and held to the face with the nondominant hand to create an airtight seal (Fig. 9–10). Mask straps or a two-person approach may improve the mask seal. The patient is ventilated by squeezing the hand ventilator with the dominant hand or with the help of an assistant. An oral airway may facilitate ventilation. Inadequate ventilation mandates airway control by tracheal intubation, laryngeal mask airway, percutaneous jet ventilation, cricothyroidotomy, or tracheotomy.

Ventilation by mask is continued until the patient is fully oxygenated. If a rapidly reversible condition such as a narcotic overdose is the cause of the patient's lack of airway maintenance, mask ventilation can be continued until the patient has regained the ability to protect his or her own airway. Otherwise, intubation is indicated to better secure the airway and protect against aspiration. If the mask airway is adequate, intubation should be an orderly procedure performed by an experienced individual. If intubation is problematic, mask ventilation is continued between intubation attempts. If a patient cannot be intubated after multiple attempts, a tracheotomy is required, preferably in the controlled environment of the operating room. Mask ventilation may result in gastric distention, which can be alleviated by the placement of a nasogastric tube.

INTUBATION

OROTRACHEAL INTUBATION

The orotracheal route is generally the preferred method for intubation of the trachea (Fig. 9–11). Indications for orotracheal intubation include airway obstruction, apnea, hypoxia, hypoventilation, prevention of aspiration, need for hyperventilation (e.g., a head injury), and therapy requiring intubation. Benefits of orotracheal intubation over mask ventilation include increased ability to keep the airway patent, to

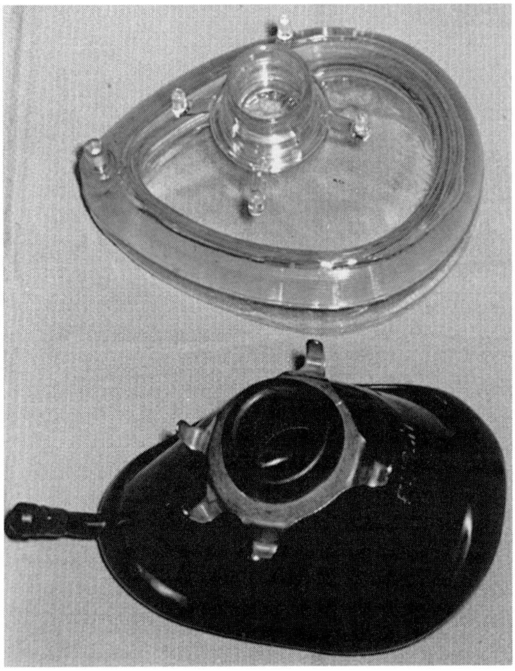

Figure 9–9. Face masks for ventilation.

deliver oxygen, and to ventilate the patient. In addition, with intubation, there is a decreased risk of aspiration. Contraindications to orotracheal intubation include trismus, severe facial trauma, continued seizures, and severe obstruction of the glottic larynx.

In the emergency setting, the most experienced intubator should perform intubation. Before intubation, 100% oxygen should be delivered for several minutes to preoxygenate the patient. Preoxygenation allows for at least 5 minutes of apnea before oxygen desaturation below 90% occur.[14]

A Yankauer handpiece should be available to suction secretions. Orotracheal intubation requires a laryngoscope for visualization of the larynx. Commonly used laryngoscopes consist of a battery handle to which a flanged blade with a lightbulb is attached (Fig. 9–12). The tip of the curved MacIntosh blade is placed into the vallecula. The tongue, the larynx, and the epiglottis are elevated, not levered, thus exposing the glottis (Fig. 9–13). A straight Miller blade is placed beneath the epiglottis, which is lifted to expose the glottis (Fig. 9–14). Once the glottis is visualized, an appropriately sized endotracheal tube is placed, under direct vision, between the vocal cords and into the trachea.

A variety of endotracheal tubes in different sizes, both cuffed and uncuffed, should be available (Fig. 9–15). Standard endotracheal tubes are made of polyvinyl chloride, which is slightly stiff but softens at body temperature. An endotracheal tube with a 7.5- or 8.0-mm internal diameter (I.D.) is usually appropriate for male patients and one with a 7.0- or 7.5-mm I.D. for female patients. Once the endotracheal tube has been placed, the cuff is inflated with enough air to create a seal. Adequate ventilation of the patient and proper positioning of the tube in the trachea are confirmed. The chest should be auscultated, and equal breath sounds should be noted. The endotracheal tube is secured with tape and an orotracheal airway is placed to prevent the tube from being bitten and thus obstructed. A chest radiograph should be obtained.

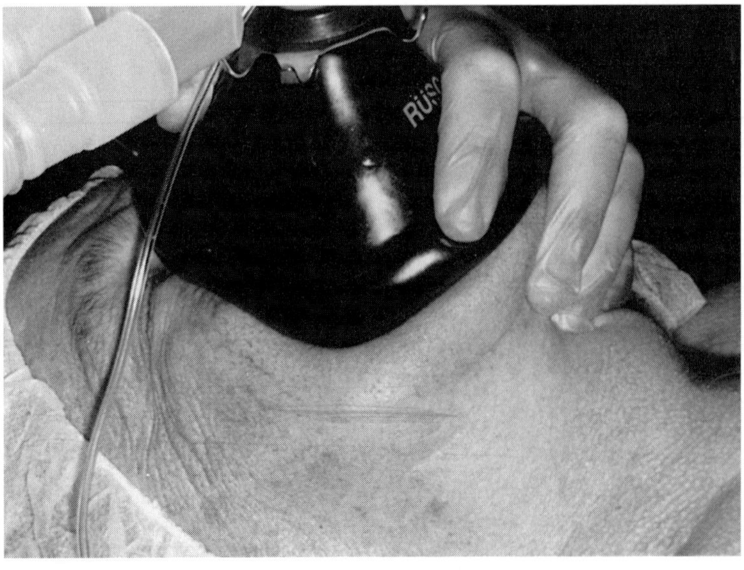

Figure 9–10. Face mask ventilation. The mask is held to the face to create an airtight seal.

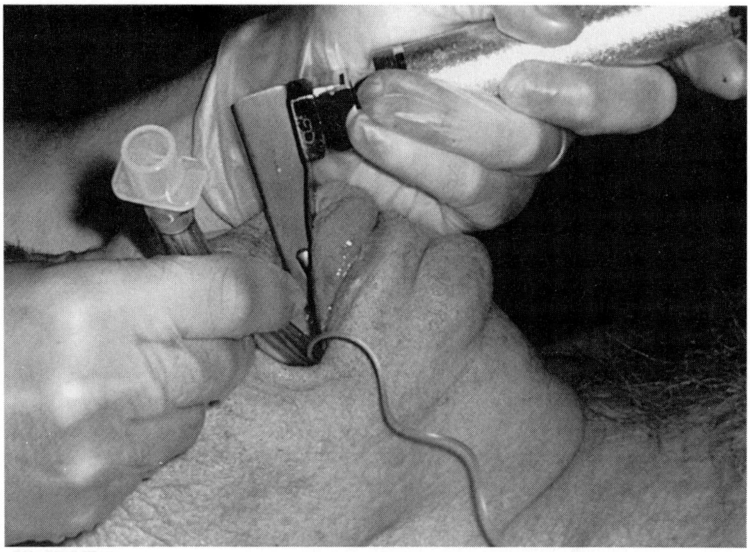

Figure 9–11. Orotracheal intubation.

Cricoid pressure may aid visualization of the vocal cords during laryngoscopy. In addition, a flexible stylet can be placed within the endotracheal tube to allow curvature of the tube, which helps in placing the tip of the endotracheal tube into the glottis (Fig. 9–16). Care must be taken that the stylet does not protrude beyond the tip of the endotracheal tube.

All trauma patients and those who have recent or unclear histories of oral ingestion should be considered to have stomach contents. Cricoid pressure (the Sellick maneuver) during mask ventilation and intubation (Fig. 9–17) is recommended in these patients to reduce the risk of aspiration of refluxed gastric contents.[15] If intubation is unsuccessful, mask ventilation should be resumed between intubation attempts. Repeated inability to intubate requires another method of intubation, cricothyroidotomy, or tracheotomy.

Complications of orotracheal intubation include tooth injury, hemorrhage, perforation, laryngeal injury, esophageal intubation, recurrent laryngeal nerve injury, and tracheoesophageal fistula.

RAPID-SEQUENCE INTUBATION

An awake or agitated patient who requires emergent endotracheal intubation should be given a rapid-sequence intubation.[16] In rapid-

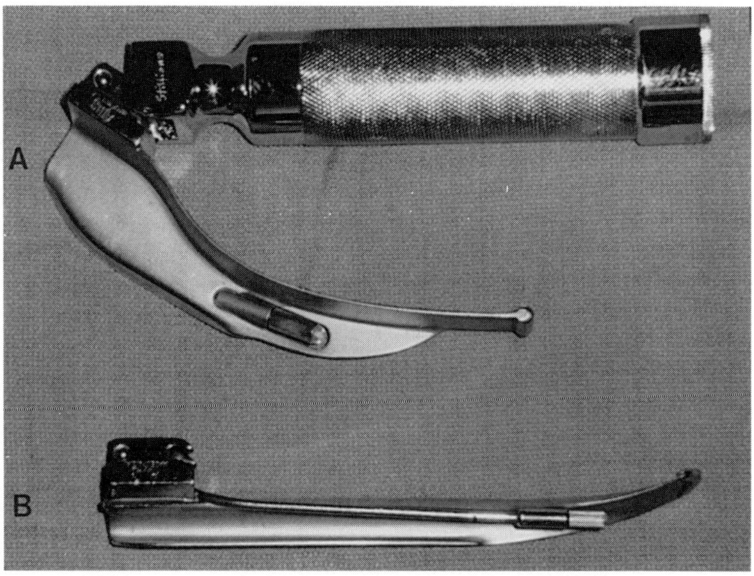

Figure 9–12. Laryngoscope for intubation. A: Curved MacIntosh blade. B: Straight Miller blade.

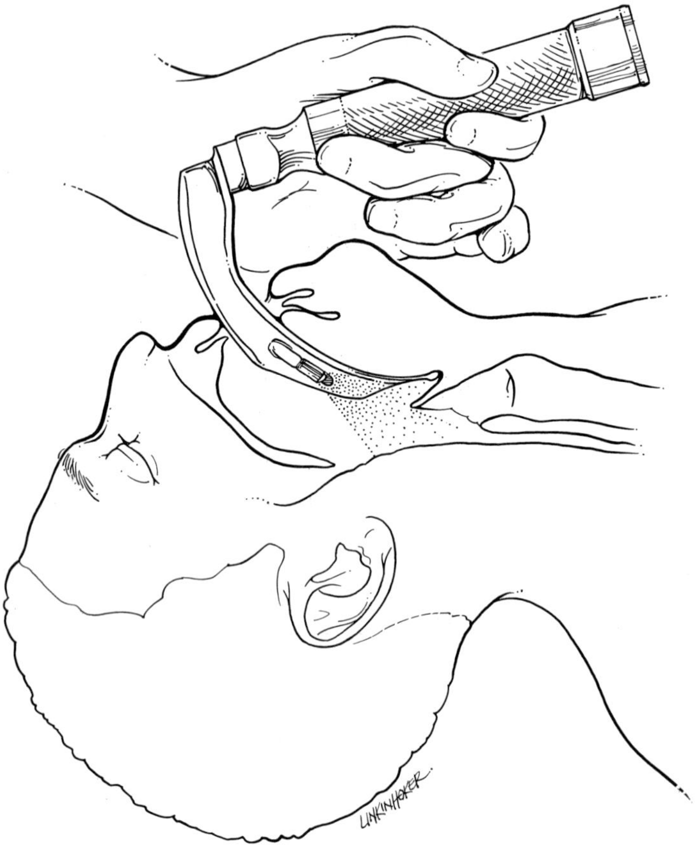

Figure 9–13. Placement of a MacIntosh laryngoscope blade during intubation. Note the placement of the tip of the blade into the vallecula.

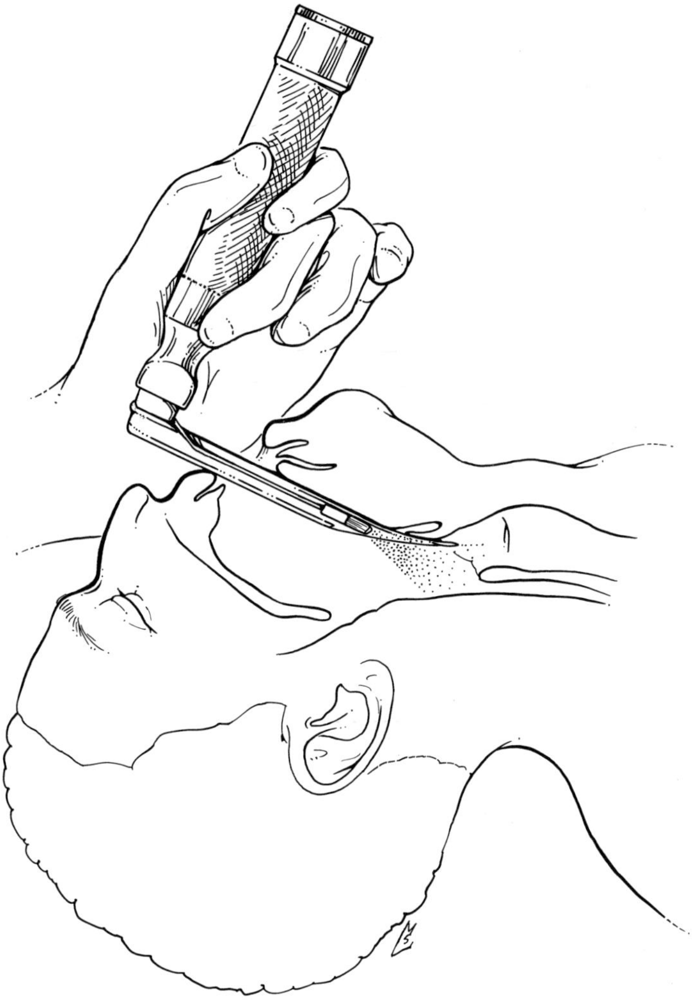

Figure 9–14. Placement of a Miller laryngoscope blade during intubation. The tip of the blade is placed beneath the epiglottis.

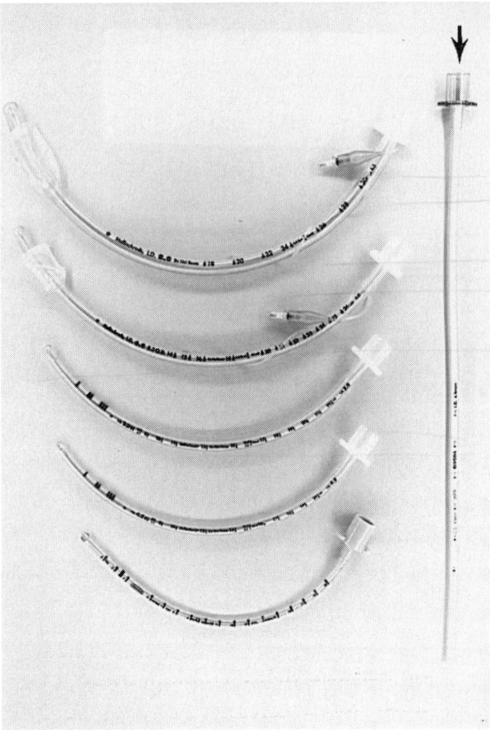

Figure 9–15. Endotracheal tubes of different sizes and lengths, cuffed and uncuffed. An epiglottis tube is indicated by the arrow.

sequence intubation, a rapid-onset paralytic agent such as succinylcholine (1 to 2 mg/kg) is administered along with a short-acting sedative such as thiopental (3 to 6 mg/kg) to induce unconsciousness. The Sellick maneuver is then performed to prevent aspiration (see Fig. 9–17). This maneuver causes the cricoid cartilage to occlude the esophageal introitus and prevents regurgitation of gastric contents into the hypopharynx. The patient is immediately intubated after paralytic relaxation occurs. After intubation, mechanical ventilation is begun and a longer-acting paralytic agent with a sedative can then be administered.

NASOTRACHEAL INTUBATION

Nasotracheal intubation is one option for intubation in a breathing patient. This can be accomplished either without visualization, which is known as "blind" nasotracheal intubation, or with guidance from a fiberoptic bronchoscope.[17] With blind nasotracheal intubation, the tube is directed into the laryngeal introitus with guidance from the intensity of breath sounds heard at the open end of the tube. Use of the nasotracheal approach to intubation requires familiarity with the technique. A contraindication to blind nasotracheal intubation is apnea.[17]

Nasotracheal intubation is of value for emergency airway control in a patient with suspected cervical spine injury because it eliminates the need to manipulate the cervical spine and in a patient in whom oral cavity access is limited by trismus, injury, edema, or hematoma. Suspected injury of the base of the cranium is a contraindication to nasotracheal intubation so as to avoid intracranial tube placement. Complications of nasotracheal intubation include epistaxis, nasal or pharyngeal injury, submucosal dissection, intracranial placement, nasal pressure necrosis, and esophageal intubation.

RIGID ENDOSCOPIC INTUBATION

Rigid endoscopic intubation relies on the use of a closed laryngoscope, which is used for direct laryngoscopy, to facilitate intubation or on the use of a rigid bronchoscope to allow direct airway intubation and ventilation. A laryngoscope such as the Holinger anterior commissure laryngoscope (Fig. 9–18A) or the larger-diameter Dedo operating laryngoscope (Fig. 9–18B) may aid in visualizing the larynx in cases in which visualization with an open-blade laryngoscope is

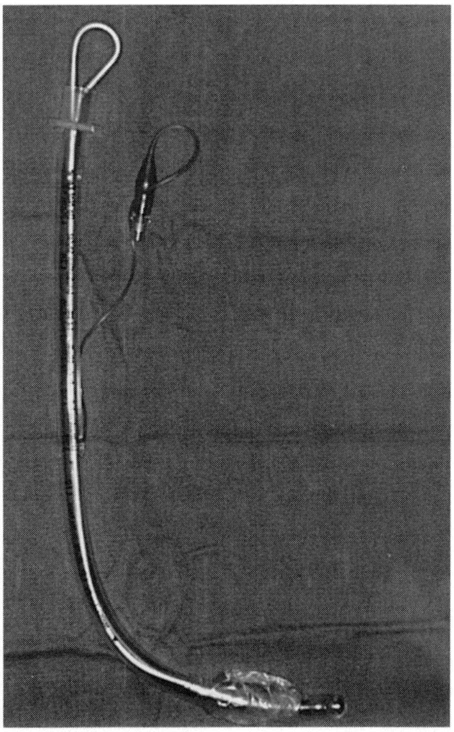

Figure 9–16. An endotracheal tube with a flexible stylet. The stylet allows for endotracheal tube curvature to assist in the placement of the tube.

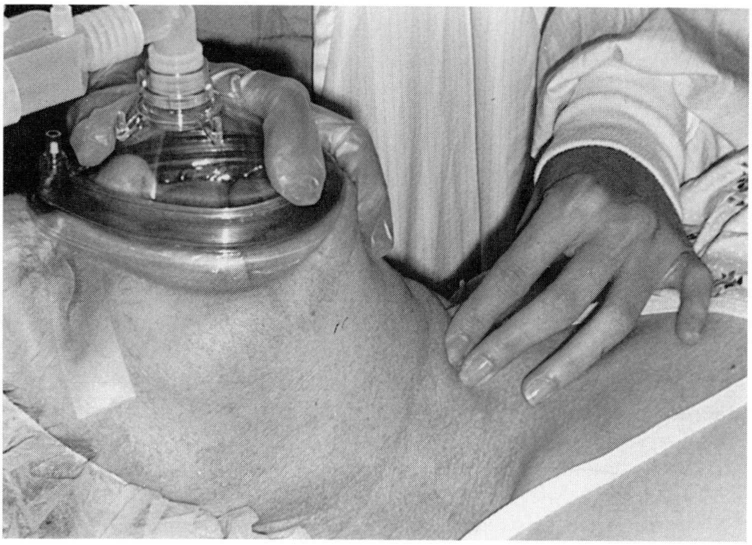

Figure 9–17. Cricoid pressure (Sellick maneuver) during mask ventilation to reduce the risk of aspiration. This maneuver may also assist in visualizing the glottis during intubation.

problematic. Unlike blade laryngoscopes, these closed-tube laryngoscopes displace tissues circumferentially, thus improving visualization of the larynx and facilitating suctioning. These laryngoscopes are useful in situations such as the presence of obstructing oropharyngeal or supraglottic masses or tumors and the inability to visualize the glottis because of anatomic distortion or tumor, friable or bleeding tumors, or fixed glottic, subglottic, or tracheal lesions. The rigid bronchoscope can be used in the presence of the same indications and is preferred for airway management in cases of tracheal or bronchial foreign bodies and selected obstructing tracheal tumors.

The Holinger anterior commissure laryngoscope is an excellent instrument for visualizing the glottis because of its configuration, with a narrow waist and anteriorly flared tip (Fig. 9–18A). Its design improves ease of placement at the glottis. Once the glottis is visualized with the laryngoscope, there are two options for intubation. The first option is to intubate through the laryngoscope. The trachea can be intubated directly through the laryngoscope and the patient can then be ventilated. Because of the relatively narrow lumen of the Holinger anterior commissure laryngoscope, however, it will accommodate only up to a 5-mm I.D. uncuffed endotracheal tube. Another option is to place a

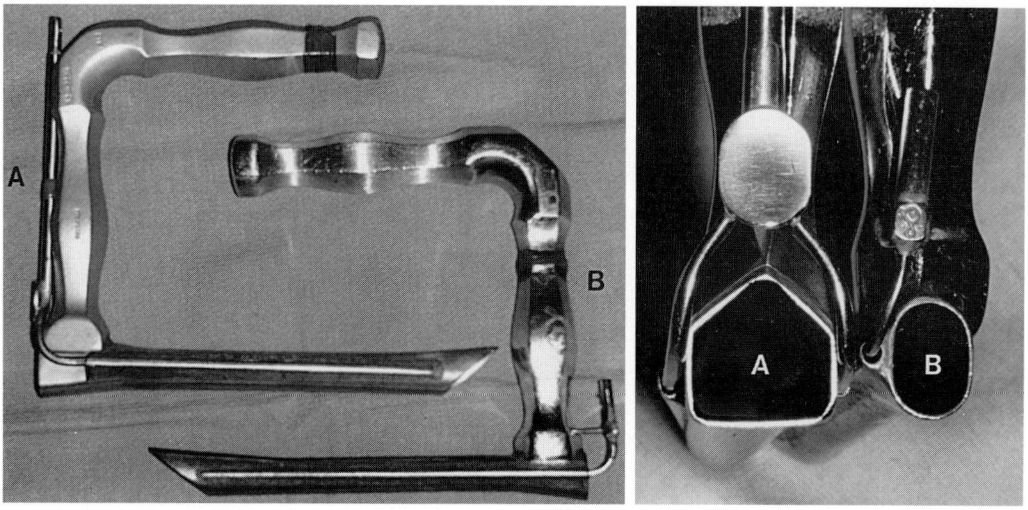

Figure 9–18. Laryngoscopes for rigid endoscopic intubation. A: Dedo laryngoscope; note the large-diameter lumen. B: Holinger laryngoscope; note the narrow waist and the anteriorly flared tip.

gum elastic bougie (an Eschmann stylet) through the laryngoscope into the trachea (Fig. 9–19A). The laryngoscope is removed, leaving the Eschmann stylet in place (Fig. 9–19B) and the patient is then intubated over the Eschmann stylet (Fig. 9–19C).[18, 19] The Eschmann stylet accommodates endotracheal tubes of 6 mm I.D. and larger.

On the other hand, the Dedo operating laryngoscope provides a larger-diameter lumen than the Holinger anterior commissure laryngoscope. Although glottic visualization may be more difficult in some cases with a Dedo laryngoscope than with a Holinger anterior commissure laryngoscope, its wider lumen allows for direct placement of up to 7.5-mm I.D. cuffed endotracheal tubes through the laryngoscope for intubation (Fig. 9–18A). Once an endotracheal tube has been placed into the trachea through the laryngoscope, the tube cuff can be inflated and the patient ventilated (Fig. 9–20A). Once the patient has been stabilized, the respiratory circuit adapter is removed from the endotracheal tube and the tube is grasped with alligator forceps (Fig. 9–20B). The laryngoscope is removed while the endotracheal tube is held in position with the forceps. The tube adapter is then replaced, the endotracheal tube cuff inflated, and the patient ventilated. Having a variety of endotracheal tube sizes available is important when using this intubation method. The choice of tube is determined by the location and degree of obstruction and the need for an endotracheal tube cuff.

Another alternative for ventilation, once the glottis is exposed with a closed laryngoscope or rigid bronchoscope, is jet ventilation. A jet ventilation adapter can be attached to the end of the laryngoscope and used to ventilate the patient (Fig. 9–21). Alternatively, a flexible-tube jet ventilator can be passed into the trachea through the laryngoscope and jet ventilation can be performed.

A rigid bronchoscope can be used to intubate the trachea directly. This method may be beneficial for the bypass of tracheal obstructions and for the management of foreign bodies in the airway. The bronchoscope is placed, under direct vision, through the glottis and into the trachea. For ventilation, the end of the bronchoscope is occluded with an eye piece and the respiratory circuit is attached to the ventilation

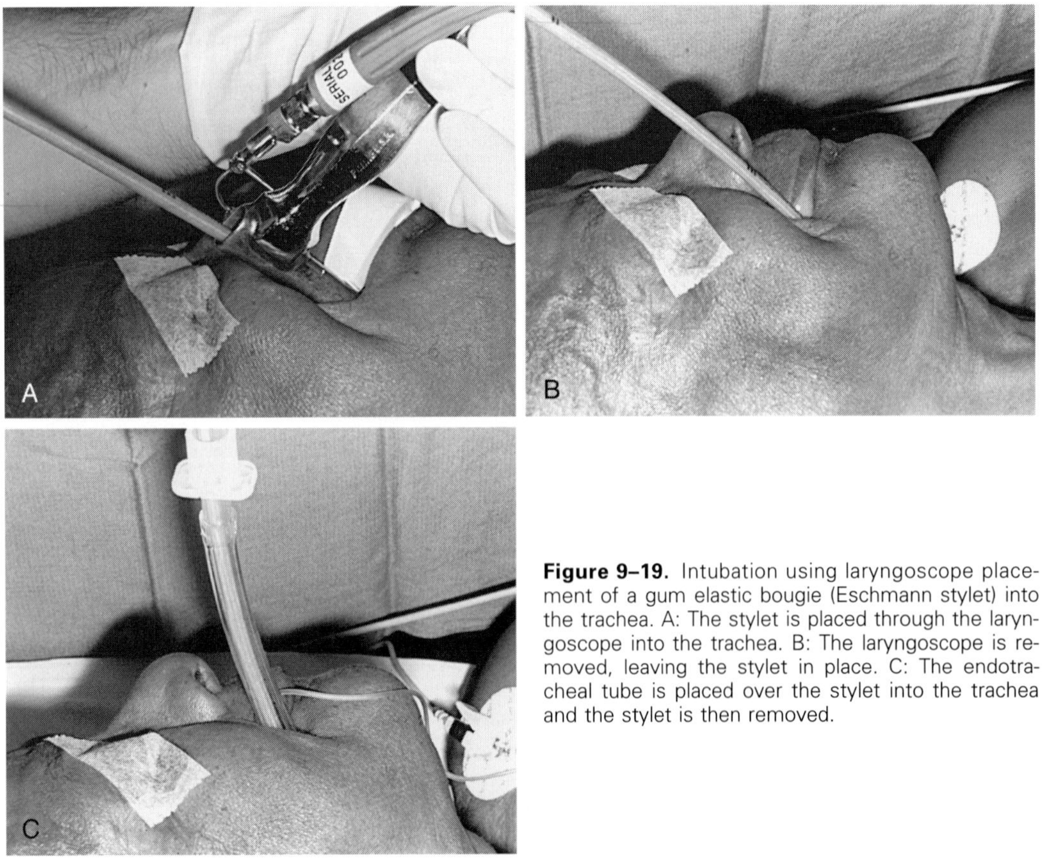

Figure 9–19. Intubation using laryngoscope placement of a gum elastic bougie (Eschmann stylet) into the trachea. A: The stylet is placed through the laryngoscope into the trachea. B: The laryngoscope is removed, leaving the stylet in place. C: The endotracheal tube is placed over the stylet into the trachea and the stylet is then removed.

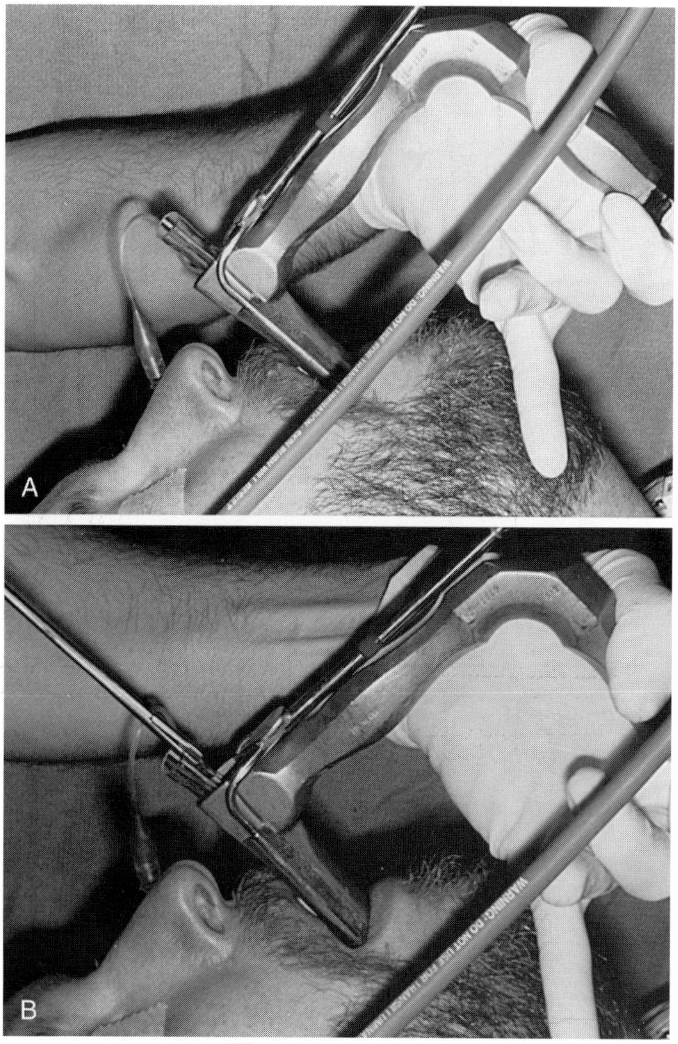

Figure 9–20. Rigid endoscopic intubation through a Dedo laryngoscope. A: The endotracheal tube is placed into the trachea through the laryngoscope. B: The endotracheal tube is grasped with alligator forceps and held in position as the laryngoscope is removed.

side port of the bronchoscope (Fig. 9–22). An Eschmann stylet can also be placed through the bronchoscope and used to facilitate the insertion of an endotracheal tube after the bronchoscope has been withdrawn, as described above.

FIBEROPTIC INTUBATION

Intubation under the guidance of a flexible bronchoscope is a safe method of intubating an awake patient with upper airway compromise.[20–22] Indications for fiberoptic intubation include trismus, oral cavity obstruction due to tumor, edema, or hematoma, upper airway neoplasms, infections, and cervical spine trauma. It is also a commonly performed method of airway control in the setting of an anticipated difficult airway such as in a morbidly obese patient with obstructive sleep apnea.

Awake fiberoptic intubation can be performed via an oral or a transnasal route. The transnasal route is easier and is better tolerated by the patient; it is indicated if the oral route is obstructed. Although fiberoptic intubation can be performed in an unconscious patient who is able to be ventilated but not intubated, soft tissue collapse and secretions make this approach problematic, and other methods of intubation are generally preferred.

To perform fiberoptic intubation, the patient's nose is topically decongested and anesthetized. In addition, the pharynx is anesthetized with lidocaine or benzocaine spray. Having the patient sit rather than lie in a supine position facilitates visualization of the larynx by the intubator, who faces the patient. Passage of successively larger, lubricated (2% lidocaine jelly) nasopharyngeal airways through the larger nasal cavity helps to dilate the nasal passage. A

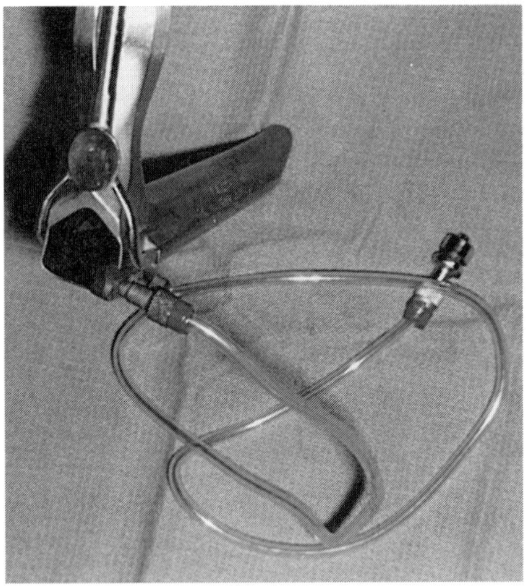

Figure 9–21. A jet ventilator adapter attached to a laryngoscope for jet ventilation.

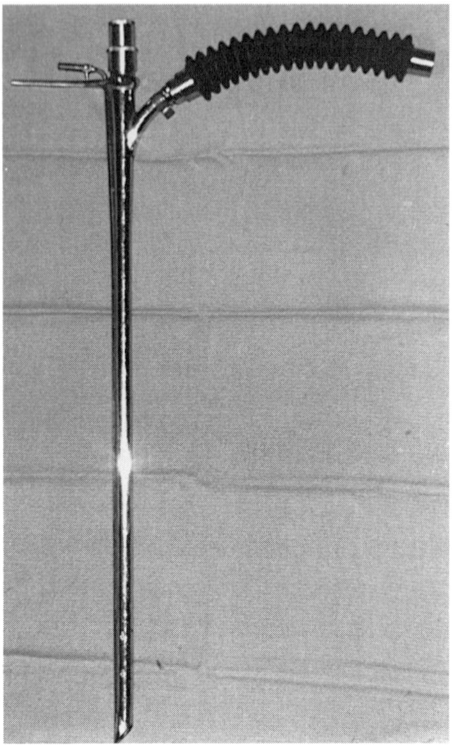

Figure 9–22. A rigid bronchoscope with respiratory circuit attached to a bronchoscope side port for ventilation.

nasotracheal tube (7 mm I.D. or larger), warmed and softened by soaking in warm saline, is then passed through the nose and nasopharynx into the oropharynx. Care must be taken to avoid passage of the tip of the endotracheal tube too far into the pharynx, which may elicit gagging.

A lubricated fiberoptic bronchoscope is then passed through the endotracheal tube (Fig. 9–23), taking care not to pass it through the Murphy eye of the endotracheal tube, and any secretions are suctioned. The glottis is visualized and the larynx is anesthetized with several applications of 2 mL 1% lidocaine delivered through the bronchoscope side port. The suction port is temporarily occluded during lidocaine instillation. The fiberoptic bronchoscope is then advanced through the glottis and into the midtrachea. The endotracheal tube is advanced over the fiberoptic bronchoscope into the trachea. The position of the endotracheal tube above the carina is confirmed visually. If there is difficulty in advancing the endotracheal tube into the larynx, the tube should be rotated and gen-

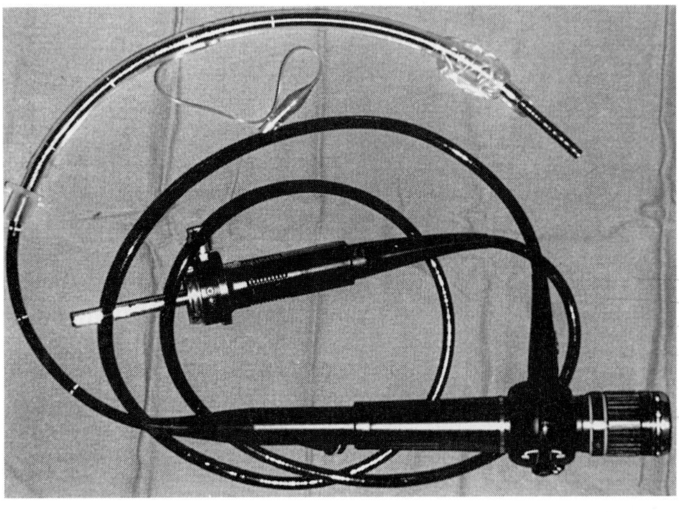

Figure 9–23. A flexible bronchoscope is placed through an endotracheal tube for fiberoptic intubation.

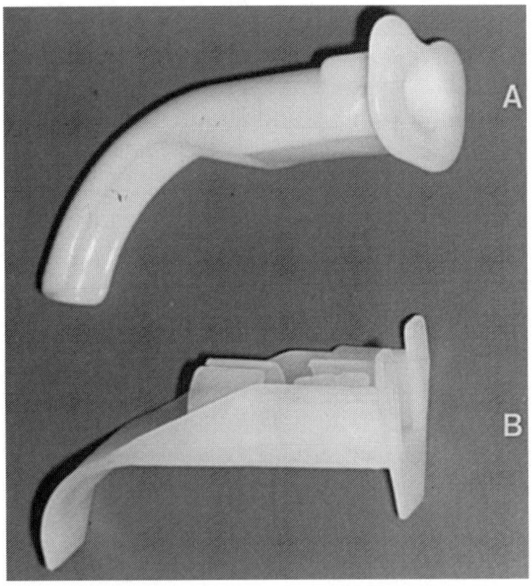

Figure 9–24. Oral airways for oral fiberoptic intubation. A: Closed-tube oral airway. B: Ovassapian oral airway.

tly readvanced. Continued inability to advance the tube may necessitate the use of a smaller tube.

Oral fiberoptic intubation is an alternative to nasotracheal fiberoptic intubation if the nasal cavity or nasopharynx is obstructed or if there is active nasal hemorrhage. This method requires good oropharyngeal anesthesia and a cooperative patient, as gagging may make this technique difficult. An oral airway guide for fiberoptic intubation facilitates orotracheal fiberoptic intubation (Fig. 9–24). The airway is inserted into the patient's mouth. A lubricated endotracheal tube is placed into the airway guide, and the fiberoptic endoscope is introduced through the endotracheal tube into the oropharynx. The glottis is visualized and the endoscope is advanced into the trachea. An advantage of the Ovassapian airway guide (Fig. 9–24B) is that it can be removed easily without disconnecting or removing the endotracheal tube.

Fiberoptic intubation requires skill, time, and the patient's cooperation. Complications include hemorrhage, esophageal intubation, laryngospasm, and other potential complications of intubation.[21, 23] Failure to intubate by this method is most commonly related to inability to visualize the airway because of blood or secretions.[22, 24]

RETROGRADE INTUBATION

Retrograde intubation is a technique of tracheal intubation that is performed by puncturing the cricothyroid membrane with a needle, passing a flexible guide wire through the needle cephalad, and retrieving the wire through the mouth or nose.[25] An endotracheal tube is then passed over the guide wire into the larynx. The guide wire is removed and the endotracheal tube is advanced into the trachea. An alternative retrograde technique is to load a flexible bronchoscope with an endotracheal tube and advance the bronchoscope over the guide wire, which is passed through the suction channel of the bronchoscope.[26] Retrograde intubation is reserved for cases in which other methods of intubation have failed. Complications of this technique are unusual but include airway injury and failure to intubate.

DIGITAL INTUBATION

Digital, or tactile, intubation is a method of intubation that may be useful if the glottis cannot be visualized by laryngoscopy.[27] To perform digital intubation, an endotracheal tube with a stylet that is bent at the end is directed, under digital guidance, past the epiglottis into the glottic aperture. The stylet is removed before the tube is advanced into the trachea. This technique should be reserved for patients who are unconscious so as to avoid bite injury to the intubator. Complications include those associated with standard endotracheal intubation.

LARYNGEAL MASK AIRWAY

The laryngeal mask airway (LMA) is a ventilation device consisting of a tube with an inflatable silicone mask (Fig. 9–25).[28] The deflated mask is placed into the pharynx and positioned

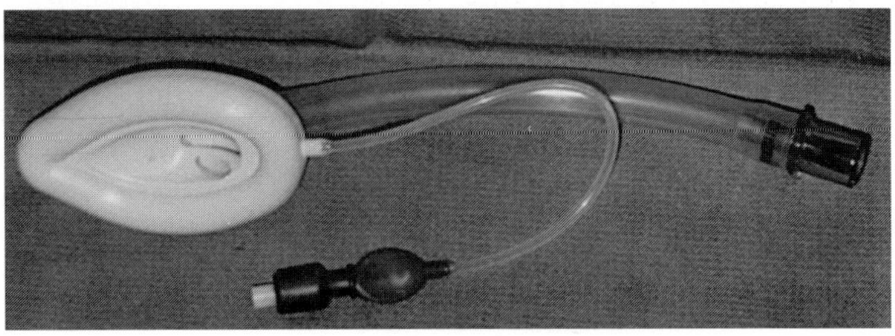

Figure 9–25. Laryngeal mask airway.

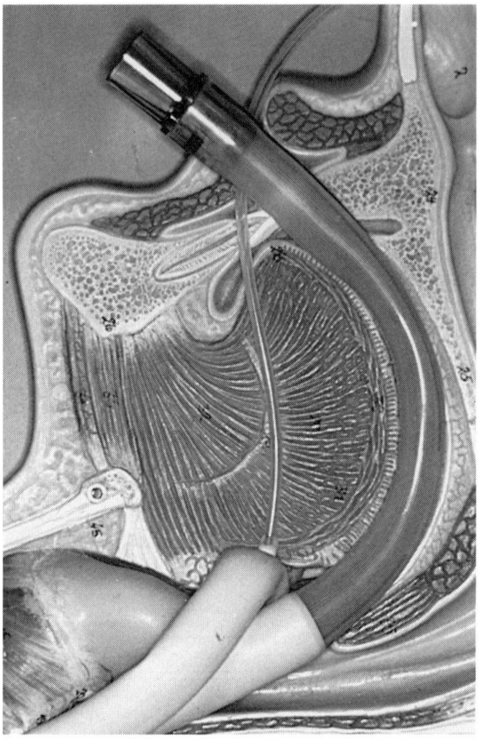

Figure 9–26. Laryngeal mask airway in position in the pharynx.

above the larynx. The mask cuff is inflated without holding the device. This creates an air seal in the pharynx above the larynx (Fig. 9–26). Although most commonly used for nonemergent airway control during general anesthesia, the LMA is an alternative for temporary emergency supraglottic airway control if standard mask ventilation is inadequate and intubation is unsuccessful. After the airway is stabilized with the LMA, an endotracheal tube is placed. Intubation with a small (less than 6.0 mm I.D.) endotracheal tube directly through the LMA can be performed. Alternatively, an Eschmann stylet can be placed through the LMA into the trachea and the LMA then exchanged for an endotracheal tube over the stylet. In addition, fiberoptic visualization of the airway through the LMA can be performed and may facilitate passage of a stylet into the trachea.[29]

The LMA is not as effective as an endotracheal tube in preventing pulmonary aspiration of gastric contents. Contraindications for an LMA include severe trismus, obstruction of the glottic or subglottic larynx, pharyngeal or supraglottic mass or abscess, and laryngospasm.

OTHER DEVICES

Several other commercially available devices for the management of the emergency airway or to facilitate intubation include the Esophageal-Tracheal Combitube, the light wand, and the Bullard laryngoscope. These devices are not universally available and familiarity with a particular device is necessary in order for it to be effective. These instruments should be considered to be adjuncts to the management of the emergency airway and not first-line methods of airway control. They are discussed here to alert the reader to their availability. It is beyond the scope of this chapter to consider the uses, benefits, and limitations of each of these devices in detail, and the reader is directed elsewhere for more in-depth understanding of their use.[30]

ESOPHAGEAL-TRACHEAL COMBITUBE

The Esophageal-Tracheal Combitube (Kendall, Mansfield, MA) is a device consisting of a double-lumen tube with two inflatable cuffs, one proximal and one distal (Fig. 9–27). The tube is advanced without visualization into the trachea or the esophagus. If the tube is placed into the trachea, the distal cuff is inflated and the patient is ventilated through the tracheal lumen, as with a standard endotracheal tube. If the esophagus is intubated, the proximal cuff, which seals the pharynx, and the distal cuff, in the esophagus, are inflated. The patient is ventilated through the esophageal lumen via side holes in the tube between the cuffs. This device is intended primarily for resuscitation by individuals not trained in endotracheal intubation. It has had high rates of success when used by paramedics for emergency airway management.[31]

LIGHT WAND

The light wand (Trachlight, Laerdal Medical, Wappingers Falls, NY), also known as the lighted stylet, is an intubating stylet with a handle and a fiberoptic light source at its tip.[32, 33] An endotracheal tube is placed on the device and the tip of the endotracheal tube is then directed toward the glottis (Fig. 9–28). The light on the stylet transilluminates the neck and directs placement of the endotracheal tube into

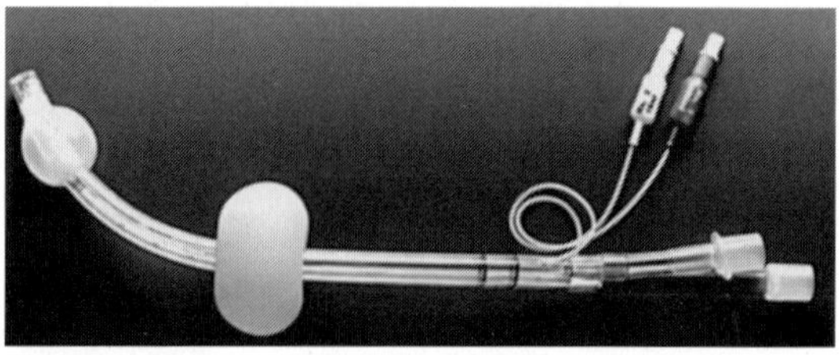

Figure 9–27. Esophageal-Tracheal Combitube. (Courtesy of Kendall, Mansfield, MA.)

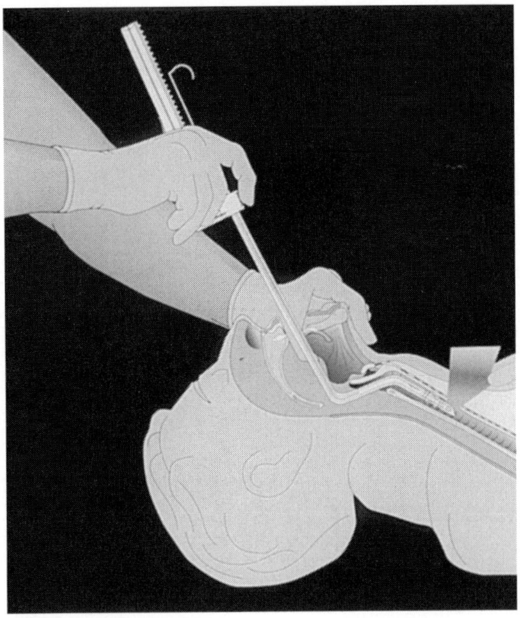

Figure 9–28. Intubation with a lighted intubating stylet (Trachlight). (Courtesy of Laerdal Medical, Wappingers Falls, NY.)

the larynx. The endotracheal tube is then advanced into the trachea.

BULLARD LARYNGOSCOPE

The Bullard laryngoscope (Circon, Stamford, CT) is a rigid, curved fiberoptic laryngoscope with an attachable endotracheal tube stylet designed to allow indirect visualization of the glottis (Fig. 9–29).[34, 35] The blade of the laryngoscope is placed into the oropharynx, the tongue and epiglottis are lifted, and the glottis is visualized. The endotracheal tube is then advanced over the stylet into the trachea.

PERCUTANEOUS TRANSTRACHEAL JET VENTILATION

A less invasive alternative to surgical cricothyroidotomy is percutaneous needle cricothyroidotomy with a large-bore intravenous catheter (12- or 14-gauge).[36] An intravenous catheter is too small to allow for spontaneous ventilation. Instead, ventilation of the patient is accomplished by intermittent delivery of high-pressure (50 psi) oxygen through a system with a manual flow interrupter and Luer-Lok connector (Fig. 9–30).

Indications for percutaneous transtracheal jet ventilation are the same as those for cricothyroidotomy. Contraindications include laryngotracheal pathology such as laryngeal fracture, subglottic stenosis, extrinsic tracheal compression, traumatic tracheal transection, obscured anatomic landmarks, for example by tumor or hematoma. Familiarity with the technique is also necessary for safe use.

The procedure is performed by first palpating the cricothyroid membrane (Fig. 9–31A). A 12- or 14-gauge angiocath attached to a syringe filled with several mL of saline is inserted through the cricothyroid membrane, and intraluminal placement is confirmed by aspiration of air into the syringe (Fig. 9–31B). The angiocath is directed caudally and the needle is removed from the angiocath. The catheter is then connected to the jet ventilator circuit and the patient is ventilated (Fig. 9–31C). Care must be taken to stabilize the catheter at the neck so as to avoid the dislodgment or kinking of the catheter. This is best done by an assistant. Adequate ventilation is confirmed by observing the chest rise and fall and by end-tidal carbon dioxide readings, if available. Adequate expiration, which is passive, must be allowed.

In cases of complete respiratory obstruction, a second catheter can be placed as an expiratory outlet, or surgical cricothyroidotomy must be performed.[1] In thin individuals in whom the

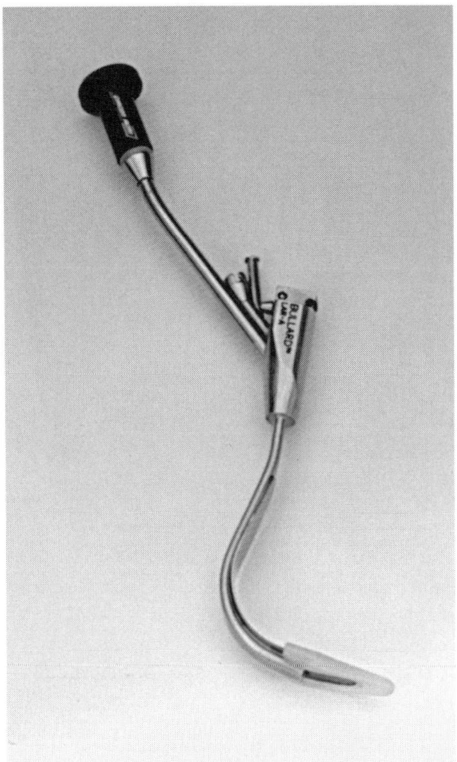

Figure 9–29. Bullard laryngoscope. (Courtesy of Circon, Stamford, CT.)

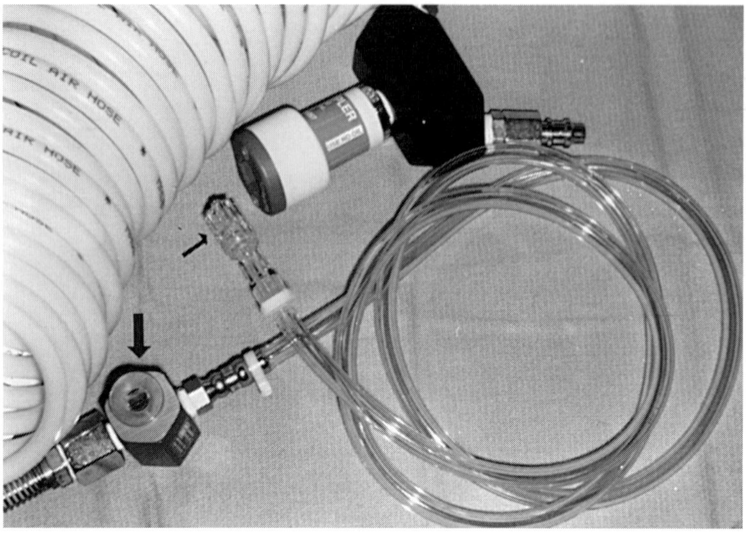

Figure 9–30. Jet ventilation delivery system with manual flow interrupter (large arrow) and Luer-Lok connector (small arrow).

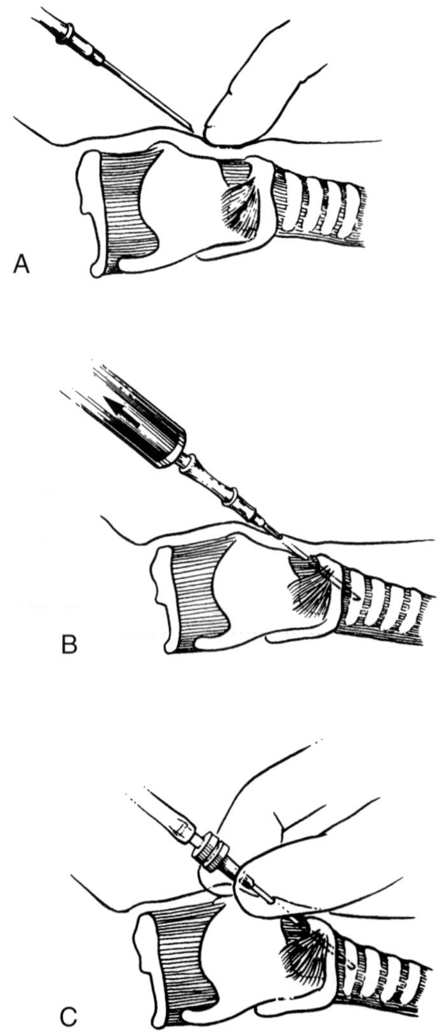

Figure 9–31. Percutaneous transtracheal jet ventilation. A: Palpation of cricothyroid membrane. B: Placement of angiocath through cricothyroid membrane and confirmation of intraluminal placement by aspiration of air into syringe. C: Catheter connected to jet ventilator circuit and stabilized. (From Cummings CW et al.: Atlas of Laryngeal Surgery. St. Louis, CV Mosby, 1984.)

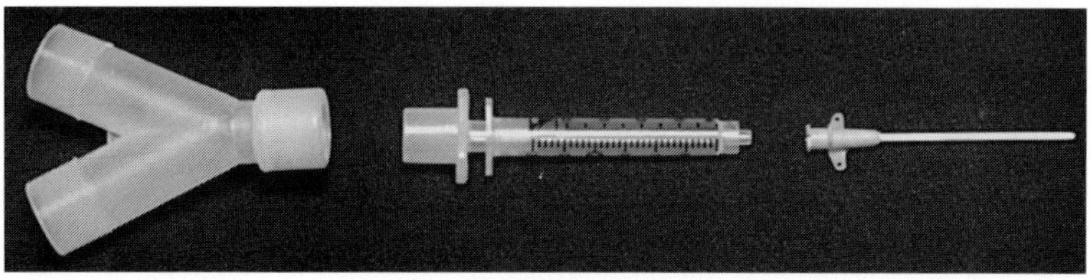

Figure 9–32. Connection between angiocath and respiratory circuit with a 7-mm endotracheal tube connector and the barrel of a 3-mL syringe.

trachea is easily palpated, catheter placement into the trachea is an alternative to cricothyroid membrane placement.

In order to be an effective alternative for emergency airway control, the equipment for transtracheal jet ventilation must be readily available. An alternative setup for oxygen delivery to the catheter can be constructed using equipment readily available in a hospital crash cart. The barrel of a 3-mL syringe and the connector of a 7.0-mm I.D. endotracheal tube fit together and can create a secure connection between the catheter and a bag-valve hand resuscitator (Fig. 9–32).[37] Transtracheal ventilation with the hand resuscitator allows for adequate short-term oxygenation and ventilation. Definitive airway control by intubation or tracheotomy should then be performed in an orderly fashion.

Potential complications of transtracheal ventilation include inability to ventilate due to catheter kinking, catheter displacement, hypercapnia, subcutaneous emphysema, pneumomediastinum, pneumothorax, pulmonary barotrauma, infection, and tracheal or esophageal perforation.

EMERGENCY CRICOTHYROIDOTOMY

Inability to mask-ventilate, intubate, or control the airway by an alternative technique mandates a surgical airway such as cricothyroidotomy or tracheotomy. All physicians should be capable of performing one of these procedures. Failure to attempt surgical access to the airway in the face of inability to control the airway by other methods will result in the death of the patient. It is better to attempt a surgical airway and fail than not to attempt one and lose the opportunity for the patient to live. Thus, the procedure must be performed when indicated without concern for operative complications or mortality.

Indications for emergency surgical airway access include maxillofacial trauma, laryngeal or pharyngeal edema, mass lesions of the pharynx and larynx, and bilateral vocal cord motion impairment. This procedure is most commonly performed in the emergency department, operating room, or intensive care unit.

Cricothyroidotomy has several advantages over tracheotomy for emergency airway control (Table 9–2). Cricothyroidotomy is technically easier and has a lower rate of significant complications than tracheotomy. Surgical landmarks for cricothyroidotomy are more readily identifiable than are those for tracheotomy. Even an inexperienced individual can perform cricothyroidotomy. For these reasons, many consider cricothyroidotomy to be the surgical procedure of choice for airway control. In our institution, cricothyroidotomy is performed twice as frequently as tracheotomy to obtain emergency surgical airway access.

Cricothyroidotomy refers to a surgical opening in the cricothyroid membrane, which is identified by palpating the cricothyroid space between the thyroid and cricoid cartilages (Fig. 9–33A). The skin overlying the cricothyroid space is injected with local anesthetic if the patient is conscious. The neck is prepared with an antiseptic solution. The thyroid cartilage is stabilized with the nondominant hand and an incision is made with a scalpel through the skin, subcutaneous tissue, and cricothyroid membrane (Fig. 9–33B). An endotracheal tube or tracheotomy tube is then inserted through the cricothyroidotomy incision and passed caudally into the trachea (Fig. 9–33C). Small-diameter tubes (e.g., a no. 4 tracheotomy tube) make intubation easier, as the cricothyroid space is approximately 9 mm wide.[38] The endotracheal or tracheotomy tube cuff is inflated and the patient is ventilated. If an endotracheal or tracheotomy tube is not readily available, the handle of the scalpel can be inserted through the

Table 9–2. *Advantages of Cricothyroidotomy Over Tracheotomy for Emergency Airway Control*

It is quicker.
It is simpler.
Identification of anatomic landmarks is easier.
There is a lower rate of significant complications.
It is easier for an inexperienced individual to perform.

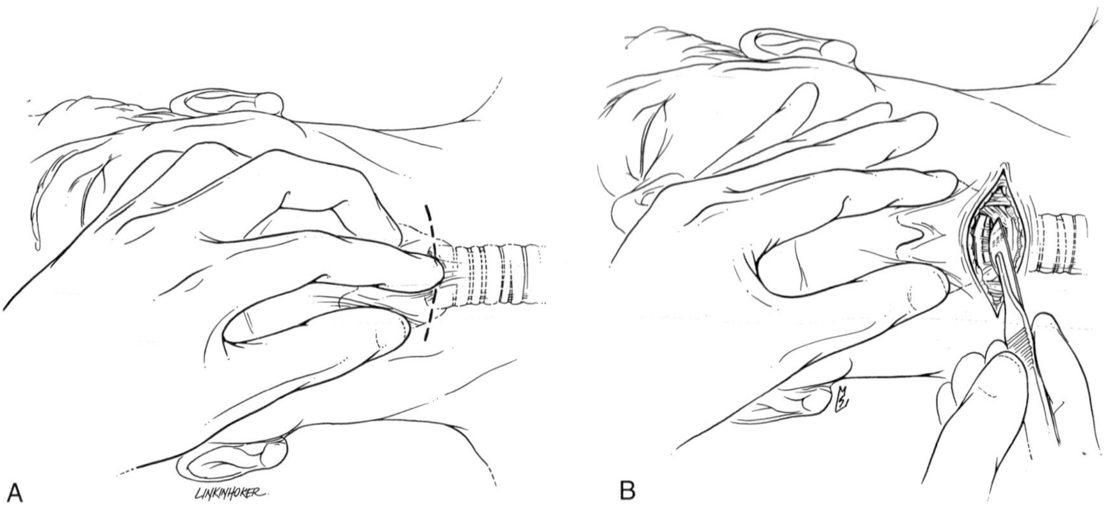

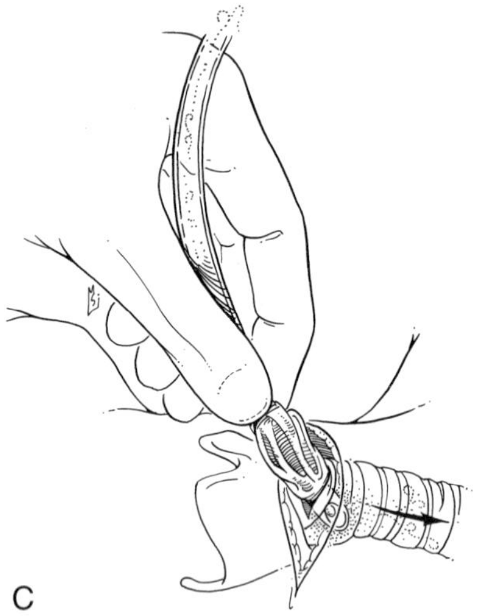

Figure 9–33. Emergency cricothyroidotomy. A: The cricothyroid membrane is palpated. B: A horizontal incision is made through the skin, subcutaneous tissues, and cricothyroid membrane. C: The endotracheal tube is passed into the trachea via the cricothyroidotomy incision.

cricothyroid membrane incision and rotated 90 degrees to maintain the airway.

Once the airway has been secured and the patient stabilized, the neck wound should be inspected and active hemorrhage controlled. The cricothyroid artery, a branch of the superior thyroid artery, runs transversely across the superior aspect of the cricothyroid membrane. In addition, anterior jugular veins and thyroid pyramidal lobes may traverse this area.

In general, direct laryngoscopy should be performed after emergency cricothyroidotomy to assess internal laryngeal injury. Any cartilage injury should be repaired. Unless decannulation is expected within several days, conversion to a formal tracheotomy and closure of the cricothyroidotomy in the operating room is recommended to avoid such complications of cricothyroidotomy as subglottic injury with stenosis.

Contraindications to cricothyroidotomy include inability to identify surgical landmarks and subglottic stenosis or mass. Cricothyroidotomy should also be avoided in children because of the small size of the pediatric cricothyroid space; instead, a tracheotomy is preferred.[39] Complications of emergency cricothyroidotomy include hemorrhage, infection (cellulitis, perichondritis), vocal cord injury, thyroid or cricoid cartilage injury, dysphonia, tracheal or esophageal injury, recurrent laryngeal nerve injury, subglottic stenosis, and subcutaneous emphysema. In addition, anatomic confusion may result in inadvertent entry through the thyrohyoid membrane.[40]

EMERGENCY TRACHEOTOMY

Emergency tracheotomy is an alternative to cricothyroidotomy for surgical airway access. It is the procedure of choice in a child, in a patient with unidentifiable cricothyroid membrane, and in a patient with subglottic stenosis or obstruction. In addition, surgeons familiar with tracheotomy may opt for tracheotomy over cricothyroidotomy in a patient who has favorable anatomy. A contraindication to emergency tracheotomy include obscured anatomic landmarks due to hematoma or tumor.

Emergency tracheotomy is performed after extending the neck, provided this maneuver is not contraindicated. The larynx is stabilized with the nondominant hand, and the cricoid cartilage is palpated. A vertical midline incision is made through the skin and subcutaneous tissues from the level of the cricoid cartilage, extending 4 to 5 cm inferiorly (Fig. 9–34A). The incision is then carried down between the strap muscles to the trachea (Fig. 9–34B). Hemorrhage may obscure the structures, but dissection can be guided by palpation. Care must be taken to avoid personal injury or injury to an assistant, if present, with the scalpel. The tracheal rings are divided vertically in the midline and opened with a finger or instrument (Fig. 9–34C). The cricoid cartilage and first tracheal ring are left intact if possible. An endotracheal tube is then placed into the trachea and directed caudally (Fig. 9–34D). Care must be taken to avoid mainstem bronchus intubation by maintaining the tip of the endotracheal tube in the trachea. The endotracheal tube cuff is inflated and the patient is ventilated. Once the airway has been stabilized, the wound is thoroughly inspected and any active bleeding is controlled. The specific location of tracheal entry should be determined. Esophageal injury requires appropriate repair. A chest radiograph should be obtained to rule out a pneumothorax.

Complications of emergency tracheotomy include hemorrhage from major blood vessels (the carotid and innominate arteries) or minor blood vessels (the anterior jugular vein, thyroid vessels, and thyroid gland), pneumothorax,

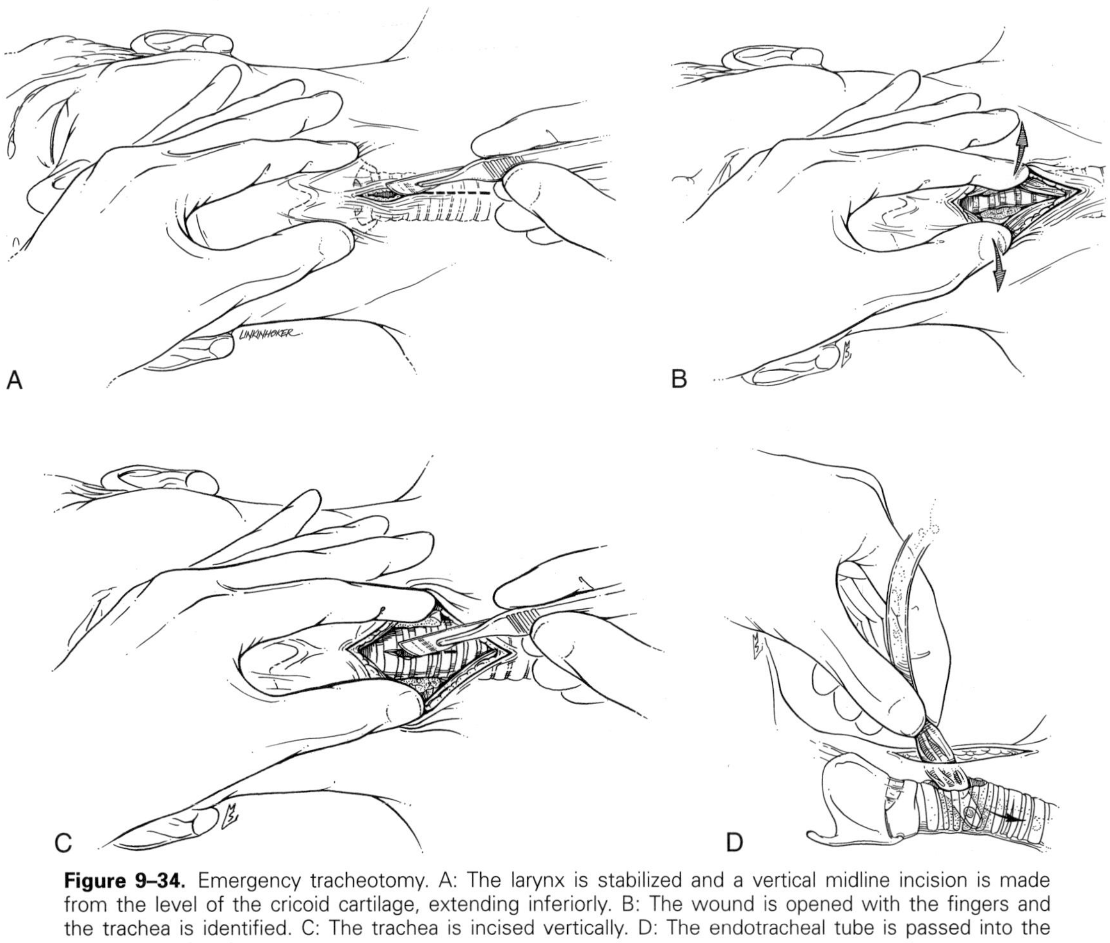

Figure 9–34. Emergency tracheotomy. A: The larynx is stabilized and a vertical midline incision is made from the level of the cricoid cartilage, extending inferiorly. B: The wound is opened with the fingers and the trachea is identified. C: The trachea is incised vertically. D: The endotracheal tube is passed into the tracheotomy incision.

pneumomediastinum, tracheoesophageal fistula, recurrent laryngeal nerve injury, cricoid cartilage injury, subglottic stenosis, tracheotomy tube obstruction or displacement, tracheal stenosis, and infection.

AWAKE TRACHEOTOMY

Indications for awake tracheotomy include impending airway obstruction, active hemorrhage in the oral cavity, oropharynx, or nasopharynx, and stenosis superior to the 4th or 5th tracheal ring. To perform an emergent awake tracheotomy, the midline lower neck is anesthetized with 1% lidocaine, and the neck is prepared with an antiseptic solution and sterilely draped without covering the patient's face (Fig. 9–35). Supplemental oxygen is delivered by face mask, so particular care must be taken to avoid an intraoperative fire if electrocautery is utilized. The patient is reassured during the procedure and additional local anesthesia is administered as necessary. Tracheotomy is performed in a timely fashion as described earlier. An endotracheal tube is introduced if general anesthesia is to be administered. Otherwise, a tracheotomy tube is inserted and the flanges of the tube are secured to the neck with sutures and twill ties.

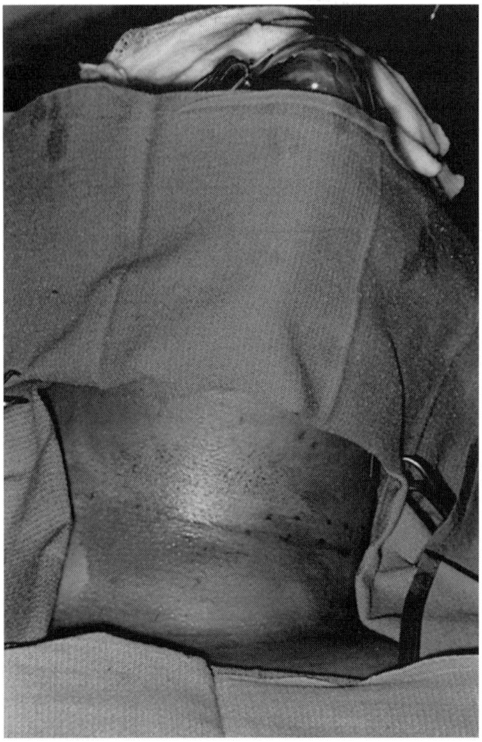

Figure 9–35. The neck is draped for an awake tracheotomy. Moist gauze covers the eyes of the patient.

VENTILATION

After the airway has been controlled, adequacy of ventilation should be assessed. A number of conditions can compromise ventilation, including intrinsic pulmonary disease or injury (e.g., pulmonary contusion), bronchospasm, bronchial obstruction (e.g., blood clots, vomitus, or foreign bodies), pneumothorax, and trauma (e.g., flail chest). In addition, respiratory paralysis can occur due to spinal cord injury proximal to C-4.

Visual inspection, palpation, and auscultation of the chest are important to clinically assess the adequacy of ventilation. Decreased unilateral breath sounds suggest hypoventilation of one lung. Main-stem bronchial obstruction, main-stem intubation, pneumothorax, or hemothorax should be considered.

A tension pneumothorax requires immediate attention. Signs of a tension pneumothorax include contralateral tracheal deviation, unilateral decreased breath sounds, distended neck veins, and cyanosis. Treatment involves immediate insertion of a large-bore needle into the 2nd intercostal space in the midclavicular line of the affected hemothorax. A finger from a sterile glove can be placed on the needle to create a flutter valve. A chest tube is then placed, once the tension pneumothorax has been relieved and ventilation and circulation are established. A simple pneumothorax is relieved by placement of a chest tube in the 4th or 5th intercostal space.

An open pneumothorax can compromise ventilation by creating a sucking chest wound. The chest wound should be occluded with a sterile occlusion dressing and taped closed on three sides to create a flutter valve.

Outcomes

Outcomes after emergency airway intervention depend on the rapidity of the intervention and on protection of the patient against hypoxemia. Delay in relief of upper airway obstruction can result in anoxic brain injury. Failure to establish an airway results in progressive hypoxemia, systemic deterioration, and death.

A low threshold for establishing a surgical airway usually results in a favorable outcome. In our experience, emergency cricothyroidotomy and tracheotomy are uniformly successful when a surgical airway is necessary. Underlying medical problems, however, are responsible for fatal outcomes in some of these patients.

All patients who have required intervention for relief of upper airway obstruction should be carefully observed after the airway has been established for possible adverse sequelae, which can include pneumothorax, aspiration pneumonia, and postobstructive pulmonary edema.

POSTOBSTRUCTIVE PULMONARY EDEMA

Pulmonary edema may develop in up to 10% of patients after relief of acute upper airway obstruction.[41] Postobstructive pulmonary edema is precipitated by reversal of postanesthetic laryngospasm in more than 50% of cases.[42–44] Other causes include relief of obstruction due to upper airway neoplasms, infections (e.g., epiglottitis), strangulation, or hanging. Pulmonary edema may also occur after relief of the chronic airway obstruction associated with airway tumors, obstructing goiters, bilateral vocal cord paralysis, and tonsillar hypertrophy.[43, 44]

The proposed pathophysiologic mechanism for postobstructive pulmonary edema is as follows. Forced inspiration against an obstruction causes a marked decrease in intrathoracic pressure. The decreased intrathoracic pressure increases venous return to the right heart, with an increase in pulmonary artery microvascular hydrostatic pressure.[43, 44] The increased hydrostatic pressure in the pulmonary capillaries results in a transudation of fluid from the capillary space to the pulmonary interstitial space, which results in pulmonary edema.[43] A proposed contributory mechanism is increased pulmonary permeability due to injury of the pulmonary capillary endothelium.[44]

Postobstructive pulmonary edema usually manifests itself within minutes of relief of acute upper airway obstruction, but its onset may be delayed for hours in some cases.[42, 44] Signs of postobstructive pulmonary edema include respiratory distress, hypoxia, frothy pink pulmonary secretions, and bilateral rales on chest auscultation. Chest radiographs reveal bilateral pulmonary infiltrates (Fig. 9–36).

The treatment of postobstructive pulmonary edema depends on its severity. Some patients respond favorably to supplemental oxygen by face mask, restriction of intravenous crystalloids, and diuresis. Most patients, however, require intubation and mechanical ventilation with a positive end-expiratory pressure (PEEP) and high FIO_2.[42, 44] The benefit of intravenous corticosteroids has not been established for this problem.

In most patients, the pulmonary edema resolves within 24 to 48 hours and recovery is uneventful.[42, 44] Progressive respiratory failure and death, however, can occur if there is a delay in the recognition of the problem or a delay in therapeutic intervention.[44]

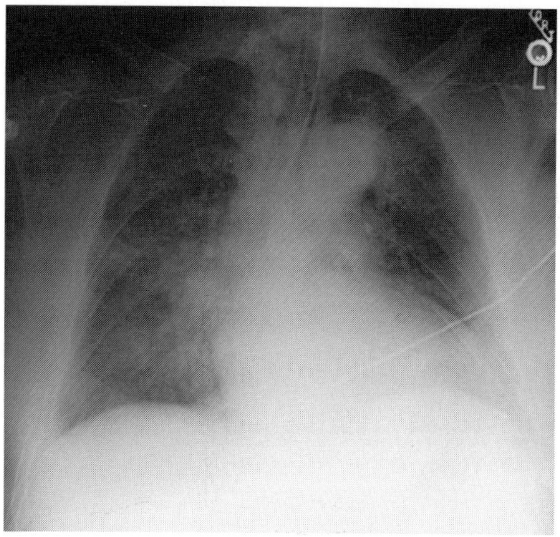

Figure 9–36. Chest radiograph showing the typical bilateral pulmonary infiltrates of postobstructive pulmonary edema.

OBSTRUCTING UPPER AIRWAY NEOPLASMS

Upper airway obstruction may be caused by a variety of neoplasms involving the pharynx, larynx, and trachea. Neoplasms may be intrinsic to the airway, such as squamous cell carcinoma (Fig. 9–37), or extrinsic, such as thyroid carci-

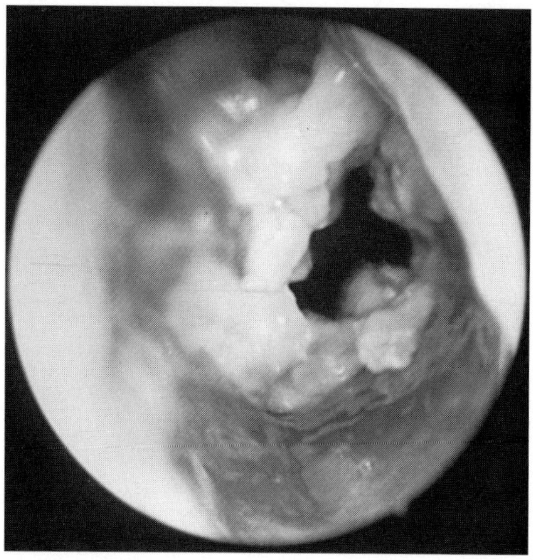

Figure 9–37. Squamous cell carcinoma of the subglottic larynx.

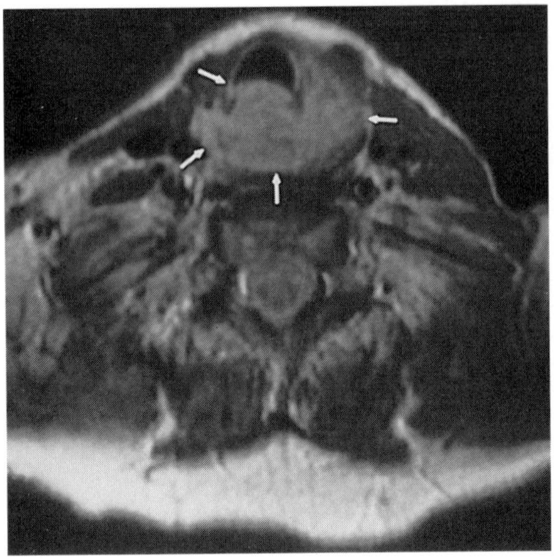

Figure 9–38. Medullary carcinoma of the thyroid with trachea and recurrent laryngeal nerve invasion (arrows).

noma (Fig. 9–38), and may cause airway compression, airway invasion, or vocal cord paralysis. In addition, respiratory papillomatosis may cause obstruction of the larynx or trachea (Fig. 9–39). Management of the airway in these situations requires careful planning, including consideration for subsequent treatment of the offending tumor.

Presentation

Patients with upper airway obstruction caused by tumor usually have progressive airway compromise related to the growth of the neoplasm and the gradual narrowing of the airway. Precipitous obstruction may occur in some patients due to hemorrhage, edema, infection, tumor necrosis, or vocal cord paralysis. Edema may occur during radiation therapy. Shortness of breath is a common complaint, and other symptoms, which vary with the tumor's location and the extent of the disease, are usually present. Common symptoms include pain, dysphagia, hoarseness, odynophagia, hemoptysis, and otalgia. Stridor is a common sign, as is increased respiratory effort. Active bleeding may be present. The neck may reveal obvious masses that can be noted visually or by palpation. The larynx or trachea may be deviated. Signs of cachexia or dehydration may be evident.

Evaluation

The degree of airway compromise and the need for immediate airway control should be determined. Vital signs and a focused history must be obtained. The head and neck are to be thoroughly examined, and mirror or fiberoptic lar-

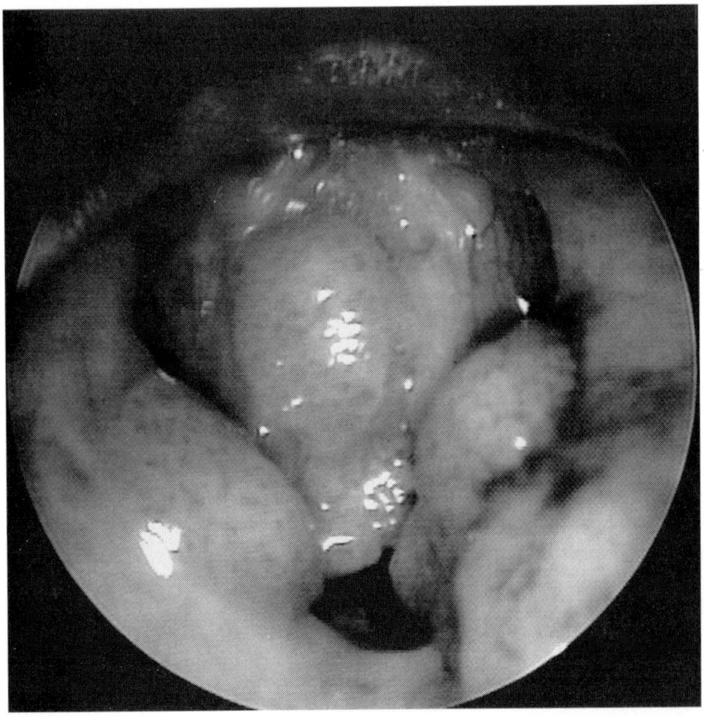

Figure 9–39. Obstructing laryngeal respiratory papillomatosis. (Courtesy of Haskins K. Kashima, M.D.)

yngoscopy should be performed. The location and extent of tumor should be determined. Vocal cord motion should be assessed. The chest should be auscultated and a chest radiograph obtained.

A CT scan is useful for the evaluation of glottic and subglottic laryngeal neoplasms, trachea neoplasms, and extrinsic tumors. A decision to obtain a CT scan must be carefully made, as the airway may deteriorate with time or become compromised when the patient assumes a supine position. A patient who is being imaged by CT scan should be closely observed by qualified personnel for these reasons. Flow-volume loops may aid in assessing the degree of obstruction. The clinical evaluation, however, should be the primary guide for airway management.

Priorities

A patient with severe airway obstruction (in extremis) requires immediate airway control by intubation or by the creation of a surgical airway. The approach to a patient with a mild or moderate airway obstruction requires a judgment about whether a patient may be treated with conservative measures and intensive care unit monitoring or should be taken directly to the operating room for expeditious intubation or tracheotomy. If conservative airway management is planned, the patient should be given humidified oxygen by face mask. Other measures include intravenous corticosteroids and antibiotics to reduce swelling and to resolve bacterial suprainfection. Heliox may improve respiration in some patients. The patient should be observed in an intensive care unit and airway intervention promptly performed if the patient's airway status worsens.

Some patients are best managed in the operating room in a timely fashion. A primary airway management plan, as well as contingency plans, should be developed by the surgeon and thoroughly communicated to the anesthesiologist. Airway management equipment should be readied for use (Table 9–3).

Table 9–3 *Adult Emergency Airway Cart*

Equipment
Dedo laryngoscope, Holinger laryngoscope
Laryngeal suction tips
Rigid bronchoscope (6 × 35) with adapter
Bronchoscope suction tips
Fiberoptic bronchoscope
Light source and fiberoptic cables
Tracheotomy set
Local anesthetic set (lidocaine with 1/100,000 epinephrine)
Jolly tube
Alligator forceps
Tooth guard
Fiberoptic bronchoscope
Jet ventilation setup
Eschmann stylet
Scalpel handle, no. 15 scalpel blade
Cup forceps, straight and up-biting
Assorted laryngeal mask airways
Assorted endotracheal tubes, epiglottitis endotracheal tubes
Assorted tracheotomy tubes
Mayo scissors
Kelly clamp
Towels, towel clip
Procedures Possible
Rigid laryngoscopy
Rigid bronchoscopy
Cricothyroidotomy and tracheotomy
Jet ventilation
Laryngeal mask airway

Awake fiberoptic intubation or rapid-sequence induction with rigid endoscopic intubation are often good options in this setting. A trachcotomy can be performed if it is to be part of the overall treatment plan. After intubation, direct laryngoscopy or tracheoscopy can be performed to assess the tumor. A biopsy should be obtained for pathologic evaluation.

Exophytic tumors and obstructing respiratory papillomatosis (Fig. 9–39) can be debulked, which may open the airway sufficiently to permit extubation. Also, tumor bleeding may resolve after debulking. Tumor debridement may be accomplished with cupped forceps, a carbon dioxide laser, or a powered debrider. Cupped forceps are quick and simple. The carbon dioxide laser is slower and carries the risks of laser injury or airway fire but has the advantage of providing hemostasis. Recently, powered debriders designed for laryngeal or tracheal use have become available (Fig. 9–40). These instruments allow rapid, safe, and thorough removal of bulky tumors.[45]

Another option is awake tracheostomy followed by endoscopy to assess tumor location and extent. In general, we recommend avoidance of tracheotomy for obstructing laryngeal carcinomas because of concern for an increased risk of peristomal tumor recurrence in this setting (Fig. 9–41). In addition, if laryngectomy is subsequently performed, a prior tracheotomy makes creation of the tracheostoma difficult because of inflammation and scarring.

A proposed mechanism that can be used for peristomal recurrence after tracheotomy per-

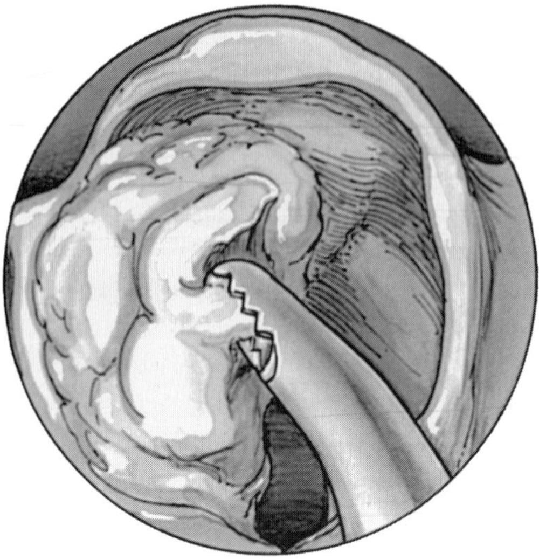

Figure 9–40. Laryngoscopic laryngeal tumor debulking with powered debrider. (Courtesy of Xomed, Jacksonville, FL.)

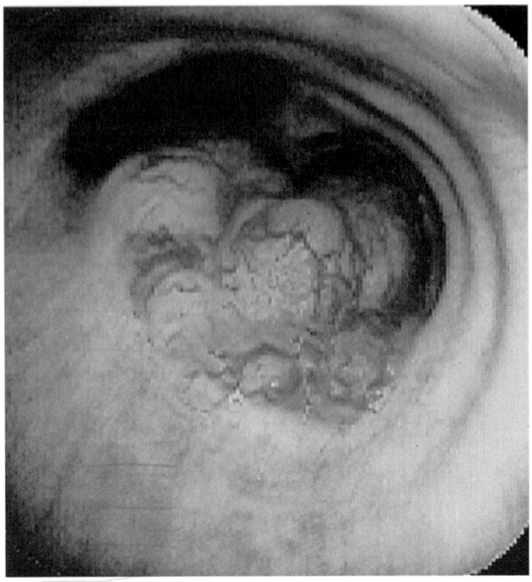

Figure 9–42. Obstructing intrinsic tracheal neoplasm.

formed for airway obstruction caused by laryngeal carcinoma is tumor cell implantation in the tracheotomy wound. Although this mechanism is possible, a patient who requires emergency tracheotomy for laryngeal carcinoma usually has a more advanced tumor than a patient without airway compromise. Thus, more advanced tumors may be responsible for peristomal recurrence. Many studies have shown that tumor-related factors are more strongly associated with the development of peristomal recurrence than is tracheotomy. Such tumor-related factors include subglottic tumor extension and extralaryngeal tumor spread.[46–48]

Obstructing intrinsic tracheal tumors (Fig. 9–42) present potentially difficult management problems because bypass of the obstruction by intubation or tracheotomy may not be possible. Passage of a long, cuffless endotracheal tube (epiglottitis tube) past the tumor may be possible (see Fig. 9–15). Endoscopic airway control with a rigid bronchoscope may be necessary to allow ventilation and tumor debulking. Extrinsic tracheal compression by tumor (Fig. 9–43) is best managed by intubation with an appropriately sized endotracheal tube and treatment of the extrinsic tumor mass. Airway invasion may necessitate resection and reconstruction of the trachea.

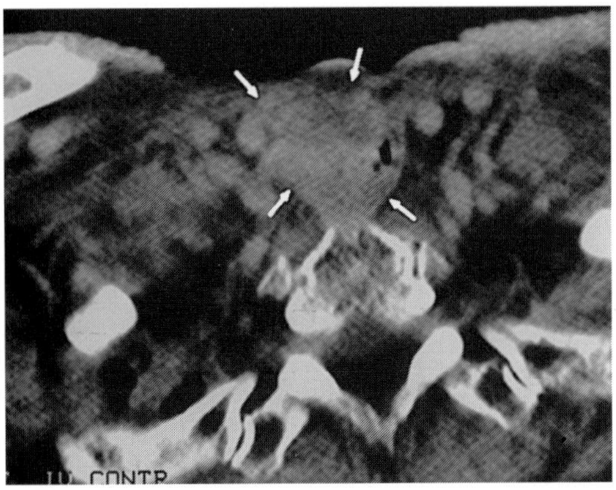

Figure 9–41. Computed tomography scan demonstrating peristomal recurrence of laryngeal carcinoma (arrows).

Outcomes

Successful airway management in cases of obstructing neoplasms depends on a thorough understanding of airway tumors and their treatment, the formulation of a rational plan for dealing with the airway, and communication among team members. Contingency airway management plans should be discussed in case the primary plan is unsuccessful. In general, airway control is usually successful when this approach is used. Complications include tumor hemorrhage or dislodgment and the other potential complications of intubation, rigid endoscopy, and tracheotomy previously discussed. Failure to control the airway can result in asphyxia, anoxia, and death. By using the approach outlined, we have had no deaths of patients with obstructive upper airway neoplasms secondary to loss of airway.

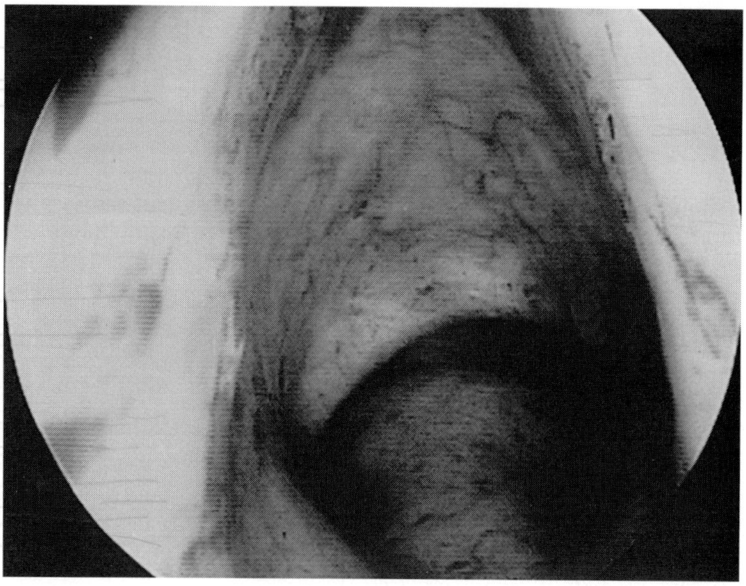

Figure 9–43. Extrinsic tracheal compression by lymphoma.

PHARYNGEAL AND LARYNGEAL FOREIGN BODIES

Foreign body obstruction of the pharynx and larynx can result in acute upper airway obstruction. Foreign body obstruction usually occurs during food ingestion, with meat being the most common cause of obstruction in adults.[49] Other food items, dentures, and ingested foreign bodies are also possible causes. Acute upper airway obstruction due to food may occur in a restaurant, hence the appellation café coronary.[13] Obstruction involving food is commonly associated with alcohol ingestion, dentures, conversation while eating, or poor chewing of food.[13]

Complete upper airway obstruction by a foreign body results in cessation of ventilation and aphonia. The patient may grasp the neck in the universal distress sign of choking (see Fig. 9–7), and anoxia and loss of consciousness may occur. The Heimlich maneuver should be performed in order to expel the foreign body from the airway (see earlier discussion). A finger-sweep maneuver should be used to sweep the pharynx and remove the foreign body in an unconscious patient. If the foreign body can be visualized, a clamp or other instrument may aid in retrieval. Care must be taken to prevent the foreign body from being forced deeper into the airway.[49]

Tracheal and bronchial foreign bodies more commonly occur in children than in adults; management of foreign bodies in children's airways is discussed in Chapter 21.

ANGIOEDEMA

Angioedema refers to nonpitting and nonpruritic edema of the subcutaneous and submucosal tissues. The facial skin, extremities, genitals, and upper aerodigestive tract are usually affected. Angioedema that involves the oral cavity, oropharynx, or larynx can cause acute upper airway obstruction. Airway obstruction related to angioedema can be rapid in onset and is life threatening.[50]

Angioedema can be an allergic reaction—mediated by immunoglobulin E (IgE)—and it occurs in patients with IgE antibodies who come into contact with an allergen.[51] Some drugs, including morphine, codeine, and iodinated contrast agents, may cause angioedema by initiating direct histamine release.[51] Angioedema can also be hereditary, acquired, or idiopathic.

The most common type of hereditary angioedema (85%) is caused by a genetic deficiency in the serum inhibitor of the first component of complement, C1 esterase inhibitor (C1 INH) and is transmitted by an autosomal dominant trait (type I).[52] Other, less common, types of hereditary angioedema are caused by a dysfunctional C1 INH (type II) or a C1 INH that binds to albumin, forming an inactive complex (type III).[52]

Acquired angioedema is caused by increased catabolism of C1 INH (type I) or by the presence of antibodies to the C1 INH (type II). Type II acquired angioedema is frequently associated with B-cell lymphoproliferative disorders.

Idiopathic, or sporadic, angioedema is usually associated with a causative factor such as medication, minor trauma, temperature, infection, foods, insect bites, or connective tissue diseases. Medications that commonly cause angioedema include angiotensin-converting enzyme (ACE) inhibitors, aspirin, nonsteroidal anti-inflammatory drugs, and penicillin.

ACE inhibitors are common antihypertensive agents; they include enalapril, captopril, benzepril, cilazapril, fosinopril, lisinopril, perindopril, quinapril, and ramipril. Angioedema occurs in approximately 0.1% to 0.2% of patients using these medications. The mechanism of angioedema related to ACE inhibitors is thought to be caused by the action of the ACE inhibitors, which not only block the conversion of angiotensin I to angiotensin II but also prevent the breakdown of bradykinin, a powerful vasodilator. ACE inhibitor–associated angioedema occurs more commonly in African American patients than in other patients.[53]

In hereditary and acquired angioedema, the absence of C1-INH or the loss of its activity results in increased vascular permeability due to the release of vasoactive substances.

Presentation

Hereditary angioedema is characterized by recurrent episodes of angioedema beginning in the second decade of life. Usually, a positive family history is present. Trauma and surgical procedures commonly precipitate episodes of angioedema in cases of the hereditary form of angioedema.[54] In contrast, acquired angioedema usually has an onset after the fourth decade of life and usually occurs in patients who do not have positive family histories of angioedema.[52] Angioedema associated with ACE inhibitors usually occurs within months after initiating the medication, but onset can range from hours to years.[53, 55]

Symptoms of angioedema include swelling, dyspnea, odynophagia, and dysphagia. Pruritus may be a symptom of angioedema not related to ACE inhibitors.[56] The predominant sign of angioedema is nonpitting edema of the face, lips, oral cavity, oropharynx, and larynx. The tongue (Fig. 9–44), soft palate, and supraglottic larynx are the sites most commonly affected.[56, 57] The edema may be significant, causing stridor and upper airway obstruction, and it may evolve rapidly. Other signs include drooling and altered voice.

Evaluation

In the case of a patient with angioedema, a thorough history should be taken to determine its cause. A prior history of angioedema, causative factors such as medications and trauma, and family history should be sought. The sites of the angioedema and the extent of the airway compromise should be determined. A thorough head and neck examination, including fiberoptic laryngoscopy, should be performed. The chest should be auscultated and vital signs should be determined and monitored because bronchospasm, hypotension, and anaphylactic shock may be heralded by angioedema.

Laboratory evaluation should include determination of levels of complement and C1 esterase and a complete blood cell count. Low levels of C1 esterase and C4 suggest hereditary angioedema.

Priorities

The severity of upper airway impairment should be determined. Airway management is the first priority for angioedema. A patient with severe airway compromise requires immediate airway control by intubation, cricothyroidotomy, or tracheotomy. Edema of the oral cavity, especially the tongue, and of the oropharynx usually eliminates orotracheal intubation as an option for airway control, so the nasotracheal route is usually the preferred method of intubation. Significant edema of the supraglottic larynx and inability to adequately visualize the glottis are contraindications to nasotracheal intubation. Under these conditions, tracheotomy is indicated.

A patient with mild to moderate oral cavity angioedema may benefit from the placement of a nasopharyngeal airway.[58] A patient with mild to moderate upper airway angioedema should be hospitalized and carefully observed in an intensive care unit until the edema has resolved. Progression of airway obstruction mandates control of the airway.

Medications to reduce angioedema include subcutaneous epinephrine (0.3 to 1.0 mL of a 1:1000 solution), H_1 antihistamines (e.g., 25 to 50 mg of intravenous diphenhydramine four times a day), H_2 antihistamines (e.g., 300 mg of cimetidine four times a day), and intravenous corticosteroids (8 to 12 mg of intravenous dexamethasone). Epinephrine and antihistamines are most effective in a patient with allergic or drug-induced angioedema. A patient with hereditary

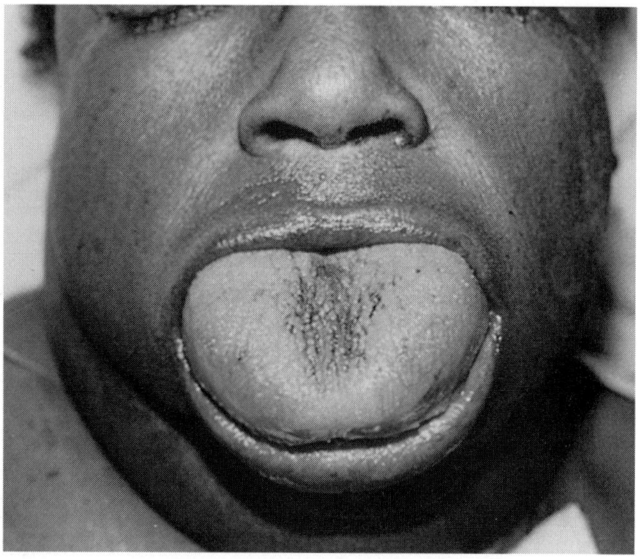

Figure 9–44. Angioedema of the tongue. (Courtesy of M. Boyd Gillespie, M.D.)

angioedema can be given C1 INH concentrate intravenously. An alternative to C1 INH concentrate is fresh-frozen plasma, but this carries with it the usual risks of blood product administration. For angioedema, related to ACE inhibitors, the causative medication should be discontinued and avoided. In a patient with acquired angioedema, the underlying disorder should be treated.

Danazol, a synthetic androgen, stimulates the hepatic synthesis of C1 INH and has been recommended as prophylactic therapy for patients with hereditary and type I acquired angioedema.[54] Patients with hereditary angioedema who must have oral surgery or other upper aerodigestive tract procedures should have prophylactic C1 INH replacement therapy. An alternative prophylactic therapy for patients with either acquired or hereditary deficiencies in C1 INH is epsilon-aminocaproic acid, an antifibrinolytic agent that inhibits the complement system.[59]

Outcomes

Angioedema usually resolves within 24 to 48 hours. Extubation should be performed only after significant resolution of upper airway edema has occurred.

Untreated angioedema is associated with a high rate of mortality (10% to 30%).[55, 60] Because of increased recognition of angioedema and its causes and treatment, however, present outcomes for patients with angioedema are excellent.[56] Continued use of an ACE inhibitor after even one episode of angioedema is associated with a markedly increased rate of recurrent angioedema.[53]

SUPRAGLOTTITIS

Supraglottitis, or epiglottitis, is an infection of the supraglottic larynx and contiguous structures and may cause life-threatening upper airway obstruction. Supraglottitis can affect both children and adults. Management of supraglottitis in children is discussed in Chapter 21.

Supraglottitis is most commonly a bacterial infection, although in immunocompromised patients, *Candida albicans* may be the pathogen. Proper diagnosis and treatment of supraglottitis is necessary to prevent fatal airway compromise.

Presentation

Adult supraglottitis occurs in both men and women and is fairly evenly distributed across adult age groups.[61] Most patients have been healthy previously. In contrast to children, who are more likely to have respiratory symptoms, the most common presenting symptoms of supraglottitis in adults are sore throat, which is usually severe, and odynophagia.[62, 63] Only one half to one third of adult patients complain of dyspnea.[61, 63] Other symptoms include fever, chills, otalgia, cough, hoarseness, dysphagia, and headache. The duration of symptoms prior to presentation may range from hours to days. Respiratory symptoms may progress rapidly.

Signs of supraglottitis include muffled voice, pharyngitis, tender cervical lymphadenopathy, drooling, erect posture, stridor, and agitation.[63, 64] Most patients have fever and tachycardia. Airway compromise may be precipitous and can result in complete airway obstruction and death.

Other infections may coexist with supraglottitis or may develop after supraglottitis has been diagnosed. These infections include peritonsillar abscess or cellulitis and pneumonia.[61]

Evaluation

Patients with unexplained sore throat and odynophagia, with or without dyspnea, should be suspected of having supraglottitis. A thorough history, a head and neck examination, and vital signs should be obtained.

Lateral soft tissue radiographs of the neck are commonly performed in emergency departments to evaluate patients with suspected supraglottitis. Most radiographic signs of supraglottitis are qualitative.[65] Radiographic signs include obliteration of the vallecula (the vallecula sign), thickening of the epiglottis (the thumb sign), swelling of the arytenoids and aryepiglottic folds, narrowing of the pharyngeal airway, and prevertebral soft tissue swelling (Fig. 9–45).[65, 66]

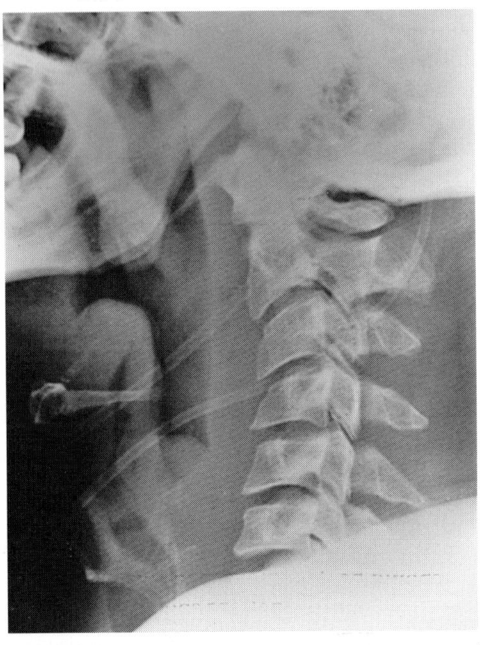

Figure 9–45. Lateral neck radiograph demonstrating marked soft tissue swelling of the epiglottis and aryepiglottic folds in a patient with supraglottitis.

Any patient with the clinical or radiographic suspicion of supraglottitis should undergo indirect laryngoscopy. Mirror or fiberoptic indirect laryngoscopy is the best method of diagnosing supraglottitis, and it can be performed in adults without risk of airway compromise. Diffuse supraglottic inflammation and edema are the most common findings.[64] A complete blood count and serum electrolyte level should be obtained. The white blood cell count is frequently elevated in the range of 14,000 to 20,000.

Bacterial blood cultures should be obtained and are positive in 10% to 40% of patients.[64] The most commonly isolated bacteria include *Hemophilus influenzae*, *Streptococcus pneumoniae*, α-hemolytic *Streptococcus* species, and *Staphylococcus aureus*.[61] *Serratia marcescens* and *Candida albicans* are less common pathogens. Cultures obtained directly from the epiglottis give a higher positive yield (75%) than do blood cultures.[61]

Priorities

The primary priority in the management of a patient with supraglottitis is the maintenance of an adequate airway until the inflammatory edema resolves with antibiotic therapy.[67] A patient with supraglottitis should be hospitalized; because precipitous airway compromise can occur, there should be a low threshold for control of the airway in any patient with supraglottitis. Airway compromise related to supraglottitis requires airway intervention. A patient with severe airway compromise requires immediate airway control by intubation or cricothyroidotomy. A stable patient with dyspnea or stridor should undergo fiberoptic nasotracheal intubation in a controlled setting such as the operating room where the necessary personnel are available to secure the airway surgically if necessary.

Airway management in a patient without signs or symptoms of airway obstruction must be individualized and must be based upon clinical and laryngeal findings.[67] Close airway observation in an intensive care unit with the capacity for immediate airway intervention, should it be necessary, is a reasonable approach for a patient without respiratory complaints or signs of airway obstruction. Humidified oxygen should be administered via face mask. Intravenous fluids should be administered. A tracheotomy set should be at the bedside. Serial laryngeal examinations should be performed.[67]

Intravenous antibiotics such as cefuroxime 1.5 g every 6 to 8 hours should be administered.

Alternatively, ampicillin and chloramphenicol can be given. Broad-spectrum antibiotics are appropriate for the immunocompromised patient. Antibiotics should be altered according to culture results and antibiotic sensitivities when these results are available.

Intravenous corticosteroids may reduce inflammatory edema in patients who are under close airway observation. The benefit of corticosteroids for supraglottitis, however, is unproven, and giving corticosteroids does not appear to shorten hospital stays.[61]

Outcomes

An appropriate index of suspicion and proper diagnostic evaluation are necessary to promptly diagnose and treat supraglottitis and thus reduce the morbidity and mortality related to this condition. Most adult patients with supraglottitis can be managed safely and effectively without performing airway intervention. Symptoms or signs of airway obstruction, however, predict the need for airway control in most patients.[61, 64]

A mortality rate of approximately 1% has been observed as a result of adult supraglottitis.[61] The absence of symptoms or signs of airway obstruction may delay the diagnosis of supraglottitis.[62] Death due to airway obstruction can result from this delay in diagnosis or from other factors, including misdiagnosis, failed intubation, and failure to perform a timely tracheotomy.[62] Other complications of supraglottitis include respiratory arrest, sepsis, adult respiratory distress syndrome, pulmonary edema, and pneumothorax.[63]

THE DIFFICULT AIRWAY: ANTICIPATED AND UNANTICIPATED OBSTRUCTION

Airway obstruction can occur during the induction of general anesthesia. This situation is best avoided by recognizing the presence of a potentially difficult airway and paying careful attention to the management of such a patient. A difficult airway is defined as a clinical situation in which a conventionally trained anesthesiologist experiences difficulty with mask ventilation, tracheal intubation, or both.[68]

Identification of a patient with a difficult airway relies upon a careful airway history to detect medical, surgical, and anesthesia-related factors that could indicate the presence of a difficult airway.[68] In addition, a physical examination should be conducted to detect any characteristics that indicate the presence of a difficult airway.[68] It is beyond the scope of this chapter to discuss airway rating systems such as the Mallampati classification that may predict the likelihood of a difficult airway, and the reader is directed elsewhere for discussion of them.[69–71]

Conditions associated with the presence of a difficult airway include prior difficult intubation, obesity, pregnancy, congenital or acquired deformities, trauma, infections, and neoplasms.[69] A well-developed strategy for the intubation and extubation of the airway should be made for these patients.[68] Assistance and specialized equipment for difficult airway management (see Table 9–3) should be readily available.

The American Society of Anesthesiologists has developed an algorithm for the management of the difficult airway (Fig. 9–46).[68] Awake fiberoptic intubation is a reasonable primary plan for most patients. An alternative plan, which is useful for some head and neck surgery patients, is an awake tracheotomy performed under local anesthesia, especially if the surgical procedure includes a tracheotomy. Alternative plans should be considered, including rigid endoscopic intubation, laryngeal mask airway, transtracheal jet ventilation, and a surgical airway.

Unanticipated inability to mask-ventilate or intubate a patient after induction of general anesthesia is estimated to occur in as many as 1.0% to 3.5% of intubations.[71] Failure to be prepared for this situation may result in the death of the patient. Thus, both anesthesiologists and surgeons should be skilled in managing this uncommon event. We have found that having an emergency airway cart available in the operating room (Fig. 9–47; see Table 9–3) and having identifiable experts in managing difficult airways—anesthesiologists and head and neck surgeons—who can be summoned for assistance is extremely beneficial for the management of the unanticipated difficult airway.

Useful techniques for control of an airway that fails after induction of general anesthesia include rigid endoscopic intubation, the laryngeal mask airway, and transtracheal jet ventilation.[72] If these methods fail, a surgical airway should be created.

When there has been a problem with airway management related to anesthesia, this information should be documented in the patient's medical record and the patient should be informed[73] and encouraged to enroll in Medic Alert and carry an emergency medical information card or wear a Medic Alert bracelet.

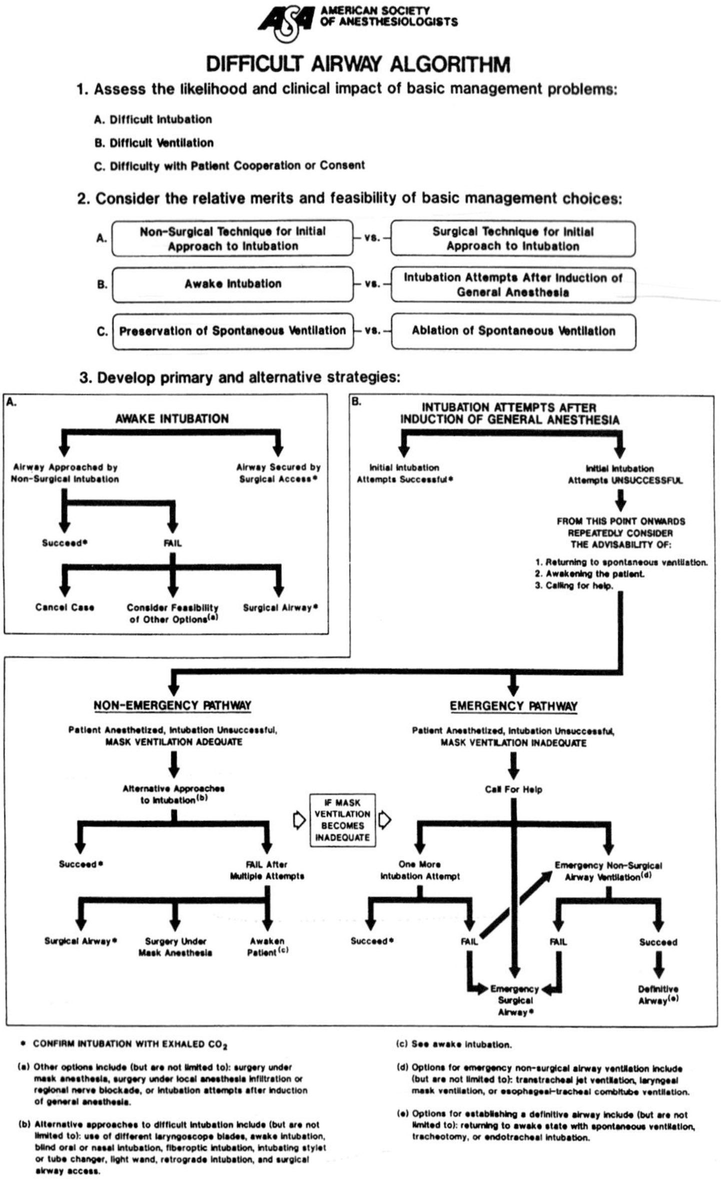

Figure 9–46. American Society of Anesthesiologists' difficult airway algorithm. (From Caplan RA, Benumof JL, Berry FA, et al. Practice guidelines for management of the difficult airway: a report by the American Society of Anesthesiologists Task Force on Management of the Difficult Airway. Anesthesiology 1993; 78:597–602.)

Extubation of a patient with a difficult airway must be carefully considered. As is necessary for intubation, a plan for airway management during emergence from anesthesia and extubation must be in place. This plan should include the possibility of extubation when the patient is awake and options for management if airway obstruction occurs after extubation. The operating room team must maintain vigilance after extubation and during recovery from anesthesia so as to prevent postanesthetic airway obstruction (see later section). Emergency airway equipment should remain available during a patient's emergence from anesthesia.

TRAUMA

A trauma patient may have an obstructed airway due to direct airway injury, neck hematoma resulting from blunt or penetrating neck injury, the presence of a foreign body, or generalized hypotonia with tongue prolapse. The method of intervention in such a patient is determined by the type and degree of injury and the location of the obstruction. If respiratory efforts are present, a jaw-thrust maneuver or an oropharyngeal or nasopharyngeal airway may relieve tongue obstruction. A patient with a mandibular fracture may benefit from a chin-lift

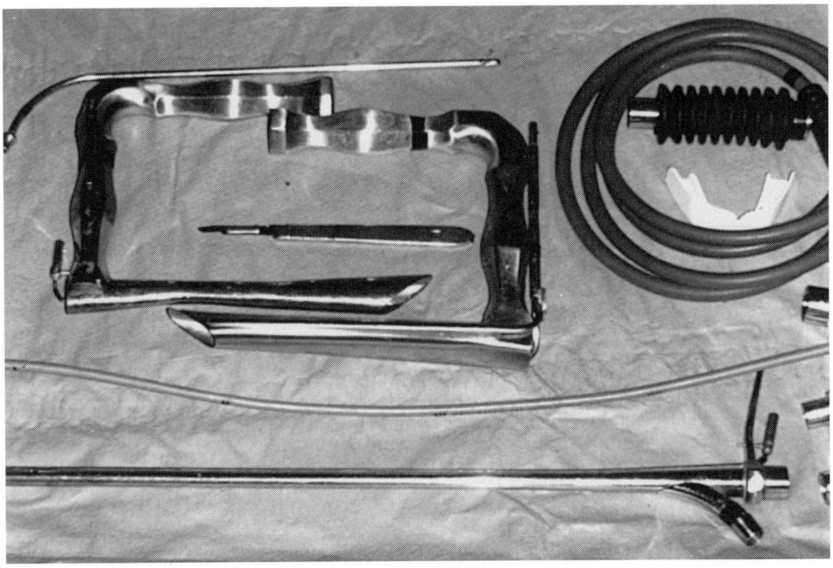

Figure 9–47. Emergency airway cart equipment, including scalpel, laryngoscopes, rigid bronchoscope, and Eschmann stylet (see Table 9–3).

maneuver. A foreign body obstructing the oral cavity or oropharyngeal area, such as dentures, teeth, or blood, should be removed. Absence of respiration or severe upper airway injury (Fig. 9–48) necessitates airway control by intubation or the creation of a surgical airway. In addition, airway intervention may be indicated in a trauma patient who has inadequate ventilation or hypoxemia, who requires airway protection because of altered mental status, or who requires hyperventilation for the treatment of intracranial injury.[74, 75]

In any patient who has sustained trauma, particularly head and neck trauma, a cervical spine injury should be suspected. The incidence of cervical spine injury in major trauma is approximately 4%.[76] In addition, cervical spine injury should be suspected in a patient with an altered mental status, flaccidity, priapism, diaphragmatic breathing, or hypotension.[77]

Secondary neurologic injuries occur more commonly if a patient has an undiagnosed cervical spine injury.[78] Thus, the cervical spine must be controlled in such a patient to prevent spinal cord injury. The neck should be immobilized and the head maintained in the neutral position. Immobilization of the neck can be achieved by using forehead tape, bilateral sandbags, and a Philadelphia collar, or with in-line stabilization by an assisting individual.[79] The cervical spine should remain immobilized until a spinal injury is ruled out radiographically and clinically. Axial traction should not be used as a stabilization method as traction may cause significant distraction and subluxation of an unstable spine.[80]

Radiographs of the cervical spine from C-1 to T-1 should be obtained in any patient suspected of having sustained a cervical spine injury. Views should include lateral, anteroposterior, and odontoid (open mouth).[81] A CT scan is indicated if all the cervical vertebrae are not visualized in standard radiographs.[82]

Although cervical spine considerations are important, airway management remains the primary consideration in a trauma patient. At present, controversy exists, as no data from clinical studies demonstrate a safety advantage in a particular technique of intubation for patients with suspected or confirmed cervical spine injuries. The most commonly recommended methods of intubation in a case of cervical spine injury include nasotracheal (fiberoptic or blind) intubation and orotracheal intubation with manual in-line stabilization of the head and neck by a second individual.[76, 79] Neither of these techniques appears to increase the incidence of secondary neurologic deficits in such a patient.[76, 83–85] Other options include retrograde intubation and the use of the light wand.[86] The choice of technique of intubation is usually determined by the expertise of the intubator and by factors unique to the patient. Failure of these techniques requires the creation of a surgical airway.

The approach to securing the airway in a patient with a penetrating laryngotracheal in-

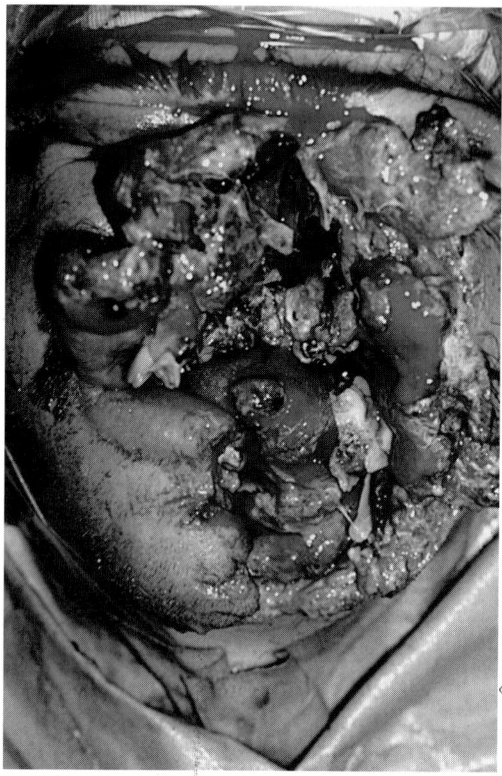

Figure 9–48. Self-inflicted shotgun injury with massive upper airway injury (Courtesy of John L. Frodel, Jr., M.D.)

jury is controversial, too. Some experts recommend tracheotomy to avoid potential exacerbation of the injury during intubation.[87] Others recommend an individualized approach based on the severity of the injury.[88, 89] A patient with a minor laryngeal hematoma or a laceration without significant laryngeal fracture can usually be safely intubated, whereas a patient with a more severe laryngeal injury, such as a large laceration, a displaced laryngeal fracture, and vocal cord immobility, is probably best managed by tracheotomy.[89] The management of laryngeal injuries is covered in Chapter 11 and the management of penetrating neck injuries discussed in Chapter 12.

TRACHEAL OBSTRUCTION

Obstruction of the trachea in an adult can be caused by a variety of conditions: stenosis related to endotracheal intubation or tracheotomy, intrinsic tracheal neoplasms, extrinsic neoplasms invading the trachea, respiratory papillomatosis, or extrinsic compression by a goiter (Fig. 9–49), tumor, abscess, or hematoma, tracheomalacia, granulation of tissue, trauma, or foreign body.[90] Tracheal stenosis usually occurs at the site of the tracheotomy or at the level of the endotracheal tube or tracheotomy tube cuff.[91, 92]

Tracheal obstruction caused by stenosis, neoplasm, or goiter usually develops slowly but may manifest suddenly.[91] In contrast, obstruction caused by a foreign body, tracheomalacia, extrinsic compression due to neck hematoma, or hemorrhage within an established goiter usually evolves rapidly.

Symptoms of tracheal obstruction include dyspnea, cough, hemoptysis, and difficulty in clearing secretions. Physical examination reveals stridor, which is primarily expiratory. Breath sounds may be diminished. Diagnosis of tracheal obstruction is aided by such imaging studies as chest radiographs and CT scans (see Fig. 9–49). Flow volume loops show decreased inspiratory and expiratory airflows. Flexible or rigid endoscopy provides definitive information regarding the extent and character of the obstruction. Rigid bronchoscopy is generally the preferred diagnostic technique because it provides an adequate channel for ventilation, and dilation of the stenosis can be performed.[92]

Obstructing tracheal lesions are potentially difficult airway management problems because bypass of the obstruction by tracheotomy may not be possible, depending on the location of the obstruction in the trachea. The airway is managed, in most cases, by tracheal intubation. Endotracheal tubes in a variety of sizes, both cuffed and uncuffed, should be available. Intubation under rigid endoscopic guidance allows proper endotracheal tube selection and placement beyond the site of obstruction. Rigid bronchoscopy may be required to maneuver past the obstruction. Ventilation can also be accomplished with the rigid bronchoscope through its ventilation side port. Rigid bronchoscopy is the method of choice for the removal of tracheal and bronchial foreign bodies, which are discussed in Chapter 10. Tracheal obstruction caused by neck hematoma (e.g., after thyroidectomy) should be relieved by opening the surgical wound and evacuating the hematoma.

Once the airway is secured and the patient stabilized, management is directed at the cause of obstruction. A compressing goiter requires thyroidectomy. An intrinsic neoplasm should be biopsied and evaluated by histopathology. Neoplasms, papillomas, and granulation tissue should be debulked or excised with cupped forceps, laser, or powered debrider.[45, 93–95] Defini-

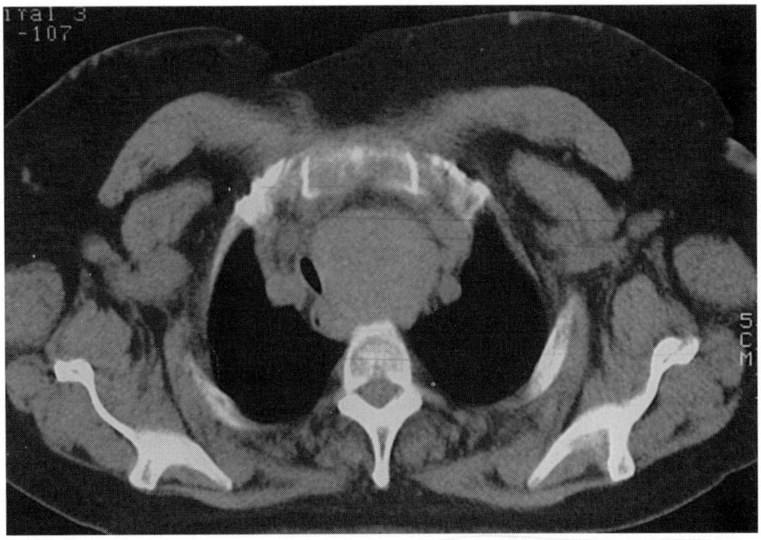

Figure 9–49. Substernal goiter with tracheal displacement and compression.

tive treatment of tracheal neoplasms is determined by tumor type and extent of disease.

Some stenotic tracheal lesions can be treated with excision and primary tracheal reanastomosis.[96] Proximal tracheal stenosis may respond to endoscopic excision or external incision with T-tube placement.[92, 97, 98] A more distal tracheal or bronchial lesion may benefit from the placement of a Silastic silicone stent.[99]

POSTOPERATIVE UPPER AIRWAY OBSTRUCTION

A variety of problems can cause upper airway obstruction after head and neck surgery. This section concerns causes of upper airway obstruction that are commonly encountered after surgical procedures are performed on the head and neck.

Laryngospasm

Laryngospasm is spasm of the laryngeal muscles with resultant laryngeal airway closure. Spasm of both the intrinsic and extrinsic laryngeal muscles may contribute to laryngeal obstruction.[100] The exact mechanism of laryngospasm is unclear, but it is thought to be a reflex response to laryngeal or pharyngeal stimulation by irritants such as blood, saliva, secretions, or instruments.[100]

Laryngospasm can cause airway obstruction after extubation and is estimated to occur in approximately 1% of general patients.[101] The incidence of laryngospasm is probably higher in patients undergoing head and neck surgery for a variety of reasons, including the presence of blood in the upper airway, laryngeal instrumentation, and avoidance of muscle relaxants.[102]

Signs of laryngospasm include lack of airflow despite respiratory efforts. Mask ventilation is usually not possible. Treatment includes 1.5 to 2.0 mg/kg of intravenous lidocaine with continued mask ventilation and reintubation if necessary. Succinylcholine may be used if lidocaine fails to relieve the obstruction. Laryngospasm is best avoided by clearance of blood and secretions from the upper airway and avoidance of instrumentation of the upper airway after extubation. Both topical and intravenous lidocaine may be beneficial for prophylaxis against laryngospasm because it blocks the afferent pathway of the laryngeal reflex.[103] Laryngospasm is also discussed in Chapter 8.

Potential complications of laryngospasm include cardiac arrest and aspiration. In addition, a patient who experiences laryngospasm should be carefully monitored for the development of postobstructive pulmonary edema (see earlier section), as laryngospasm is the most common cause of this complication.[44]

Upper Airway Edema

Upper airway edema may occur after head or neck surgery and may be caused by trauma resulting from intubation or endoscopy, by the trauma of the surgical procedure, or by interruption of lymphatic or venous drainage. Edema usually manifests 24 to 48 hours postoperatively.

The location and the severity of the edema

determine the degree of airway obstruction. The location and severity of the edema also determine treatment. Intravenous corticosteroids, humidified mist oxygen, and close observation in an intensive care unit may be appropriate for mild or moderate edema. Tongue and soft palate edema may be successfully bypassed with a nasopharyngeal airway. Edema may evolve, and significant airway obstruction due to edema requires airway control by intubation. The endotracheal tube is removed once the edema has resolved. Subglottic edema may make intubation difficult, and tracheotomy may be required.

Neck Hematoma

A hematoma that occurs after neck surgery is an uncommon postoperative complication and is usually related to inadequate hemostasis at the time of surgery. A hematoma that occurs after a thyroidectomy can cause airway obstruction due to tracheal compression and increased venous pressure, with resultant laryngeal and upper airway edema,[104] but this occurs in less than 1% of cases.[105]

Lateral neck hematomas may cause pharyngeal compression; upper neck (e.g., submandibular) hematomas may cause elevation of the floor of the mouth and posterior tongue displacement. Significant hematomas may occur in both drained and undrained neck wounds. Neck hematomas may also occur in connection with trauma or central venous access procedures.

Emergent treatment of a postoperative neck hematoma consists of immediately opening the wound, evacuating the hematoma, and providing an adequate airway. Relief of tracheal compression usually results in a satisfactory airway. Significant upper airway edema, however, may accompany neck hematoma, and emergency airway intervention may then be necessary. Once an adequate airway has been ensured, the patient should be returned to the operating room for wound exploration, control of bleeding vessels, and wound closure.

Bilateral Vocal Cord Paralysis

Bilateral vocal cord paralysis can result in acute upper airway obstruction postoperatively. The most common cause of this problem is thyroidectomy; the approximate incidence is 1 in 400 cases. Most cases of bilateral vocal cord paralysis are temporary. This complication can occur in any case that places both recurrent laryngeal nerves at risk or in a case in which one vocal cord has preexisting paralysis and the contralateral, functioning recurrent laryngeal nerve is placed at risk. Laryngeal edema may accompany bilateral vocal cord paralysis and contribute to the degree of airway obstruction.[104, 106]

Bilateral vocal cord paralysis can cause upper airway obstruction when the vocal cords fail to abduct after extubation. Inspiratory stridor is a typical sign. Airway obstruction may not be immediate after extubation because of the stenting effect of the endotracheal tube. The vocal cords usually assume a paramedian position, with resultant glottic obstruction.

Airway obstruction due to bilateral vocal cord paralysis requires immediate establishment of an airway. This is usually best accomplished by orotracheal intubation. If both recurrent laryngeal nerves were identified and protected intraoperatively, then reextubation in a controlled setting in several days should be considered. Intravenous corticosteroids may be administered in the interim. If at the time of reextubation, bilateral vocal cord paralysis and upper airway obstruction persist, a tracheotomy is indicated.

Tracheomalacia

Tracheomalacia is weakness of the cartilaginous trachea caused by the effect of chronic pressure by a long-standing goiter. Tracheomalacia may result in tracheal collapse and airway obstruction following thyroidectomy. Airway obstruction due to tracheomalacia, however, is a rare occurrence after thyroidectomy,[107, 108] but it can arise suddenly and progress rapidly.[107]

Airway obstruction resulting from tracheomalacia should be managed by reintubating the patient. The patient is then extubated several days later under controlled conditions. The development of paratracheal fibrosis usually results in satisfactory tracheal support. An alternative approach to emergency airway management for tracheomalacia is tracheostomy.

Tracheostomal Obstruction

A narrowing of the tracheostoma, or tracheostomal stenosis, can occur after total laryngectomy and can result in progressive airway obstruction (Fig. 9–50). Crusts, dried blood, or edema can also result in acute obstruction (Fig. 9–51). In addition, granulation tissue at the tracheostoma

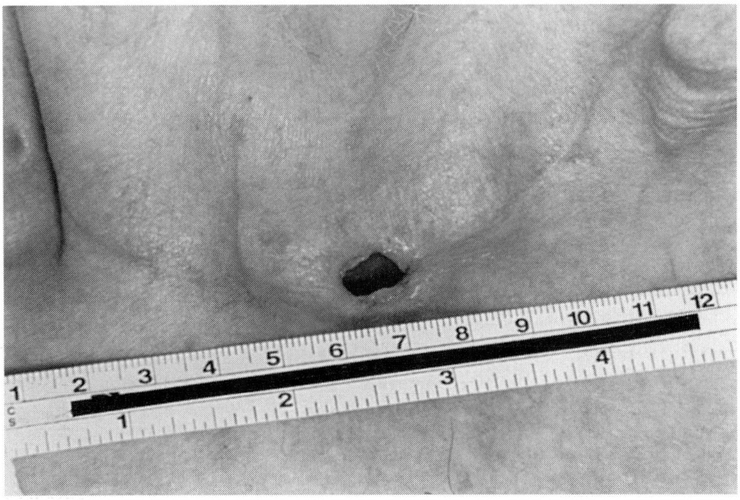

Figure 9–50. Tracheostomal stenosis after total laryngectomy.

or within the trachea may contribute to airway narrowing. Management of airway obstruction following laryngectomy should include removal of obstructing crusts and granulation tissue and control of bleeding with suction and cautery (e.g., silver nitrate).

A tracheostomal stent or laryngectomy tube should be placed to open the stoma if it has narrowed. A shortened nasopharyngeal airway works well for this purpose if other tubes are not available. Alternatively, an endotracheal tube can be placed temporarily, but ventilator assistance may be necessary, depending on the diameter of the endotracheal tube. If tube or stent insertion is difficult, the tracheostoma can be incised in four quadrants with a scalpel. The stoma can be progressively dilated with serial insertion of larger tubes. Tracheostomal revision surgery or maintenance of a stomal tube or stent is indicated for long-term management of tracheostomal stenosis.

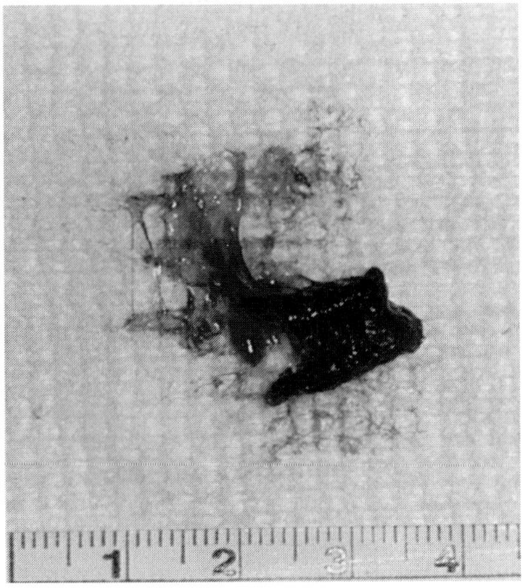

Figure 9–51. Obstructing tracheal plug removed with a hemostat from the trachea of a laryngectomy patient.

Obstructive Sleep Apnea

The prevalence of obstructive sleep apnea (OSA) in middle-aged adults is estimated to be approximately 4% in men and 2% in women.[109] The diagnosis of OSA is made by polysomnography. Risk factors include obesity (as defined by a body mass index greater than 28 kg/m^2), a history of snoring or daytime sleepiness, male gender, and a positive family history.[110] The presence of any of these risk factors should increase the suspicion of undiagnosed OSA.

Any patient with OSA should be considered to have a difficult airway. Obesity, a high apnea-hypopnea index, large neck circumference, and skeletal deficiency correlate with intubation complications in these patients.[111, 112] Sedatives, narcotics, and anesthetic agents can cause muscular relaxation with resultant soft palate and tongue collapse against the posterior pharynx as well as collapse of the pharyngeal walls. Awake fiberoptic intubation is a low-risk method of intubation for a patient with OSA as it allows the patient to maintain airway tone during intubation.

Most airway emergencies related to OSA occur postoperatively, and sedating drugs and airway edema are usually responsible.[113] In addition, perioperative mortalities related to OSA are most commonly due to airway loss.[113]

The same level of vigilance with regard to the airway should be exercised at the time of emergence from anesthesia. Postoperative extubation should be performed only when upper airway tone and consciousness have been restored. Extubation in the operating room provides a satisfactorily controlled environment for airway intervention after extubation, should it be necessary. The anesthesiologist and surgeon should be prepared to reestablish an airway and have a plan of action ready, should airway obstruction occur after extubation.

The use of an airway protocol in OSA patients appears to minimize risks to the airway that are attendant upon general anesthesia and upper airway surgery in these patients.[112] The administration of narcotics intraoperatively appears to increase the risk of postoperative airway complications in patients with OSA,[111] so intraoperative narcotics should be avoided.

AIRWAY FIRES

Intraoperative airway fires can occur due to accidental ignition of the endotracheal tube with a heat source.[114, 115] This problem can occur during tracheotomy, during laser procedures on the pharynx and larynx, or during any procedure in which a heat source such as electrocautery or laser contacts a fuel (such as the endotracheal tube) in an oxygen-rich environment.[116] Other materials in the airway may serve as fuels for fires intraoperatively, including gauze, nasogastric tubes, and flexible endoscopes.[117] Surgical drapes, skin preparation agents, gloves, the patient's hair, and other materials may also serve as fuels during head and neck surgery and emergency airway procedures.[116, 118]

Managing an endotracheal tube fire requires immediate action. The breathing circuit should be disconnected from the endotracheal tube and the endotracheal tube removed from the patient. The airway should then be reestablished and the patient ventilated with air until it is established that no remnant of the endotracheal tube is burning in the airway. The patient is then ventilated with 100% oxygen. The airway should be thoroughly examined endoscopically and any products of combustion removed.[114] A chest radiograph should be obtained to rule out a pneumothorax. The patient should be monitored closely in an intensive care unit. Antibiotics and corticosteroids are recommended to reduce edema and infection.[114] Positive-pressure ventilation may be required. Serial endoscopic examinations of the airway should be performed to assess injury progression and to remove airway crusts and sloughed tissue.

The management of other burning materials such as gauze in the airway or on the patient requires immediate disconnection of the breathing circuit, removal of the burning material, and resumption of ventilation. The patient is carefully examined for burn injuries and treated accordingly.

Fortunately, surgical airway fires are uncommon and can be prevented by carefully controling heat sources in the operating room and preventing contact between them and potential fuels.[116] Fire during a tracheotomy can be avoided by judicious use of electrocautery and avoidance of tracheal entry by means of electrocautery. In addition, thorough communication between the anesthesiologist, who usually controls the oxygen source, and the surgeon, who usually controls the heat source, is important to further minimize the risk of intraoperative fires.

FUNCTIONAL LARYNGEAL DYSKINESIA

Functional laryngeal dyskinesia, also known as psychogenic upper airway obstruction[119] or functional laryngeal obstruction,[120] is a condition that can mimic laryngeal airway obstruction or asthma.[121] This disorder, however, is characterized by signs and symptoms of airway obstruction that are without anatomic cause. It can affect both adolescents and adults and is more common in female patients. A precipitating psychological or psychosocial event can be identified in many cases.

Patients with functional laryngeal dyskinesia complain of dyspnea. Some patients also complain of throat pain. All patients have stridor. Adduction of the vocal cords during inspiration is the usual finding on laryngoscopy. Arterial blood gases usually reveal mild hypocapnia, and chest radiographs are typically normal.

Careful laryngoscopy lasting several minutes and including distraction techniques such as having patients cough, sniff, or count may allow visualization of vocal cord abduction.[121] Visualization of normal vocal cord abduction allows exclusion of vocal cord paralysis or fixation as diagnoses.

Emergency airway intervention by intubation or tracheotomy is not unusual for patients with functional laryngeal dyskinesia as a result of misdiagnosis. A high index of suspicion is required to promptly recognize and treat this disorder. Treatment consists of reassurance, supportive therapy, and psychological counseling.

Recurrent episodes of functional laryngeal dyskinesia are unusual but can occur.

REFERENCES

1. Weymuller EA. Acute airway management. In Cummings CW et al., eds. Otolaryngology: Head and Neck Surgery, 3rd ed. St. Louis, Mosby–Year Book, 1998, pp. 2368–2381.
2. Miller RD, Hyatt RE. Evaluation of obstructing lesions of the trachea and larynx by flow-volume loops. Am Rev Resp Dis 1973;108:475–481.
3. Acres JC, Kryger MH. Clinical significance of pulmonary function tests: upper airway obstruction. Chest 1981;80:207–211.
4. Kashima HK. Documentation of upper airway obstruction in unilateral vocal cord paralysis: flow-volume loop studies in 43 subjects. Laryngoscope 1984;94:923–937.
5. Bass H. The flow-volume loop: normal standards and abnormalities in chronic obstructive pulmonary disease. Chest 1973;63:171–176.
6. Hawkins DB, Crockett DM, Shum TK. Corticosteroids in airway management. Otolaryngol Head Neck Surg 1983;91:593–596.
7. Boorstein JH et al. Using helium-oxygen mixtures in the emergency management of acute upper airway obstruction. Ann Emerg Med 1989;18:688–690.
8. Orr JB. Helium-oxygen gas mixtures in the management of patients with airway obstruction. Ear Nose Throat J 1988;67:866–869.
9. Skrinskas GJ, Hyland RH, Hutcheon MA. Using helium-oxygen mixtures in the management of acute upper airway obstruction. Can Med Assoc J 1983;128:555–558.
10. Harrison RR et al. Mouth-to-mask ventilation: a superior method of rescue breathing. Ann Emerg Med 1982;11:74–76.
11. Heimlich HJ. A life-saving maneuver to prevent foodchoking. JAMA 1975;234:398–401.
12. Heimlich HJ, Hoffman KA, Canestri FR. Food-choking and drowning deaths prevented by external subdiaphragmatic compression. Ann Thorac Surg 1975;20:188–195.
13. Haugen RK. The café coronary: sudden deaths in restaurants. JAMA 1963;186:142–143.
14. Fugimori M, Virtue RW. The value of oxygenation prior to induced apnea. Anesthesiology 1960;21:46–49.
15. Sellick BA. Cricoid pressure to control regurgitation of stomach contents during induction of anesthesia. Lancet 1961;2:404–406.
16. Dufour DG, Larose DL, Clement SC. Rapid-sequence intubation in the emergency department. J Emerg Med 1995;13:705–710.
17. Iserson KV. Blind nasotracheal intubation. Am Emerg Med 1981;10:468–471.
18. Kidd JF, Dyson A, Latto IP. Successful difficult intubation use of the gum-elastic bougie. Anaesthesia 1988;43:437–438.
19. McCarroll SM et al. The gum-elastic bougie: old but still useful. Anesthesiology 1988;8:643–644.
20. Messeter KH, Petersson KI. Endotracheal intubation with the fiberoptic bronchoscope. Anaesthesia 1980;35:294–298.
21. Ovassapian et al. Fiberoptic nasotracheal intubation: incidence and causes of failure. Anesth Analg 1983;62:692–695.
22. Mlinek EJ et al. Fiberoptic intubation in the emergency department. Ann Emerg Med 1990;19:359–362.
23. Delaney KA, Hessler R. Emergency flexible fiberoptic nasotracheal intubation: a report of 60 cases. Ann Emerg Med 1988;17:919–926.
24. Afilalo M et al. Fiberoptic intubation in the emergency department: a case series. J Emerg Med 1993;11:387–391.
25. Butler FS, Cirillo AA. Retrograde tracheal intubation. Anesth Analg 1960;39:333–338.
26. Bissinger U, Guggenberger H, Lenz G. Retrograde-guided fiberoptic intubation in patients with laryngeal carcinoma. Anesth Analg 1995;81:408–410.
27. Stewart RD. Tactile orotracheal intubation. Ann Emerg Med 1984;13:175–178.
28. Pennant JH, White PF. The laryngeal mask airway: its uses in anesthesiology. Anesthesiology 1993; 79:144–163.
29. Hasham F, Kumar CM, Lawler PGP. The uses of the laryngeal mask airway to assist fiberoptic orotracheal intubation. Anesthesia 1991;46:891.
30. Gonzales RM et al. Recent advances in airway management in anesthesiology: an update for otolaryngologists. Am J Otolaryngol 1996;17:145–160.
31. Atherton GL, Johnson JC. Ability of paramedics to use the Combitube in prehospital cardiac arrest. Ann Emerg Med 1993;22:1263–1268.
32. Vollmer T et al. Use of a lighted stylet for guided orotracheal intubation in the prehospital setting. Ann Emerg Med 1985;14:324–328.
33. Verdile VP et al. Nasotracheal intubation using a flexible lighted stylet. Ann Emerg Med 1990;19:506–510.
34. Gorback M. Management of the challenging airway with the Bullard laryngoscope. J Clin Anesth 1991;3:473–477.
35. Cooper S, Benumof J, Ozaki G. Evaluation of the Bullard laryngoscope using the new intubating stylet: comparison with conventional laryngoscopy. Anesth Analg 1994;79:965–970.
36. Weymuller EA et al. Management and difficult airway problems with percutaneous transtracheal ventilation. Ann Otol Rhinol Laryngol 1987;96:34–37.
37. Richtsmeier WJ, Eisele DW, MacMurray A. Transtracheal ventilation with crash cart equipment. Otolaryngol Head Neck Surg 1990;102:191–192.
38. Caparosa RJ, Zavatsky AR. Practical aspects of the cricothyroid space. Laryngoscope 1957;67:577–591.
39. Tucker JA. Obstruction of the major pediatric airway. Otolaryngol Clin North Am 1979;12:329–341.
40. Erlandson MJ et al. Cricothyroidtomy in the emergency department revisited. J Emerg Med 1989;7:115–118.
41. Tami TA et al. Pulmonary edema and acute upper airway obstruction. Laryngoscope 1986;96:506–509.
42. Willms D, Shure D. Pulmonary edema due to upper airway obstruction in adults. Chest 1988;94:1090–1092.
43. Guffin TN et al. Acute postobstructive pulmonary edema. Otolaryngol Head Neck Surg 1995;112:235–237.
44. Goldenberg JD et al. Negative-pressure pulmonary edema in the otolaryngology patient. Otolaryngol Head Neck Surg 1997;117:62–66.
45. Flint PW. Powered surgical instrumentation for laryngeal surgery. Otolaryngol Head Neck Surg (in press).
46. Rubin J, Johnson JT, Myers EN. Stomal recurrence after laryngectomy: interrelated risk-factor study. Otolaryngol Head Neck Surg 1990;103:805–812.
47. Esteban F et al. Risk factors involved in stomal recur-

rence following laryngectomy. J Laryngol Otol 1993;107:527–531.
48. Yotakis J et al. Evaluation of risk factors in stomal recurrence after laryngectomy. Clin Otolaryngol 1996;21:135–138.
49. Emergency Cardiac Care Committee and Subcommittees, American Heart Association. Guidelines for cardiopulmonary resuscitation and emergency cardiac care, II: Adult Basic Life Support. JAMA 1992;268: 2184–2198.
50. Barna JS, Frable MAS. Life-threatening angioedema. Otolaryngol Head Neck Surg 1990;103:795–798.
51. Megerian CA, Arnold JE, Berger M. Angioedema: 5 years' experience with a review of the disorder's presentation and treatment. Laryngoscope 1992; 102:256–260.
52. Karlis V et al. Hereditary angioedema. Oral Surg Oral Med Oral Pathol Oral Radiol Endod. 1997;83:462–464.
53. Brown NJ, Snowden M, Griffin MR. Recurrent angiotensin-converting enzyme inhibitor–associated angioedema. JAMA 1997;278:232–233.
54. Heymann WR. Acquired angioedema. J Ann Acad Dermatol 1997;36:611–615.
55. Slater E et al. Clinical profile of angioedema associated with angiotensin-converting enzyme inhibition. JAMA 1988;260:967–970.
56. Agah R, Bandi V, Guntupalli KK. Angioedema: the role of ACE inhibitors and factors associated with poor clinical outcome. Intensive Care Med 1997; 23:793–796.
57. Gunkel AR et al. Angioneurotic edema as a reaction to angiotensin-converting enzyme inhibitors. Am J Otolaryngol 1996;17:87–91.
58. Gannon TH, Eby TL. Angioedema from ACE inhibitors: a cause of upper airway obstruction. Laryngoscope 1990;100:1156–1160.
59. VanDellen RG. Long-term treatment of C1 inhibitor deficiency with epsilon-aminocarproic acid in two patients. Mayo Clin Proc 1996;71:1175–1178.
60. Moore GP, Hurley WT, Pace SA. Hereditary angioedema. Ann Emerg Med 1988;17:1082–1086.
61. Hebert PC et al. Acute epiglottitis in a Canadian setting. Laryngoscope 1998;108:64–69.
62. Deeb ZE. Acute supraglottitis in adults: early indicators of airway obstruction. Am J Otolaryngol 1997;18:112–115.
63. Kucera CM et al. Epiglottitis in adults and children in Olmsted County, Minnesota, 1976–1990. Mayo Clin Proc 1996;71:1155–1161.
64. Frantz TD, Rasgon BM, Quesenberry CP. Acute epiglottitis in adults. JAMA 1994;272:1358–1360.
65. Ducic Y et al. Description and evaluation of the vallecula sign: a new radiologic sign in the diagnosis of adult epiglottitis. Ann Emerg Med 1997;30:1–6.
66. Nemzek WR et al. A reappraisal of the radiographic findings of acute inflammation of the epiglottis and supraglottic structures in adults. Am J Neuroradiol 1995;16:495–502.
67. Barrow HN, Vastola AP, Wang RC. Adult supraglottitis. Otolaryngol Head Neck Surg 1993;109:474–477.
68. Caplan RA et al. Practice guidelines for management of the difficult airway: a report by the American Society of Anesthesiologists Task Force on Management of the Difficult Airway. Anesthesiology 1993;78:597–602.
69. Ovassapian A, Mesnick PS. Evaluation of the patient with a difficult airway. In Longnecker DE et al., eds. Principles and Practice of Anesthesiology, 2nd ed. St. Louis, Mosby–Year Book, 1998, pp. 219–231.
70. Norton ML, Brown ACD. Evaluating the patient with a difficult airway in anesthesia. Otolaryngol Clin North Am 1990;23:771–785.
71. Norton ML. The difficult airway. In Norton ML, ed. Atlas of the Difficult Airway. St. Louis, Mosby–Year Book, 1996, pp. 3–16.
72. Sofferman RA, Johnson DL, Spencer RF. Lost airway during anesthesia induction: alternatives for management. Laryngoscope 1997;107:1476–1482.
73. Mark JJ et al. The difficult airway: mechanisms for effective dissemination of critical information. J Clin Anesth 1992;4:247–251.
74. Ligier B, Breslow MJ, Dorman T. Airway management in the trauma patient. In Cameron J, ed. Current Surgical Therapy. St. Louis, Mosby–Year Book, 1995, pp. 794–780.
75. Ampel L et al. An approach to airway management in the acutely head-injured patient. J Emerg Med 1998;6:1–7.
76. Criswell JC, Parr MJA, Nolan JP. Emergency airway management in patients with cervical spine injuries. 1994;49:900–903.
77. Nicholls BJ, Cullen BF. Anesthesia for trauma. J Clin Anesth 1988;1:115–129.
78. Reid DC et al. Etiology and clinical course of missed spine fractures. J Trauma 1987;27:980–986.
79. Wood PR, Lawler PGP. Managing the airway in cervical spine injury. Anesthesia 1992;47:792–797.
80. Bivens HG et al. The effect of axial traction during orotracheal intubation of the trauma victim with an unstable cervical spine. Ann Emerg Med 1986;15:417–420.
81. Freemyer B et al. Comparison of five-view and three-view cervical spine series in the evaluation of patients with cervical trauma. Ann Emerg Med 1989;18:818–821.
82. Schleehaulf K et al. Computed tomography in the initial evaluation of the cervical spine. Ann Emerg Med 1989;18:815–817.
83. Suderman VS, Crosby ET, Lui A. Elective oral tracheal intubation in cervical spine-injured adults. Can J Anesth 1991;38:785–789.
84. Meschino A et al. The safety of awake tracheal intubation in cervical spine injury. Can J Anesth 1992;39: 114–117.
85. Crosby ET. Tracheal intubation in the cervical spine-impaired patient. Can J Anesth 1992;39:105–109.
86. Barriot P, Riou B. Retrograde technique for tracheal intubation in trauma patients. Crit Care Med 1988;16:712–713.
87. Schaefer SD. The acute management of external laryngeal trauma: a 27-year experience. Arch Otolaryngol Head Neck Surg 1992;118:598–604.
88. Gussack GS, Jurkovich GJ. Treatment dilemmas in laryngotracheal trauma. J Trauma 1988;28:1439–1444.
89. Grewal H et al. Management of penetrating laryngotracheal injuries. Head Neck 1995;17:494–502.
90. Coulson AS, Rossiter SJ, Guernsey JM. Progressive tracheal obstruction. J Thorac Cardiovasc Surg 1974;67:733–743.
91. Attar S et al. Tracheal obstruction. Ann Thorac Surg 1973;16:555–567.
92. Streitz JM, Shapshay SM. Airway injury after tracheotomy and endotracheal intubation. Surg Clin North Am 1991;71:1211–1230.
93. Mathisen DJ, Grillo HC. Endoscopic relief of malignant airway obstruction. Ann Thorac Surg 1989; 48:469–475.
94. Beamis JF et al. Endoscopic laser therapy for obstruct-

ing tracheobronchial lesions. Ann Otol Rhinol Laryngol 1991;100:413–419.
95. Stanopoulos IT et al. Laser bronchoscopy in respiratory failure from malignant airway obstruction. Crit Care Med 1993;21:386–391.
96. Grillo HC. Primary reconstruction of airway after resection of subgottic laryngeal and upper tracheal stenosis. Ann Thorac Surg 1981;33:3–18.
97. Shapshay SM et al. Endoscopic treatment of subglottic and tracheal stenosis by radial laser incision and dilation. Ann Otol Rhinol Laryngol 1987;96:661–664.
98. Montgomery WW. Silicone tracheal T-tube. Ann Otol Rhinol Laryngol 1974;83:71–75.
99. Wasserman K et al. Emergency stenting of malignant obstruction of the upper airways: long-term follow-up with two types of silicone prostheses. Ann Otol Rhinol Laryngol 1998;107:149–154.
100. Fink BR. The etiology and treatment of laryngeal spasm. Anesthesiology 1956;17:569–577.
101. Olsson GL, Hallen B. Laryngospasm during anesthesia: a computer-aided incidence study in 136,929 patients. Acta Anaesth Scand 1984;28:567–575.
102. Tyler EP. Complications of anesthesia for otolaryngology-head and neck surgery. In Weissler MC, Pillsbury R, eds. Complications of Head and Neck Surgery. New York, Thieme Medical, 1995, pp. 371–388.
103. Staffel JG et al. The prevention of postoperative stridor and laryngospasm with topical lidocaine. Arch Otolaryngol Head Neck Surg 1991;117:1123–1128.
104. Wade JSH. Respiratory obstruction in thyroid surgery. Ann Royal Coll Surg Engl 1980;62:15–24.
105. Lacoste L et al. Airway complications in thyroid surgery. Ann Otol Rhinol Laryngol 1993;102:441–446.
106. Martis C, Athanassiades S. Post-thyroidectomy laryngeal edema. Am J Surg 1971;122:58–60.
107. Green WER et al. Tracheal collapse after thyroidectomy. Br J Surg 1979;66:554–557.
108. Geelhoed GW. Tracheomalacia from compression goiter: management after thyroidectomy. Surgery 1988;104:1100–1108.
109. Young T et al. The occurrence of sleep-disordered breathing among middle-aged adults. N Engl J Med 1993;328:1230–1235.
110. Strohl KP, Redline S. Recognition of obstructive sleep apnea. Am J Respir Crit Care Med 1996;154:279–289.
111. Esclamado RM et al. Perioperative complications and risk factors in the surgical treatment of obstructive sleep apnea syndrome. Laryngoscope 1989;99:1125–1129.
112. Riley RW et al. Obstructive sleep apnea surgery: risk management and complications. Otolaryngol Head Neck Surg 1997;117:648–652.
113. Fairbanks DNF. Uvulopalatopharyngoplasty complications and avoidance strategies. Otolaryngol Head Neck Surg 1990;102:239–245.
114. Aly A, McIlwain M, Duncavage JA. Electrosurgery-induced endotracheal tube ignition during tracheotomy. Ann Otol Rhinol Laryngol 1991;100:31–33.
115. Burgess GE, LeJune FE. Endotracheal tube ignition during laser surgery of the larynx. Arch Otolaryngol 1979;105:561–562.
116. deRichemond AL, Bruley ME. Head and neck surgical fires. In Eisele DW, ed. Complications in Head and Neck Surgery. St. Louis, Mosby–Year Book, 1993, pp. 312–322.
117. Gupte SR. Gauze fire in the oral cavity: a case report. Anesth Analg 1972;51:645–646.
118. Bowdle TA et al. Fire following use of electrocautery during emergency percutaneous transtracheal ventilation. Anesthesiology 1987;66:697–698.
119. Geist R, Tallett S. Diagnosis and management of psychogenic stridor caused by a conversion disorder. Pediatrics 1990;86:315–317.
120. Sim T et al. Functional laryngeal obstruction: a somatization disorder. Am J Med 1990;88:293–295.
121. Ferris RL, Eisele DW, Tunkel DE. Functional laryngeal dyskinesia in children and adults. Laryngoscope 1998;108:1520–1523.

CHAPTER 10

Foreign Bodies in the Upper Aerodigestive Tract

David M. Huchton, MD, and
Bernard R. Marsh, MD

Foreign bodies in the upper aerodigestive tract continue to be a challenge. There has been a rapid proliferation of new instrumentation whose proper role in foreign-body work has yet to be established. Flexible instruments are very popular, but in the hands of physicians with little training in their specific use in foreign-body work, they may result in unnecessary morbidity. Modern instrumentation can never replace knowledge of the lessons learned and techniques pioneered by the old masters of endoscopy such as Chevalier Jackson. For successful management of foreign bodies, nothing can substitute for the practice essential for developing sound, basic endoscopic techniques using time-honored methods.

FOREIGN BODIES IN THE AIRWAY

Complete obstruction of the airway by a foreign body (at the laryngeal inlet, trachea, or carina) is seldom observed in a hospital setting. Such victims rarely make it to the hospital alive. If they do, the object has necessarily become partially obstructive. Care is rendered in a "thoughtfully urgent" rather than an emergent manner.

Coughing, gagging, and throat clearing are reflexes of children and adults alike and are indications of incomplete obstruction. Overzealous attempts by emergency personnel to aid these victims are unnecessary and potentially catastrophic. A finger swiped through a choking child's mouth or probing the pharynx blindly may transform a partial obstruction into a complete obstruction. Likewise, inverting a child and delivering back blows may drive a tracheobronchial foreign body into the conus elasticus, converting partial into complete obstruction.[1]

Complete airway obstruction in a young child is heralded by the inability to cough, speak, or cry. In an older child or adult, the neck may be clutched reflexively as well.

Foreign Bodies in the Airways of Children

The most common pediatric airway foreign body is vegetable matter. Nuts, especially peanuts, account for one third of cases. Carrot and apple bits, sunflower and watermelon seeds, popcorn kernels, and dried beans account for much of the remainder of vegetable matter found in the airway. Dried peas, beans, and corn are of special concern, as they can swell as they acquire moisture in the airway and can progress from causing partial obstruction to causing complete obstruction in a matter of hours. Roasted peanuts can produce a remarkable inflammatory reaction in a short period.[2]

Metallic objects such as safety pins and straight pins are becoming less common, but radiolucent plastic objects and toy parts are becoming more prevalent, and because of their inert nature, they frequently produce more indolent symptoms.

Children under the age of 3 years are at the highest risk because of their tendency to explore the environment with their mouths and also because their posterior dentition and sensory reflexes are not fully developed.[1] Almost 75% of pediatric foreign bodies occur in children under the age of 3, and 85% occur before age 5 (Fig. 10–1).

Teeth can be aspirated, too, and should be suspected, especially in the setting of trauma with the finding of newly lost teeth not otherwise discovered.

Bulky or multiple upper esophageal foreign bodies may also obstruct the airway posteriorly by compression and must always be considered, especially in a small child (Fig. 10–2).

PRESENTATION

Three stages may be recognized in a patient with a foreign body in the airway:[1]

1. Violent paroxysms of coughing, gagging, choking, and possibly transient complete obstruction occur upon aspiration of the foreign body.
2. A period of asymptomatic or silent foreign-body residence in the airway usually follows. This period often leads to delay in diagnosis, as the patient, physician, or parents are falsely reassured by the victim's ease.
3. Complications resulting from the foreign object in the airway ensue. They may take the form of pneumonia, atelectasis, wheezing or asthma, a crouplike infection, a lung abscess, or hemoptysis. Fever, cough, malaise, and generalized fatigue and toxicity may also be present.

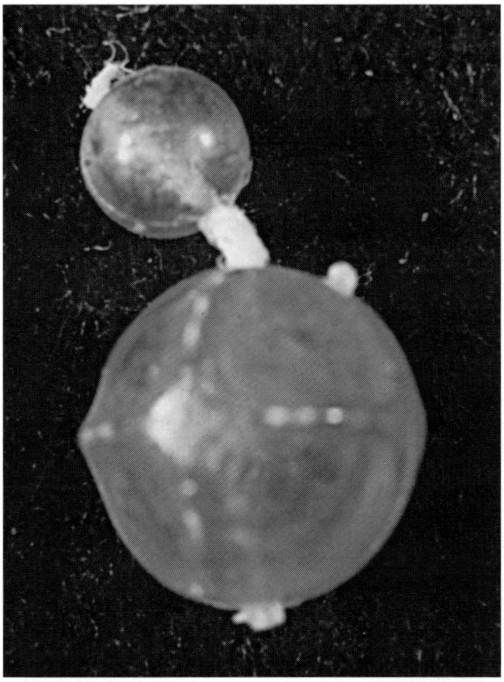

Figure 10–1. Inert plastic beads removed from a child's right mainstem bronchus. They resulted in little symptomatology and minimal acute mucosal reaction.

A negative history may be misleading; the parent may not recall or may minimize the initial event, and the child may be embarrassed to admit the occurrence. A positive history should be taken seriously, even if given by a young child who describes an event unwitnessed by others.

It is important to remain vigilant with children who have recurrent crouplike illnesses, recurrent pneumonia, or new-onset asthma. Resolution followed by recurrence after antibiotics or steroids should further heighten one's index of suspicion.

Dyspnea may be severe if a foreign object is lodged in the larynx or trachea or at the carina but may be less so in cases of bronchial obstruction. Laryngeal foreign bodies cause stridor, hoarseness, cough, pain, and sometimes dysphagia. They are commonly aligned in the anteroposterior sagittal plane between the vocal cords.

Tracheal foreign bodies cause three classic sounds, as described by Chevalier Jackson: the audible slap and palpatory thud with coughing or deep inspiration and the asthmatoid wheeze on expiration. Esclamado and Richardson found aspiration and choking to be present in 90% of children with tracheal foreign bodies, stridor in 60%, wheezing in 50%, and cough in 40%.[3]

Esophageal foreign bodies may compress the airway, resulting in dyspnea, dysphagia, odynophagia, a change in diet in older children, and failure to thrive in younger children.

EVALUATION

Posteroanterior and lateral chest and soft tissue neck radiographs should be obtained. The abdomen should be included as well.

Expiratory and inspiratory posteroanterior chest radiographs may be valuable in grossly localizing a bronchial foreign body. With expiration, the air distal to the foreign body will be trapped, resulting in obstructive emphysema and hyperinflation of that lung, which causes a mediastinal shift to the opposite side. In the

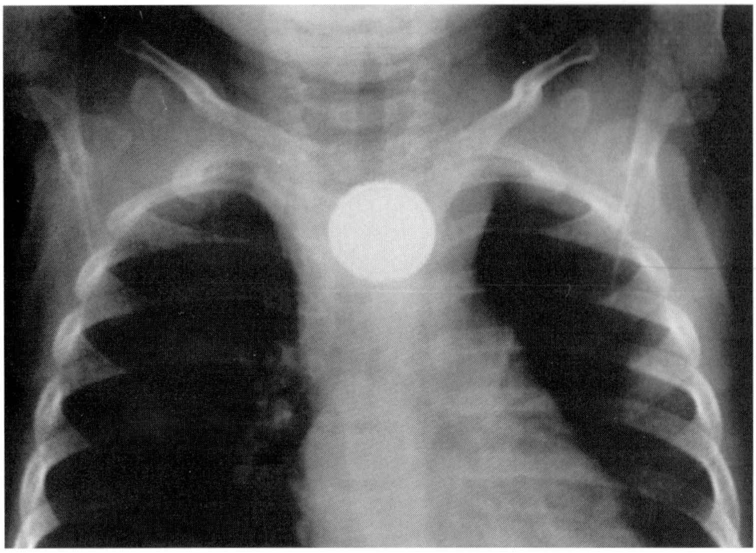

Figure 10–2. Esophageal foreign body with deviation of air column.

very young, fluoroscopy may yield the same findings (Figs. 10–3 and 10–4).

A barium esophagram is seldom indicated in the event of suspected esophageal obstruction and airway compromise. The barium may be aspirated and may complicate the operative evaluation later.[4]

PRIORITIES

Key factors in successful management of airway foreign bodies are the following:

1. A surgical team experienced in the management of foreign bodies in the airway and the resulting complications,
2. An anesthesia team likewise experienced,
3. Nurses and technicians with some familiarity with the necessary equipment, and
4. The availability of appropriate equipment for the task at hand.[2]

It is important to remember that the therapy for partially obstructive airway foreign bodies is to be thoughtfully urgent rather than emergent.

Prior to the patient's arrival, the equipment

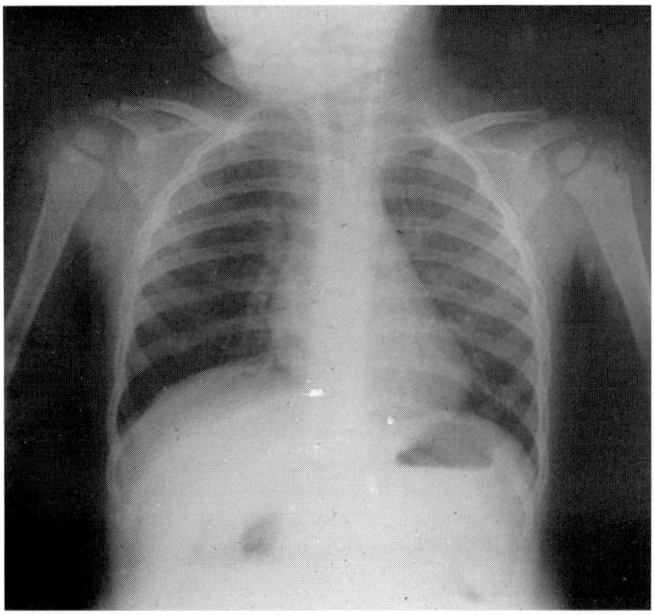

Figure 10–3. Normal-appearing chest radiograph after right mainstem foreign body aspiration.

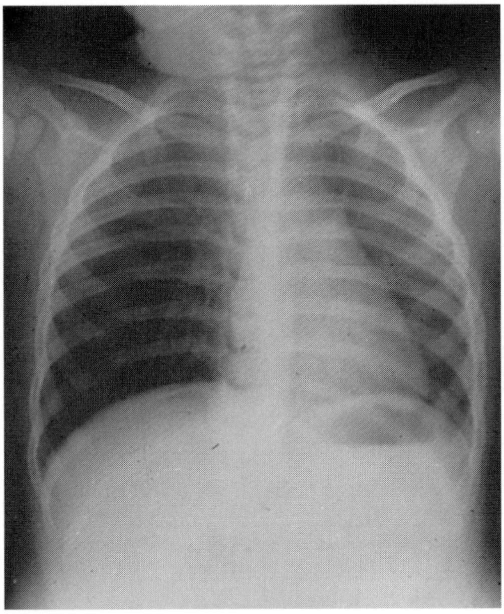

Figure 10–4. Expiratory phase radiograph revealing air trapping in right lung fields distal to foreign body.

should be carefully inspected. If possible, a duplicate foreign body should be obtained and studied in light of the planned retrieval instruments to determine which instrument is most suitable for the specific requirement. Two light sources should be available. The bulbs should be checked before anesthesia is administered and one light source should remain illuminated before anesthesia is induced; bulbs tend to burn out when turned on rather than during use.

Before proceeding, one should select a bronchoscope and telescope of the anticipated size and of at least one size smaller, in addition to a diagnostic laryngoscope and an esophagoscope. In a well-developed 2-year-old child, Storz 3.5 × 26 and 4 × 30 bronchoscopes are reasonable choices.

Finally, prior to commencing the procedure, equipment for an airway emergency should be on hand, including jet ventilation materials. The anesthesia team should be familiar with its use.

The preoperative discussion with the family should include information about the risks of complete airway obstruction, esophageal perforation, rupture of the bronchi or trachea, pneumothorax, and failure of extraction as well as the possibility of proceeding to thoracotomy for removal.

General anesthesia is usually used for airway foreign-body work in children. If there is concern about a laryngeal foreign body, examination with a flexible laryngoscope under local anesthesia may assist in planning the ultimate anesthetic management. A laryngeal foreign body with an adequate airway allows induction of general anesthesia followed by direct visualization with laryngoscope and extraction of the object. Rarely, a tracheotomy is required for severely impacted foreign bodies.[5]

For tracheobronchial foreign bodies, anesthesia with spontaneous respiration can be employed rather than paralysis, as the patient can still breathe on his or her own, even with temporary loss of the airway. Vigorous bagging should be avoided if possible as it may drive bronchial foreign bodies into a distal position not readily accessible by endoscopy.

Rigid bronchoscopy is usually the method of choice for visualization and extraction of foreign bodies in the airway. It offers several advantages over flexible bronchoscopy and other techniques. Ventilation can be provided through the bronchoscope, rigid telescopes may be used, and a wide variety of sizes and types of retrieval forceps are available. Also, the object may be partially or completely sheathed within the bronchoscope on removal. This is particularly useful in the extraction of pins, needles, and other sharp objects; it also helps to prevent stripping off the object as the glottis is passed. Insertion of the bronchoscope may be facilitated by exposure of the larynx with the anesthesia laryngoscope, and visualization may be improved by simultaneously inserting the rigid telescope within the bronchoscope as it is inserted. Once in the airway below the glottis, the ventilatory circuit can be connected.

The bronchoscope is secured with the left hand, scissoring the upper lip away from the scope with the fingers and resting the scope on the thumb, which is also used to gently advance the tube under visualization. The right hand is used to direct head and neck orientation, guide the scope in the airway, and apply instruments when appropriate. In children, foreign bodies in the airway usually lodge in the main bronchi. Once the foreign body has been localized, forceps spaces are identified, and the bronchoscope is withdrawn slightly to allow for the opening of the jaws of the forceps prior to application. Optimal technique is paramount here, as inadvertent distal displacement may complicate management and require thoracotomy for extraction.

Optical pediatric forceps are particularly valuable in most cases of children with vegetable matter in a main bronchus. These forceps allow direct visualization of the application of the forceps to the foreign body. Smaller children and

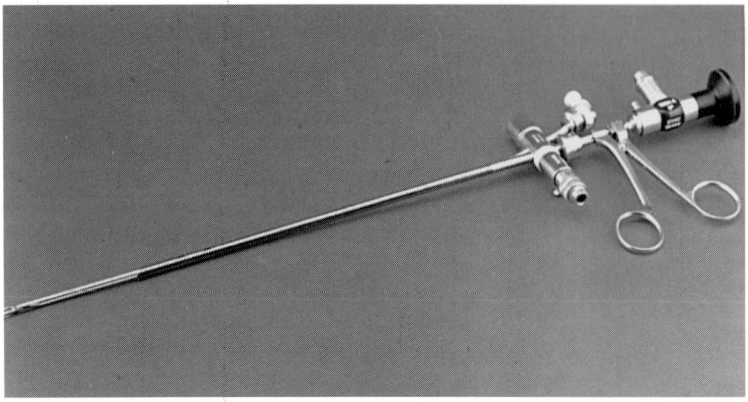

Figure 10–5. Pediatric double-action optical forceps, passed through a ventilating bronchoscope.

more distal bronchi may not allow ready passage of these forceps (Fig. 10–5).

Double-action, forward-grasping forceps are available in fenestrated, alligator, nonfenestrated, and fine/miniature varieties. These forceps have the advantage of very good control at the time of application onto the object, and they can be used to dilate a distal bronchus with discernible forceps space prior to dilation and extraction. A disadvantage of these forceps, compared to the passive-action Jackson forward-grasping forceps, is that they generate more force on application and can fragment vegetable or other matter between the jaws. This risk generally applies to less experienced surgeons, which points up the importance of practice and training in the animal laboratory prior to clinical exposure (Fig. 10–6).

Care should be taken to rotate the scope if that is necessary to pass the foreign body at its widest dimension in the sagittal plane at the glottis. If the foreign body does strip off into the airway, it may result in complete obstruction, necessitating prompt revisualization, forceps application, and extraction. If it descends into the main bronchi, it may well pass into the normal bronchus, as edema at the original site may diminish air flow.[1]

Following the extraction of a foreign body, the bronchoscope should be reinserted to verify absence of additional foreign material. Once that has been verified, the patient is usually orotracheally intubated by the endoscopist or anesthesiologist until fully awakened, and then extubated.

Pins, nails, and sharp-pointed objects are commonly found in a point-up orientation. Disimpaction of the point may be necessary prior

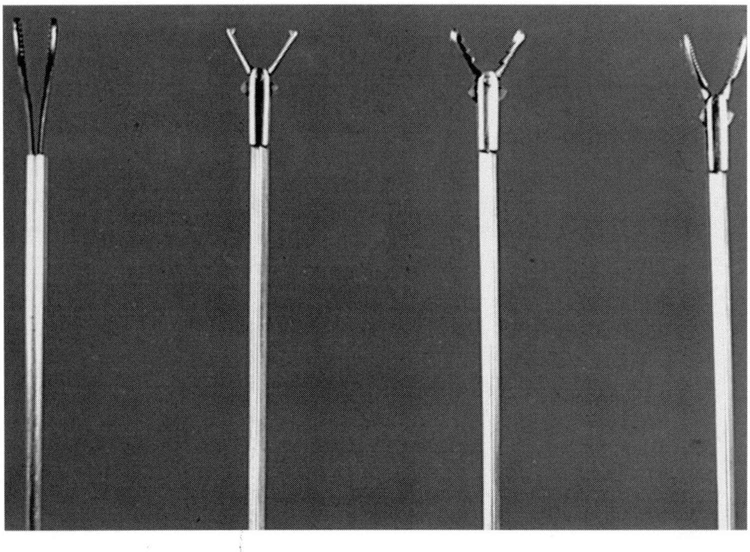

Figure 10–6. Examples of various forceps (from left to right): Jackson fenestrated forceps, double-action rotation forceps, double-action small alligator forceps, double-action fenestrated forceps.

to removal and may require displacement slightly more distally prior to regrasping and removal.

Fiberoptic Bronchoscopic Applications. Flexible instrumentation is becoming more popular for diagnostic and therapeutic use in the upper airways, and as flexible forceps instrumentation improves and becomes more diverse, a knowledge of this modality broadens the armamentarium from which the surgeon may draw in approaching the problem of foreign bodies in the airway. However, Marsh describes several criteria that should be considered before using flexible equipment for foreign-body work.[2] These criteria include the following:

1. The staff is trained in rigid and flexible techniques,
2. The use of rigid technique is inappropriate for anatomic or medical reasons,
3. The patient is older than 10 years of age,
4. The foreign body is segmented,
5. The object is small and nonobstructive,
6. Flexible instrumentation appropriate to the foreign body is available, and
7. The foreign body is unimpacted.

If these conditions pertain, then one may proceed either through the endotracheal tube or directly, without intubation. Once introduced, the scope should be suctioned clear of debris and the forceps then passed through the instrument port, visualizing the object throughout. It is usually necessary to advance the forceps some distance from the tip of the scope to manipulate the forceps and visualize its application to the foreign body. Once that has been achieved, an assistant should grip the handle with appropriate firmness and, in conjunction with the endoscopist, proceed with the extraction of the object. The foreign body should remain in view at all times to enable immediate discovery of inadvertent loss of the object from the jaws of the forceps.

Two contraindications to the use of flexible instrumentation bear stressing: (1) the presence of large, impacted foreign bodies, especially when associated with granulation or extensive edema, as these predispose to dislodgement or failure to extract the object; (2) the presence of sharp, impacted foreign bodies that require sheathing to protect against soft-tissue injury during extraction.

The Fogarty Catheter. The use of a Fogarty catheter for the removal of foreign bodies in the airway is mentioned only to point out its *very* limited role. The uninflated catheter and balloon are passed distal to the object. The balloon is inflated and used to pull the foreign object out as it is advanced forward by the retracted catheter.[6]

This technique provides very little control of the foreign body, and complications during its use have been reported, including reaspiration of a retrieved foreign body.[7] It should be considered only when established techniques have failed and preferably is performed by an experienced endoscopist aware of the potential risks.

OUTCOME

Along with the complications described in the preoperative discussion with the family, traumatic laryngitis and laryngeal edema may occur. They are treated with humidity, steroids, and racemic epinephrine nebulization.

If a child has had pneumonia preoperatively, antibiotics are continued postoperatively. Likewise, antibiotics are initiated if purulent bronchitis is encountered intraoperatively. Atelectasis is treated with chest physiotherapy. If the foreign body is a sharp, contaminated object, tetanus prophylaxis is warranted if preventive inoculations are not up to date.

If the patient is improving, nontoxic, and stable on the day following operation, discharge home is warranted.

Foreign Bodies in the Airways of Adults

The adult population affected by foreign bodies in the airway is usually older than 50 and the risk increases with denture wear (which impairs the gingival and palatal sensation of a food bolus), alcohol use, and neurologic deficiencies.

The most common oropharyngeal foreign bodies are fish and chicken bones. Aspiration into the tracheobronchial tree is uncommon and usually consists of food. Teeth are occasionally aspirated and should be suspected and sought in a setting of trauma, intoxication, or lost, unaccounted for teeth (Figs. 10–7 and 10–8).

The aspiration of a tracheoesophageal speech prosthesis is a special circumstance occasionally encountered by the head and neck surgeon. Flexible instrumentation is often effective for such extraction (Fig. 10–9).

Most inhaled foreign bodies enter the right main-stem bronchus if they pass the glottis. The right main-stem bronchus is shorter, wider, and less angulated from the direction of the trachea.

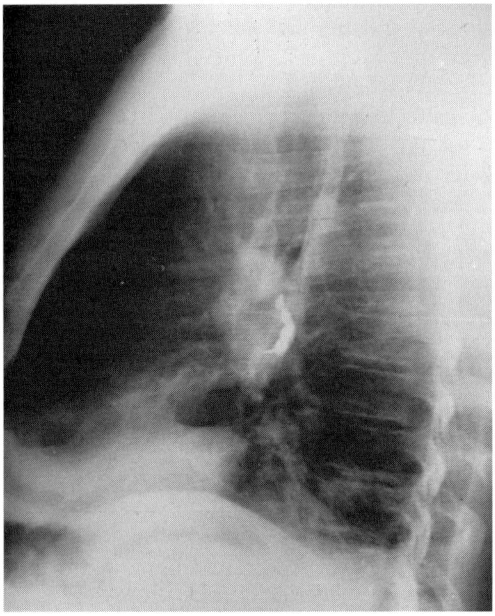

Figure 10–7. Right main-stem partial dental bridge prosthesis aspirated by an adult.

PRESENTATION

The three stages of foreign-body aspiration—the acute event, the silent period, and the phase of complications—occur commonly in adults as

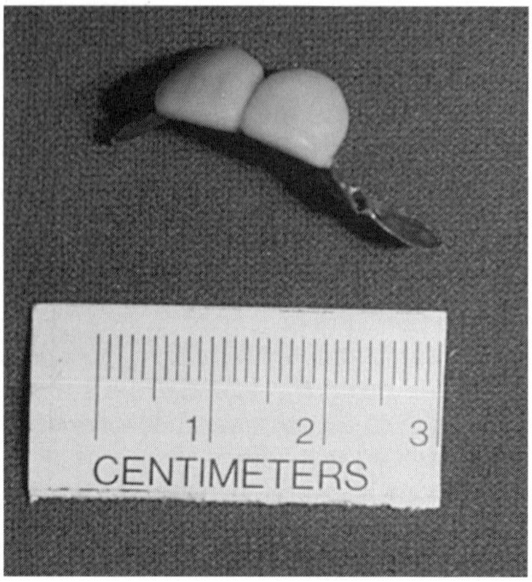

Figure 10–8. Close-up view of partial dental prosthesis after extraction.

in children. Adults are likely to provide a more detailed history when able, but in acutely intoxicated patients or those with severe neurologic debility, no history may be available, and only a high index of suspicion may lead to the proper diagnosis.

Stridor, hoarseness, cough, and odynophonia may occur in laryngeal, tracheal, or bronchial

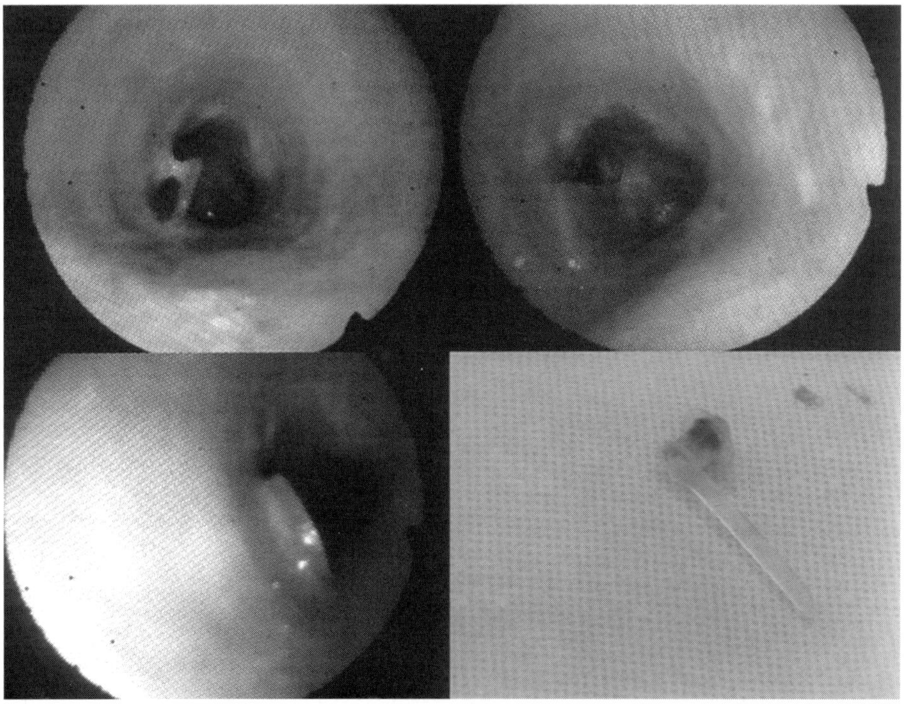

Figure 10–9. Voice prosthesis aspirated by an adult after a laryngectomy. Successful removal from left main-stem bronchus employed a fiberoptic bronchoscope with intravenous sedation via the tracheal stoma.

foreign bodies, and dysphagic symptoms ensue in cases of large esophageal foreign bodies.

EVALUATION

There is no substantial difference in radiographic evaluation of foreign-body aspiration by children and adults. Adults, however, are less likely to require fluoroscopy to document the ball valve air trapping that commonly occurs with lobar or segmental bronchial obstructions.

PRIORITIES

There is no substitute for experienced surgery and anesthesia teams, appropriate and functional equipment, and operative support staff to provide care of and assistance with this equipment. In fact, the argument has been made that, given the expense of maintaining this equipment and the experience necessary for safe treatment, the treatment of foreign bodies in the airway might best be relegated to regional, tertiary care centers.

Equipment should be inspected, practice with a variety of scopes and forceps should be applied to duplicate objects, and discussion with the anesthesia team about unexpected eventualities should precede the administration of anesthesia. Adult-sized bronchoscopes, telescopes, esophagoscopes, laryngoscopes, and forceps should be assembled before a patient is anesthetized.

Preoperative discussion with a patient and the family is no different from that with a pediatric patient. The assessment and stabilization of the patient's medical condition may prove to be more complex in the adult population because of neurologic, psychiatric, and complex medical comorbidities that are likely to complicate the overall picture.

General anesthesia is usually advocated in adults. However, sedation with local anesthesia can be used successfully with flexible instrumentation in some cases. Decisions about instrumentation and anesthesia can be individualized according to specific patient requirements and the endoscopist's preference.

The operative technique employed does not substantively differ from that described for the pediatric patient.

OUTCOMES

Complications and postoperative care are the same as those for the pediatric population. As these patients may have more extensive comorbid conditions, a longer hospital stay may be required.

FOREIGN BODIES IN THE ESOPHAGUS

A Foreign Body in the Esophagus of a Child

Coins are the most common foreign body seen in children, especially in children under 3 years of age, and 95% of pediatric esophageal foreign bodies lodge in the cervical esophagus[4]; the majority of them lodge at the level of the cricopharyngeus muscle. If the foreign body lodges, it raises the suspicion of a congenital esophageal malformation, and a follow-up esophagram should be obtained 2 to 3 weeks after an acute event and extraction.[1]

Ingestion of metallic foreign bodies has been supplanted in frequency by ingestion of plastic foreign bodies, largely due to the change in toy construction and composition. However, plastic pieces are usually quite inert, which often results in delayed diagnosis by which time the object may have caused a very serious complication such as esophageal erosion or a tracheoesophageal fistula.

The safety pin has become a fairly rare object of accidental ingestion, as disposable diapers have virtually replaced cloth diapers secured with safety pins. Nonetheless, the management of this and other sharply pointed ingested foreign bodies, including tacks, screws, staples, pins, nails, and glass, remains an important aspect of the study of foreign bodies in the aerodigestive tract, as urgent attention and extraction are required. Any signs or symptoms indicating esophageal perforation must prompt rapid operative intervention.

Other objects that require urgent attention are disk batteries such as those in small clocks, calculators, hand-held video games, and other small appliances and obstructive meat or other food boluses. Maves and associates demonstrated that prompt removal of ingested disk batteries is absolutely necessary, as they begin mucosal injury within 1 hour, erode into the muscular layer within 4 hours, and can perforate through the wall within 8 to 12 hours.[8] As with foreign bodies in the airway, a careful, thoughtful urgency should be the standard in their management.

PRESENTATION

In young children, a history is commonly absent. Young children explore the environment and objects with their mouths, and inadvertent swallowing of objects frequently ensues. Complete esophageal obstruction results in the pooling of secretions, drooling, coughing and aspiration, and the subjective sense of something being stuck, if the patient is old enough to describe this sensation. Dysphagia with or without odynophagia accompanies an incomplete obstruction. Older children may alter their diets to primarily liquids, and younger children may exhibit progressive failure to thrive.

Esophageal foreign bodies may be large enough or may have resulted in enough edema or erosion that airway symptoms such as dyspnea or recurrent aspiration with cough are present.

EVALUATION

Posteroanterior and lateral chest, abdominal, and soft tissue neck radiographs should be obtained when the diagnosis is entertained.

For suspected esophageal foreign bodies, the retropharyngeal space and mediastinum should be carefully assessed for air, and the airway assessed for deviation. Nonopaque foreign bodies may deviate the air column.

Barium-impregnated cotton or an esophagram is not indicated in the event of suspected esophageal obstruction. The barium may be aspirated and, if pooled in the hypopharynx, may complicate the operative evaluation later. It also delays safe retrieval, as the child's NPO status has been violated by the study.

If radiographic analysis is unrevealing but symptoms persist or progress, esophagoscopy should be performed. Many items are very difficult to demonstrate radiographically, including fish bones and pieces of wood, glass, plastic, and aluminum. Left in situ, they can cause life-threatening morbidity.

PRIORITIES

Once there are compelling reasons to suspect the presence of a foreign body in the esophagus, expeditious but safe esophagoscopy should be performed. It begins with the four-component approach, as described above.

For esophagoscopy, either rigid or flexible instrumentation may be employed safely; there are proponents of both techniques. The variety of forceps is broader for rigid scopes, and the protective sheathing action of the rigid esophagoscope over the foreign body upon retraction lessens the risk of esophageal tear or perforation. Special considerations, such as anatomic problems (conditions precluding mobilization of the head and neck during esophagoscopy), multiple, small foreign bodies (some of which might hide under uninflated mucosal folds), and complex foreign bodies with a sharp end pointing up (requiring gastric version), are relative indications for flexible over rigid esophagoscopy.

Instrumentation considerations aside, preoperative planning is identical to that for extraction of a foreign body from the airway. Appropriate, functioning instruments should be checked and arranged for ease of availability, and practice on a duplicate object helps in choosing forceps. A laryngoscope may suffice for visualization of a high esophageal foreign body. A Jesberg esophagoscope should be available as well.

Preoperative consent from the family should include discussion of the risks, as in cases of foreign bodies in the airway, but should also include mention of the risk of esophageal tear or perforation, which could require an external esophagotomy repair.

General anesthesia with endotracheal airway control is recommended in all patients 10 years of age and under. If flexible esophagoscopy is to be employed, intravenous sedation may be considered and has been successfully employed by others. We prefer general anesthesia even if flexible instruments are employed so as to allow for airway control and the prevention of aspiration in the event of inadvertent loss of an extracted object into the airway.

The patient is placed in a supine position, and the movable headpiece of the bed is elevated slightly. The eyes are protected by tape and a head drape, and the upper teeth are protected by a tooth guard or moist gauze. The head is extended, and the mouth scissored open with the thumb and middle finger of the left hand.

The scope is introduced into the mouth at a right angle and then directed downward over the base of tongue into the right pyriform sinus, lateral to the right arytenoid. The scope is gently advanced with the left thumb and guided by the right hand. Perforation almost always occurs in the cervical esophagus, so care must be exercised when performing this technique.

If it is necessary to proceed below the cervical esophagus, the head and shoulders are allowed to fall back so as to straighten the thoracic vertebrae. In the lower third of the esophagus, the scope should be angled toward the left anterior superior iliac spine to follow the course of the esophagus toward the gastroesophageal junction. The esophagoscope is withdrawn slowly and carefully, inspecting for unseen foreign matter and for mucosal tears or lacerations.

After the foreign body has been extracted, the scope should be reinserted to assess for esophageal pathology or anatomic lesions predisposing to impaction, especially in cases of obstruction by food.

If the foreign body is a coin, a double-action or alligator forceps usually provides the most secure grip on the object. One should be aware of the possibility of catching mucosa along with the coin. If the coin is not seen on endoscopy, an intraoperative radiograph may confirm its passage into the stomach. If this occurs, it may be safely allowed to pass through the gastrointestinal tract with no further intervention.

A safety pin with the pointed end up or a double- or multiply pointed object with the sharp ends up is usually best managed by using a flexible esophagoscope. The spring or central axis is grasped with the flexible forceps and the object is dragged into the gastric lumen and allowed to turn 180 degrees. The foreign body is then extracted with the sharp end trailing. If a complex object is fairly large and has multiple sharp points, an overtube inserted with the flexible scope protects the mucosa during its extraction (Fig. 10–10).

Disk batteries are also readily retrieved with double-action or alligator forceps. Extraction is as with bronchoscopic extraction of a foreign body. Foreign bodies can strip off the ends of the forceps, however; if these make their way into the gastric lumen, they usually pass through the gastrointestinal tract without complication. However, if a disk battery transits into the stomach, the stool should be examined by the parents until passage is confirmed, and any symptoms of bowel inflammation or perforation warrant immediate reevaluation.

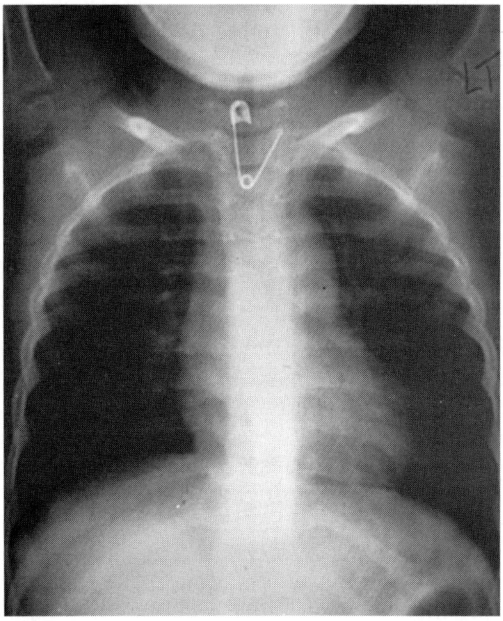

Figure 10–10. Cervical esophageal safety pin, removed using the gastric version technique.

OUTCOME

In uncomplicated extractions, the diet may be advanced rapidly, and discharge can occur the same day. If the object was sharp, close observation for 24 hours is warranted. If there is reason to suspect esophageal perforation, a contrast esophagram should be obtained postoperatively. Any symptoms of cervical esophageal perforation or mediastinitis are to be appropriately and rapidly evaluated and treated accordingly (see Chapter 20.). Routine postoperative antibiotics or steroids are not recommended.

A Foreign Body in the Esophagus of an Adult

Meat impaction is the most common esophageal obstruction in an adult. Predisposing factors include altered mental status, intoxication, neurologic conditions, esophageal anomalies such as stricture, and diminished sensation, as with dentures. With any meat impaction, there may be associated bony fragments.

Most other esophageal foreign bodies are secondary to inadvertent swallowing of objects in the mouth, such as coins, aluminum can pull tabs, toothpicks, buttons, and pieces of plastic, glass, or wood (Fig. 10–11).

If an object does not pass into the stomach and beyond, it has, in 90% of cases, become stuck at the cricopharyngeus muscle; otherwise, it may be stuck at a site of esophageal anatomic narrowing, such as a web or stricture. Plain radiographs are often not revealing. A barium study is indicated if symptoms are persistent but mild, but barium-impregnated cotton is to be avoided. Reexamination in 24 to 48 hours is warranted, but if symptoms persist or progress, esophagoscopy should ensue expeditiously.

PRESENTATION

Unless intoxication or neurologic status precludes taking a history, adults can usually pro-

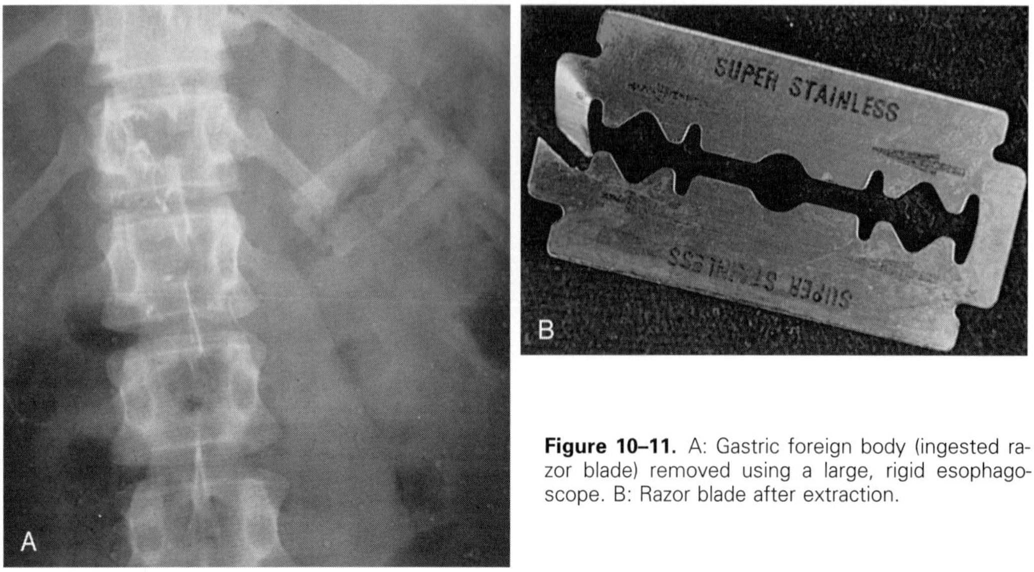

Figure 10–11. A: Gastric foreign body (ingested razor blade) removed using a large, rigid esophagoscope. B: Razor blade after extraction.

vide valuable information such as the timing, material, and likely location of an esophageal foreign body.

Troublesome dysphagia, odynophagia, and pooling or drooling of secretions usually ensue. Complete obstruction of salivary passage can be caused by meat impaction.

EVALUATION

In an adult, evaluation is identical to the evaluation performed in the case of a foreign body in the esophagus of a child.

PRIORITIES

General endotracheal anesthesia is used when performing the rigid technique; intravenous sedation may be used for flexible esophagoscopy. For meat impaction, large double-action or forward-grasping meat forceps are ideal for extraction. An attempt may be made to remove the bolus all at once, but usually the bolus cannot be pulled into the scope and is best removed by securing it at the end of the scope and removing the complex as a unit. Alternatively, the meat may be removed piecemeal. Undue force should not be used, as a radiolucent bone fragment may be abutting the esophageal wall, ready to perforate if attempts at extraction are too vigorous. Once the meat impaction has been removed, reinsertion of the scope and inspection for a stricture or other lesion is warranted.

OUTCOME

A follow-up esophagram in 1 to 2 weeks is indicated.

Postesophageal Foreign Bodies

Pointed objects such as bones and pieces of wood, plastic, or aluminum that tranverse the esophagus and enter the stomach are likely to pass through the gastrointestinal tract without complication. Serial radiographs should be obtained for radiopaque objects to assess their transit. The transit of a smooth object may be verified simply by examining the stools until it passes.

Long objects are likely not to traverse the duodenum in children under 2 years of age and should be extracted from the stomach. Likewise, sharp objects such as straight pins and objects that have remained in the stomach longer than a week should be endoscopically removed.

Oropharyngeal Foreign Bodies

It is common for fish bones to lodge in the oropharynx, and they are often radiolucent. They may be very distressing to the patient. If the pain is unilateral, the bone may be lodged within a tonsillar crypt. Adequate lighting, suction, topical anesthesia, and an operating microscope, if necessary, usually allow identification and extraction of a fish bone in the tonsil, vallecula, or base of the tongue.

Some foreign bodies may require a mirror or a flexible laryngoscope or bronchoscope for identification. They can usually be extracted while the patient is awake and providing his or her own lingual retraction with a sweetheart tongue depressor. Chicken, beef, and pork bones may lodge in the oropharynx or vallecula and can be extracted in a similar fashion. If they descend to the cervical esophagus, prompt esophagoscopy and extraction are warranted, as they result in perforation with some regularity if left untreated.

Nonendoscopic Methods of Esophageal Foreign-Body Retrieval

The use of papain and other meat tenderizer preparations has previously been advocated as an alternative to operative intervention. This practice has resulted in necrosis of the esophagus as well as erosion into major blood vessels, both of which may cause death. The practice is mentioned only so as to be condemned.

Placing a transoral or transnasal uninflated Foley or other balloon catheter and passing it distal to the foreign body and then inflating the balloon, in the hope of extracting the object on retraction of the catheter, is also an unsafe practice. Complications such as laryngospasm, epistaxis, mucosal lacerations, esophageal perforations, and aspiration of the uncontrolled dislodged foreign body illustrate the dangerous nature of this practice when performed by those not trained in controlled endoscopic techniques. Control is once again paramount in the care of a patient with a foreign body in the upper aerodigestive tract.

Other Techniques of Evaluating Esophageal Foreign Bodies

For cases of witnessed aspiration of small, metallic, blunt foreign bodies that by symptomatology are likely to be in the esophagus, many reports in the pediatric literature advocate diagnosis by means of noninvasive metal detectors.[9, 10] They may be employed in a clinic or in urgent or emergent care settings on an outpatient basis. Once diagnosed, the passage of these objects into the stomach may be followed by serial examinations with the metal detector. If they make no progress over several hours, radiographic imaging and further invasive therapy are then applied as appropriate. This technique should not be used in cases of swallowed disk batteries or sharp, pointed objects. Although we have no first-hand experience with this technique, it has been safely employed and reported by many primary care providers.

CONCLUSION

Fortunately, in most cases, the ingestion or aspiration of a foreign body is not an immediate threat to life. A deliberate but expeditious preoperative evaluation should be undertaken, including a careful history. Most of these events occur in children, however, so a negative or incomplete history is frequently encountered. Therefore, a high level of suspicion must be maintained. Radiographic studies should be carefully evaluated, duplicate foreign bodies obtained for practice, and all members of the team apprised of the concerns of each case and the planned approach. Good working order of the instruments must be verified. Reasonably prompt endoscopic removal under maximally safe conditions should be the principal objective.

REFERENCES

1. Holinger LD. Foreign bodies of the airway and esophagus. In Holinger LD, ed. Pediatric Laryngology and Bronchoesophagology. Baltimore, Williams & Wilkins, 1996.
2. Marsh BR. Foreign bodies in the air and food passages. In Myers E, ed. Advances in Otolaryngology: Head and Neck Surgery, vol. 6. St. Louis, Mosby, 1992.
3. Esclamado RN, Richardson MA. Laryngotracheal foreign bodies in children. Am J Dis Child 1987;141:259.
4. Marsh BR. Upper gastrointestinal tract endoscopy for foreign bodies. In Cameron JL, ed. Current Surgical Therapy, 4th ed. Toronto, BC Decker, 1992.
5. Marks SC, Marsh BR, Dudgeon DL. Indications for open surgical removal of airway foreign bodies. Ann Otol Rhinol Laryngol 1993;102:690–694.
6. Hunsicker RC, Gartner WS. Fogarty catheter technique for removal of endobronchial foreign bodies. Arch Otol 1977;103:103–104.
7. Carpenter RJ, Snyder GG. A complication in the use of a Fogarty catheter for foreign body removal during bronchoscopic management. Otol Head Neck Surg 1981;89:998–1000.
8. Maves MD, Carithers JS, Birck HG. Esophageal burns secondary to disc battery ingestion. Ann Otol Rhinol Laryngol 1984;93:364.
9. Ros SP, Cetta F. Successful use of a metal detector in locating coins ingested by children. J Pediatr 1992;120:752.
10. Carraccio C, Sacchetti A, Lichenstein R. A new way to locate swallowed coins. Contemp Pediatr 1996;13:49–54.

CHAPTER 11

Acute Laryngeal Trauma

Paul F. Castellanos, MD

INTUBATION INJURY

It is important to state at the outset that injury to the larynx in the process of securing the airway is seldom the result of negligence.[1–3] The interval between the induction of general anesthesia and intubation of the airway is brief and fraught with hazard. Some of these hazards can be anticipated and overcome. Others, even when anticipated, result in poorer outcomes owing primarily to host factors.[4] Airway classifications that relate to oral aperture, oropharyngeal patency, and other elements of upper airway physiognomy have been devised to alert the anesthesiologist to the need for extraordinary measures to secure the airway.[5–8] Host factors are the most important elements that may predispose toward acute and chronic iatrogenic laryngeal injury as a result of intubation.[4,9] Problems with access, the inability to mask-ventilate after induction, and functional laryngeal narrowing caused by edema and induration are among the many ways a patient's anatomy may impede swift and atraumatic intubation.[6] Compression and erosion of the airway by the endotracheal tube in the face of tissue edema, high tissue fluid pressures, relative ischemia, and diminished repair mechanisms predispose a patient to complications such as secondary vocal fold fixation,[10] granulomata,[11] web formation, and acquired glottic and subglottic stenosis.[3] Reflux laryngitis also carries significant risk for acute as well as chronic injury (Fig. 11–1).[12] Systemic diseases such as diabetes mellitus are also associated with the airway complications during intubation[4] and after prolonged intubation.[9]

Presentation

Intubation injury of consequence is very rare.[1,2,10] Endotracheal tube technology and techniques of orotracheal intubation are associated with an incidence of significant intubation injury of between 0.5% and 6%.[1,2] Subclinical injury, however, occurs frequently, as judged by the high rate of transient oropharyngeal and voice complaints that follow general anesthetics—the rate is estimated to be as high as 69%.[1] Acute injury can occur after even brief intubation because of traumatic introduction of the intubating laryngoscope, the endotracheal tube, or both.[13] Use of either straight or curved laryngoscope blades can result in the disruption of the soft tissues of the larynx. If, for example, an intubating laryngoscope is introduced into the postcricoid space, it may be "toed in" as it is withdrawn in order to expose the endolarynx, creating a risk of subluxation of either arytenoid anteromedially.[14–16] This situation would cause severe hoarseness and may progress to airway compromise if there is enough associated edema.[14–16] The endotracheal tube itself can traumatize the vocal folds by tearing blood vessels or epithelium or by avulsing the vocal fold in the coronal plane, particularly when a stylet is used (Fig. 11–2). Arytenoid disruption in the posterolateral orientation can be the direct result of such trauma.

Intubation for any length of time results in some degree of airway injury, given the delicacy of laryngeal and tracheal tissues. Furthermore, prolonged intubation nearly always results in gross injury to the larynx, subglottis, and trachea. As long as extubation can be accomplished

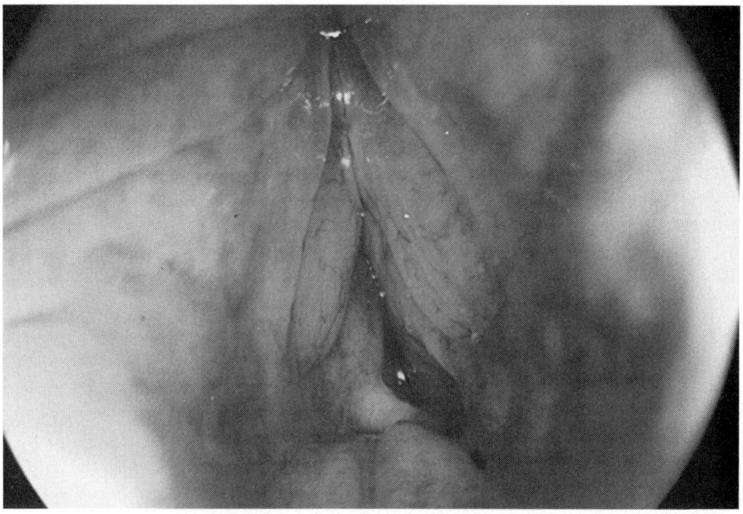

Figure 11–1. The larynx of a patient with postintubation bilateral vocal cord paralysis and reflux laryngitis. After many months of intensive proton pump inhibitor therapy and a short course of systemic steroids, his larynx improved to the point where he could tolerate tracheostomy plugging.

within 1 to 2 weeks, the granulation tissue and the focal ulcerations that have formed tend to heal spontaneously.[3] A "tube cast" of granulation tissue may appear within the glottis following an intubation as short as 2 days. Granular tissues that mature into intubation granulomas can progress after extubation if the predisposing factors of reflux and chronic inflammation persist. Bilateral granulation tissues may come into contact, become epithelialized, and form a synechia (Fig. 11–3). Over time, these bridges of tissue will bind the vocal folds even closer and cause secondary stenosis. A circumferential subglottic epithelial injury can cause the formation of a cicatrix that will result in stenosis or even in complete subglottic fusion (Fig. 11–4). Benjamin refers to this as a laryngeal "bed sore."[3]

Evaluation

The choice of the type of exam should be directed by the severity of the presenting symptoms. Endoscopy is indicated in patients with substantial or persistent hoarseness following endotracheal tube intubation. Fiberoptic evaluation using a nasopharyngoscope is an excellent modality for the primary assessment of the lar-

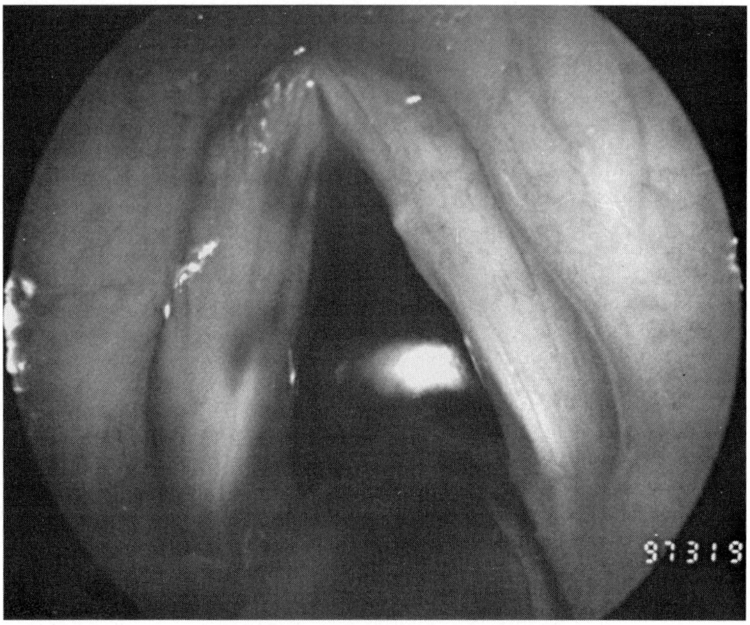

Figure 11–2. The larynx of a patient with chronic vocal nodules and reflux laryngitis. No reports of difficulty with intubation were noted by the anesthesiologist, but her larynx had this appearance immediately after the intubation. The hemorrhage required evacuation after 1 month, as her voice failed to improve, and the volume of the left vocal fold had not spontaneously reverted to normal.

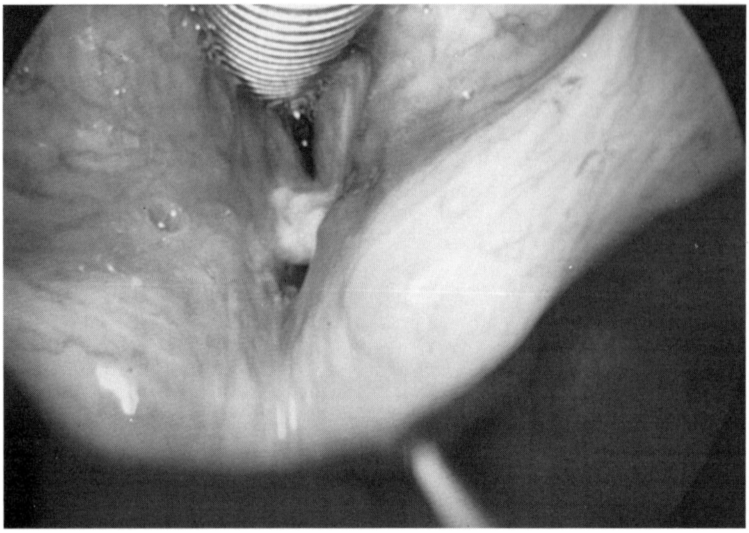

Figure 11–3. The larynx of a 16-year-old male who had been followed at another institution for bilateral posterior glottic granulomata a year earlier. He presented to the author with obstructive sleep apnea and dyspnea on exertion. After resection of his glottic synechia, all of his symptoms resolved.

ynx. Although a large series was reported using only indirect laryngoscopy at the bedside,[2] the fiberoptic technology offers a more detailed examination. Rigid laryngoscopy is also indicated in any patient with a history of airway obstruction after intubation.[2] The procedure should include palpation of the arytenoids to evaluate the potential for ankylosis or dislocation.[13] Serial exams are also of benefit as they can demonstrate improvement and obviate the need for operative intervention.

Unlike its place in other forms of laryngeal trauma, the role of radiographic imaging in the assessment of intubation injury is very limited. The reason is that the tissue changes that occur in this type of injury are usually very subtle and thus do not appear on imaging studies. A negative computed tomography (CT) scan therefore does not rule out significant injury. Suspected arytenoid subluxation is one clinical situation in which a CT scan may be useful.[17]

Pulmonary function tests may indicate upper airway obstruction. Specifically, flow-volume loops may demonstrate the effects of a narrow laryngeal aperture, collapse of the involved soft tissues, or laryngospasm. This study may prompt an airway consultation but does not replace a visual exam of the airway by any other modality.

Intubation injury can produce airway com-

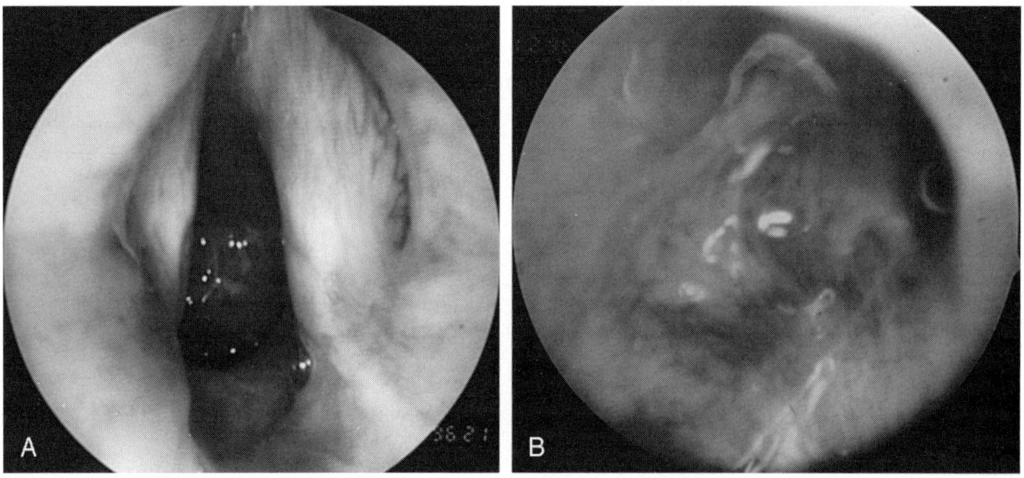

Figure 11–4. A: Glottis. B: Subglottis. The patient had sustained a closed head injury several months earlier. He was unable to voice, on digital occlusion of his tracheostomy cannula. Laryngoscopy performed at the time of tracheostomy revealed subglottic granulation and complete obstruction. He was known to have gastroesophageal reflux.

promise. In the case of a difficult intubation, the injury may be an arytenoid dislocation, but more commonly the injury is associated with hemorrhage into the vocalis muscle or a hematoma into the subepithelium of Reinke's space. These injuries usually produce voice change rather than airway obstruction. The conditions associated with airway obstruction after intubation include severe laryngeal or tracheal edema, bilateral, true vocal-fold midline motion restriction, and extensive laryngeal hemorrhage. Laryngospasm is also a cause of airway obstruction postextubation, but it is usually immediately recognized by the anesthesiologist and resolves quickly with positive-pressure mask ventilation. The other causes just listed usually present more mildly, and the airway deteriorates as the dilating effects of the endotracheal tube abate.

Priorities

In a patient who is persistently stridorous on extubation, the airway should be secured with caution and speed. A suspension laryngoscopy in the operating theater may be indicated if airway compromise requires reintubation. A complete assessment of the nature and severity of the injury may be encumbered by the endotracheal tube. Therefore, a reasonable option may be to perform a tracheostomy to allow the removal of the tube from the injured larynx and thus allow a more thorough exam. This should be considered seriously if a patient has failed more than one attempt at extubation. The placement of an endolaryngeal stent made in the form of a larynx cast such as the Montgomery stent[18] or a soft glove finger are among the appropriate options if mucosal tears are extensive. Stenting is indicated too, if the injuries involve either commissure. Open repair may also be necessary in some cases (see Priorities in the Blunt and Penetrating Trauma section for a more detailed discussion of stenting). Sometimes the arytenoid is degloved or even subluxed during intubation. Degloving superficial to the perichondrium usually heals spontaneously, but subluxation carries a far poorer prognosis for recovery and a strong chance of persistent voice problems.[14] If an arytenoid is found to be dislocated, an attempt should be made to reduced it. Sataloff and colleagues describe a detailed technique for reduction of a dislocated arytenoid, along with results of this procedure.[13, 19]

A subepithelial hematoma is a relatively benign injury that can have dramatic consequences to the voice. It may warrant operative intervention if spontaneous resorption is not evident on repeat endoscopy. The collection of fluid in Reinke's space is detrimental to the normal synchronous vibration of the vocal folds. This condition can result in diplophonia based on the asymmetry in weight or vibratory characteristics among the vocal folds. If the blood resorbs slowly, it might be replaced by scar, preventing the normal flow of an epithelial wave through the involved area. This also results in a poor voice, more typically described as coarse or harsh rather than diplophonic. The treatment consists only of evacuation of the accumulated blood and focal cautery of the feeding vessel or vessels in the acute setting. Later, this area may take on the nature of a unilateral polyp and as such would also warrant resection of the excess epithelium. Deep scarring from an intramuscular hemorrhage is more apt to result in a poor voice that may warrant further more involved attempts at restoration, such as fat grafts or collagen injections.[20]

Outcomes

The incidence of postintubation laryngeal injury is 69% according to a study that evaluated a large number of intubated patients. This must mean that the vast majority of intubation injuries resolve with little or no intervention. The incidence of vocal fold hemorrhages that result in polyps requiring surgery is not identified in the literature but can be presumed to be small. A normal voice is usually restored after polyp resection. A poor voice outcome is a multifactorial process.[21] The true denominator of epithelial injuries or vocal fold motion restriction associated with intubation trauma is unknown. At the University of Maryland Shock Trauma Center, less than 5% have residual poor voices after such trauma. Poor voice is most often the result of persistent motion restriction from either nerve dysfunction or arytenoid fixation. The role played by laryngopharyngeal reflux as a cofactor is also unclear in the literature. It is a very common element, in the author's experience, and is known to be a factor in idiopathic hoarseness[22] and difficult intubations.[23]

BLUNT AND PENETRATING TRAUMA

The distinction between blunt and penetrating trauma to the larynx lies primarily in the associated injuries. Blunt trauma is apt to produce multiple fractures of the lamina, whereas penetrating injury may result in only a single element of disruption in the endolarynx. Penetrating injury is more apt to cause associated vascular and esophageal or pharyngeal injuries. The stratification system of laryngeal fractures used at the Maryland Shock Trauma Center is based on the large series published by Schaefer in 1982 and 1989.[24, 25] This system divides laryngeal fractures into four grades, or levels, of severity by elements that are morphologically distinct and prognostically significant. Type I injuries are based in the soft tissue and involve little or no discernible cartilaginous injury. This may include occult, or greenstick, fractures that spontaneously return to the normal anatomic position. These injuries have little risk of airway obstruction and can be treated expectantly, with supportive measures. Type II injuries are more severe and involve mucosal or epithelial tears, hematoma, and laryngeal framework fractures that are minimally displaced or nondisplaced. Type III fractures demonstrate gross framework distortion. These injuries are much more dangerous and generally require awake tracheostomy and open reduction, with repair of the soft-tissue defects. Type IV injuries are the most extreme, with severe airway disruption necessitating prompt surgical intervention. Bent and colleagues further separated the worst of the Schaefer type IV injuries into a type V injury that involves cricotracheal separation.[26] This is a dire airway emergency and can rapidly lead to death with little perturbation.

Presentation

There is a wide spectrum of presentations by patients with laryngeal fractures. They can appear at ease, with few if any complaints referable to the neck or larynx; or they can present with acute or impending airway obstruction (see the Priorities section). They may not be hoarse and may deny hemoptysis, shortness of breath, odynophagia, or odynophonia, although these are among the most common presenting symptoms. Although the presence of such symptoms implies a laryngeal fracture, their absence should not rule out an airway injury in the face of a mechanism of injury that could produce one. High-speed motor vehicle accidents, strangulation injuries, neck gunshot or stab wounds, and "clothesline" injuries often require evaluation for laryngeal injury. A seat belt mark, bruising over the neck, a blunting of the thyroid ala notch (the Adam's apple), subcutaneous emphysema, and focal tenderness (by gentle palpation) are among the signs that indicate an airway injury. If any are present, a full evaluation is commonly necessary.

Sometimes laryngeal fractures are initially undiscovered because of the gravity and extent of the associated injuries (Fig. 11–5). If the trauma victim's airway was secured by intuba-

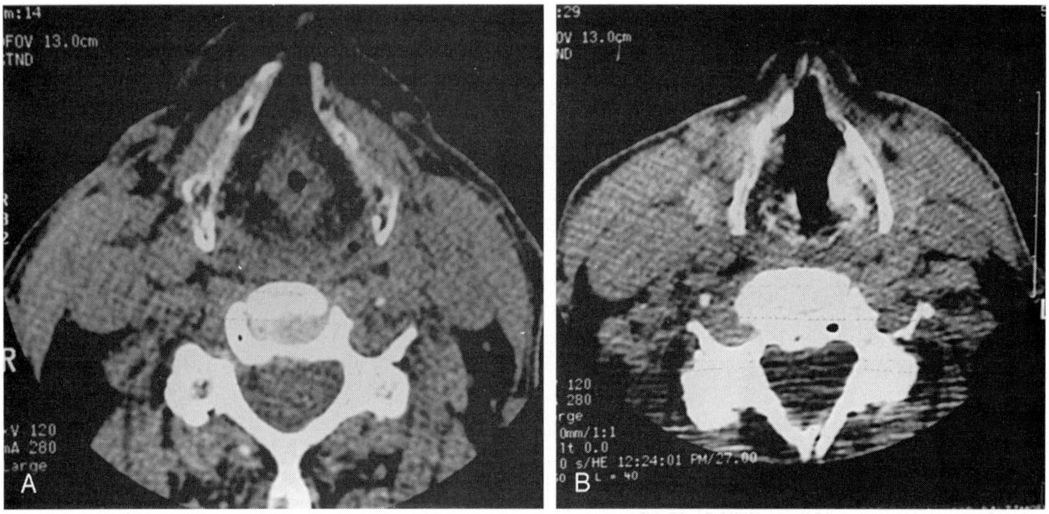

Figure 11–5. CT images of a 72-year-old male who sustained blunt polytrauma in a motor vehicle accident. His persistent hoarseness and breathiness prompted a consultation a year after his injury. A: Evidence of a left thyroid lamina greenstick fracture is seen. B: An anterior commissure rupture is also present. He required an open laryngotracheoplasty to restore his voice.

tion in the field or on arrival at the emergency department, the features of laryngeal injury described above may be all but undetectable. The patient may be unconscious or sedated. In such cases, the timely workup of a laryngeal fracture may be prompted by the mechanism of injury and nothing else.

Evaluation

Each of the diagnostic studies outlined in this section has advantages and limitations. The care of a patient with a possible airway injury must not be predicated on the availability of these modalities but rather on the needs of the patient and the training of the most able clinician at the scene.

THE FIBEROPTIC NASOPHARYNGOSCOPE

The fiberoptic nasopharyngoscope is the mainstay in the evaluation of a patient with a possible airway injury. It has several advantages over the other modalities as well as some limitations. This scope provides a direct view, although it is relatively low in resolution. Newer video-tipped scopes may obviate this limitation. Unfortunately, the added need for video equipment to view the image reduces portability. Another limitation is the need for topical anesthesia to perform an atraumatic evaluation. Inherent in the procedure is the risk of stimulating coughing, gagging, or laryngospasm that may render the patient's airway obstructed. This risk should be anticipated by the clinician and, if possible, should be explained to the patient. Formal informed consent is rarely possible, however, under the typical circumstances.

Nasopharyngoscopy reveals the features of the fracture and allows classification of the injury and planning for the next level of assessment or intervention. Many elements of laryngeal structure and function can be assessed by this technique, including upper airway patency, vocal fold motion, the presence of hematoma, cartilage disruption, and commissure abnormalities. A test of supraglottic sensation, however, should be avoided since this may precipitate laryngospasm. This information is particularly valuable in a patient with supraglottic avulsion injuries in which the superior laryngeal nerves are at risk, but it should be conducted only after the airway has been secured. If the larynx appears to be normal but other signs of aerodigestive tract injury are present, such as subcutaneous emphysema, it is important to continue the evaluation. Examination of the subglottis and trachea is rarely prudent unless the airway is secured and the lumen is well anesthetized. In some cases the patient has been previously intubated and a laryngeal fracture is suspected because of the presence of subcutaneous emphysema. A fiberoptic scope can be passed through the endotracheal tube, which can then be gradually withdrawn, leaving the endoscope in place. The airway can be inspected with the endoscope acting as a stylet to allow for the ready replacement of the endotracheal tube. This procedure is performed under general anesthesia with the aid of a neuromuscular blockade and should be done only by an experienced airway clinician.

RADIOGRAPHIC IMAGING

A plain film of the airway remains the radiographic mainstay in the evaluation of neck injury for a possible laryngeal fracture (Fig. 11–6). Available in most emergency facilities, it can be obtained at the bedside without the necessity for significant head repositioning. Frontal and lateral views will reveal many aspects of the airway quickly and atraumatically. Free air in the soft tissues of the neck is the sine qua non of upper aerodigestive tract injury. Irregularities of the air column approaching the glottis can indicate a paraglottic hematoma or soft-tissue disruption. Irregular calcification of the thyroid lamina makes the detection of nondisplaced fractures difficult.

A CT scan affords greater spatial resolution of the various structures of interest. Spiral scanning technology can provide resolution down to millimeters in a matter of a few seconds and requires little cooperation from a patient who may be in pain or emotional distress. Furthermore, the study can reveal the dissection pattern of any free air present and can identify related injuries to the mediastinum and upper chest. The calcification pattern of the thyroid cartilage is never uniform. Thus, fracture fragments may not be easily distinguished. Surrounding soft tissue emphysema may enhance visualization of the fracture by creating air contrast (Fig. 11–7). Subacute injuries may manifest fluid accumulation and even early abscess formation such as may result from pyriform sinus avulsion or rupture. Arytenoid avulsion or dislocation can sometimes be detected on a CT scan.[17]

A magnetic resonance imaging (MRI) study has little value in the initial evaluation of the airway. On an MRI the air-filled lumen of the

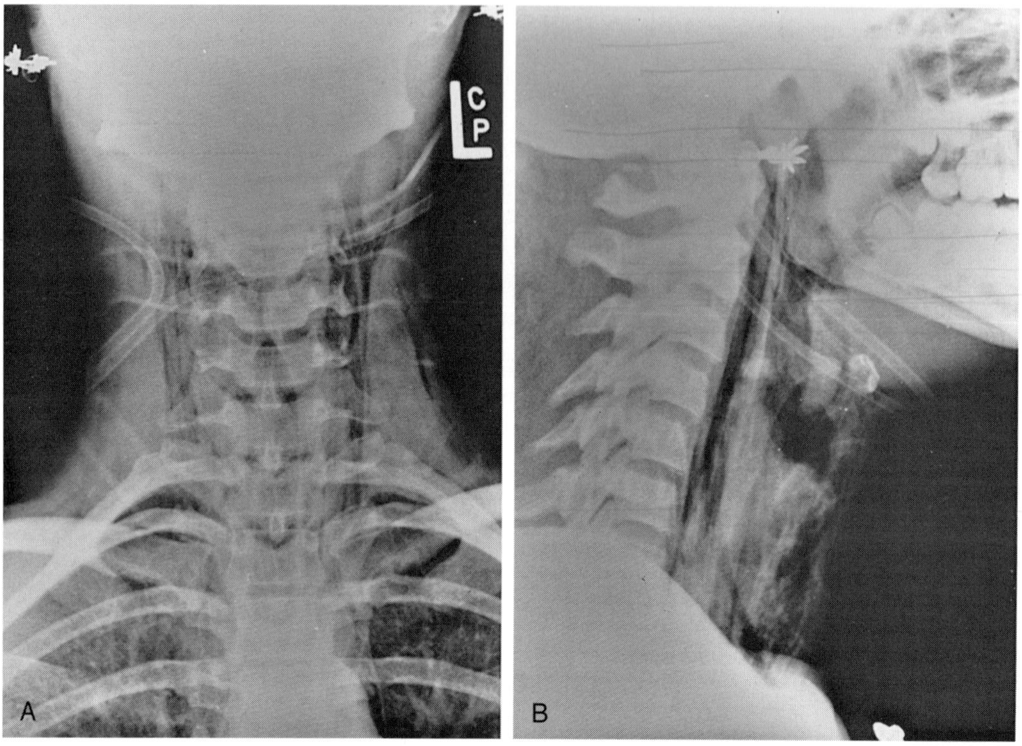

Figure 11–6. A and B: Plain films of a 16-year-old female's neck after she sustained a blunt clothesline injury while riding a motor scooter in the dark. These films were taken immediately before her airway was surgically secured. She was transferred after emergent bronchoscopic intubation and tracheostomy. Notice the free air in the paralaryngeal soft tissues and the subtle evidence of cartilage disruption. At the time these images were taken, the patient was not complaining of any airway distress and had a normal voice.

larynx and trachea is a moving signal void that is therefore difficult to differentiate from the surrounding soft tissues. Diffuse edema may appear bright in the T1 mode but offers little detail of the extent of injury. Furthermore, MRI is often poorly tolerated in stressful circumstances, especially by a patient who is already very anxious. If, however, the patient is intubated, an MRI can distinguish between the laryngeal soft tissues and the airway lumen when they are filled with secretions or blood. This situation is common in a patient with a laryngeal fracture who is intubated. A CT scan cannot resolve these features well, as they are radiographically isodense. Multiplane images are also possible with MRI, offering another dimension of visualization. Some centers offer three-dimensional reconstructions based on spiral CT scans, but this service is rarely available on an emergency basis, given the labor-intensive nature of the software packages currently needed for this process.[27]

Radiographic evaluation of the esophagus is indicated when the neck cannot be extended because of known or suspected cervical spine injury. Diatrizoate (Hypaque) or diatrizoate meglumine (Gastrografin) is preferable for the diagnosis of an esophageal perforation because it is less toxic to the mediastinum than barium. Barium is relatively inert in the airway whereas Hypaque and Gastrografin are associated with acute pneumonitis. Therefore, the risk of aspiration should also be considered when choosing a radiopaque fluid and the method of its delivery.[28, 29] The use of low-osmolarity, nonionic contrast materials such as iohexol has also been advocated when the extent of injury is difficult to predict or the chance of mediastinal and respiratory contamination is high.[29] Some authors recommend nonbarium esophagography initially, with a second evaluation using barium to exclude undiagnosed injury,[28, 30, 31] but others refute the benefit.[29]

RIGID LARYNGOSCOPY

Rigid laryngoscopy is the gold standard for the evaluation of the larynx. It also carries a potential risk for further soft tissue disruption. Unlike the traditional diagnostic laryngoscopy, which is

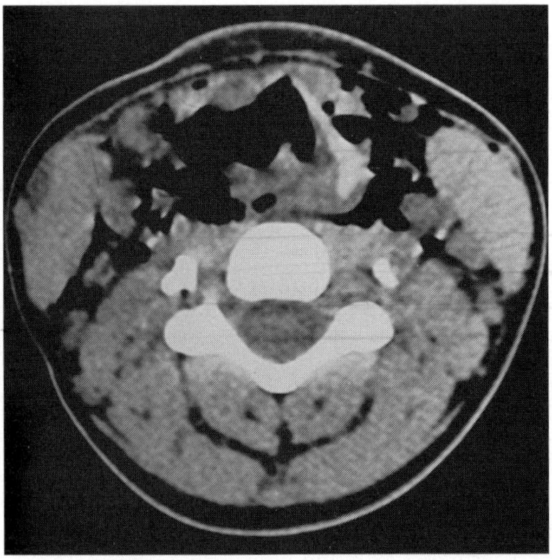

Figure 11–7. A CT scan of the patient depicted in Figure 11–6. Note the increased definition of the gross airway disruption and the extensive dissection of air through the soft tissues. The tracheostomy had already been performed at this point.

considered minimally morbid, laryngoscopy in the case of a presumed laryngeal fracture must be performed with the maximum of caution. If the laryngeal injuries are extensive, normal anatomic landmarks may not be identifiable. The surgeon may consider postponing endoscopic evaluation until after the inflammation has subsided or may convert to open exploration of the injury.[32] The later is the author's personal preference because delaying the definitive repair can increase granulation and the difficulty of the repair.[26]

Once the extent of injury has been estimated by direct laryngoscopy, the surgeon may consider suspending the larynx to complete the exam. This enables bimanual instrument use and high magnification. Standard laryngoscopes may distract thyroid laminar fractures by the force of the suspension apparatus. To avoid this distraction, a vallecular scope such as a Lindhölm laryngoscope (Karl Storz, Germany) can be used. If properly placed, this scope should apply distracting forces only to the hyoid bone, which should not result in significant morbidity.

ESOPHAGOSCOPY AND BRONCHOSCOPY

The esophagus should be evaluated as part of the evaluation of all significant neck injury because as many as 20% of significant esophageal perforations are devoid of signs or symptoms on presentation.[30] The sensitivity and specificity of esophagoscopy and esophagography are largely equivalent. Both have a spectrum of iatrogenic complications and limitations that must be part of the algorithm used in choosing one over the other (see Radiographic Imaging).[33, 34] Thus imaging as the initial evaluation is particularly reasonable if the neck cannot be manipulated due to known or suspected spinal injury. It is also appropriate if the index of suspicion for vascular or airway injury is low and thus the patient's neck is unlikely to be explored. Some authors advocate beginning with esophagography and following with rigid esophagoscopy if the result of imaging is at all equivocal.[30] Resorting to esophagoscopy is a reasonable option at the outset if the patient is already in need of rigid endoscopy and has no contraindication to neck extension. Flexible esophagoscopy is an option that has the benefit of avoiding cervical extension.[33] However, this modality does require the insufflation of air that theoretically may worsen soft tissue emphysema and its associated problems.

Bronchoscopy is also an important element of a complete evaluation because the discovery of a laryngeal fracture does not exclude tracheal injury. Flexible technology has no particular limitations in the lungs, as described for esophagoscopy above. It has the added benefit of being able to be introduced through an existing endotracheal tube. If it is going to be performed in a patient who is not intubated, it is incumbent on the airway clinician to be ready to secure the airway emergently should the evaluation result in obstruction. Atomized lidocaine through a nebulizer circuit is an excellent way to gently anesthetize the airway. Coughing can be largely avoided if a low concentration is used to begin the process and gradually increased (1%, 2%, then 4%). Gentle technique is also crucial.

EXPLORATORY SURGERY

In a case of severe crush injury with or without spinal injury, the surgeon may opt to explore the neck and repair the fracture fragments by open inspection. This is a particularly attractive option when laryngoscopy poses a significant risk of further disruption. The surgeon's understanding of the endolaryngeal injury will be very limited, however, and the choice of incisions for entry into the larynx will of necessity be dictated by the superficial aspects of the injury. The pharynx and the cervical esophagus can also be assessed by using an open approach, but there is a significant chance that a small rent will not be visible. The use of methylene blue–stained saline or dilute peroxide has been advocated as a means of discovering such tears. It is essential, however, that this fluid be delivered without entering the disrupted larynx, as the cytotoxic effects of peroxide can adversely affect tissue healing. A red rubber catheter can be passed into the esophageal inlet from above or directly through the open larynx to avoid this risk.

Priorities

AIRWAY EXTREMIS

The first task for a clinician presented with an airway injury is to determine whether the patient is in a state of respiratory extremis. If so, the patient is in emergent need of a secure airway. The most qualified person at the scene must determine the appropriate means of establishing airway access. The nuances of management of a laryngeal fracture are not relevant in a life-and-death situation. The spectrum of options even includes attempting intubation in the face of a probable laryngeal fracture if a surgical airway is beyond the capacity and training of the clinician.

If possible, the clinician should consider producing a surgical airway to avoid iatrogenic airway injury resulting from intubation. This operation may be a cricothyroidotomy or a tracheostomy. The procedure should take only seconds to perform initially, without regard to hemostasis or aseptic technique, to establish an airway and resuscitate the patient. Creating a surgical airway can be impeded by body habitus, obesity, extensive soft tissue injury of the neck, and subcutaneous emphysema. If at all possible, positive-pressure mask ventilation should be avoided, given the high risk of producing or increasing soft tissue emphysema that may lead to pneumothorax and pneumomediastinum.

If the patient's airway is deteriorating, there may not be time to fully assess the injury prior to securing the airway. Even a gentle fiberoptic evaluation may result in the need for a surgical airway. Being prepared for a possible fiberoptic intubation is prudent under such circumstances. There is little indication for sending a patient at risk of impending airway obstruction for diagnostic radiographs without airway access options on hand or immediately available. Transport time to the operating theater carries the same risk of deterioration. The patient should be accompanied by a clinician and assistants capable of performing a surgical airway should the need arise.

TYPE I FRACTURES

Type I fractures have a high likelihood of spontaneous recovery with little or no intervention. The majority of patients with this type of fracture are probably not diagnosed because of the minor airway or voice symptoms. A patient who presents with hoarseness and vocal fold ecchymosis should be evaluated with a spiral CT scan, placed on systemic steroids, and observed in a monitored setting. Serial fiberoptic studies can be performed to determine whether the process is progressing or resolving. Substantial edema on presentation suggests mucosal lacerations that have not been identified and upgrades the diagnosis to a type II injury. In most cases, a laryngeal fracture of any grade is an indication for absolute voice rest and minimal activity. Such a patient rarely requires NPO status for longer than 24 hours, as there will be demonstrable improvement or deterioration within that time. Bed rest is appropriate for the first 48 hours to reduce the risk of expanding the hemorrhage by straining or coughing that is provoked by a Valsalva maneuver.

TYPE II FRACTURES

Type II fractures are defined by the presence of mucosal lacerations and minimally distracted cartilage fragments. Therefore, the stability of the airway is significantly lower than that found in a type I injury. Odynophagia and sometimes odynophonia are features of this level of injury. A patient should remain in a monitored setting long enough to ensure airway stability—an average of 3 to 4 days. During this time, systemic steroids are administered and cool, humidified air is delivered through a face tent. The patient should have bed rest and absolute voice rest. Stool softeners are administered for constipation that results from inactivity or the narcotics used for pain control.

Like type I injuries, some type II fractures heal well with only the supportive measures described. A subset of patients with type II injuries require open repair. If a vocal fold is ruptured or if a depressed greenstick fracture of the lamina deforms one vocal fold, operative intervention may be warranted. A tracheostomy to secure the airway initially is reasonable but not always necessary. If the patient needs further endoscopic or surgical repairs, a tracheostomy serves to obviate secondary injury from intubation through the damaged or recently reconstructed larynx. If there are areas of exposed cartilage, granulation tissue may form and convert to granuloma. Depending on the location, this may become an important process and require more than one endoscopic resection. The same tendencies of untoward healing associated with granulation tissue described previously for prolonged or traumatic intubation apply here, as do the indications for the removal of such tissue if it does not spontaneously resolve.

Systemic steroids increase the risk of gastritis. A high-stress state is associated with an increased risk of gastroesophageal reflux[35] and acid hypersecretion.[36, 37] It stands to reason that disrupted tissues and exposed cartilage are more vulnerable to the effects of acid and enzymes if exposed to them by the reflux. Gaynor[9, 12] has implicated acid reflux in intubation-related disease. By extension, traumatized airway tissues present a reasonable indication for aggressive antireflux measures such as postural adjustment, bolus tube feeding, and medication with proton pump inhibitors to suppress acid production.

TYPE III FRACTURES

Type III laryngeal fractures are airway emergencies of distinct urgency, and they require a rapid and concerted effort by all involved to secure the patient's airway and then to effect a definitive repair. In the absence of a clinician trained in the techniques of awake surgical airway access, orotracheal intubation should be attempted by the most experienced intubationist. Great care must be employed to avoid iatrogenic disruption of the fractured and avulsed fragments. Some extension of these injuries is to be expected under such conditions and is an acceptable risk in the face of impending airway loss and death.

The Awake Tracheostomy. The gold standard in the treatment of a type III larynx injury is awake tracheostomy, preferably in the operating theater, without sedation or manipulation of the airway prior to securing it from below. Sedation presents several problems. First, the patient may already have taken sedatives or hypnotics that would interact with these agents and result in the potential loss of respiratory drive, in emesis with aspiration, in coughing and gagging, and in the loss of a valuable cushion of time for generating surgical access. Second and perhaps more important, respiratory decompensation induced by sedation may necessitate the need for positive-pressure mask ventilation. Though sometimes necessary, this type of ventilation is very dangerous and should be avoided because of the risk of extravasation of pressurized air into the soft tissues of the neck, the chest, and the mediastinum. A tension pneumothorax or pneumomediastinum can result. Subcutaneous emphysema is often clinically evident on initial presentation in the emergency department. Air extravasation may also arise from swallowing, coughing, or mask ventilation in the field. Any deterioration of the patient's respiratory status in the face of positive airway pressure should be assumed to be a tension pneumatic process. If a cricothyroidotomy is being considered, it is important to remember that this level of the airway might be involved in the injury. A traditional tracheostomy may be a superior airway in this situation. Hemostasis is believed to be more difficult to achieve through a "slash tracheostomy," as it has been termed, than through a cricothyroidotomy, but bleeding can be controlled once the airway is secure and the patient is placed under general anesthesia. If the procedure is performed in the operating theater, a monopolar cautery device can be employed to reduce bleeding. It is important to inject local anesthesia to the level of the pretracheal fascia so that the patient is comfortable and not prone to coughing. Coughing and the Valsalva maneuver can produce high pressures that promote extravasation of air into the soft tissues and result in pneumothorax, as is described with positive-pressure ventilation (Fig. 11–8). Therefore, it is wise to delay administering local anesthetic into the tracheal lumen until immediately prior to surgical penetration, as the topical anesthesia can cause initial irritation of the respiratory epithelium and generate a vigorous cough reflex. It is also prudent to inform the anesthesiologist when entry into the airway is imminent so the appropriate medications are ready for prompt initiation of general anesthesia.

Suspension Laryngoscopy. Once the airway has been secured, the surgeon's attention can be focused on a detailed airway assessment and repair, beginning with an atraumatic approach to rigid laryngoscopy. If the disruption is found to be extensive on the initial views, further rigid evaluation may worsen the injury. In this situation, an open exploration should be undertaken. If, however, the extent of injury is clear on the initial laryngoscopy and the vital structures such as the cricoarytenoid joint complexes and the anterior commissure can be safely visualized, the airway surgeon should proceed with a suspension study. A vallecular scope is a reasonable instrument to avoid suspension forces against injured tissues. A thorough evaluation of the fractured larynx is possible with the benefit of binocular microscopy or optical telescopes. The

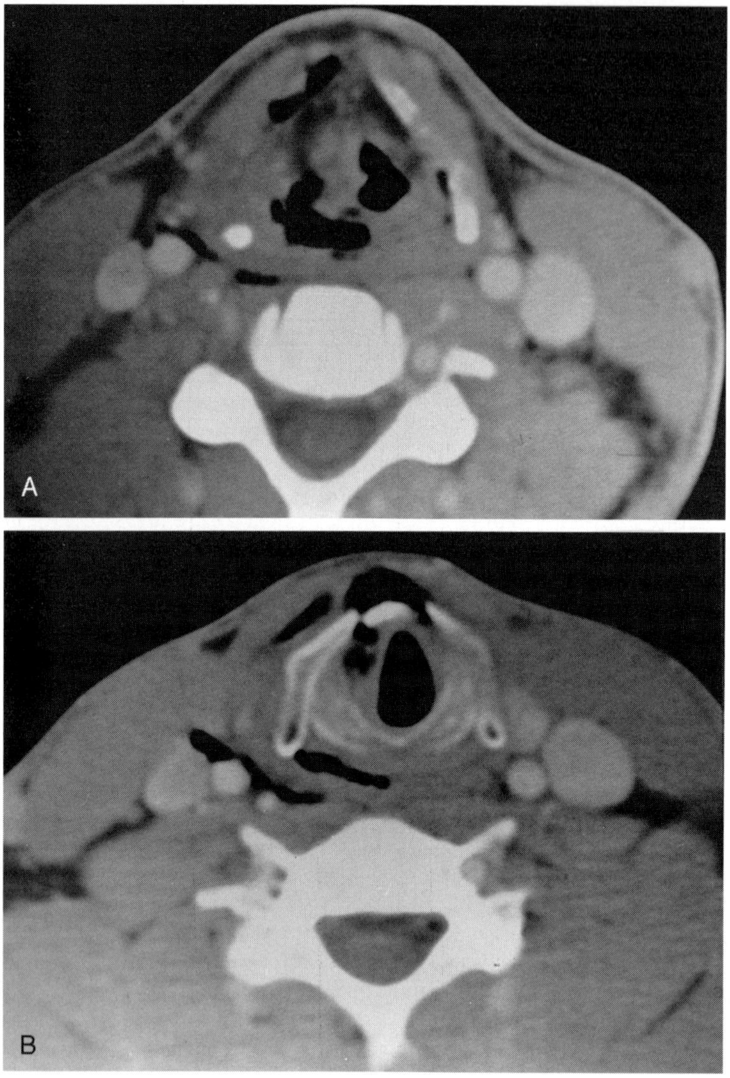

Figure 11–8. A CT scan of a 26-year-old male who was kicked in the neck during a martial arts sparring match. Although he was acutely short of breath and had hemoptysis, his symptoms rapidly cleared and he sought medical attention only because of pressure from his family. Note the air extravasation into the neck soft tissues. He had a normal voice and no airway complaints at the time of his awake tracheostomy. On surgical exploration, his membranous and cartilaginous anterior commissure was found to be completely detached from the rest of his larynx.

stability and mobility of the cricoarytenoid joint complexes should be assessed by gentle palpation. At the Maryland Shock Trauma Center, many type III laryngeal fractures have presented with mucosal avulsion along the ventricular spaces. This region may represent a zone of structural vulnerability that, in essence, acts as a kind of anatomic crumple zone (Fig. 11–9). By shearing above the level of the vocal folds, the anterior commissure is commonly spared, along with the posterior attachments of the arytenoids. This unit includes the inferior cartilaginous rim of the thyroid lamina in continuity with the anterior commissure and cricothyroid joints (see below). The functional unit of the larynx and the glottis proper seems to stay intact despite the supraglottic avulsion. This finding is significant as the anteroposterior support of the commissure is the most important structural feature of normalcy that must be restored.

Open Reduction and Internal Fixation. The techniques of open reduction and internal fixation (ORIF) are many and varied. The overall purpose is to restore to normal anatomic position the cartilaginous and mobile components of the larynx with as little risk of iatrogenic complication as possible. The specific targets are (1) to reconstruct the inferior cartilage rim so that there is anteroposterior strength, necessary because the inferior rim of the lamina acts as a cartilaginous bridge between the cricothyroid joints and the anterior commissure and is crucial for maintaining solid and symmetrical vocal fold tension; (2) to suspend the anterior commissure in its anatomic location, while

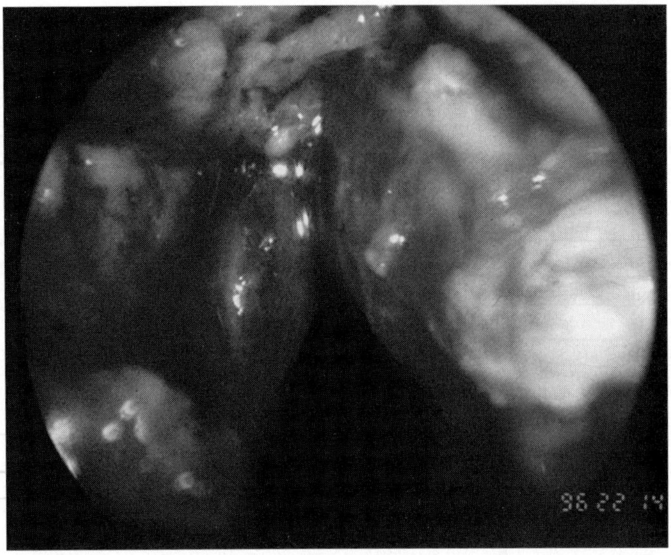

Figure 11–9. A direct laryngoscopic view, using a carefully placed suspension laryngoscope, of the patient depicted in Figures 11–6 and 11–7. The injury is about 14 hours old at this point and has already begun to granulate. Purulence was found in a pocket anterior to the larynx during the repair.

matching the vocal fold levels; (3) to protect the glottis and subglottis from fusion by repairing mucosal tears or by using a stent when necessary; and (4) to suspend the epiglottis anteriorly in order to prevent retroversion and secondary airway obstruction. The lamina may need rigid support, even if the fracture is only of the greenstick type. The two vocal folds may be functionally under different tensions if this symmetry is not restored, and this causes diplophonia and a poor voice.

One approach to ORIF is to use nonabsorbable suture such as Prolene or stainless steel to reapproximate cartilage fragments that are distracted or unstable. Titanium miniplates can restore strength in areas of strain such as along the inferior rim of the lamina and the anterior commissure. This area is thick and calcified enough in most adults to hold a screw. Self-tapping "emergency" screws are optimal to engage as much cartilage as possible in the threads. A 23-gauge needle is sufficient for tapping a hole prior to placing the screw. If stripping occurs, another hole should be used rather than a larger screw, as this may itself produce a stress fracture (Fig. 11–10). Debridement of cartilage fragments and torn mucosa should be performed judiciously. An aggressive approach

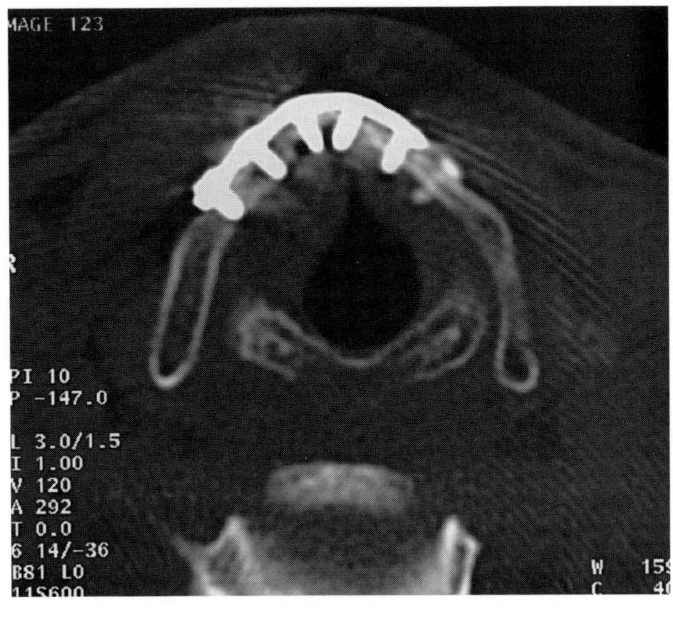

Figure 11–10. CT scan of the patient depicted in Figure 11–8 after repair at 3 months. A titanium plate was placed along the inferior thyroid lamina to secure the anterior commissure to the two main cartilaginous fragments. Notice the persistent asymmetry of the right supraglottis where the avulsion was nearly complete.

usually results in strictures that later require more complicated reconstruction, including tissue grafting, and in general poorer results.[38] Although it is tempting to restore all internal mucosal tears to anatomic normalcy, the benefits of opening the larynx to access these mucosal tears must be weighed against the risk that greater deficits will be generated, particularly by reducing the integrity of the cartilaginous framework. If this framework has been crushed, it is not likely to be further impaired by the laryngofissure. The author's preference is to use absorbable monofilament on a small taper needle (RB-1) to restore any tension-holding elements such as the anterior commissure or the petiole of the epiglottis. A buried suture technique avoids the granulation reaction that otherwise can persist for a very long time with the use of slowly absorbed sutures such as polydioxanone or Maxon. For simple epithelial reapproximation, mild chromic or catgut material can be used as the epithelial edges heal very quickly under most circumstances. Exposed cartilage should be covered with surrounding soft tissues if at all possible, as granuloma often forms in areas of denuded cartilage and that is likely to warrant further surgical intervention.

It is also possible to access the endolarynx through the ventricular sulci, even if a lateral thyrotomy is necessary. An oblique cartilage incision can be created from the anterior notch to about a centimeter above the cricothyroid joint. This approach does not risk the integrity of the anteroposterior support, but care must be taken to avoid injury to the adductor division of the recurrent laryngeal nerve, which lies within the fascia of the thyroarytenoid muscle, just deep to the inner perichondrium of the thyroid lamina.

There are some benefits to stenting, but stents also increase the tendency to form granulation tissue and thus can promote the untoward healing they were intended to prevent.[39] Most stent materials are far closely matched, anatomically, to the contours of the larynx than is an endotracheal tube. A finger cot is soft and relatively innocuous in its effect on the delicate tissues of the glottis. Despite this, after about 3 to 4 weeks of stenting, the benefits are outweighed by the encroaching granular reaction.[18, 40] This process thereafter becomes the basis for motion restriction in the arytenoids and web formation at the commissures.

TYPE IV FRACTURES

The most dangerous airway injuries are designated type IV. They include the complete laryngotracheal dissociation that can result from high-speed motor vehicle accidents, the classic clothesline injuries that occur in individuals on motorcycles, and stab injuries. The majority of these injuries are associated with such extensive polytrauma that they are most commonly diagnosed in a postmortem state. Type IV injuries in life cause the most precarious of airway states. All of the elements described above for type III injuries apply, with an emphasis on the hazards associated with orotracheal intubation. The glottis may be successfully intubated, but the tube may just as easily pass into the soft tissues of the neck. Any airway patency present prior to the intubation may therefore be lost. The intubationist, having seen the tube pass through the glottis, may not believe the clinical evidence of respiratory deterioration, thus extending the time it takes to determine that ventilation is not effective. This situation can be corrected only by surgical access of the most rapid sort. Sometimes, such a patient may even be breathing through the soft tissue injuries in the neck, the so-called self-trached patient (Fig. 11–11). Adding to the danger inherent in caring for such a patient is the potential of presentation with a normal voice and no shortness of breath. Extremis may develop after a coughing spell or laryngospasm resulting from endoscopic evaluation. Therefore, the endoscopy of a patient with suspected airway injury should be performed by an experienced airway physician prepared for an abrupt conversion from assessment to intervention. A patient with complete tracheal transection may have associated bilateral recurrent laryngeal nerve injury and thus may require more extensive attention to the restoration of the airway and the voice. These considerations may even be at odds if the folds come to the midline, as the patient may one day require a lateralization or cordotomy procedure.

Outcomes

There is little in the literature that reviews the outcomes of laryngeal fractures other than in retrospect or in small series. Leopold, in 1983, published a quasi meta-analysis of published reports prior to that time in order to evaluate the various treatment approaches used.[41] The 1989 Schaefer and Close update on laryngeal fractures is one of the few prospective studies of the results of treatment strategies.[25] Based on it and the study by Bent and colleagues,[26] several basic principles can be stated. Overall, the treatment of laryngeal fractures has improved over

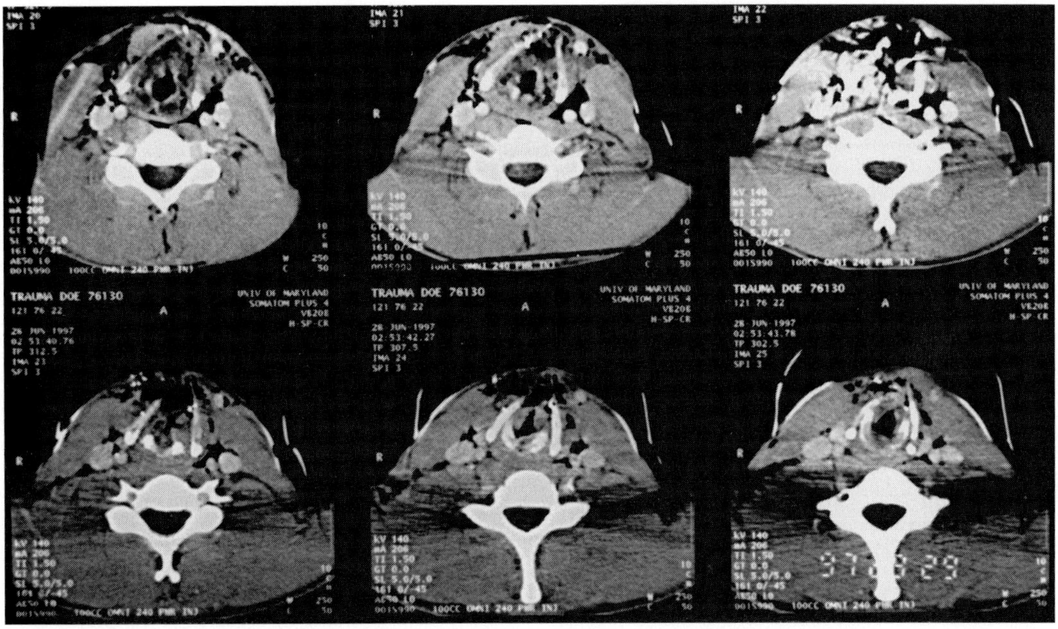

Figure 11–11. This patient with a type IV laryngeal fracture was shot in the neck through the larynx. He was found to be passing air through the wound. Notice, in the lower central panel, that his vocal folds appear to be attached to each other despite the fact that the cartilaginous anterior commissure was obliterated.

the past several decades; there has been complete abandonment of total laryngectomy as a necessary treatment in severe cases. The consensus is that injuries should be repaired as early as possible to achieve the greatest degree of primary healing.[25, 26, 41] Olson and others have advocated delayed repair in order to allow the tissue edema to subside.[42] The stated benefit is to reduce the need for endolaryngeal stenting. The worst voice and functional results are associated with stent use, both in the literature and in the author's experience.[26, 41] This is likely to be in part due to the degree of injury that prompts the use of stents more than to the deleterious effects of the stent itself (Fig. 11–12). Another, similar principle is that if no open repair is needed, the functional recovery will be best.[26, 41] This is also likely to be based on the fact that the more minor fractures are amenable to medical care and thus tend to recover completely. Even the worst grades of injury reported in the Schaefer and Close report had good voice and airway outcomes.[25] Of 29 patients, 9 were thought to have fair to good voices and none had poor voices. Only 2 of 30 (7%) in the same report had poor (glottic) airways, and 28 of 30 (93%) had good airways. These statistics agree closely with outcomes at the author's institution, and they compare favorably with reports of outcomes prior to 1984, as described by Leopold, in which results indicated 16% with poor voice and 8% with poor airway (tracheostomy-dependent) among patients treated within 24 hours. The numbers jump to 47% with poor voice

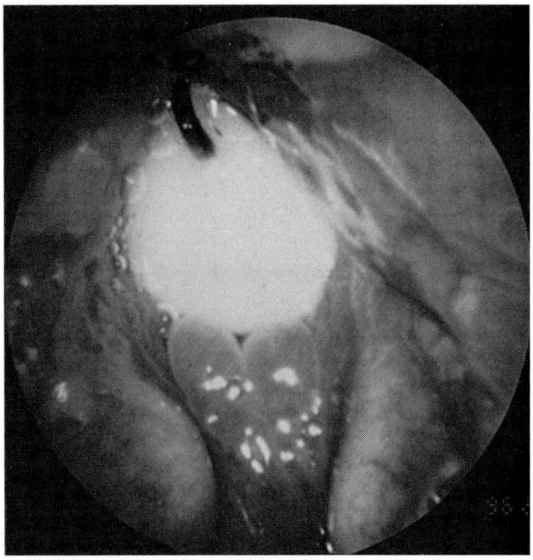

Figure 11–12. The suspension laryngoscopic view of a patient with a Montgomery stent in place at 3 weeks, just prior to removal. The stent is encased in a channel of granulation tissue. Despite this, the patient healed well and without web formation, requiring only one further procedure for laser treatment of granulation tissue.

and 47% with tracheostomy dependence when repair is delayed for 8 days.

REFERENCES

1. Kambic V, Radsel Z. Intubation lesions of the larynx. Br J Anaesth 1978;50:587–590.
2. Peppard SB, Dickens JH. Laryngeal injury following short-term intubation. Ann Otol Rhinol Laryngol 1983;92:327–330.
3. Benjamin B. Prolonged intubation injuries of the larynx: endoscopic diagnosis, classification, and treatment. Ann Otol Rhinol Laryngol Suppl 1993;160:1–15.
4. Reissell E et al. Predictability of difficult laryngoscopy in patients with long-term diabetes mellitus. Anaesthesia 1990;45:1024–1027.
5. Randell T. Prediction of difficult intubation. Acta Anaesthesiol Scand 1996;40:1016–1023.
6. Ganzouri AR et al. Preoperative airway assessment: predictive value of a multivariate risk index. Anesth Analg 1996;82:1197–1204.
7. Tse JC, Rimm EB, Hussain A. Predicting difficult endotracheal intubation in surgical patients scheduled for general anesthesia: a prospective blind study. Anesth Analg 1995;81:254–258.
8. Mallampati SR et al. A clinical sign to predict difficult tracheal intubation: a prospective study. Can Anaesth Soc J 1985;32:429–434.
9. Gaynor EB, Greenberg SB. Untoward sequelae of prolonged intubation. Laryngoscope 1985;95:1461–1467.
10. Cavo JW. True vocal cord paralysis following intubation. Laryngoscope 1985;95:1352–1359.
11. Feder RJ, Michell MJ. Hyperfunctional, hyperacidic, and intubation granulomas. Arch Otolaryngol 1984; 110:582–584.
12. Gaynor EB. Gastroesophageal reflux as an etiologic factor in laryngeal complications of intubation. Laryngoscope 1988;98:972–979.
13. Sataloff RT et al. Arytenoid dislocation. J Voice 1988;1:368–377.
14. Stanley RB, Colman MF. Unilateral degloving injuries of the arytenoid cartilage. Arch Otolaryngol Head Neck Surg 1986;112:516–518.
15. Hoffman HT et al. Arytenoid subluxation: diagnosis and treatment. Ann Otol Rhinol Laryngol 1991; 100:1–9.
16. Quick CA, Merwin GE. Arytenoid dislocation. Arch Otolaryngol 1978;104:267–270.
17. Dudley JP, Mancuso AA, Fonkalsrud EW. Arytenoid dislocation and computed tomography. Arch Otolaryngol 1984;110:483–484.
18. Montgomery WW, Montgomery SK. Manual for use of Montgomery laryngeal, tracheal, and esophageal prostheses: update 1990. Ann Otol Rhinol Laryngol Suppl 1990;150:2–28.
19. Sataloff RT, Bough IDJ, Spiegel JR. Arytenoid dislocation: diagnosis and treatment [Review]. Laryngoscope 1994;104:1353–1361.
20. Benninger MS et al. Vocal fold scarring: current concepts and management. Otolaryngol Head Neck Surg 1996;115:474–482.
21. Baker BM et al. Persistent hoarseness after surgical removal of vocal cord lesions. Arch Otolaryngol 1981;107:148–151.
22. McNally PR et al. Evaluation of gastroesophageal reflux as a cause of idiopathic hoarseness. Digest Dis Sci 1989;34:1900–1904.
23. Cantillo J et al. Difficult intubation from gastroesophageal reflux disease in adults. J Clin Anesth 1998;10:235–237.
24. Schaefer SD. Primary management of laryngeal trauma. Ann Otol Rhinol Laryngol 1982;91:399–402.
25. Schaefer SD, Close LG. Acute management of laryngeal trauma: update. Ann Otol Rhinol Laryngol 1989;98:98–104.
26. Bent JP, Silver JR, Porubsky ES. Acute laryngeal trauma: a review of 77 patients. Otolaryngol Head Neck Surg 1993;109:441–449.
27. Castelijns JA, van den Brekel MW, Niekoop VA, Snow GB. Imaging of the larynx [Review]. Neuroimaging Clin North Am 1996;6:401–415.
28. James AEJ et al. Barium or Gastrografin: which contrast media for diagnosis of esophageal tears? Gastroenterology 1975;68:1103–1113.
29. Brick SH et al. Esophageal disruption: evaluation with iohexol esophagography [Comments]. Radiology 1988;169:141–143.
30. Weigelt JA et al. Diagnosis of penetrating cervical esophageal injuries. Am J Surg 1987;154:619–622.
31. Michel L, Grillo HC, Malt RA. Esophageal perforation [Review]. Ann Thorac Surg 1982;33:203–210.
32. Olson NR. Wound healing by primary intention in the larynx. Otolaryngol Clin North Am 1979;12:735–740.
33. White RK, Morris DM. Diagnosis and management of esophageal perforations. Am Surg 1992;58:112–119.
34. Kelly JP et al. Management of airway trauma. II: Combined injuries of the trachea and esophagus. Ann Thorac Surg 1987;43:160–163.
35. Marrone GC, Silen W. Pathogenesis, diagnosis and treatment of acute gastric mucosal lesions [Review]. Clin Gastroenterol 1984;13:635–650.
36. Bricker SR, McLuckie A, Nightingale DA. Gastric aspirates after trauma in children. Anaesthesia 1989; 44:721–724.
37. Burgess P et al. Effect of ranitidine on intragastric pH and stress-related upper gastrointestinal bleeding in patients with severe head injury. Digest Dis Sci 1995;40:645–650.
38. Goldenberg D et al. Severe laryngeal injury caused by blunt trauma to the neck: a case report. J Laryngol Otol 1997;111:1174–1176.
39. Hawkins DB. Glottic and subglottic stenosis from endotracheal intubation. Laryngoscope 1977;87:339–346.
40. Montgomery WW, Montgomery SK. Manual for use of Montgomery laryngeal, tracheal, and esophageal prostheses. Ann Otol Rhinol Laryngol Suppl 1986;125:1–16.
41. Leopold DA. Laryngeal trauma: a historical comparison of treatment methods [Review]. Arch Otolaryngol 1983;109:106–112.
42. Olson NR. Surgical treatment of acute blunt laryngeal injuries. Ann Otol Rhinol Laryngol 1978;87:716–721.

CHAPTER 12

Penetrating Trauma of the Neck

Shelly J. McQuone, MD
David W. Eisele, MD

Penetrating neck trauma is a life-threatening emergency because of the potential injury to vital structures of the neck and thorax, including major blood vessels and nerves, the aerodigestive tract, the lungs, and the spinal cord. Successful management of penetrating neck trauma depends on prompt recognition of injury, appropriate diagnostic evaluation, and proper surgical intervention. A thorough understanding of the anatomy of the neck and chest and the mechanisms of penetrating injury to these areas is necessary to care optimally for patients with neck trauma.

The majority of penetrating neck injuries in civilians presenting to major trauma centers result from gunshot or stab wounds inflicted during violent interpersonal exchanges. These injuries may also result from occupational accidents or recreational accidents such as hunting and gun cleaning. Rarely, motor vehicle accidents result in penetrating neck trauma, but more commonly they cause blunt injury. Animal bites can involve the neck (the management of potential infection from these injuries is reviewed in Chapter 13).

The amount of injury produced by a penetrating projectile is related to a variety of factors, including the characteristics of the weapon, the characteristics of its projected missiles, and the distance from the victim. The size of the bullet, its caliber, reflects the diameter of the muzzle bore. The shape and design of the missile also affect the degree of tissue injury. Some bullets are coated with metal jackets to decrease resistance, whereas others have soft tips that expand on contact to increase injury to soft tissue. A particularly important determinant of injury is the kinetic energy delivered to the tissue, which is determined by the formula $KE = \frac{1}{2}MV^2$, where M = mass and V = velocity. Because the velocity value is squared in this equation, high-velocity injuries carry the greatest potential for tissue damage. Tissue damage results from direct injury and from injury transmitted to surrounding tissue, which is called temporary cavitation. Temporary cavitation occurs with the impact of high-kinetic energy missiles and accounts for injury of anatomic structures adjacent to the area penetrated by the projected missile. High-velocity injuries are characterized by loss of tissue, rather than simple damage to tissues as is associated with low-velocity injuries. Firearms with muzzle velocities greater than 1,000 feet per second (or greater than 600 feet per second, by some criteria) are considered high-velocity weapons. These include many military and civilian rifles, as well as some shotguns. Handguns and most shotguns are low-velocity weapons, as are stabbing weapons such as knives, ice picks, razors, and glass. Because of the greater velocity involved and the associated risk of cavitation, gunshot wounds are more likely to injure vessels, nerves, and the aerodigestive tract than are stab wounds. In addition, transcervical gunshot wounds are more than twice as likely to injure vital structures of the neck than those not crossing the midline.[1]

This chapter reviews the presentation, evaluation, and management of penetrating neck trauma. Various diagnostic modalities and the management of specific injuries are addressed, and the long-standing controversy of mandatory vs. selective exploration is discussed.

PRESENTATION

Penetrating neck trauma may be isolated or may occur in association with other injuries. The presentation by patients with penetrating neck trauma is highly variable and is determined by the mechanism, severity, and location of injury, which may predict the anatomic structures injured. A combined review of 16 series determined the most common sites of cervical injury in penetrating trauma.[2] Vascular injury occurs in more than 20% of patients. Approximately 9% of patients suffer injury to the internal jugular vein, another 9% experience injury to the carotid system, 2% of patients have subclavian vessel injury, and only 1% of patients sustain injury to the vertebral artery. The larynx and trachea are injured in 10% of patients, and the pharynx and esophagus are injured in another 10% of patients. Other structures at risk for injury include cranial nerves VII, IX, X, XI, and XII, the brachial plexus, cervical nerves (including the phrenic nerve), the thoracic duct, and the lungs. The cervical spine and spinal cord are reportedly injured in almost 3% of patients with gunshot wounds.

Trauma to the neck is classified as immediately life-threatening or not immediately threatening to life. The presentation of an immediately life-threatening injury is quite dramatic. Significant neurologic deficit, including paralysis and impaired mental status, may be apparent because of lack of cerebral oxygenation. Severe respiratory compromise is associated with such intrathoracic injuries as hemothorax or pneumothorax. Signs of life-threatening injury include shock (discussed in Chapter 3), significant hemorrhage, expanding cervical hematoma, and the signs of respiratory and neurologic compromise previously mentioned.

The presentation of patients without life-threatening injury is more variable and usually affords time for a more thorough history, physical examination, and diagnostic evaluation. A description of the weapon used and the history of the attack may be useful. The position of the victim relative to the assailant can be important. An overhand, downwardly directed stab, for example, is more likely to slide behind the clavicle and injure the subclavian vessels than is a horizontally directed bullet.

Symptoms in patients without life-threatening injuries include pain, respiratory distress, dysarthria, hoarseness, dysphagia, odynophagia, hemoptysis, hematemesis, drooling, and fever. Patients might also complain of weakness or sensory loss in the face, tongue, shoulder, or upper extremities. Like the symptoms of penetrating neck trauma, the signs are extremely variable and depend on the structures involved. A vascular injury might produce a hematoma of the neck or oropharynx, a pulse deficit, a carotid bruit or thrill, tachycardia, or hypotension. An injury of the upper aerodigestive tract might present with signs such as stridor, subcutaneous emphysema, or air bubbling from an open wound. Cranial nerve palsies, Horner's syndrome, hemiplegia, and quadriplegia are associated with injury to neural structures, including the cranial nerves, brachial plexus, sympathetic chain, and spinal cord.

EVALUATION

The evaluation of a patient with a penetrating neck trauma begins with the principles of the Advanced Trauma Life Support guidelines outlined by the American College of Surgeons.[3] An initial assessment of the patient's airway, breathing, circulation, and cervical spine is vitally important, as is assessment of the patient's neurologic status. Penetrating trauma to the neck often occurs in a victim who has experienced multiple traumas, so associated injury is common. The unclothed patient must be fully examined for identification of all entrance and exit wounds. Vital signs are determined and serially monitored.

A thorough head and neck examination is conducted, with specific attention to the signs of injury. A careful clinical examination is usually an accurate predictor of the extent of injury in a patient with penetrating neck trauma. Neurologic evaluation, including cranial nerve assessment, is essential, especially as cranial nerve compromise may herald the involvement of adjacent vital structures in an otherwise stable patient. Bilateral auscultation of the chest and palpation of peripheral pulses, especially of the upper extremities, should be performed as well. The wounds should be identified and inspected, but not probed. Probing a penetrating neck wound could potentially dislodge a blood clot and lead to severe hemorrhage.

Inspection of the wound should determine its depth in relation to the platysma muscle. The layers of the deep cervical fasciae lie below this muscle, protecting the vital structures of the neck. Consequently, wounds superficial to the platysma have no potential for serious injury, whereas wounds deep to the platysma muscle require further evaluation (Chapter 19 includes a complete review of the fascial layers of the neck.)

Laboratory evaluation of a patient with a deep penetrating neck wound includes hematocrit and typing and screening of a blood sample. A patient should undergo plain radiographs of both the neck and chest to detect retained foreign bodies such as bullet or knife fragments and to identify a pneumothorax, hemothorax, or pneumomediastinum. Cervical spine films are essential and cervical immobilization should be maintained until the cervical spine is radiographically cleared. Injury to the cervical spine, although rare, is more common with a gunshot wound than with a stab wound, especially in the case of a high-velocity injury.[4]

The extent of the diagnostic evaluation is based in part on the anatomic location of the neck wound. The neck is commonly divided horizontally into three zones (I, II, and III) to aid in predicting the structures at risk for injury and in selecting appropriate further diagnostic modalities (Fig. 12–1).

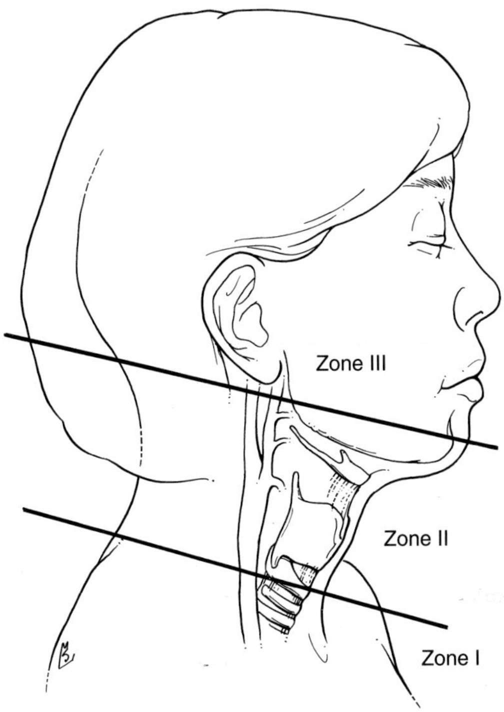

Figure 12–1. Cervical zones I, II, and III.

Zone I extends from the sternal notch to the inferior border of the cricoid cartilage and contains the apices of the lung, the trachea, the esophagus, the common carotid arteries, the internal jugular veins, the subclavian vessels, the innominate artery, the brachial plexus, and the spinal cord. Zone I is protected by the sternum and clavicle, which create significant obstacles to surgical exploration of this zone.

Zone II extends from the inferior border of the cricoid cartilage to the angle of the mandible. The larynx, trachea, esophagus, carotid arteries, internal jugular veins, vertebral arteries, spinal cord, and cranial nerves may be involved in injury to this region. Zone II is the most exposed region of the neck and therefore is the most commonly injured area in cases of penetrating neck trauma.[5] Because this region is easily accessed surgically, great controversy exists regarding mandatory vs. selective surgical exploration.

Zone III extends from the angle of the mandible to the base of the skull. The important structures found in zone III include the distal internal carotid arteries, internal jugular veins, vertebral arteries, branches of the external carotid arteries, pharynx, and spinal cord. Zone III is surrounded by skeletal structures, including the skull base and the mandible, which account for its lower susceptibility to injury but also result in extremely difficult surgical access when exploration is warranted.

Classification of the location of a neck wound according to zone, along with recognition of the associated symptoms and signs described previously, facilitates the development of a management strategy for penetrating neck trauma. A patient with a life-threatening injury manifested by hemodynamic instability, exsanguinating hemorrhage, rapidly expanding hematoma, or rapidly evolving neurologic deficit demands immediate surgical exploration without further diagnostic evaluation. A stable patient merits consideration of further diagnostic evaluation (Fig. 12–2).

Zone I

Vascular damage is the most common zone I injury. Angiography is an extremely sensitive, specific, and accurate means of identifying and assessing vascular injury in the neck and is commonly recommended for every patient with a zone I injury. A patient with such symptoms requires surgical exploration, and angiography provides the benefit of accurate preoperative knowledge of the extent of injury. This informa-

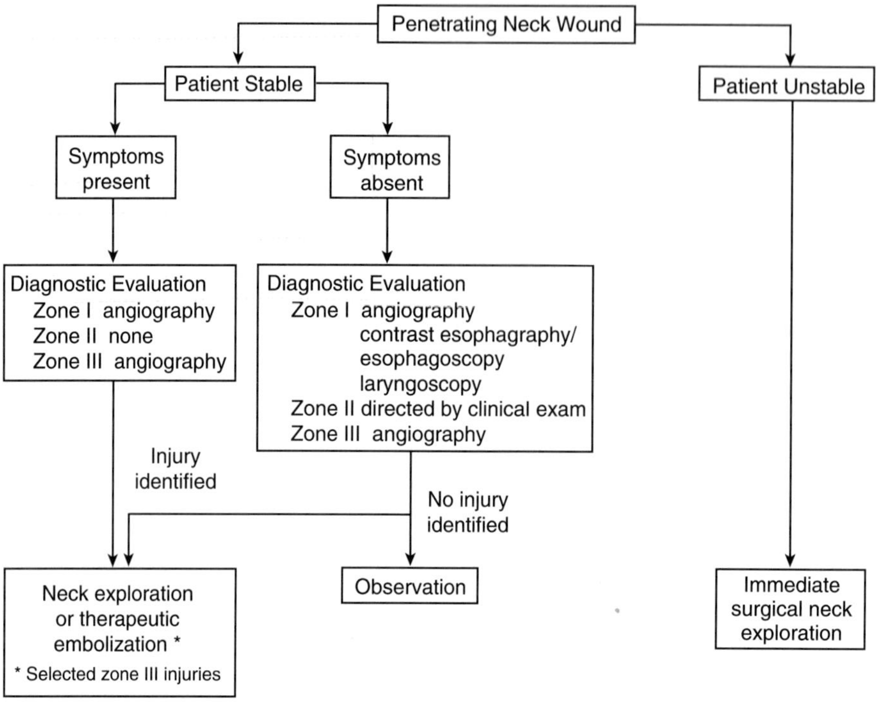

Figure 12–2. Algorithm for the management of penetrating neck trauma.

tion facilitates the planning of the surgical approach, which may require median sternotomy or thoracotomy. In addition, approximately 30% of patients without symptoms suffer vascular injury in zone I.[6, 7] If an injury is identified angiographically in an asymptomatic patient, surgical exploration and repair are warranted. Many reports have shown that an asymptomatic patient with a negative arteriogram can be safely observed and have a good outcome.[8]

Some authors do not recommend arteriography for a patient with a zone I neck trauma because angiography is an invasive and costly procedure with potentially adverse effects and because a patient evaluated clinically who undergoes surgical exploration for positive clinical findings appears to have an outcome equivalent to that of a patient who has undergone routine angiography.[9]

In recent years, color Doppler sonography, or color-flow Doppler (CFD), has been proposed as a safe and cost-effective alternative to traditional angiography.[10, 11] CFD is associated with more than a 90% sensitivity and specificity,[10] and its proponents believe that CFD may supplant angiography as the standard diagnostic modality for assessing vascular trauma in the neck. CFD is not yet widely available, and further studies that directly compare it to angiography are warranted.

A patient with a zone I injury is also at risk for tracheal and esophageal injuries. Damage to the upper aerodigestive tract at the level of zone II generally produces symptoms within hours, whereas injury to the trachea or esophagus in zone I may be clinically silent until the development of significant complications such as mediastinitis and sepsis. Therefore, the aerodigestive tract should be evaluated in any patient with a zone I injury, but the means of esophageal evaluation remains controversial. Both contrast esophagraphy with Gastrografin and esophagoscopy (either flexible or rigid) demonstrate sensitivities of 80% to 90% in identifying esophageal injury.[12] The combination of contrast imaging and endoscopy appears to increase the sensitivity for injury identification to nearly 100%. Some trauma centers advocate combined modality evaluation in all patients because of the grave consequences of a missed zone I esophageal injury, whereas others recommend thorough clinical examination combined with single-modality evaluation.

Bedside flexible fiberoptic laryngoscopy should be performed in a patient with a zone I neck injury. This evaluation can identify impaired vocal fold function and the presence of blood or edema in the upper respiratory tract. These findings warrant direct operative laryngoscopy with tracheoscopy and bronchoscopy in order to more thoroughly evaluate the airway. Although flexible laryngoscopy can be normal in the presence of a tracheal injury, clinically significant tracheal disruption rarely remains silent. Most experts currently advocate careful observation without endoscopy in asymptomatic patients who have normal flexible fiberoptic examinations.

Zone III

Zone III injuries, like zone I injuries, pose significant risk for vascular injury, and surgical exposure is difficult because of surrounding skeletal structures. Many vascular injuries at this level, however, are amenable to definitive treatment with interventional radiographic embolization techniques[2] and thus may not require surgical exploration. A symptomatic patient with a zone III injury should undergo angiography and definitive treatment with embolization by an interventional radiologist. If this technology is not available, or if the injury is not amenable to embolization, surgical exploration is required.

As many as 25% of patients with arterial injuries to zone III are asymptomatic at presentation.[13] Routine arteriography is advocated, therefore, in every stable patient with a zone III injury. An asymptomatic patient with a positive angiogram is treated as described previously.

CFD is an alternative means of detecting vascular damage in zone III, but it is a less sensitive modality for assessing the vertebral system than is four-vessel angiography.[11] Clinically significant vertebral arterial injury is extremely rare in an asymptomatic patient.

At the level of zone III, the pharynx is accessible to physical examination, and undetected injury is uncommon. Further diagnostic evaluation of the pharynx is not necessary in an asymptomatic patient with a zone III injury.

Zone II

Because zone II of the neck is readily accessible surgically, a patient with signs or symptoms of significant vascular or upper aerodigestive tract injury does not require further diagnostic evaluation prior to surgery. Preoperative angiography in a symptomatic patient with a zone II injury has not demonstrated any advantage over clinical evaluation alone.[14]

The central controversy in the management of penetrating trauma to the neck involves an asymptomatic patient with a zone II injury. Prior to the Vietnam War, the mortality rate of patients with penetrating neck wounds approached 15%.[2] By the end of the war, mortality rates had decreased to 3% to 6%,[2] and this reduction was attributed largely to the policy of mandatory surgical exploration of all neck wounds penetrating the platysma muscle. The success of this philosophy during the war led to its popularization in the management of civilian injuries, and until the 1980s most trauma surgeons advocated mandatory neck exploration.[15, 16] Mandatory surgical exploration of the neck in victims of penetrating neck trauma, however, fails to reveal an identifiable injury in 50% to 90% of cases.[17, 18] Recognition of this substantial number of negative neck explorations led many trauma surgeons to advocate a policy of selective neck exploration.[5, 19–26]

Arguments in favor of mandatory neck exploration include the small but significant incidence of injury missed by diagnostic evaluation and the increased requirements for hospitalization and serial evaluations in nonoperated patients. Morbidity resulting from a negative neck exploration is generally very low, and cosmetic deformity is usually minimal. In addition, the imaging and endoscopic modalities employed as alternatives to surgery are expensive.

Proponents of selective exploration policies argue that the few clinically significant injuries missed during diagnostic evaluation would have been detected during subsequent serial physical examinations. They note that an operation requiring a general anesthetic is expensive, is often unnecessary, and subjects the patient to avoidable potential iatrogenic morbidity and scarring. Outcomes appear to be equal with both policies, but the current trend clearly favors selective management.[15, 19–26]

The definition of selective operative management of zone II injuries varies, however, especially when applied to patients without any specific signs or symptoms. Some clinicians believe that all such patients warrant evaluation by esophagoscopy or contrast esophagraphy, laryngoscopy, and angiography, whereas others believe that a 48- to 72-hour period of careful monitoring in a hospital setting without any additional diagnostic evaluation is adequate.

Sometimes, a patient demonstrates clinical findings suggestive of, but not specific to, injury to particular structure. If the patient is stable, a directed examination is proposed, based on the physical examination and the anatomic path of the projectile. A patient with hematemesis or dysphagia, for example, should undergo contrast esophagraphy or esophagoscopy. A patient with vocal fold paralysis, hoarseness, laryngeal tenderness, or hemopysis warrants further evaluation with direct laryngoscopy and bronchoscopy.

The role of angiography in an asymptomatic patient with a zone II injury remains controversial. Some reports find no difference between clinical examination and angiography in detecting vascular injury in zone II.[14] Other studies suggest that angiography is superior to clinical evaluation in select cases.[13] A patient with a projectile in close proximity to the major vessels or a patient with signs or symptoms of injury to structures adjacent to the vessels such as Horner's syndrome might benefit from angiography.

Although computed tomography (CT) imaging is not routinely employed in evaluating a victim of penetrating neck trauma, selected cases of suspected laryngeal injury that appear normal on flexible fiberoptic laryngoscopy might warrant CT evaluation. Stabilization of the airway prior to imaging is essential in such a patient (laryngeal trauma is thoroughly reviewed in Chapter 11).

PRIORITIES

Life-threatening injuries are treated according to basic principles of trauma management. Airway control is the first priority, and intubation (nasotracheal, transoral, or via tracheostomy) is often indicated. Approximately 10% of patients with penetrating neck trauma experience significant airway compromise.[26] A patient with penetrating neck trauma should initially be presumed to have associated cervical spine injury, and in-line cervical stabilization should be maintained while the airway is secured. Hemorrhage from the neck should be controlled by direct pressure. The wound should not be probed, and penetrating objects remaining in the neck should not be removed. A blood clot or retained foreign body may temporarily tamponade a hemorrhage. Several large-bore intravenous catheters are placed, and volume resuscitation is undertaken as appropriate (see Chapter 3). After the patient is stabilized, evaluation can proceed as discussed previously.

In a case of massive hemorrhage, further diagnostic evaluation is deferred and the patient is taken directly to the operating room. A high-velocity rifle injury to the neck is associated with an extremely high likelihood of mortality, and a surviving victim is a candidate for neck exploration based on this mechanism of injury. In a candidate for surgical exploration, adequate exposure of vital structures of the neck is essential. A transverse midneck incision placed in a natural skin crease can be employed and extended by a posterior, vertical half-H limb if necessary. An apron incision is an appropriate choice for a transcervical injury. Exposure of distal vascular injuries at the skull base in an emergency situation remains challenging. Vertical or midline mandibular osteotomy or suboccipital craniotomy may be required[27] (Figs. 12–3 and 12–4) in addition to standard transcervical access (Fig. 12–5). Neurosurgical consultation is indicated for a patient who may require a craniotomy. Proximal and distal control of damaged vessels should be carefully undertaken, and blind clamping of vessels should be avoided because of the risk of injury to adjacent structures.

An injury that does not present an immediate threat to life is managed according to the depth and location of the wound. A neck wound superficial to the platysma muscle may be reapproximated without additional diagnostic evaluation. A neck wound that violates the platysma is classified by zone, and the diagnostic strategy presented earlier is followed (see Fig. 12–2).

Management of Specific Injuries

VASCULAR INJURY

An injured vein in the neck can be safely ligated. If both internal jugular veins are damaged, an attempt should be made to repair one or both of them to avoid complications arising from venous outflow obstruction due to bilateral juglar vein occlusion (see Chapter 19). An injury to the external carotid arterial branches can safely be suture-ligated, as collateral circulation to the areas supplied by these vessels is good.

An injury to the common or internal carotid system is more complicated. Because of the risk of neurologic compromise resulting from impaired carotid artery flow, repair should be undertaken for all carotid arterial injuries. Control of the hemorrhage proximal and distal to the injury with vessel loops or vascular clamps is imperative. When the internal carotid artery is injured at the skull base, the distal vessel may not be accessible for circumferential control. A no. 4 Fogarty catheter may be passed beyond the injury. Inflation of the balloon occludes the lumen and controls the bleeding while repair is performed. Alternatively, a Pruitt-Inahara shunt may be passed over the Fogarty catheter beyond the injured segment, allowing removal of the

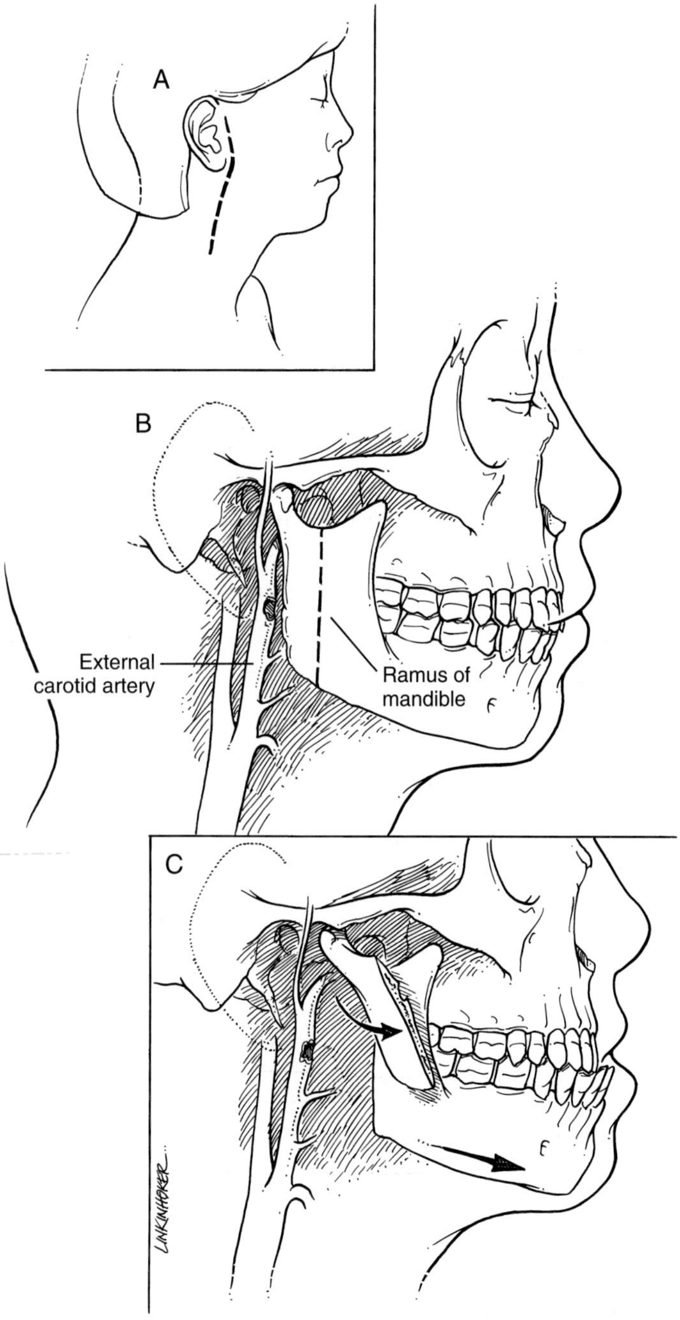

Figure 12–3. Surgical access to the carotid arterial system by division of the mandible.

catheter so that repair or shunting of the vessel can be undertaken.[29]

Primary repair of the carotid artery is performed whenever possible, using monofilament suture. Consultation with a vascular surgeon should be obtained in a case of complex or extensive damage to the carotid artery. An injury not amenable to primary closure may require end-to-end anastomosis, a patch, or interposition grafting. Graft materials include autogenous veins, such as the saphenous and cephalic veins, and prosthetic materials such as Gore-Tex. (Fig. 12–6). Internal carotid injury may also be repaired by transposition of the external carotid artery to the internal carotid system (Fig. 12–7). The carotid artery should be ligated only when damage is irreparable, access for repair is impossible, or the patient has suffered profound neurologic damage manifested by coma and fixed, dilated pupils. In these

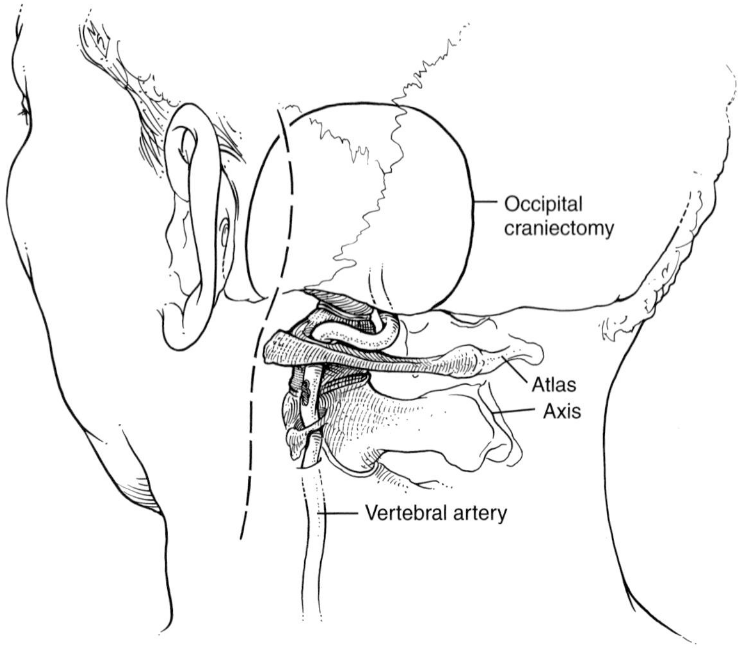

Figure 12–4. Occipital approach to the injured vertebral artery by craniectomy.

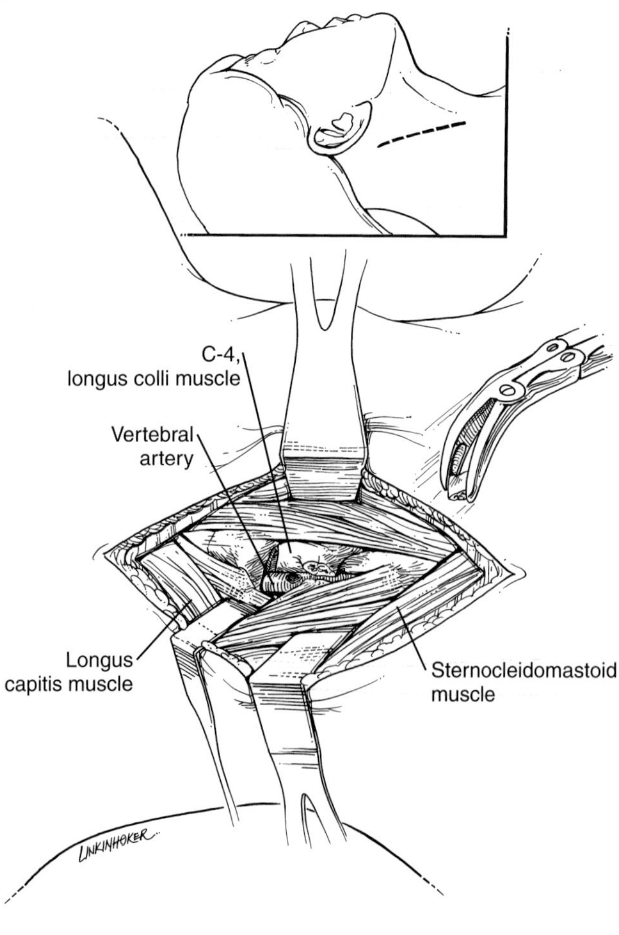

Figure 12–5. Transcervical approach to the injured vertebral artery.

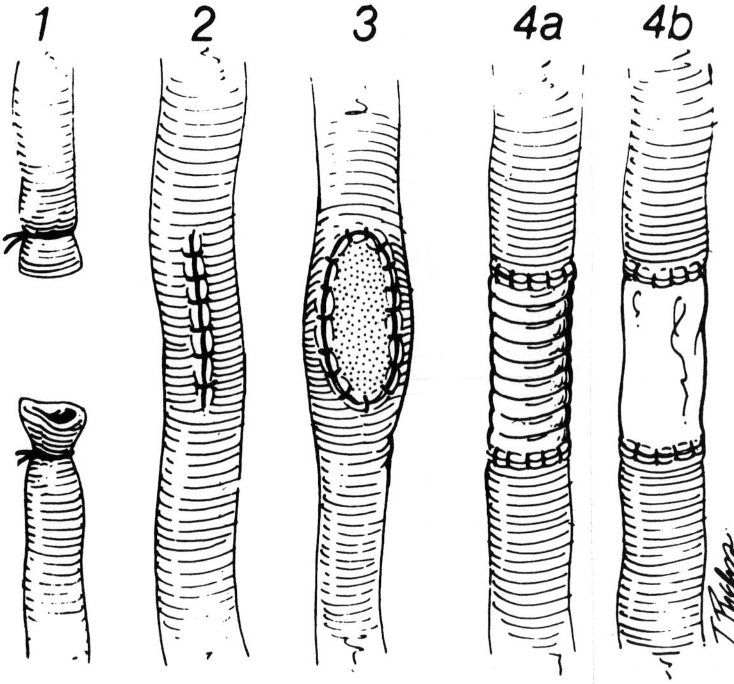

Figure 12–6. Types of vascular repair: 1, ligation; 2, primary repair; 3, patch angioplasty; 4a, prosthetic material; 4b, vein graft. (From Dichtel WJ, et al. Lateral mandibulotomy: a technique of exposure for penetrating injuries of the internal carotid artery at the base of the skull. Laryngoscope 1984;94:1142).

cases, the vessel is ligated, oversewn, and buttressed with surrounding muscular tissue.

Carotid artery repair in the setting of neurologic impairment remains controversial. The possibility of converting an ischemic infarction to a more severe hemorrhagic infarction by restoration of cerebral blood flow in a neurologically compromised patient has been raised. Concern about hemorrhagic infarction after revascularization led to initial recommendations against routine restoration of carotid arterial flow.[30] Recent literature disputes the concept of hemorrhagic infarction after revascularization and supports attempts to reestablish blood flow through the carotid arteries in most patients with neurologic deficits.[30] Severe ischemic injury in a neurologically impaired victim may be a contraindication to revascularization, but it is difficult to quantitate brain ischemia expeditiously. CT imaging displays significant ischemic changes in only 50% of patients within 3 to 6 hours after cerebral ischemia.

Only about 4% of patients with penetrating neck trauma sustain injury to the subclavian vessels,[2] but the mortality rate of patients with such injuries is high. The prognosis for subclavian venous injury is worse than that of subclavian arterial injury because of the usually fatal

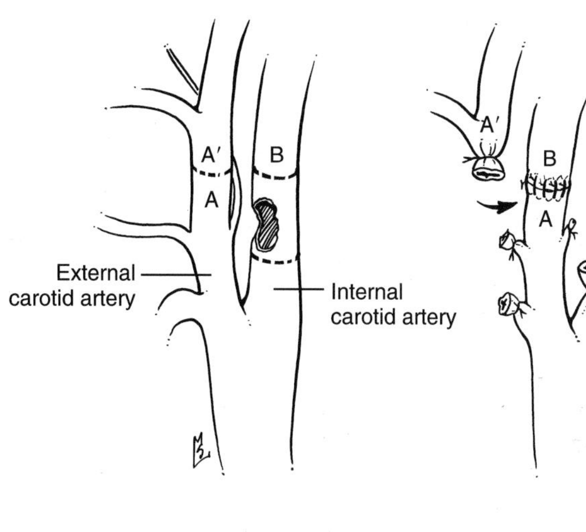

Figure 12–7. Bypass of an internal carotid arterial injury with the external carotid system.

complication of air embolism. Because access to the major vessels in zone I is limited, a median sternotomy or thoracotomy is usually required for vascular control and repair. In cases of severe hemorrhage, the balloon tamponade technique discussed for carotid injuries can be employed transcervically until adequate surgical access is achieved. Alternatively, an Allis clamp can be applied to an injured vein and twisted to stop the bleeding (see Chapter 19). Ligation of the subclavian artery should be avoided, as the risks of ligation include upper extremity claudication and ischemia and subclavian steal syndrome if the vessel ligated is proximal to the vertebral artery.

Injury to the vertebral artery resulting from a penetrating neck injury was believed to be extremely rare. Routine use of four-vessel angiography, however, has identified a higher frequency of such an injury. Damage to the vertebral artery is more likely to occur in a patient with a gunshot wound than in one with a stab wound,[30] and two thirds of these patients have associated injuries of the cervical spine.[30] The advent of embolization techniques by interventional radiologists has had a dramatic impact on the management of vertebral arterial injury, as most of these lesions are amenable to therapeutic embolization. Surgery for vertebral arterial injury is reserved for extremely distal injuries not amenable to embolization, for cases in which embolization has failed, and for injuries that present with life-threatening hemorrhage.

PHARYNGOESOPHAGEAL INJURY

An injury to the oropharynx or upper hypopharynx is managed differently from an injury to the inferior hypopharynx or cervical esophagus. Pharyngeal tissues superior to the level of the arytenoid cartilage are not subjected to the dependent drainage of salivary secretions and therefore do not generally require closure. Such an injury is managed by withholding oral intake and administering intravenous antibiotics.

An inferior hypopharyngeal or cervical esophageal injury should be repaired primarily, with a two-layer, watertight closure. A muscular flap based on the adjacent strap muscles or sternocleidomastoid muscle can be used to reinforce the closure. Often the repair can be accomplished transcervically, but if the injury extends inferiorly, thoracic surgical consultation is indicated for consideration of median sternotomy or thoracotomy. Drains should be placed in the neck at the time of repair, oral intake is withheld postoperatively, and parenteral antibiotics are administered. If the diagnosis of an esophageal injury is delayed beyond 24 hours, primary repair is not recommended. In this patient, a controlled pharyngocutaneous fistula is created in the neck using drains to divert salivary flow away from vital structures and prevent abscess formation. In a case of extensive esophageal injury, diversion with a cervical esophagostomy may be warranted, along with inferior esophageal ligation and placement of a feeding gastrostomy tube. Such a patient may be a candidate for esophageal reconstruction at a later time.

LARYNGOTRACHEAL INJURY

A patient with a laryngotracheal injury has a high incidence of concomitant esophageal injury and must be thoroughly evaluated for trauma to the digestive tract. Such a patient is not usually a candidate for endotracheal intubation and often requires a tracheostomy for airway control. A patient with small wounds limited to the trachea and without associated tissue loss may avoid tracheostomy.[28] A stab wound to the trachea should be closed primarily in two layers, an initial layer to approximate mucosal edges and a second layer to secure the position of the cartilagenous rings. If the trachea is transected, end-to-end anastomosis can be performed. Reapproximation must be performed without tension, and if a segment of trachea is lost, the remaining trachea can be mobilized. Tracheal loss of less than 2 or 3 cm can generally be handled by reapproximation without significant dissection. Longer segments require suprahyoid or infrahyoid release maneuvers, which can provide an additional 4 to 6 cm of tracheal mobilization. In a case of extensive tissue loss in which primary reanastomosis is not possible, musculofascial flaps and synthetic materials have been employed.[26] (The management of acute laryngeal trauma is a complex topic that is thoroughly reviewed in Chapter 11.)

NERVE INJURY

Diagnosis of injury to the cranial nerves, brachial plexus, or cervical nerve branches as a result of penetrating trauma to the neck is made on clinical examination. Repair is recommended when injury involves cranial nerves VII, XI, or XII, a division of the brachial plexus, or the phrenic nerve. A hand-held nerve stimulator may aid in intraoperative identification of distal nerve ends if exploration is undertaken within 3 days of injury. The edges of a transected nerve should be freshened and epineural repair performed with several interrupted, fine, monofilament sutures. Loss of a nerve segment is more likely to occur with a gunshot wound than with a stab wound, and in such a case, nerve grafting can be performed using the great auricular or sural nerve. It is also reasonable to repair an injury to the vagus nerve or recurrent laryngeal nerve if it is recognized intraoperatively, but synkinetic laryngeal movement is the expected outcome in such a case.

CERVICAL SPINE INJURY

Debridement of devitalized tissue and removal of bone fragments should be undertaken transcervically in a case of cervical spine injury. Parenteral antibiotics are recommended if there is an associated pharyngeal injury in order to reduce the risk of osteomyelitis due to salivary contamination. Neurosurgical or orthopedic surgical consultation is advised for the management of cervical spine injury.

THORACIC DUCT INJURY

Injury to the thoracic duct is rare and is usually associated with trauma to the left subclavian vein. If an injured thoracic duct is identified intraoperatively, it should be ligated. More commonly, this kind of injury is not recognized initially and presents with chyle leaking through a drain or a transcutaneous fistula or accumulating subcutaneously as a chylocele.

INTRATHORACIC INJURY

A high index of suspicion for associated intrathoracic injury must be maintained in every patient with a penetrating trauma of the neck. If a pneumothorax is present, a chest tube is placed. Associated thoracic injury requires consultation with a thoracic surgeon.

OUTCOMES

As noted previously, the pre-Vietnam War mortality rate from penetrating neck trauma approached 15%. The current overall mortality rate from penetrating trauma to the neck in civilian practice is currently 3% to 6%.[2] Mortality resulting from these injuries depends on the structures injured. Hemorrhage from vascular injury remains the leading overall cause of death in neck trauma. Zone I neck injuries demonstrate higher mortality rates (12%) than injuries involving the more superior zones[31]; this is most likely related to the significant risk of major vascular damage with zone I neck injuries.

Likelihood of mortality is also influenced by the characteristics of the weapon. High-velocity rifle injuries and close-range shotgun injuries to the neck are associated with extremely high mortality rates. Most victims of such trauma do not survive to reach a hospital and therefore are not included in reported series concerning penetrating neck trauma.

Morbidity resulting from penetrating neck trauma is related primarily to the injury itself. Transient cerebral ischemia or permanent stroke can result from vascular injury associated with severe hemorrhage. Airway obstruction can result from laryngotracheal injury. Hemiplegia or quadriplegia can result from spinal cord injury, and isolated neurologic deficits can result from injury to any of the nerves mentioned above.

Esophageal trauma is the most commonly missed injury resulting from penetrating neck trauma. Delay in diagnosis of digestive tract injury is associated with severe complications and increased mortality rates.[31] The majority of these complications are infections, including neck abscess, mediastinitis, and osteomyelitis of the cervical spine. (The reader is referred to Chapter 19 for a complete review of the management and complications of neck infections.) Fistulous tracts, including pharyngocutaneous fistulas and tracheoesophageal fistulas, can also develop in patients with unrecognized digestive tract injuries.

Surgical exploration of a neck in which no injury is found commonly occurs in centers that practice mandatory neck exploration, and it occurs infrequently in centers that perform selective neck explorations. Potential morbidity resulting from any negative neck exploration includes cosmetic deformity and the possible iatrogenic surgical complications of neck exploration.

CONCLUSION

Penetrating injuries to the neck are life-threatening emergencies that demand immediate, skilled evaluation and management. The extent of injury is determined by the type of weapon employed, the history of the attack, and the location of the injury. This information, in combination with a careful clinical examination, can be used to predict the anatomic structures potentially damaged. Adjunctive diagnostic modalities such as angiography, contrast esophagography, and endoscopy are invaluable in identifying the presence and precise location of an injury. These diagnostic strategies are used to direct management and to select patients for surgery and, when used appropriately, can significantly reduce the number of negative neck explorations performed without increasing morbidity or mortality. Techniques such as color Doppler sonography and angiographic embolization are also important diagnostic and therapeutic aids, when they are available. Surgery remains the mainstay of treatment for patients with recognized injury to cervical structures that result from penetrating neck trauma. Surgery is also indicated for unstable patients when time does not permit diagnostic evaluation and for patients who present to hospitals in which adjunctive diagnostic modalities are not available.

REFERENCES

1. Demetriades D et al. Transcervical gunshot injuries: mandatory operation is not necessary. J Trauma 1996;40:758–760.
2. McConnell DB, Trunkey DD. Management of penetrating trauma to the neck. Adv Surg 1994;27:99–119.
3. American College of Surgeons Committee on Trauma. Advanced Trauma Life Support Course. Chicago, American College of Surgeons, 1993.
4. Demetrius D et al. Management options in vertebral artery injuries. Br J Surg 1996;83:83–86.
5. Obeid FN et al. A critical reappraisal of a mandatory exploration policy for penetrating wounds of the neck. Surg Gynecol Obstet 1985;160:517–522.
6. Rao PM et al. Cervical vascular injuries: a trauma center experience. Surgery 1993;114:527–531.
7. Mansour MA et al. Validating the selective management of penetrating neck wounds. Am J Surg 1991;162:517–521.
8. Hiatt JR, Busuttil RW, Wilson SE. Impact of routine arteriography on management of penetrating neck injuries. J Vasc Surg 1984;1:860–866.
9. Rivers SP et al. Limited role of arteriography in penetrating neck trauma. J Vasc Surg 1998;8:112–116.
10. Demetriades D et al. Penetrating injuries of the neck in stable patients: physical examination, angiography, or color-flow Doppler. Arch Surg 1995;130:971–979.
11. Montalvo BM et al. Color Doppler sonography in penetrating injuries of the neck. Am J Neuroradiol 1996;17:943–951.
12. Noyes L, McSwain N, Markowitz I. Panendoscopy with arteriography versus mandatory exploration of penetrating wounds of the neck. Ann Surg 1996;204:21.
13. Scalfani SJA et al. The role of angiography in penetrating neck trauma. J Trauma 1991;31:557–563.
14. Jarvik JG et al. Penetrating neck trauma: sensitivity of clinical examination and cost-effectiveness of angiography. Am J Neuroradiol 1995;16:647–654.
15. Saletta JD et al. Penetrating trauma of the neck. J Trauma 1996;16:579–587.
16. Kenefick TC. Gunshot wounds to the head and neck. J Laryngol Otol 1976;90:335–344.
17. Bishra RA et al. The necessity of mandatory exploration of penetrating zone II neck injuries. Surgery 1986;100:655–660.
18. Jurkovich GJ et al. Penetrating neck trauma: diagnostic studies in the asymptomatic patient. J Trauma 1985;25:819–822.
19. Velhamos GC et al. Selective surgical management in penetrating neck injuries. Can J Surg 1994;37:487–491.
20. Narrod JA, Moore EE. Initial management of penetrating neck wounds: a selective approach. J Emerg Med 1984;2:17–22.
21. Ngakane H, Muckart DJ, Luvuno FM. Penetrating visceral injuries of the neck: results of a conservative management policy. Br J Surg 1990;77:908–910.
22. Wood J, Fabian TC, Mangiante EC. Penetrating neck injuries: recommendations for selective management. J Trauma 1989;29:602–605.
23. Massac E Jr, Siram SM, Leffall LD Jr. Penetrating neck wounds. Am J Surg 1983;145:263–265.
24. Cabasares HV. Selective surgical management of penetrating neck trauma: 15-year experience in a community hospital. Am Surg 1982;48:355–358.
25. Pate JW, Casini M. Penetrating wounds of the neck: explore or not? Am Surg 1980;46:38–43.
26. Lundy LJ Jr et al. Experience in selective operations in the management of penetrating wounds of the neck. Surg Gynecol Obstet 1978;147:845–848.
27. Dichtel WJ et al. Lateral mandibulotomy: a technique of exposure for penetrating injuries of the internal carotid artery at the base of the skull. Laryngoscope 1984;94:1140–1144.
28. Grewal H et al. Management of penetrating laryngotracheal injuries. Head neck 1995;17:494–502.
29. Perry M. Injuries of the carotid and vertebral arteries. In Bongard FS, Wilson SE, Perry MO, eds. Vascular Injuries in Surgical Practice. Norwalk, CT, Appleton Lange, 1991.
30. Demetriades D et al. Complex problems in penetrating neck trauma. Surg Clin North Am 1996;76:661–683.
31. Rao PM et al. Penetrating injuries of the neck: criteria for exploration. J Trauma 1983;23:47–49.
32. Bladergroen MR, Lowe JE, Postlewalt MD. Diagnosis and recommended management of esophageal perforation and rupture. Ann Thorac Surg 1986;42:235–239.
33. Shama DM, Odell J. Penetrating neck with tracheal and esophageal injuries. Br J Surg 1984;71:534–538.

CHAPTER 13

Penetrating Trauma of the Face

G. Richard Holt, MD

As with a penetrating trauma to the neck, a facial injury assumes a level of importance proportional to the cause and location of the wound. Penetrating forces vary tremendously in the energy imparted to the tissues, primarily as a product of their own velocities at the time of impact as well as of the shape and stability of the object and the resistance of the target tissues. For instance, a .22 caliber bullet carries less velocity at tissue impact than a .357 caliber bullet so consequently, the .22 caliber missile is more likely to gyrate through the tissues without significant osseous injury.

At the other end of the spectrum is the knife wound, which may cause little soft tissue damage in terms of volume, yet manages to transect all of the major vessels and nerves in its path. Additionally, in the cases of some penetrating injuries, it may be difficult to discern just what course occurred in the tissues, as the angle of attack with respect to the plane of the face is unknown.

In a case of massive soft tissue trauma, the initial challenge may be to sort out which tissues are missing and which are still present, albeit in different forms or locations. With lesser degrees of injury by penetration, the history of the injury based on the patient's history and on indirect evidence becomes very important in reconstructing the angle and depth of penetration. Additionally, a complete head and neck examination is vitally important, with special attention being paid to neurologic findings. The ultimate goal is to have the best possible understanding of the mechanics of the penetrating force as well as knowledge of its course in the facial tissues prior to formulating a surgical plan. A complete knowledge of head and neck anatomy and physiology is essential to diagnosing and managing penetrating wounds of the face.

ANIMAL AND HUMAN BITES

Dog, cat, and human bites account for 99% of bite wounds; facial bites in general account for less than 1% of all emergency department visits. Lacerations caused by bites occur three times more frequently than puncture wounds. In the past, animal bites were treated similarly to human bites—that is, very few were closed primarily. Copious irrigation was performed, the wound was minimally debrided, and delayed primary closure was performed as opposed to healing by secondary intention. This usually resulted in scars that were less than ideal or even unacceptable. Scar revision was a necessity, and functional disturbances caused by scarring were common.

The current standard of care has progressed significantly, particularly with respect to animal bites, based primarily on emergent wound care and use of antibiotics.[1] Human bites remain problematic, and primary closure is selected only in the most favorable circumstances. Most bites are contaminated by a polymicrobial population, including anaerobic and aerobic organisms. Thus, it is common to utilize broad-spectrum antibiotics with excellent anaerobic and microaerophilic efficacy. An overriding concern in animal bites is the risk for the rabies virus, whereas in human bites one must be concerned about hepatitis B and C, herpes, and the HIV viruses.

Evaluation

Bite wounds are usually a combination of penetration and avulsion caused by the tearing action of the teeth on tissue (Fig. 13–1). Tissue loss is minimal unless a piece is missing from a protruding structure such as the ear or nose. Depth of penetration is variable and is dependent upon the resistance of the skin as well as on the force of jaw contracture of the animal or human.

In general, human bites are less likely to penetrate deeply into facial tissue than animal bites, owing to the length and shape of the anterior teeth. Additionally, humans are loath to draw much blood during a bite because of an aversion to the blood of another in the mouth and because of fear of blood-borne diseases. All in all, human bites are significantly less common than animal bites because of the availability of other, more sophisticated instruments of injury such as knives, guns, and wooden beams. Human bites are often associated with lovers' quarrels and usually involve a single region of injury (ear, nose, or lip), whereas animal bites may have recurring attack patterns in multiple sites. It is good practice to treat a human bite as a possible HIV exposure, and an HIV test should be performed on the patient as well as on the attacker.

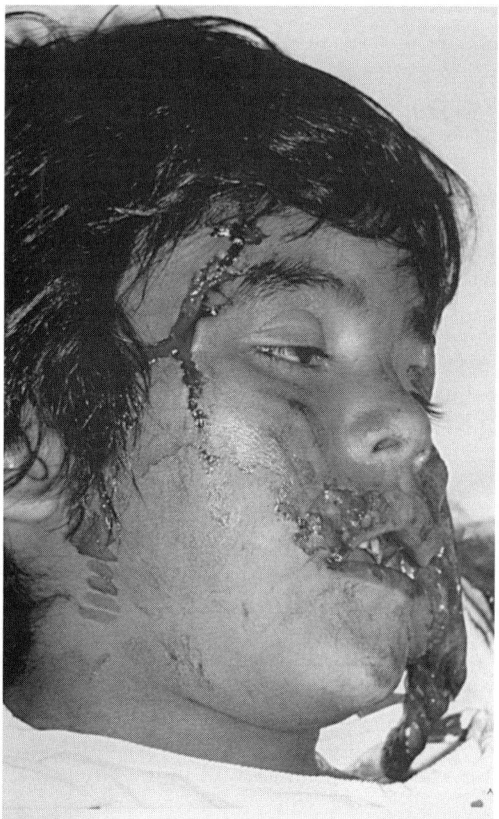

Figure 13–1. A dog bite to the face, with multiple avulsive injuries to the lip, cheek, and forehead.

The level of penetration should be assessed and estimated, paying particular attention to damage to underlying structures, such as muscles, ducts, and neurovascular bundles. With animal bites, an initial deep penetration may be masked by an avulsive injury of more superficial tissues, so that exploration of the wound after anesthetization is warranted. It should always be kept in mind that a bite by an older dog might result in the implantation of a loose tooth deep in the wound.

Because a tremendous amount of force can be delivered to the tissues by a bite, it is also possible for bony injury to occur. When a small child is attacked by a large-mouthed dog, fractures of the skull or jaw must be ruled out by computed tomography (CT) scans, if indicated. Microscopic injury to adjacent tissues is to be expected, and one must assess tissue viability based not only on the initial evaluation, but also on an evolving evaluation throughout the emergency care process. Because of the short distance from the face to the neck, it must be considered that some injury could coexist in the neck in children, and a thorough assessment of that possibility should be made.[2]

Priorities

The most urgent priorities are to assess the airway (especially in bites involving the neck and the floor of the mouth), the risk for a life-threatening incident, and the neurologic status. Fortunately, most penetrating wounds caused by bites involve soft tissue only, but certain vascular regions are at risk because of their superficial location over bony prominences, such as the superficial temporal, facial, and angular arteries. Included in neurologic concerns are facial nerve function, vision and ocular movement, and tongue motion. Consultations with the appropriate consulting physicians should be obtained, including the pediatric service if the victim is a child. Monitored CT scanning is mandatory if physical findings raise a concern about neurologic or osseous damage.

After the patient has been stabilized and adequately evaluated, tetanus prophylaxis and intravenous antibiotics should be administered. If the patient has not previously received the tetanus series, it should be begun right away and should be given early in the emergency visit so it is not forgotten. If rabies is a possibility, the patient should receive the first dose of immunoglobulin on the day of the injury, followed by the vaccine at days 0, 3, 7, 14, and 28. Because 90% of the rabies risk can be reduced by cleansing the wound with povidone, this should be done. For any significantly penetrating soft tissue bite, it is recommended that an intravenous bolus of a second-generation cephalosporin be administered. If penicillin sensitivity cross-reaction is a major concern with a cephalosporin, parenteral ciprofloxacin is a good choice. Alternatively, clindamycin can be considered. This parenteral dose should be given in advance of any surgical care, so that blood levels can be determined. If the wounds are considered severe, consideration should be given to continued parenteral antibiotic therapy, either on an inpatient basis or at home, with intravenous therapy. Usually, after the wounds have been cared for emergently, the patient may be discharged with oral antibiotics, which are effective against a wide variety of organisms, including anaerobes. Good choices include Augmentin, cephalexin, clindamycin, and ciprofloxacin.

The main key to successful management of penetrating wounds made by human or animal bites is copious irrigation with either sterile saline or tap water from a clean outlet, in order to decrease the bacterial load in the tissues.[3] Several liters of saline irrigation are adequate, but the author prefers a solution of saline and povidone (2:1); usually about 1.5 liters are used. For larger wounds, a bulb syringe or intravenous tubing irrigation suffices, but for smaller penetrations or puncture wounds, a plastic intravenous catheter on a 20-mL syringe works quite well.

Debridement of the wounds is the second most important step in caring for soft tissue wounds. Anesthesia can be obtained by administering regional nerve blocks (infraorbital, mental, supratrochlear, and supraorbital) as well as by means of local infiltration after the blocks have been effected. If the procedure is likely to take longer than 1 to 1½ hours, 0.25% Marcaine can be added to the local anesthetic solution to prolong its effect. It is also helpful, particularly with children, to buffer the anesthetic solution with sodium bicarbonate (10% of the total volume) to reduce local wound infiltrative discomfort. In extensive wounds, and in many children, a general anesthetic may be warranted (and humane).

For small, punctate penetration wounds caused by animal or human bites, the author prefers to excise the puncture tract with a 2-, 3-, or 4-mm dermatologic punch, with the goal of removing damaged and contaminated tissue. This converts such a track to a clean, cylindric wound that can be irrigated and loosely closed with one or two dermal sutures after instillation of antibiotic ointment within its depth.

Flaps or tissue should be minimally debrided, and the surrounding tissue to which the flap will be sutured should be slightly elevated to facilitate a dermal closure. The wound should be irrigated and closed rather loosely with 4-0 or 5-0 chromic catgut suture (or Vicryl suture if some tension exists), followed by loosely placed epidermal sutures of 6-0 polypropylene or 5-0 fast-absorbing catgut (in children). Bactroban ointment can be applied topically to the wound and used for approximately 1 week postoperatively. It may not be wise to apply a Steri-Strip to a bite wound, as it is important to observe the wound for infection and to allow a slight laxity of the wound's margins for seepage of serous fluid.

Human bites not deemed safe to close primarily may be packed open with frequent dressing changes and application of topical antimicrobials, then closed in a delayed fashion 2 to 4 days after wounding (if clean) or left to heal by secondary intention. The latter course of healing will probably require subsequent scar revision. Replacement of completely avulsed tissue is not generally productive unless the facial part is an entire ear, nose, or lip, in which case microvascular reanastomosis should be attempted if possible.

Outcomes

When the above wound care precautions are appropriately adhered to, most penetrating wounds caused by animal and human bites heal reasonably well. However, the patient and family should be prepared for a less than ideal result from the beginning and should understand that subsequent scar revision is likely to be required (Fig. 13–2). This procedure might include one or more of the following: excision of the scar and reapproximation, steroid injections, dermabrasion, laser resurfacing, and reorientation of the scar. There is some clinical evidence that the use of silicone gel or sheeting may affect the subsequent scar in a positive manner. For

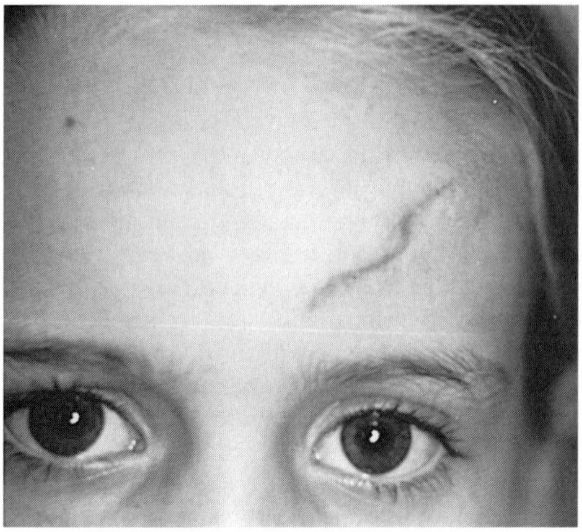

Figure 13–2. Poor cosmetic scar result after a dog bite to the forehead of a young girl. Narrowing, reorientation, and dermabrasion will be required to improve the result.

movable areas such as the lips, the gel is more practical. Scar revision is a process that may extend over several years and involve multiple procedures, and such a possibility should be explained very early in the counseling process, usually in the emergency room.

In addition to caring for the physical sequelae of an animal bite, attention must be paid to the psychologic impact of the injury on the child, particularly if it was caused by a family pet. The child may blame himself or herself, especially if the animal is euthanized, and the surgeon should be supportive and seek counseling for the family if the child becomes withdrawn or generally fearful.

LATERAL FACIAL PENETRATING INJURIES

The cheek is a common site for penetrating injuries because of its large surface area. Both penetrating and avulsive injuries may be seen, although the relative resistance of cheek tissue and the fact that it is tethered between the fixed points of the zygoma, ear, and mandible may favor a reduced risk for major avulsion. Knife wounds, gunshot wounds, and automobile accidents account for the majority of the penetrating injuries to the cheeks; animal bites are less common.

Evaluation

Penetrating wounds to the lateral face are of considerable concern because of the risk to the parotid gland, facial nerve, and facial vasculature. Fortunately, because of the thickness of the parotid gland and the superficial musculoaponeurotic system, the facial nerve is injured only in cases of very deep penetration. However, in the usual cases of knife and gunshot wounds, it is rare to not have sufficient penetration to involve at least one branch of the nerve.

Facial nerve testing is usually limited to the peripheral trunk and branches after their exit from the stylomastoid foramen (see Chapter 22 for proximal facial nerve lesions). Therefore, elicitation of voluntary motion in the conscious patient can determine which, if any, branches are involved. Electrical stimulation of the facial nerve peripherally in the emergency room is helpful, however, in unconscious or uncooperative patients.

Wound inspection before irrigation may reveal a salivary leak from the body of the gland or from the parotid duct anterior to the masseter muscle. Because the duct and the buccal branch of the facial nerve are closely aligned in their courses, both structures may be injured. Even in the presence of an intact nerve, severance of a specific facial mimetic muscle such as the zygomaticus or depressor labii inferioris, may mimic facial paralysis.

In the lateral face, just anterior to the jaw and auricle, the superficial temporal artery and internal maxillary artery can be injured. Active bleeding may be encountered, or an expanding hematoma may be present in the pterygomaxillary space. Severe epistaxis may occur as a result of injury to an internal maxillary artery, which requires an emergent arteriogram and vascular embolization or occlusion. A gunshot wound to the lateral face can also directly injure the mandible, maxilla, and internal carotid artery. If such damage is suspected by virtue of the location of the entry wound and the likely course of the penetration as well as other signs found on physical examination, the patient should undergo angiography (if stable) and a CT scan to assess osseous damage. Foreign bodies may be present deep in the wound and yet remain undetected to the examining surgeon. Radiographic evaluation can be helpful to identify such objects (Fig. 13–3).

Neurologic injuries can be present in cases of sufficient penetration and can involve the nerves of the orbit, the sympathetic chain, and even the spinal cord, nerve roots, and intracranial contents via the infratemporal fossa.[4] A cervical spine injury should be deemed present until they are ruled out by radiographic studies and the patient has been stabilized appropriately.

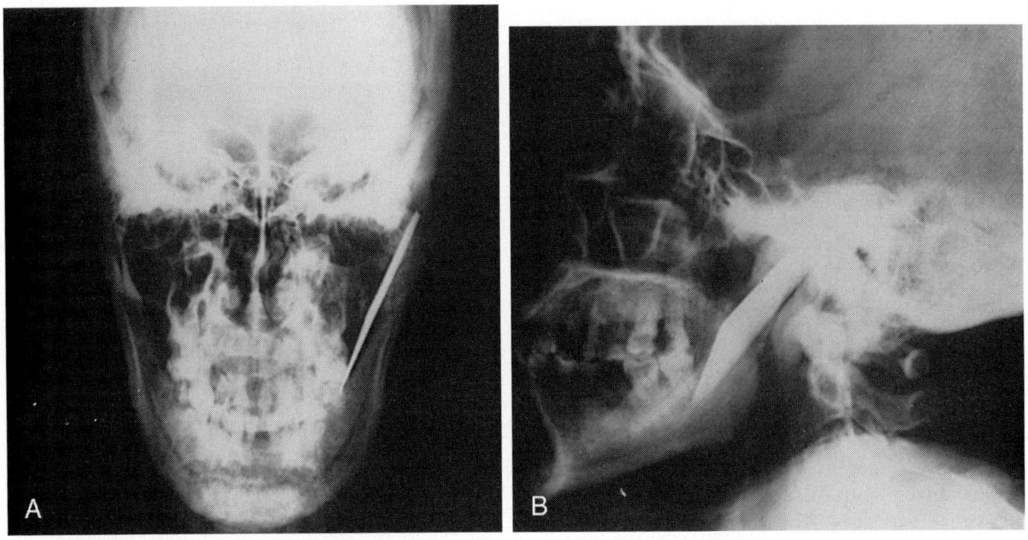

Figure 13–3. Plain facial radiographs demonstrating broken penknife blade behind left zygoma and embedded in mandible. A: Anteroposterior view. B: Lateral view.

Cranial nerves IX, X, XI, and XII can be at risk at the skull base.

Priorities

The airway becomes an issue if there is a spinal cord injury, an expanding hematoma in the lateral pharyngeal space, penetration of the brain stem, or damage to the tongue, palate, or floor of the mouth. The latter includes fractures of the mandible or maxilla by a gunshot wound. The airway should be secured with an endotracheal tube or tracheostomy, as indicated.

As mentioned above, bleeding from a vessel such as the superficial temporal or facial artery can usually be controlled by compression. It is not wise to clamp these vessels randomly in a facial wound, unless absolutely necessary, because of the risk to the facial nerve and its branches. Injury to larger vessels such as the internal maxillary or internal carotid artery or the jugular vein requires arteriography for precise diagnosis and either embolization or emergent exploration to repair or ligate the vessel.

Injury to a peripheral nerve such as the facial nerve should be explored as soon as feasible and the extent of injury should be identified. If exploration is performed within 72 hours of the injury, it is possible to utilize the nerve stimulator intraoperatively to assist in the identification of the distal branches of the severed nerve or nerves. The use of loupe magnification (×4.0 to 4.5) or the operating microscope is essential in identifying the nerve endings in the traumatized tissues and in facilitating the repair of the nerve. It is unusual to be able to perform a primary anastomosis of a nerve severed by a traumatic penetration, as it is necessary to trim the ends of the cut nerve sharply in order to obtain undamaged neural bundles for repair. Thus, a cable or interposition graft is required. This graft can be obtained from a sensory nerve such as the greater auricular nerve or, if that is not available due to the trauma, from the sural nerve. Unfortunately, these nerves are not similar to the facial nerve and its branches in cross-sectional diameter, so one or more fascicles must be stripped from the donor nerve and sutured into position. No tension should be placed on the interposed graft. The nerve should not be too long, or the reaxonization will be delayed. An epineural closure should be performed using 8-0 or 9-0 nylon sutures, or if a single fascicle is used, only a few fine nylon sutures at the periphery are needed. The wound should be copiously irrigated again after closure to reduce the risk of local infection and inflammation in response to foreign materials or nonviable tissue.

It is usually necessary to perform a superficial parotidectomy to expose the proximal branches or trunk of the facial nerve. If the gland has been penetrated, it is wise to also debride the gland by using the parotidectomy method. The deep lobe of the parotid can usually be left intact, as it is not a likely source of leakage of saliva. If, however, the parotid duct has been severed, the surgeon has the choice of repairing the duct or removing the gland. In most cases, it is possible to perform a ductal anastomosis using 6-0 or 7-0 nylon sutures and loupe magnification. It may be necessary to cannulate the duct through Stensen's orifice, as one can perform the anastomosis circumferentially, taking care not to suture the duct closed (Fig. 13–4). Postoperatively, the wound should be compressed to reduce the stasis of saliva and the patient should consume a bland diet for 7 to 10 days.

All obviously devitalized soft tissue should be debrided, as should any suspicious, marginally vital tissue, which might include muscle—the masseter muscle and the facial muscles. The edges of the wound should also be sharply debrided, and the wound closed in layers. If a large dead space exists or if an avulsed flap has been replaced, it may be necessary to place a small drain, either suction or nonsuction. If the duct or parotid gland has been injured or removed, a suction drain may be preferred, although it is not required (Figs. 13–5 and 13–6).

If osseous trauma is present, the bone should be debrided, occlusion obtained, and internal stabilization plates applied. The care of facial fractures is beyond the scope of this chapter, but let it suffice to say that even if the wound appears to be contaminated, small plates and mandibular-maxillary fixation can still be utilized in conjunction with wound drainage, high-dose parenteral antibiotics, and copious wound irrigation.

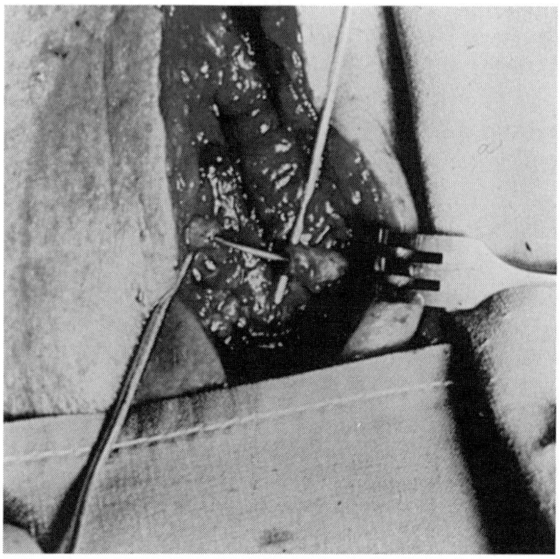

Figure 13–4. Complete severance of the right parotid duct (midportion) caused by a knife wound. The duct is cannulated via Stensen's orifice prior to reanastomosis.

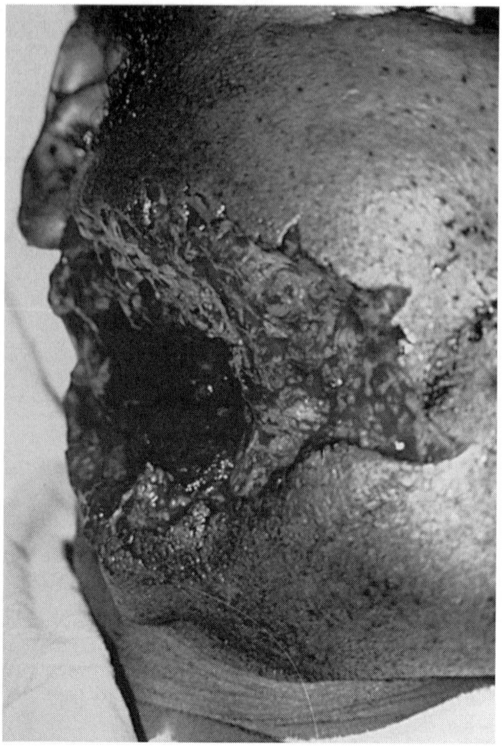

Figure 13–5. A high-velocity (military) gunshot wound to the right cheek, involving soft tissue, the masseter muscle, and the parotid gland.

Outcomes

Primary anastomosis of a facial nerve disruption should lead to recovery within 12 months. If an interposition graft is used, the length of time to potential recovery varies directly with the length of the graft and how far distally the injury is located. The longer the graft, the more likely it is that recovery time might approach 24 months; a distal injury is more likely to recover in half that time. If a long recovery time is anticipated, static rehabilitation of the face should be considered in the interim, including a gold weight on the upper eyelid, canthoplasty (in an older individual), and suspension of the nasal ala and oral commissure with Alloderm or Gore-Tex. These measures provide a pleasant appearance in repose, yet should not interfere with the chance of later motion. If recovery does not occur or is incomplete, then one has a viable static support in place. The use of transcutaneous electrical stimulation of the facial musculature in order to maintain bulk and prevent atrophy has been advocated. There is no apparent contraindication to this, and the patient may feel comfortable performing some self-assistance at home.

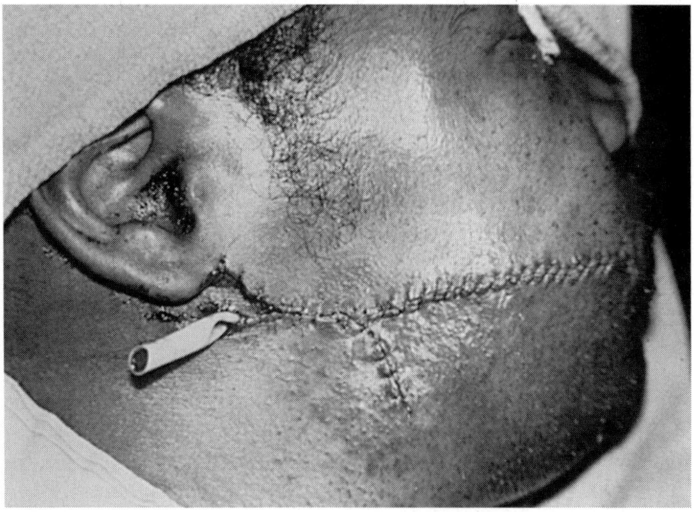

Figure 13–6. The wound shown in Figure 13–5 after debridement of the muscle and soft tissue, including superficial parotidectomy and closure under minimal tension.

If reanastomosis of the parotid duct is not successful, the duct will stenose and the gland will become engorged and inflamed. Treatment with antibiotics, massage, heat, and sialogogues may help with acute obstruction, but the gland will atrophy or will require secondary parotidectomy. Because of the protracted course of parotid inflammation after stenosis of the duct, the surgeon may elect to perform a primary parotidectomy at the time of exploration and repair of the wound so as to avoid that complication.[5]

Postrepair infections of the face are uncommon after traumatic injury repair, owing primarily to the excellent blood supply available. However, other deterrents to infection include copious irrigation in the emergency department and operating room, judicious debridement of devitalized tissue, wound drainage, if indicated, and perioperative antibiotics that continue for 7 to 10 days after repair, depending upon the extent of the tissue damage. Hypertrophic scarring is more likely to occur with traumatic injuries and can be lessened by applying silicone gel twice a day for up to 2 months after initial wound healing. If persistent cosmetic problems ensue, scars on the cheek resulting from avulsions or puncture injuries can usually be managed by reorienting the scar into the lines of relaxed skin tension, breaking up the scar with geometric, broken line closures, and dermabrasion. Makeup camouflage is also quite helpful.

MIDFACE PENETRATING INJURIES

Penetrating injuries of the midface present with bleeding, edema, difficulty with speech, and airway and muscle injury. In this area, the lips, the nose, and the periorbital structures are the main structures of concern (see Chapter 25 for a discussion of periorbital injuries). Because the lips are mobile, they are subject to stretch and avulsion injuries. Penetrations may affect the teeth, the attached gingiva, and the oral cavity. Nasal injuries occur because of the projecting position of the nose on the face, making it the first contact structure in most full-face wounding episodes.

Evaluation

Bleeding and hematoma are the main concerns in a nasal evaluation. Anterior epistaxis usually occurs as a result of trauma to the soft tissues of the nasal tip, alae, and columella, but posterior bleeding is more dangerous and may signal an injury to the greater palatine or sphenopalatine artery. Inspection after suctioning, using either a head mirror and nasal speculum or a nasal endoscope, usually identifies the source of the injury. Septal hematoma is an emergent condition and must be identified. The source of significant bleeding may best be identified by means of carotid angiography, in a stable patient. If the nasal cartilages are avulsed or separated, they require surgical reapproximation. Also at risk for damage from penetrating wounds to the nose and nasal cavity are the palate, nasopharynx, paranasal sinuses, cribriform plate, and intracranial contents. A cerebrospinal fluid leak can be identified by means of a crude filter paper test or by chemical analysis of clear drainage from the nose.

Evaluation of the lips should identify

whether the penetration involves the labial mucosa. If the penetration is close to the vermilion border, the labial artery might have been severed. The status of the orbicularis oris muscle must be ascertained, for, if separated in continuity, a deficit of closure will result. Deep penetrations may avulse teeth or implant them in the surrounding soft tissues; all teeth must be accounted for. Soft tissue wounds may be associated with alveolar or segmental fractures of the dental arches. If the tongue and floor of the mouth are involved through edema, hematoma, or laceration, the airway must be secured. Gunshot wounds are more likely to result in airway compromise than any other cause of penetrating injury.

Neural injury to the infraorbital, mental, or supraorbital nerve should be identified by pinprick tests in the areas of their distribution. These nerves may be directly injured by being penetrated and severed, may be rendered neuropraxic because of edema, or may be involved in a fracture site. CT scans confirm the form of injury.

Priorities

The airway must first be controlled if it is at risk. This may require something simple such as an oral airway or placement of a retraction suture for the tongue. If severe obstruction exists, nasal intubation, cricothyroidotomy, or tracheostomy should be performed in the emergency department to secure the airway before any other diagnostic or therapeutic procedures are performed.

Nasal bleeding requires urgent packing with either Telfa pads or Merocel sponges soaked with Otrivin and topical thrombin, or the insertion of nasal tamponading balloons. If a cerebrospinal fluid leak is suspected, the nasal packing is used only as a temporizing measure to control the bleeding until the patient can be taken to the operating room for vessel ligation or to the angiography suite for embolization. For operative control of significant intranasal bleeding, the location of the bleeding, as identified by nasal cavity endoscopy, guides the surgical approach. If the bleeding is in the inferior nasal cavity, the internal maxillary artery can be ligated through a transantral approach, using fine metallic ligature clips. The greater palatine artery can be injected via the foramen in the oral cavity for temporary control of bleeding until the internal maxillary artery can be ligated. If the bleeding is found to be located high in the nasal cavity, an external ethmoidectomy approach can be used; both the anterior and posterior ethmoid arteries are identified and clipped or cauterized with bipolar cautery bayonet forceps. The anterior ethmoid artery must be divided after ligation or cautery in order to approach the posterior ethmoid artery. The posterior ethmoid artery need not be divided after ligature or cautery.

If the alar cartilages have been split or avulsed, the cartilage should be minimally debrided and sutured into proper anatomic position using 4-0 chromic catgut. Puncture wounds of the nose generally heal well with only minimal debridement and loose closure. For through-and-through nasal punctures, only one surface, usually the skin surface, should be closed. Special care must be taken to carefully reapproximate the alar margin (rim) if it is severed, as any slight malalignment will be noticeable. The skin wounds may be closed with 6-0 polypropylene sutures.

Management of lacerations of the lip is determined by the depth of penetration. If the lip is only partially involved, dermal and skin closure are sufficient. If the muscle has been penetrated, it should be reapproximated with either 4-0 chromic catgut or 4-0 Vicryl suture, taking care to close its entire dehiscence so that a continuity defect does not occur. If the penetration is full thickness, the inner mucosal layer should be only loosely closed with buried 4-0 chromic gut sutures, so that saliva does not become entrapped, allowing an infection to ensue. Special care should be taken to reapproximate the vermilion-skin borders; loupe magnification can be quite helpful to guide the reapproximation. The vermilion border can be sutured with 6-0 silk, as the suture tails lie down gently on the vermilion surface and are not irritating to the patient's tongue.

Dental avulsions should be cleaned, replaced, and maintained in position through fixation using arch bars or interdental wiring. Alveolar fractures are also treated with interdental wiring and mandibular-maxillary fixation, often in conjunction with plastic splints to maintain the proper occlusal plane of the teeth. Avulsed attached gingiva can be reconnected with 4-0 chromic catgut. Slowly absorbed suture material such as Vicryl can certainly be utilized on the mucosa but with the understanding that it will take a longer time than chromic gut to leave the surface.

Injury to the paranasal sinuses should be treated by performing open or endoscopic exploration and removing blood clots, damaged mucosa, and devitalized bone. Enlarging the sinus ostium is important so that blood can properly and easily flow from the cavity. Packing can be used but is usually not necessary, given a widely patent ostium. Deeper penetrations into the nasopharynx may involve the anterior cervical spine or cranial cavity and thus require consultation with the neurosurgery service. CT scans are required to adequately identify the extent and depth of the penetration and the resultant injury.

Outcomes

Fortunately, penetrating wounds of the nose and nasal cavity are unusual, and with expedient control of bleeding and management of complicating factors such as hematoma or nasopharyngeal penetration, the results are generally good. Unless the penetration has involved the cranial nerves at the base of the skull, neurologic sequelae are rare. Leakages of cerebrospinal fluid are generally self-sealing, although some require repair by endoscopic nasal techniques or, more rarely, by intracranial dural patching. If cranial nerve I has been injured, the olfactory sense may not return.

Nostril stenosis is perhaps the most common complication of penetrating nasal trauma, and it may require widening of the vestibule by Z-plasty or composite grafting from the auricle. Dilations, injections of steroids, and soft nostril stents can be helpful. If the nasal valve region has been damaged, internal stenting with onlay cartilage grafting usually works well.

If sutured properly, lip penetrations heal well and the sphincter effect of the oral stoma can be maintained. If the oral commissure has been blunted, a commissuroplasty using intraoral mucosa can be performed. Notching of the lip (the "whistle deformity") because of incomplete closure of the orbicularis oris muscle can be rehabilitated by excision of the deformity and proper reapproximation of the muscle. If the vermilion border is malaligned, it must be revised and aligned as closely as possible.

SUMMARY

Penetrating injuries of the face may involve many vital functional structures as well as causing cosmetic deformities. Threats to the airway and vascular system should be dealt with emergently, followed by an accurate assessment of the extent of the damage. It is often difficult to identify the damage deep to a traumatic penetration, so the physical examination and diagnostic studies assume primary importance. Animal and human bites require particular care, including copious irrigation, debridement of devitalized tissue, and utilization of perioperative antibiotics. Concerns about virus transmission by bites must be substantiated and early precautions and treatment options exercised.

Penetrating injuries to the face require meticulous repair of neural, vascular, and muscular structures and fine plastic closure of the soft tissue wounds. Psychosocial and emotional support must also be given, as these wounds often cause significant cosmetic and functional deformities. Scar revision and functional rehabilitation may require long-term care and multiple procedures, and the patient and family should understand this possibility as early as possible in the course of the care.

REFERENCES

1. Schultz RC. Animal bites. In Facial Injuries, 3rd ed. Chicago, Year Book Medical, 1988, pp. 207–227.
2. Mutabagani KH et al. Penetrating neck trauma in children: a reappraisal. J Pediatr 1995;30:341–344.
3. Angeras MH et al. Comparison between sterile saline and tap water for the cleaning of acute traumatic soft tissue wounds. Eur J Surg 1992;158:347–350.
4. Kornblut RM, Spetka LM, Heffner DK. Penetrating injuries involving the anterior cranial fossa. Arch Otorhinolaryngol 1989;246:411–416.
5. Lewis G, Knottenbelt JD. Parotid duct injury: is immediate surgical repair necessary? Injury 1991;22:407–409.

CHAPTER 14

Emergencies in Facial Cosmetic Surgery

Stephanie A. Joe, MD, and
John L. Frodel Jr., MD

Emergencies after facial cosmetic procedures are quite rare but when they occur, they can be devastating. This is particularly true in light of the fact that essentially all of these procedures are elective in nature and the tenet "do no harm" is always of paramount importance.

This chapter is organized around procedures in facial cosmetic surgery for which incidences of postsurgical emergencies have been reported. The procedures that are addressed include rhinoplasty, blepharoplasty, rhytidectomy, otoplasty, and skin resurfacing. Most of the emergent complications that occur are associated with bleeding and hematoma formation. Delayed complications are a separate issue and are not discussed here. An additional section addresses surgical fires as they pertain to facial cosmetic procedures.

RHINOPLASTY

Emergencies in rhinoplasty, including both isolated rhinoplasty and combination septorhinoplasty, can be divided into two groups: those that occur intraoperatively and those that occur in the immediate postoperative period. Intraoperative emergencies are extremely rare and are limited to the unusual occurrence of uncontrollable epistaxis. In both circumstances, prevention is the key. Preoperative discussion and examination should elicit any history of bleeding diathesis or potential intraoperative bleeding problems.[1]

Although rarely reported, infection after cosmetic nasal surgery must be considered a potential problem. Toxic shock syndrome is the one emergent and life-threatening infection associated with nasal procedures that is mentioned with any regularity in the literature.

Bleeding or Hematoma

PRESENTATION AND EVALUATION

Regardless of the findings during preoperative evaluation, bleeding can occur in any patient. Inadvertent entry into a paranasal vessel, particularly one that is anomalous, can lead to significant intraoperative bleeding. Familiarity with the maneuvers that are associated with hemorrhage is crucial to appropriate management of such problems. Bleeding of a moderate nature is not uncommon during the performance of osteotomies, but it is during this maneuver that the most vigorous bleeding commonly occurs.

PRIORITIES

Generally, nasal bleeding during rhinoplasty can be managed by direct digital pressure for several minutes over the outside of the nose. However, persistent bleeding may require nasal packing. Nasal packing should be approached in a systematic fashion in order to avoid intranasal mucosal injuries, possible septal perforation, and subsequent nasal collapse as a result of overaggressive packing. Early postoperative bleeding is treated similarly.

Septal hematoma may occur in any patient who has had septal surgery. Diagnosis of this process can be challenging, as significant swelling usually occurs in the immediate postoperative period. If septal hematoma is suspected, previous septal incisions should be opened or a limited new incision created through the mucoperichondrial envelope to search for a hematoma.[1] Development of such a hematoma can generally be prevented by the placement of silicone splints sutured to one another through the septum or by the use of an absorbable quilting suture. Hematomas can still occur despite these preventive measures. The surgeon should be aware of this potential problem and treat it emergently if it is suspected.

OUTCOMES

The incidence of hematoma is quite low, but a patient who does develop a septal hematoma can potentially go on to develop a septal perforation, loss of cartilage, and eventual nasal collapse.[2]

Toxic Shock Syndrome

PRESENTATION AND EVALUATION

The occurrence of toxic shock syndrome after nasal surgery is unpredictable. There are no predisposing factors discernible from a patient's medical history or cost-effective preoperative laboratory studies to indicate (1) colonization by toxic shock syndrome's toxin-1–producing *Staphylococcus aureus* or (2) a patient's susceptibility to this toxin. In many cases, *S. aureus* is not even cultured. Use of prophylactic antibiotics does not ensure the impossibility of developing such an infection.[3]

Toxic shock syndrome is generally considered a rare infection. It has been linked to staphylococcal toxins that may be harbored intranasally and that proliferate in gauze packing. Its occurrence has also been linked to the use of nasal splints.[4] Prevention includes prompt removal of any packing within 24 hours postoperatively and prescription of prophylactic antibiotics. Onset is heralded by symptoms that include fever, hypotension, nausea, vomiting, rash, and diarrhea. Often, this progresses to multisystem involvement, including acute renal failure, leukocytosis, and thrombocytopenia.[2–4] Any patient with nasal packing who develops any of these symptoms should immediately be suspected of having developed toxic shock syndrome. Interestingly, the surgical site does not typically appear to be infected.

PRIORITIES

With the onset of the above symptoms, the patient is transferred to an intensive care unit. Hemodynamic stabilization and supportive care are instituted. Nasal packing is immediately removed and aggressive intravenous fluid replacement is initiated. Cultures are taken of the nose and blood to examine for the presence of *S. aureus.* If they are positive, the culture is then tested for toxic shock syndrome toxin-1. Intravenous antibiotic coverage for *Staphylococcus* species is begun. Good choices include penicillin, nafcillin, or a first-generation cephalosporin.

OUTCOMES

A patient who develops toxic shock syndrome has a prolonged hospital stay, its length determined by the rate of recovery from the acute onset. Many develop desquamation of the palms and soles during the recovery phase. Poorly responding and unresponsive cases can result in permanent organ damage or death.[3]

OPEN AGING-FACE PROCEDURES

Open aging-face procedures include principally blepharoplasty, rhytidectomy, brow lifts, and lipectomy (liposuction or open lipectomy). Although considered by some surgeons to be common, no other complication is more emergent or serious than hematoma. Its formation following either a traditional coronal brow lift or an endoscopic brow lift does not constitute an emergency, although drainage is generally recommended. With rhytidectomy or blepharoplasty, more serious complications such as skin necrosis or vision loss may occur as a result of hematoma formation.

Blepharoplasty

Complications of the blepharoplasty procedure are mentioned because of their association with vision loss. Hematoma formation and globe injury must be treated emergently to prevent eventual visual compromise.

Hematoma following blepharoplasty is, fortunately, quite unusual, but it carries with it the risk of visual loss and even blindness due to blood collection within the retrobulbar space. Fastidious hemostasis during dissection aids in preventing this complication. Thus, particular care should be taken during the dissection and removal of herniated fat from the upper or lower lid compartments.[5] Because the temporary vasoconstrictive effect of epinephrine can mask bleeding sites and lead to delayed hematoma formation, its use during blepharoplasty is sometimes avoided altogether.

Numerous cases in the literature report blindness following blepharoplasty, but it remains extremely rare.[5] Retrobulbar hemorrhage is considered the most common cause of elevated intraocular and intraorbital pressures leading to vision loss. Theoretically, acute pressure elevations are transmitted throughout the orbit, leading to optic nerve ischemia and central retinal artery compromise. Other potential sources of elevated pressures are exacerbation of acute-angle glaucoma, tight pressure dressings, and traction on periorbital fat.[5, 6]

Globe injury caused by inadvertent injection of local anesthesia and manipulation during surgery is also very rare. Transient mydriasis or ophthalmoplegia can result from the parasympathetic effects of the anesthetic. If significant volumes of it are injected, signs and symptoms similar to those seen in retrobulbar hematoma may result.[6] The treatment approach should be the same as for hematoma.

PRESENTATION AND EVALUATION

The preoperative interview should focus on any history of ophthalmologic problems and should also elicit any suspicion of potential operative or postoperative problems such as hypertension or bleeding disorders. Valsalva maneuvers are to be avoided postoperatively. In general, detection of visual compromise requires a high index of suspicion and close monitoring for complications.

An intraorbital hematoma manifests itself in acute onset of periorbital ecchymosis and edema. Pain, visual acuity changes, proptosis, chemosis, miosis, and ophthalmoplegia are present in a severe case. In addition, an afferent pupillary defect and optic disk changes can be found on fundoscopic examination.[5, 6] Most commonly, instances of vision loss occur within the first few hours postoperatively. This is a clinical diagnosis. No laboratory or radiographic studies are warranted. In fact, such studies may delay proper treatment and result in blindness.

PRIORITIES

Orbital hematoma is an emergency that requires immediate treatment. If it is suspected, all incisions should be immediately opened to decompress the wound. Bleeding vessels are controlled and cauterized under sterile conditions. If visual compromise occurs or progresses, lateral canthotomy and inferior cantholysis should be performed to further decompress the orbit.[5] These maneuvers help to alleviate the compressive effects of an expanding hematoma on the confined space of the skeletal orbit and eyelids.

In addition to the measures outlined, emergent ophthalmologic consultation is requested for full examination and pressure measurements. Intravenous diuretics and steroids are often administered to decrease intraocular pressures. One regimen is mannitol 20%, 12.5 g over 3 to 5 min; Diamox, 500 mg; and Decadron 10 mg, given as a slow intravenous push.[6]

OUTCOMES

The incidence of blindness has been reported to be 0.04%. Long-term sequelae of small hematomas can result in eyelid malposition. The inflammatory response incited during the resolution phase of an untreated hematoma can cause scarring and increase the incidence of such a problem.[6] As in all emergencies after cosmetic procedures, the final result is sacrificed. If desired, it can be addressed at a later date, long after the immediate issues have resolved.

Rhytidectomy

Branches of the superficial temporal artery are often the source of hematoma following rhytidectomy.[7] In the case of hematoma under the facelift skin flap, it is important to recognize the potentially compromised blood supply that exists in the periauricular regions. Pressure caused by an underlying hematoma as well as by biochemical breakdown products that further compromise flap vascularity may lead to further vascular compromise around the incisions and to eventual skin necrosis.[8, 9] This problem is best prevented by using careful hemostasis techniques during dissection and prior to flap closure. Some surgeons feel that the rate of hematoma formation is decreased by the use of closed suction drains under these flaps. However, the most popular form of hematoma prevention is the use of pressure dressings. Seromas are also known to occur within the same time period. These are addressed in the same manner as hematomas.[7]

Liposuction emergencies are anecdotally reported but can occur with overzealous subcutaneous cannulation in the neck region. Improper placement of the liposuction cannula in the subplatysmal plane could subject branches of the jugular chain and carotid system to injury. If such an injury occurs intraoperatively, compression should be applied to the neck. If bleeding has not stopped, the neck should be surgically explored and the bleeding vessel or vessels controlled. Hematoma formation that occurs after liposuction is treated similarly to that which occurs after rhytidectomy.

PRESENTATION AND EVALUATION

Significant hematomas usually present within the first 24 to 48 hours after surgery. Diagnosis is based on the physical examination findings of excessive facial swelling and facial ecchymosis. The patient usually complains of pain out of proportion to that expected to be experienced as a result of the surgical procedure (Fig. 14–1).

A patient with a history of hypertension, bleeding diathesis, or straining during the postoperative period is at risk.[9] Males have a greater blood supply in their thicker, more sebaceous skin and beard area. The use of longer flap techniques and male gender have also been associated with increased incidence of this complication.[10]

PRIORITIES

If a patient with a large bulky dressing complains of significant pain in the first 48 hours postoperatively, the dressing should be removed immediately and the surgical sites inspected for evidence of hematoma. With any suspicion of hematoma, the surgical incision should be opened in a controlled fashion, the wound copiously irrigated, and hemostasis obtained. This is best achieved in the operating room under general anesthesia. In a patient with persistent generalized wound bleeding, both a closed section drain and a pressure dressing should be applied, with frequent changes, until there is no further evidence of bleeding. Prophylactic antibiotics should be continued.

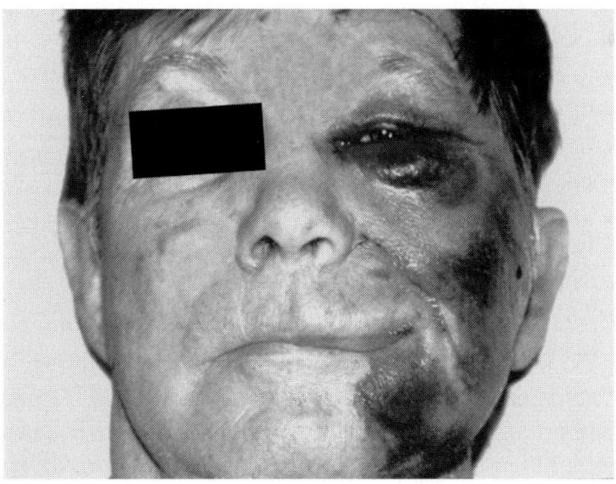

Figure 14–1. A patient who developed a hematoma after rhytidectomy. Note the swelling and significant ecchymoses.

OUTCOMES

Pressure on the flap caused by a hematoma can lead to necrosis of the flap and its eventual loss. Aside from the immediate concerns of tissue and flap loss, an untreated hematoma can incite an inflammatory response and eventually lead to infection. As a result, significant scarring and soft tissue irregularities may occur.[10] However, in the majority of cases, the long-term effects of such complications are rarely noticeable.[9] To minimize such complications, a patient is instructed about attention to wound care, local massage, avoidance of sun exposure, and the liberal use of sunscreens.

OTOPLASTY

The incidence of hematoma formation after otoplasty (cosmetic ear surgery) is 1% to 3%.[11] As in nasal septal surgery, hematomas around ear cartilage require prompt recognition and treatment. Infection in an auricular hematoma can cause necrosis not only of auricular cartilage but also of the overlying skin, and thus lead to significant scar deformity. An auricular hematoma interrupts the blood supply to the cartilage and causes necrosis of the cartilage. This, in turn, may lead to significant ear deformity or "cauliflower ear," which is extremely difficult to correct.

Infection can also cause loss of soft tissue and cartilage. Evident within the first postoperative week, skin contamination and infection can spread to the perichondrium and then to the cartilage. Rarely, suppurative chondritis occurs.

Presentation and Evaluation

Accordingly, in a patient who has undergone otoplasty, if excessive pain is noted in the early postoperative period, ear dressings should be removed and the ear and wound carefully examined. A hematoma is heralded by significant ecchymosis and edema. The detection is by clinical examination, and no other studies are necessary unless preoperative inquiry indicates a bleeding disorder.

Priorities

The postauricular incision should be opened and the wound examined. Any hematoma is evacuated. As in the treatment of hematomas found after other procedures outlined here, hemostasis is best achieved under general anesthesia. The wound is then thoroughly irrigated prior to closure. At completion of the procedure, a pressure dressing is reapplied. The bandage is removed the following day and the site again inspected for hematoma formation. Prophylactic antibiotics are continued to prevent the development of infection.

Any evidence of infection mandates empiric coverage with intravenous antibiotics. *Staphylococcus* and *Streptococcus* species are the common causative organisms. If symptoms persist, coverage for *Pseudomonas* species must be considered. Any abscess is to be cultured, drained, and irrigated.[11]

Outcomes

If left undrained or if too much time passes before it is detected, pressure necrosis results in scar formation and auricular deformity, the so-called "cauliflower ear."

SKIN RESURFACING

Skin resurfacing in a patient with an aging face can be performed using either chemical peels or laser ablative techniques. Chemical peels can be divided into three types—light, medium, and deep peels. The agents used in the first two categories are fairly safe in nature, and although complications can occur with any agent, true emergencies are rare. However, deep-peel agents containing phenol do carry with them a small risk of cardiac toxicity.[12, 13] Phenol is being used less frequently since the introduction of laser resurfacing techniques, but problems involving the use of phenol are important to understand.

When absorbed in large quantities, phenol is a potential toxin that can affect a variety of organ systems. A patient with a history of cardiac, renal, hepatic, or neural disorders should be thoroughly evaluated and apprised of the possibility of toxicity.[12, 13] All peeling agents are applied topically, so the risk of systemic absorption and subsequent problems is small. Cardiac toxicity is the one true emergency associated with phenol-containing peeling agents.

Emergent injuries related to laser use in skin resurfacing are limited to ocular injuries and fire.

Chemical Peels

CARDIAC TOXICITY

Presentation and Evaluation. Cardiac toxicity caused by phenol use can manifest as various forms of arrhythmias, including paroxysmal atrial contractions, premature ventricular contractions, and bigeminy. This is most likely to occur when too much agent is applied, particularly relative to the speed with which the face is peeled when a phenol-based agent is used. To avoid absorption of large volumes of phenol, a full-face peel should be performed gradually over an hour or longer. Also, sequential treatment of facial subunits limits skin exposure and systemic absorption. In this way, the agent is absorbed more slowly and has less risk of cardiac toxicity. Phenol is excreted slowly by the kidney, and intravenous fluids should be administered during the procedure.[12, 13]

Priorities. If cardiac toxicity does occur, the arrhythmia should be treated with standard resuscitative and pharmacologic intervention. The existing peel agent is removed with a combination of water and soap. Under no circumstances should any alcohol-based fluid be applied, as it will lead to increased absorption of the phenol-based agent.[12]

OCULAR INJURY

The other potential emergency that can occur with the use of peeling agents is entry of the agent into the eye region, which can cause chemical injury to the cornea.

Presentation, Evaluation, and Priorities. The chemical peeling procedure is done with the patient awake and, therefore, complaints can immediately be addressed. If the peeling agent enters the eye, the agent should be neutralized immediately by irrigating the eye copiously with saline. This is followed by placement of a lubricating ophthalmic ointment. Ophthalmologic consultation should be immediately obtained if a chemical burn of the eye is suspected.

Outcomes. The popularity of phenol peels has waned in the past several years with increasing use of lasers for skin resurfacing. Thus, these complications are quite rare.

Laser Resurfacing

Currently, the most popular type of laser for skin surface ablation is the CO_2 laser. One of the principal reasons for its popularity is the safety of the machine and the ease with which it is controlled. Other than the potential risk that this device could act as an igniter and cause combustion and subsequent fire, the emergencies that exist with this apparatus are limited to potential corneal injury because of an unprotected eye.

EVALUATION AND PRESENTATION

Training of all personnel in laser safety must predate the planned procedure. Intraoperatively, everyone involved with the case wears protective goggles, and the patient wears approved corneal protectors.[14] In general, local anesthesia and intravenous sedation can be used for laser resurfacing procedures, so ocular injury can be immediately signaled by the patient.

PRIORITIES

If injury to the cornea occurs, all laser work is terminated. Emergent ophthalmologic consultation is called upon for complete evaluation of any corneal or retinal injury. Antibiotic lubricating ophthalmic ointment is applied to treat a corneal injury. Further recommendations provided by the consultants are followed.

OUTCOME

Reports of emergent complications resulting from laser resurfacing are rare and sporadic (see also Chapter 25 for a discussion of corneal injury).

INTRAOPERATIVE SURGICAL FIRES

Although infrequent, fires during facial cosmetic and minor reconstructive surgeries do occur. The usual situation in which a fire occurs is in the setting of a surgical procedure being performed in the facial region under intravenous sedation. Numerous intraoperative fires in this situation have now been reported, some with devastating results. The common denominator in all such fires is the use of oxygen that is delivered through an open system to the nasal or mouth region during surgery under intravenous sedation. The three elements necessary for any fire include the following: (1) a fuel source (flammable skin preparation solution, dry gauze sponges, surgical drapes); (2) a source of ignition (electrocautery is the most common source, although lasers can also cause ignition); and (3) an oxidizer, which is almost always oxygen.[14–16] The first two of these elements are consistently present during these procedures. However, controversy remains as to the necessity of supplemental oxygen, particularly when delivered through an open source such as a cannula in the nose or mouth.

Presentation, Evaluation, and Priorities

Fires are immediately obvious—flames flare up, the surgical drapes catch fire, the patient signals pain or burning sensations. Prevention is always the key, and open communication with the anesthesiologist prior to any incision is absolutely essential. It is now quite clear that some patients do not require supplemental oxygen.[15] Accordingly, oxygen should be administered only when necessary during these procedures. Pulse oximetry is recommended to monitor patient oxygenation throughout the procedure. If oxygen delivery is essential, it should be turned off whenever electrocautery is being utilized, and a delay should be allowed for clearance of oxygen from the facial region and from under the surgical drapes immediately around the patient. It is important to understand that oxygen, which is denser than air, can collect under the drapes.[14]

If an intraoperative fire does occur, the source of ignition, usually oxygen, should be immediately turned off. Ignited materials such as gauze and drapes are immediately removed from the patient and the fire is extinguished. The patient is evaluated and treated for any burns that may have occurred. Small, manageable fires turn into life-threatening fires within seconds, and effective communication among all operating room personnel is essential to prevent disastrous results.[14, 15]

Outcomes

In many instances, injuries are limited to superficial burns that heal without sequelae after routine wound care. However, severe injuries continue to be reported sporadically (see also Chapter 7 for thermal injuries).

REFERENCES

1. Holt GR, Garner ET, McLarey D. Postoperative sequelae and complications of rhinoplasty. Otolaryngol Clin North Am 1987;20:853–876.
2. Hoffman JF, Cook TA. Complications of rhinoplasty. In Eisele DW, ed. Complications in Head and Neck Surgery. St. Louis, Mosby, 1993, pp. 471–480.
3. Jacobson JA, Kasworm EM. Toxic shock syndrome after nasal surgery. Arch Otolaryngol Head Neck Surg 1986;112:329–332.
4. Wagner R, Toback JM. Toxic shock syndrome following septoplasty using nasal splints. Laryngoscope 1986;96: 609–610.
5. Heinze JB, Hueston JF. Blindness after blepharoplasty: mechanism and early reversal. Plast Reconstr Surg 1978; 61:347–351.
6. Adamson PA, Constatinides MS. Complications of blepharoplasty. Facial Plast Surg Clin North Am 1995;3: 211–221.
7. Perkins SW et al. Prevention of seromas and hematomas after face-lift surgery with the use of postoperative vacuum drains. Arch Otolaryngol 1997;123:743–745.
8. Mulliken J. Pathogenesis of skin flap necrosis from an underlying hematoma. Plast Reconstr Surg 1979; 63:540–545.
9. Thompson DS, Ashley FL. Facelift complications: a study of 922 cases performed in a 6-year period. Plast Reconstr Surg 1993;51:417–420.
10. Adamson PA, Moran ML. Complications of cervicofacial rhytidectomy. Facial Plast Surg Clin North Am 1993;1:257–271.
11. Cheney ML, Rounds M. Otoplasty. Facial Plast Surg Clin North Am 1997;5:319–327.
12. Brody HJ. Complications of chemical peels. In Brody HJ, ed. Chemical Peeling. St. Louis, Mosby, 1992, pp. 121–145.
13. Mandy SH, Landsman L. Dermabrasion and chemical peel. In Papel ID, Nachlas NE, eds. Facial Plastic and Reconstructive Surgery. St. Louis, Mosby, 1991, pp. 198–207.
14. Ries WR, Aly A, Nachlas NE. Lasers in facial plastic surgery. In Papel ID, Nachlas NE, eds. Facial Plastic and Reconstructive Surgery. St. Louis, Mosby, 1991, pp. 312–322.
15. de Richemond AL, Bruley ME. Head and neck surgical fires. In Eisele DW, ed. Complications in Head and Neck Surgery. St. Louis, Mosby, 1993, pp. 312–322.
16. Brechtelbauer PB, Carroll WB, Baker S. Intraoperative fire with electrocautery. Otolaryngol Head Neck Surg 1996;114:328–331.
17. Chang, BW, Petty P, Manson PN. Patient fire safety in the operating room. Plast Reconstr Surg 1994;93:519–521.

CHAPTER 15

Flap Emergencies

Mark T. Brown, MD

FREE-TISSUE TRANSFER EMERGENCIES

Microvascular techniques have dramatically changed head and neck recontructive surgery, providing the reconstructive surgeon with fasciocutaneous, myocutaneous, and composite tissue options otherwise unavailable. Microvascular reliability rivals traditional methods of reconstruction. In reports from experienced centers, survival rates after surgery involving free flaps in the head and neck range from 93.5% to 95.5%.[1, 2]

Acute emergencies in microvascular surgery are typically related to arterial or venous insufficiency. Surgical technique and, to a lesser extent, pharmacologic interventions have had a significant impact on success rates, but intense and consistent postoperative monitoring of flaps is equally important. Early detection of vascular compromise and immediate return to the operating room are the keys to successful intervention.

Prevention of Flap Emergencies

Anyone who has undergone a free-tissue transfer is at risk for flap loss. There are no series that report 100% success. Therefore, every patient must understand the finite possibility of an unsuccessful outcome. It is my observation that patients previously treated with a combination of radiation and chemotherapy are at significantly increased risk for failure as opposed to patients treated with radiation alone and those who have had no prior therapy.[3] Previous therapies are therefore taken into account during preoperative counseling.

INTRAOPERATIVE STRATEGIES

Prevention of vascular compromise begins in the operating room. The purpose of every maneuver is to provide optimal vascular flow for the flap. Proper and exact suturing technique is fundamental to every microvascular effort. Tightly tied or bunched sutures cause irregularity in the suture line and damage to the endothelium, which can initiate the clotting cascade, platelet activation, and thrombus.[4] Appropriate geometry of the vascular pedicle allows the artery and vein to lie without undue tension, kinking, or twisting.[5] Straight vessels with well-crafted anastomoses are less prone to thrombosis.

Clear communication with the anesthesia team is important as well. During harvest and early perfusion, the administration of vasoconstrictive substances such as neosynephrine or ephedrine for blood pressure support is potentially fatal to a flap. Maintaining systemic pressures by nonpharmacologic means, such as lightening the level of anesthesia and giving fluid boluses, is preferred. Of course, the patient's well-being takes precedence over any reconstructive effort, and there are no restrictions in the case of extreme hypotension or vascular collapse.

In addition to refined surgical technique, antithrombotic pharmacologic measures are often used perioperatively.[6, 7] Surgeons vary greatly in their reliance upon local and systemic platelet and clotting factor inhibitors. In fact, a survey of 73 microvascular centers failed to demonstrate any common patterns of anticoagulant use. Additionally, there was no positive correlation between flap survival improvement and the use of these medications.[8] Despite the lack of objective evidence, many surgeons apply a regimen of medications directed at decreasing thrombosis and improving outcomes.

The only pharmacologic intervention proven to have any benefit in decreasing fibrin deposition at the suture line is intraluminal heparin irrigation during anastomosis.[9–13] Normal vascular endothelium has a negative charge that inhibits platelet and fibrin deposition. Intimal injury dissipates this charge, shifting the balance toward increasing thrombotic potential. Heparin is a strongly negative macromolecule that concentrates on the intima, helping to prevent this charge shift and thus inhibiting thrombosis.[14] Studies of the systemic application of heparin demonstrate the maintenance of high endothelial levels even after serum levels have diminished.[15] Irrigation of the vessels with heparinized saline or Ringer's lactate solution prior to suturing concentrates the heparin where it is needed without affecting the clotting cascade systemically. Intravenous heparin is used in trauma and replantation microvascular surgery, in which vessels are often injured, with significantly increased thrombotic potential.[16] Some data suggest that high-dose systemic heparin in association with urokinase decreases the incidence of rethrombosis of flaps during anastomotic salvage.[17] However, because vessels in the head and neck are not usually traumatized, and because of the increased risk of hematoma formation,[13, 18] systemic use of heparin is not indicated during routine head and neck reconstruction.

Dextran, a macromolecule made of glucose polymers, acts as a hemodiluter, volume expander, and platelet adhesion inhibitor when given intravenously.[13, 19, 20] All of these effects are theoretically beneficial for a flap because they improve circulation. Albeit rare in occurrence, the reported risks include acute renal failure, pseudotumor cerebri,[21] and anaphylaxis. Additionally, in my experience, the need for transfusion increases with prolonged dextran use due to hemodilution. Transfusions may increase recurrence rates of head and neck cancer.[22, 23] To avoid the need for blood products, short-term use is indicated if dextran is to be used at all. Aspirin is a very effective platelet inhibitor that has theoretic benefit. Prophylaxis against the common gastrointestinal side effects must accompany the use of aspirin. Neither agent is associated with an increased bleeding risk after microvascular surgery.[13]

POSTOPERATIVE STRATEGIES

Monitoring is critical for the early detection and diagnosis of vascular compromise, particularly in the first 72 hours postoperatively. In a large reported series, flap survival for 3 days predicts a 99.7% chance of success without anastomotic failure.[24]

The clinical examination of a flap provides the surgeon with the greatest amount of information.[25] For a flap with an exposed skin paddle, capillary refill and pinprick bleeding are the most sensitive indicators of the circulatory health of the flap. However, not all persons responsible for monitoring flaps are experienced in the clinical evaluation of blood flow. For inexperienced and ancillary personnel, the Doppler ultrasound flow meter is a useful tool. This instrument provides a reliable and reproducible auditory signal using the Doppler principle. Ultrasonic sound waves are produced and projected into the tissue. The motion and velocity of the arterial and venous blood reflect the sound back with characteristic frequencies and patterns. The status of arterial and venous flow within the flap is thus determined.[26] The key to the successful use of Doppler ultrasound is communication. Before the patient leaves the operating room, a baseline flow signal is established. The primary surgeon demonstrates the location, quality, and quantity of the signal to all other caretakers. Any subsequent staff asked to monitor the flap must hear the signal with the previously responsible person. Any change in the quality or quantity of the sound is immediately brought to the attention of the surgeon. A clinical evaluation of the flap is then performed to determine the need for exploration. Without seamless communication, flaps can be lost.

Other methods of flap monitoring described in the literature include oxygen saturation, oxygen tension, flap and arterial thermometry, laser Doppler velocimetry, radioisotope scanning, fluorescein washout, electrical impedence, and plethysmography.[25, 27] The gold standards in monitoring have remained the clinical and Doppler examinations because of their simplicity, reliability, and ease of administration.

Ideally, every flap has an externalized segment available for evaluation.[25, 28] Occasionally, though, a flap is completely buried. In this case, it is possible to assess the vascular pedicle using Doppler ultrasound through the skin. Confounding variables that make this less reliable than direct observation include signals from flow in the dermal vessels, the carotid artery, and the internal jugular vein. Clearly placing the transcutaneous monitoring site far away from the great vessels decreases the likelihood of crossover vascular sounds.

Wound infections pose a serious threat to

the survival of free flaps.[29, 30] In the head and neck, salivary fistulas present the most likely source of infection. Experimentally, in the presence of untreated infection, venous anastomoses are less resistant to thrombosis than arterial anastomoses. However, appropriate antimicrobial therapy and debridement of infected tissue significantly improves patency rates.[31] Therefore, careful closure is exceedingly important when insetting a microvascular flap in the head or neck. If an infection is suspected, rapid institution of systemic antibiotics and drainage are necessary.

Adjunctive global measures are taken to sustain the patient and the free flap postoperatively. Perfusion of the flap is maintained with adequate arterial perfusion and intravascular volume and a hemoglobin level of 7.5 to 9.0 g/dL to maximize oxygen delivery without increasing blood viscosity. Aggressive diuresis to remove excess total body fluid overload is usually not indicated. Monitoring central venous pressures and urine output allows the tailoring of fluid management to maintain adequate intravascular volume without overload and the risk of heart failure. Third-space fluid mobilization occurs on the second or third postoperative day as in abdominal surgery patients, although with lesser volumes. Careful diuresis to assist the patients during fluid shifts is permissible as long as central venous pressure levels indicate adequate intravascular volume.

Presentation

Emergencies in free-flap surgery present with compromise of either venous outflow or arterial inflow. Venous anastomoses are more susceptible to thrombosis than are arterial anastomoses. The low pressures and slow flows in the venous system create a favorable environment for the initiation and propagation of thrombus. Additionally, veins are more easily compressed and obstructed by hematomas or overlying soft tissues than are arteries.[30] Arterial compromise occurs more often because of technical error at the suture line.

Healthy capillary refill in the cutaneous paddle of a flap takes 1 to 3 sec. A well-perfused flap is warm, pink, and soft. Sticking a needle into the flap results in very slow ooze of bright red blood. Doppler signals reveal a rounded, strong, arterial pulse. The venous phase is characterized by a lower frequency hum heard under the arterial sounds.

The venous blood–congested flap appears dusky or purple. It is full and may have pitting edema. Capillary refill is rapid, less than 1 sec. A needle stick reveals dark, exuberant bleeding. The Doppler examination has a distinct arterial sound described as a "water hammer" pulse. The full force of the systolic arterial pressure is attempting to fill a system without adequate venous outflow (Fig. 15–1).

Alternatively, a flap with arterial insufficiency is pale, cool, flaccid, and without capillary refill. A needle stick results in no bleeding at all. The Doppler examination is quiet (Fig. 15–2).

Priorities

Any patient whose flap demonstrates clinical evidence of vascular inflow or outflow compro-

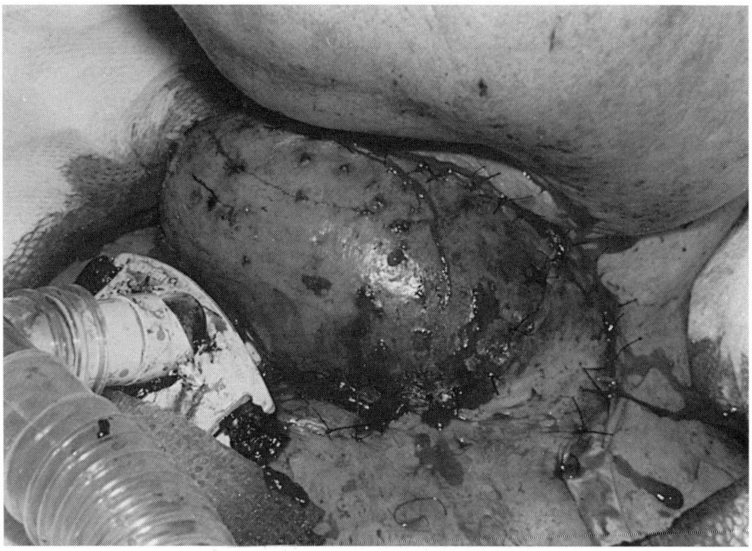

Figure 15–1. Radial forearm free flap for neopharyngeal stenosis after laryngectomy and radiation therapy. Despite venous anastomotic patency, the flap had insufficient outflow. An attempt at leech therapy failed to salvage the flap. Note the fullness and dark color of the flap relative to the surrounding neck skin. Blood is oozing from leech bites because of high venous pressures.

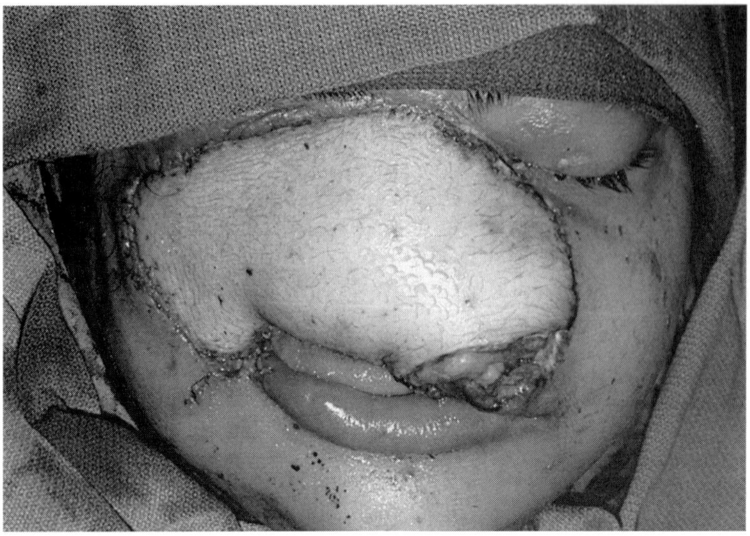

Figure 15–2. Rectus abdominis free flap for reconstruction of a midfacial defect after resection of a massive, atypical, locally aggressive melanoma. Arterial insufficiency developed 48 hours postoperatively due to an acute disruption of the arterial suture line. Note the pale color of the flap relative to the facial skin. Needle sticks to the flap resulted in no bleeding.

mise is immediately returned to the operating room for exploration of the vascular pedicle. Delayed intervention results in flap loss.

Postponement of revascularization in a flap with arterial embarrassment can result in the no-reflow phenomenon, which is similar to that seen in cerebral or myocardial ischemia.[32] The mechanism of no reflow is still unclear. Granulocyte plugging[33] or injury induced by oxygen free radicals[34] are possible causes of this phenomenon. Functionally, there appears to be an ischemia-related increase in the peripheral resistance to blood flow. This phenomenon occurs after 8 to 12 hours of ischemia in free-tissue transfer.[35] There are no limits to the number of revisions of anastomoses that may be attempted. However, if an anastomosis is patent and there is still no flow distally through the flap, no therapeutic interventions have been found to be successful in reversing the no-reflow phenomenon.

Venous congested flaps are equally at risk if delayed intervention occurs. However, irreversible damage occurs more quickly than is typically seen in arterial obstruction. Edema, progressive thrombosis of the small vessels, and hemorrhage into the flap make salvage difficult.

Once in the operating room, neck incisions are opened and a compressive hematoma is ruled out, particularly in flaps with venous outflow obstruction. The anastomosis is then observed under the operating microscope and revised as necessary.

Medical leech therapy is indicated if, despite maximizing venous outflow, the flap is still congested.[36] Leeches (*Hirudo medicinalis*) are available for immediate shipping from a number of commercial sources. They attach preferentially to venous blood–congested skin. Their teeth pierce the skin as they attach to the flap. Leech saliva, which contains hirudin (an extremely potent nonenzymatic thrombin inhibitor) and other enzymes and vasodilators, is secreted to maintain flow through the cutaneous injury.[13] The leech releases when full. Constant attention is required to remove and apply leeches as appropriate. When the flap is no longer congested, their use is no longer indicated. The reported success rate in salvaging free flaps with leeches is 83% in one series.[37] However, leech use is always considered a last resort maneuver and not a substitute for good anastomotic technique, pedicle geometry, and flap design.

Outcomes

If flap compromise is recognized promptly, a diagnosis of a correctable anastomotic problem is made, and return to the operating room is not delayed, a high percentage (33% to 100%) of flaps survive.[38–41] In the event of flap loss, which type of intervention is chosen (pedicled vs. additional free flaps) depends on the location and severity of the resultant wound[42] and the general condition of the patient. These possibilities are always discussed with the patient preoperatively. The surgeon's planning should always include alternative reconstructive strategies for use in the event of failure.

PEDICLED FLAP EMERGENCIES

Prior to the advent of microvascular techniques, pedicled flaps provided the surgeon with reli-

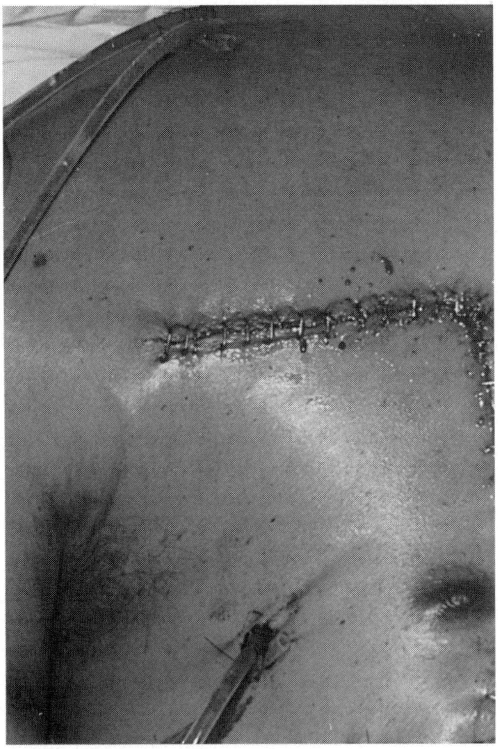

Figure 15–3. Pectoralis myocutaneous flap donor site. The skin paddle demonstrated venous congestion. Examination of the donor site (pictured) revealed a bulging and tense wound, suggesting a compressive hematoma.

able, technically uncomplicated tools for head and neck reconstruction. The most commonly used is the pectoralis major muscle or myocutaneous flap, described in 1979.[43, 44] The latissimus[45] and trapezius[46–48] muscles offer flap options as well, although with lower reliability and versatility. Pectoralis flap survival rates range from 97%[49] to 99%[50] in reported series. In contrast to free flaps, pedicled flaps may experience partial losses, which occur in 3%[50] to 29%[49] of cases. Surgical technique is the single most important factor in determining the success of pedicled flaps.

Prevention of Flap Emergencies

Knowledge of the anatomy of pedicled flaps is critical to their ultimate success. Positive identification of the vascular pedicle is crucial to its protection and preservation. The most common acute emergency in pedicled flaps is venous outflow obstruction either by constriction of the vessels by a tight closure or by compression of the vessels by hematoma.

Presentation

Flaps with venous outflow obstruction are dusky, plethoric, and edematous and have brisk capillary refill. Often, palpation of the harvest site and the path of the pedicle reveals either a closure under tension or fullness and an obvious collection (Fig. 15–3).

Priorities

A patient is urgently returned to the operating room to explore the flap pedicle and relieve the

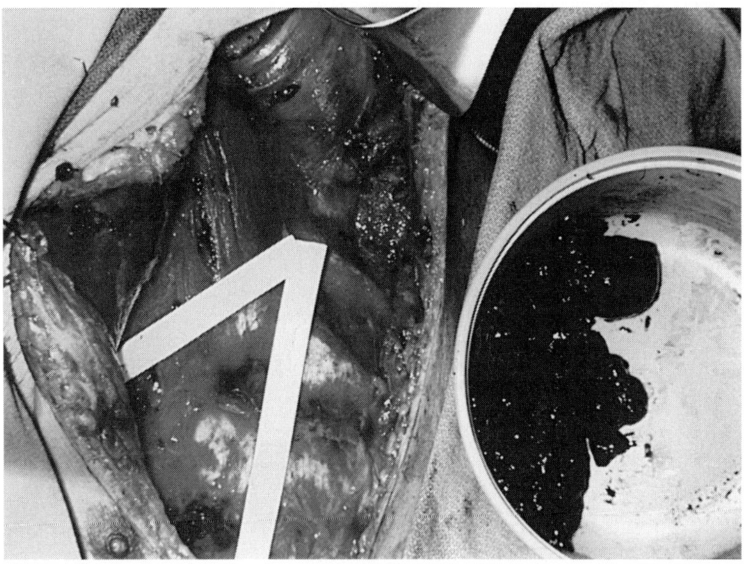

Figure 15–4. Pectoralis major donor site opened in the operating room demonstrating hematoma (in basin). The flap did well.

outflow obstruction. If a hematoma is present, it is removed and hemostasis is achieved (Fig. 15–4). If it is determined that the skin closure is too tight, relaxing incisions, wide undermining, or debridement of the flap pedicle is performed to ensure a tension-free closure.

Outcomes

All pedicled flaps that are identified as being at risk are salvageable if the patient is returned quickly to the operating room.

REFERENCES

1. Urken ML et al. Microvascular free flaps in head and neck reconstruction. Arch Otolaryngol Head Neck Surg 1994;120:633–640.
2. Schusterman MA et al. A single center's experience with 308 free flaps for repair of head and neck cancer defects. Plast Reconstr Surg 1994;93:472–480.
3. Brown MT. Personal communication.
4. Mattox DE. Microvascular anastomosis: a scanning electron microscopic study. Otolaryngol Head Neck Surg 1980;88:252–256.
5. Urken ML et al. Geometry of the vascular pedicle in free-tissue transfers to the head and neck. Arch Otolaryngol Head Neck Surg 1989;115:954–960.
6. Ketchum LD. Pharmacological alterations in the clotting mechanisms: use in microvascular surgery. J Hand Surg 1978;3:407–415.
7. Das SK, Miller JH. Current status of topical antithrombotic agents in microvascular surgery. Microsurgery 1994;15:630–632.
8. Davies DM. A world survey of anticoagulation practice in clinical microvascular surgery. Br J Plast Surg 1982;35:96–99.
9. Khouri RK et al. Thrombosis of microvascular anastomoses in traumatized vessels: fibrin versus platelets. Plast Reconstr Surg 1987;86:110–117.
10. Greenberg BM, Masem M, May JW. Therapeutic value of intravenous heparin in microvascular surgery: an experimental vascular thrombosis study. Plast Reconstr Surg 1988;82:463–470.
11. Sinclair S. The importance of topical heparin in microvascular anastomoses: a study in the rat. Br J Plast Surg 1980;33:422–426.
12. Zinberg E, Choo DI, Zotter LA. Effect of heparinized irrigating solutions on patency of experimental microvascular anastomoses. Microsurgery 1989;10:103–107.
13. Johnson PC, Barker JH. Thrombosis and antithrombotic therapy in microvascular surgery. Clin Plast Surg 1992;19:799–807.
14. Jaques LB, Hiebert LM. The close relationship of heparin and the vessel wall. Artery 1989;16:140–150.
15. Hiebert LM, Jaques LB. The observation of heparin on endothelium after injection. Thromb Res 1976; 8:195–204.
16. Elcock HW, Fredrickson JM. The effect of heparin on thrombosis at microvenous anastomotic sites. Arch Otolaryngol 1972;95:68–71.
17. Hirigoyen MB et al. Additional benefit of heparin in the thrombolytic salvage of ischemic skin flaps. Ann Plast Surg 1995;35:612–619.
18. Kroll SS et al. Anticoagulants and hematomas in free flap surgery. Plast Reconstr Surg 1995;96:643–647.
19. Batlle J et al. Effect of dextran on factor VIII/von Willebrand factor structure and function. Thromb Haemostasis 1985;54:697–699.
20. Wieslander JB et al. The influence of dextran and saline solution upon platelet behavior after microarterial anastomosis. Surg Gyn Ob 1986;163:256–262.
21. Hardin CK, Kirk WC, Pederson WC. Osmotic complications of low-molecular-weight dextran therapy in free-flap surgery. Microsurgery 1992;13:36–38.
22. McCullough TM, VanDaele DJ, Hillel A, The Department of Veterans Affairs Laryngeal Cancer Study Group. Blood transfusion as a risk factor for death in stage III and IV operative laryngeal cancer. Arch Otolaryngol Head Neck Surg 1995;121:1227–1235.
23. Wooley AL et al. Effects of blood transfusion on recurrence of head and neck cancer: retrospective review and meta-analysis. Ann Otol Rhinol Laryngol 1992;101:724–730.
24. Kroll SS et al. Timing of pedicle thrombosis and flap loss after free-tissue transfer. Plast Reconstr Surg 1996;98:1230–1233.
25. Stepnick DW, Hayden RE. Postoperative monitoring and salvage of microvascular free flaps. Otolaryngol Clin North Am 1994;27:1201–1216.
26. Moelleken BRW, Mathes SJ, Amerhauser A. Flap monitoring. Perspect Plast Surg 1990;4:94–111.
27. Machens HG et al. Techniques of postoperative blood flow monitoring after free-tissue transfer: an overview. Microsurgery 1995;15:778–786.
28. Urken ML et al. Free flap design in head and neck reconstruction to achieve an external segment for monitoring. Arch Otolaryngol Head Neck Surg 1989; 115: 1447–1453.
29. Khouri RK. Avoiding free flap failure. Clin Plast Surg 1992;19:773–781.
30. Souminen S, Asko-Seljavaara S: Free flap failures. Microsurgery 1995;16:396–399.
31. Luk KDK et al. Effect of treated infection on microvascular anastomosis. Microsurgery 1992;13:84–91.
32. Ames A et al. Cerebral ischemia. II: The no-reflow phenomenon. Am J Pathol 1968;52:437–447.
33. Schmid-Schonbein GW. Capillary plugging by granulocytes and the no-reflow phenomenon in the microcirculation. Fed Proc 1987;46:2397–2401.
34. McCord JM. Oxygen-derived free radicals in postischemic tissue injury. N Engl J Med 1985;312:159–163.
35. May JW et al. The no-reflow phenomenon in experimental free flaps. Plast Reconstr Surg 1978;61:256–267.
36. Kraemer BA et al. Use of leeches in plastic and reconstructive surgery: a review. J Reconstr Micro 1988; 4:381–386.
37. Soucacos PN et al. The use of medicinal leeches, *Hirudo medicinalis*, to restore venous circulation in trauma and reconstructive surgery. Int Angiol 1994;13:251–258.
38. Irons GB, Wood MB, Schmitt EH. Experience with one hundred consecutive free flaps. Ann Plast Surg 1987;18:17–23.
39. Harashina T. Analysis of 200 free flaps. Br J Plast Surg 1988;41:33–36.
40. Reick B, Mailender P, Machens HG. Vascular complications after free-tissue transfer. Microsurgery 1995;16:400–403.
41. Hidalgo DA, Jones CS. The role of emergent exploration in free-tissue transfer: a review of 150 consecutive cases. Plast Reconstr Surg 1990;86:492–498.
42. Oliva A et al. Salvage of wounds following failed tissue transplantation. J Reconstr Microsurg 1993;9:257–263.

43. Ariyan S. The pectoralis major myocutaneous flap. Plast Reconstr Surg 1979;63:73–81.
44. Baek S et al. The pectoralis major myocutaneous flap for reconstruction of the head and neck. Head Neck Surg 1979;1:293–300.
45. Barton FE, Spicer TE, Byrd HS. Head and neck reconstruction with the latissimus dorsi myocutaneous flap: anatomic observations and report of 60 cases. Plast Reconstr Surg 1983;71:199–204.
46. Netterville JL, Panje WR, Maves MD. The trapezius myocutaneous flap, dependability and limitations. Arch Otolaryngol Head Neck Surg 1987;113:271–281.
47. Donald PJ, Chole RA. Superior-based trapezius flap. Laryngoscope 1984;94:969–973.
48. Cummings CW, Eisele DW, Coltrera MD. Lower trapezius myocutaneous island flap. Arch Otolaryngol Head Neck Surg 1989;115:1181–1185.
49. Shah JP et al. Complications for the pectoralis major myocutaneous flap in head and neck reconstruction. Am J Surg 1990;106:352–355.
50. Baek S, Lawson W, Biller HF. An analysis of 133 pectoralis major myocutaneous flaps. Plast Reconstr Surg 1982;69:460–467.

CHAPTER 16

Oral Cavity and Dental Emergencies

Steven G. Ashman, DDS

Although many emergencies of the oral cavity are in the area of dentistry or oral and maxillofacial surgery, some hospitals do not have specialists in these areas on staff. This chapter is intended to review emergencies of the oral cavity and help guide the management of such patients.

PERIODONTAL ABSCESS

The teeth are supported in the alveolar bone of the maxilla and mandible by the periodontal membrane. This membrane is made primarily of collagenous fibers that form a suspensory ligament that attaches the tooth to the surrounding alveolar bone. Accumulations of plaque or calculus on the teeth lead to inflammation of this membrane and the loss of the alveolar bone supporting the tooth[1] (Fig. 16–1). The inflammation stems from bacteria contained in the accumulations of plaque or calculus and frequently results in an acute inflammatory episode, the periodontal abscess.[2] Patients who are at greater risk than others include those with diabetes, immunosuppression, mental impairment, alcoholism, and generalized debility. Most periodontal abscesses are mixed infections consisting of aerobic gram-positive cocci, anaerobic gram-positive cocci, and anaerobic gram-negative rods. The major pathogenic bacteria that cause periodontal infections are *Streptococcus* species, *Peptococcus* species, *Peptostreptococcus* species, *Bacteroides* species, and *Fusobacterium* species.

Presentation

The patient reports pain and swelling of the gingiva along with a bad taste and halitosis. There is commonly a history of bleeding of the gums. The patient may also report one or more loose teeth. Occasionally, there will be a history of fever.

Evaluation

The diagnosis of periodontal abscess is made by careful examination of the oral cavity. Adequate

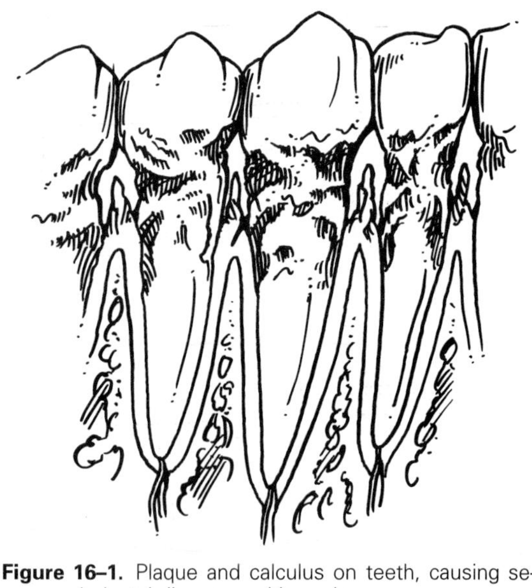

Figure 16–1. Plaque and calculus on teeth, causing severe periodontal disease and bone loss.

light and instruments such as tongue blades to retract the cheeks and tongue are needed to perform this examination. Physical findings include erythema, edema, and tenderness of the gingiva. Frank purulence can sometimes be expressed from the gingival sulcus around the affected tooth by pressing firmly on the gum. The affected tooth may show some degree of mobility. The tooth may be tender to palpation and percussion. In severe cases, the patient may present with a fever. Dental radiographs sometimes show bone loss associated with the affected teeth.

Priorities

Management of a periodontal abscess is directed toward prevention of further spread of the infection into the associated oral cavity and deep neck spaces. The patient is therefore begun on a broad-spectrum antibiotic. Penicillin is the antibiotic of choice; a penicillin-allergic patient should be started on erythromycin or clindamycin. A patient may be placed on an antibiotic mouth rinse such as chlorhexidine. If a fluctuant swelling is present in the gingiva or alveolar mucosa, an incision and drainage should be performed. The patient should be referred to a dentist for consideration of periodontal surgery or extraction. (See Chapter 19 for discussion of deep-space neck infections and their sequelae.)

Outcomes

A severe infection of a space in the head or neck region often begins as a simple periodontal abscess, so it is important to treat such an infection aggressively in order to avoid a more serious infection. It is usual for a patient to respond quickly to treatment of a periodontal abscess.

PERICORONITIS

Pericoronitis refers to a painful inflammation or infection of the tissues surrounding the crown of an unerupted or impacted tooth, the pericoronal tissues. This inflammation most often occurs in an adolescent or young adult between the ages of 15 and 25 but can occur in anyone with an unerupted tooth.[3] It commonly occurs during a time when normal oral hygiene is neglected such as in a college student around the time of final exams, in an immunocompromised patient with diabetes, immune suppression, or a debilitating disease, or in a patient who requires steroid therapy. The bacteria most often associated with this infection are *Peptostreptococcus*, *Fusobacterium*, and *Bacteroides* species.[4]

Presentation

A patient usually presents with a history of jaw pain and ear pain on the affected side. Swelling of the overlying gingiva is commonly seen. Sometimes a patient develops cellulitis and abscess in the buccal space, masticator space, or even submandibular space. Trismus due to inflammation of the medial pterygoid muscle is also a common presenting symptom, along with fever.

Evaluation

The diagnosis of pericoronitis is made by careful examination of the oral cavity. Adequate light and instruments such as tongue blades to retract the cheeks and tongue are needed to perform this examination. There may be swelling and tenderness of the buccal space, submandibular space, or masticator space. Often a portion of the impacted tooth can be seen extruding through the gingiva, with ulceration of the surrounding tissues and frank purulence within the wound. There is often erythema of the gingival tissues, and a fetid oral odor is frequently encountered. Dental radiographs demonstrate impacted teeth.

Priorities

Urgent management of a patient with a pericoronal infection is required to prevent the spread of the infection into the associated spaces. Broad-spectrum antibiotic therapy should be initiated, and as with other oral infections, penicillin is the antibiotic of choice. A penicillin-allergic patient should be started on erythromycin or clindamycin. A patient may be placed on an antibiotic mouth rinse such as chlorhexidine.[5] If a fluctuant swelling is present in the gingiva or alveolar mucosa, an incision should be performed to allow drainage. The patient should be referred to a dentist for additional treatment such as extraction of the impacted tooth, which is often delayed until the infection is brought under control to avoid spread into the parapharyngeal tissues.

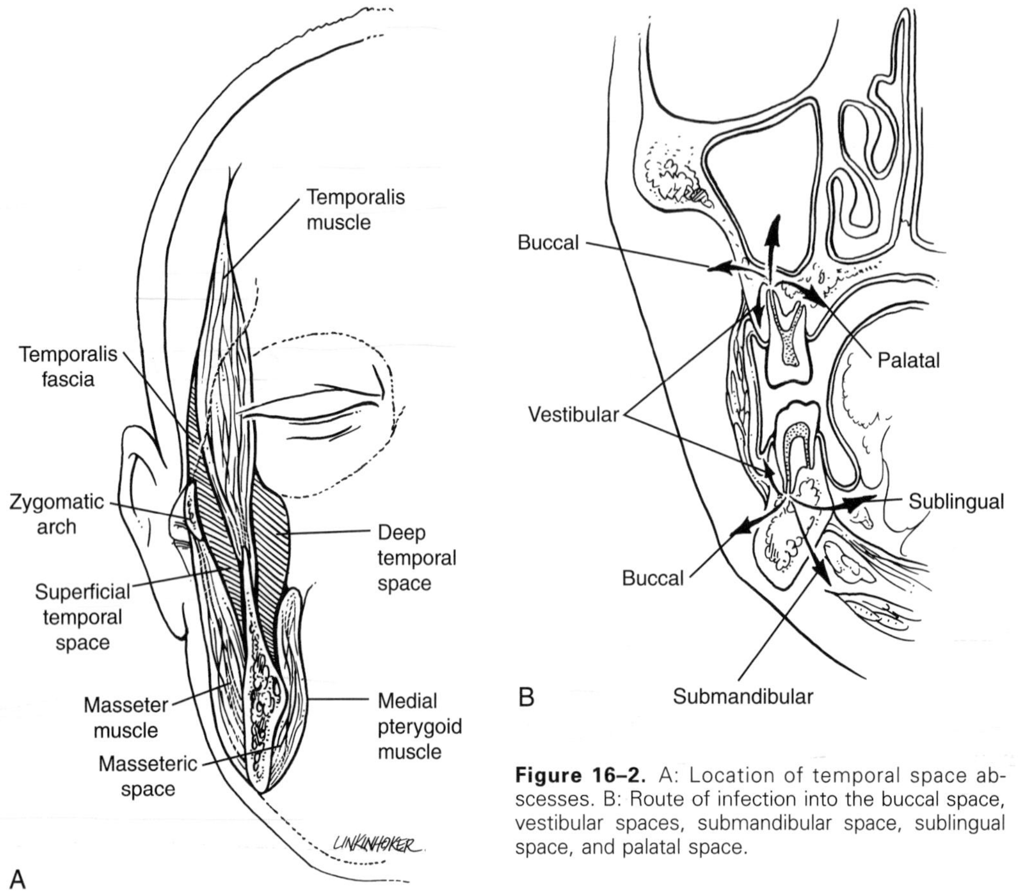

Figure 16–2. A: Location of temporal space abscesses. B: Route of infection into the buccal space, vestibular spaces, submandibular space, sublingual space, and palatal space.

Outcomes

Recovery from a pericoronal infection and removal of an impacted tooth may be prolonged because of the nature of the surgery needed to remove an impacted tooth embedded in bone. A patient is likely to have continued swelling and trismus that lasts up to 2 weeks and thus requires diet restrictions because of these sequelae. Some teeth impacted in the mandible impinge upon the neurovascular bundle of the mandible, and removal of the impacted tooth can cause injury to the inferior alveolar nerve, which results in paresthesia on the affected side. Teeth impacted in the posterior maxilla are adjacent to the maxillary sinus, and removal can sometimes violate the sinus membrane, which may cause nasal hemorrhage, maxillary sinusitis or, rarely, an oromaxillary fistula.

SEVERE ODONTOGENIC INFECTION, PERIAPICAL ABSCESS

An odontogenic infection occurs as a result of the invasion of bacteria into the pulp of the tooth through a carious lesion, which causes necrosis of the dental pulp. This necrotic tissue is confined within the rigid calcified walls of the pulp chamber and serves as an excellent culture medium for the anaerobic bacteria that have invaded the tooth. Because the blood supply is interrupted by the necrosis of the pulpal tissue, antibiotics cannot penetrate into the pulp chamber. The apex of the tooth has a narrow pulpal foramen through which the bacteria may gain access to the alveolar bone supporting the tooth. Once the infection has extended beyond the apex of the tooth, the infectious process is determined by the number of bacteria present, the virulence of the organisms, the resistance of the host, and the anatomy of the area of bone involved. Any patient with deep dental caries, deep restorations, or poor oral hygiene is at risk for development of an odontogenic infection. The result may be the formation of a mucosal fistula, a dental-cutaneous fistula, a soft tissue cellulitis, an intraoral soft tissue abscess, osteomyelitis, bacteremia-septicemia, a deep fascial-space infection, or an ascending facial-cerebral infection.[6–10] The spaces at risk for infections of odontogenic origin are the (1) canine fossa, (2) buccal space, (3) infratemporal space, (4) submental space, (5) submandibular space, (6) sublingual space, (7) masseteric space, (8) pterygomandibular space, and (9) superficial and deep temporal spaces[11] (Fig. 16–2*A* and *B*). Gram-positive cocci are the most common aerobic bacteria found in odontogenic infections, with *Streptococcus* species present 90% of the time. *Bacteroides* species are the most common anaerobic bacteria found in odontogenic infections; these are gram-negative rods. *Peptostreptococcus* species are the most common gram-negative cocci found in odontogenic infections.[12]

Presentation and Evaluation

The most common sequence of events following the necrosis of the dental pulp is the onset of severe pain localized to a specific tooth. The infection is confined to the medullary bone at the apex of the tooth. As it progresses, the infection perforates the cortex of the bone and causes swelling in the soft tissue overlying the bone in the buccal, labial, or lingual vestibules or the palatal mucosa. This is often associated with a decrease in pain due to the reduction of intrabony pressure. The overlying soft tissue eventually breaks down and a mucosal or cutaneous fistula is formed, allowing the abscess to drain naturally. If host resistance is compromised or if the bacteria causing the infection are especially virulent, the presentation of the infection is more acute. The patient may develop cellulitis and diffuse edema and erythema of the surrounding tissues. The involved area is soft, warm, and tender to the touch. The patient may be febrile and may present with trismus. Such a patient is also at risk of developing an abscess involving the fascial planes of the head and neck area (Fig. 16–3) and may present with a hard, warm, painful swelling. Fever and trismus are often associated with abscess formation.

Particular oral cavity space infections commonly produce characteristic signs and symptoms.[11]

A patient with a *canine fossa* abscess complains of a history of pain in an anterior maxillary tooth, most often the canine or lateral incisor. The tooth exhibits mobility and tenderness to percussion. The infection at the apex of the canine or lateral incisor perforates the labial cortical plate of bone above the insertion of the levator anguli oris muscle. As a result, the patient may present with edema and erythema lateral to the ala of the nose. The upper lip may

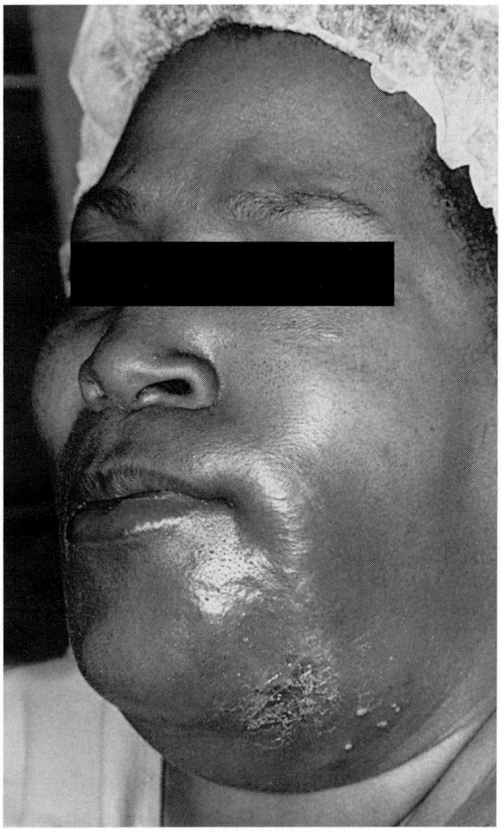

Figure 16–3. Submandibular space abscess.

also be edematous and there may be swelling in the anterior maxillary vestibule. The infection may invade more superfically and extend between the levator anguli oris and the muscles that elevate the upper lip, the zygomaticus minor, the levator labii superioris, and the levator labii superioris alaeque nasi. As a result, the inferior and superior eyelids may become edematous with cellulitis to the point where the patient may not be able to open the ipsilateral eye.

The *buccal space* lies between the buccinator muscle and the skin. It is bounded superiorly by the zygomatic arch and inferiorly by the inferior border of the mandible. Infections of this space are caused most commonly by maxillary molar teeth, although extension of infections of maxillary and mandibular bicuspid teeth and mandibular molar teeth can also lead to abscesses in this space. When the perforation of the buccal cortex of bone occurs superior to the insertion of the buccinator muscle on the maxilla or inferior to the buccinator muscle on the mandible, the infection spreads into the buccal space. This space contains the buccal fat pad, the parotid (Stenson's) duct, and the external maxillary (facial) artery. The patient presents with painful swelling of the cheek that does not extend beyond the inferior border of the mandible.[13]

The *infratemporal space* is located posterior to the maxilla. The superior and medial boundaries are the sphenoid bone. Laterally, it continues as the deep temporal space. The maxillary third molar teeth are usually the cause of the rare infection of this space.[13]

The mandibular incisor teeth are the source of infections of the *submental space*. This midline space is bounded laterally by the anterior bellies of the right and left digastric muscles. The superior wall is the mylohyoid muscle and the inferior wall is the skin and the mentalis muscle. Infections of this space can also be caused by a necrotic lymph node draining a carious tooth or a periodontal infection. The patient has hard, painful swelling in the chin and between the bone of the most anterior point of the mandible and the hyoid bone. The floor of the mouth is not raised.[13]

The medial surface of the mandible serves as a common boundary for the *submandibular and sublingual spaces* (Fig. 16–4). These spaces are separated by the mylohyoid muscle, which disappears posteriorly, allowing the spaces to communicate with each other and with the pterygomandibular space. Infections of the mandibular molar and bicuspid teeth are common sources of odontogenic infections of these spaces; the submandibular space has the skin as its inferior border and the digastric muscle as its medial border. This space contains the submandibular gland, lymph nodes, the facial vein and artery, the marginal mandibular branch of the facial nerve, the hypoglossal nerve, and the lingual nerve. The mucosa of the floor of the mouth serves as the superior border of the sublingual space. This space contains the sublingual gland, Wharton's duct, the lingual artery, and the lingual nerve. Infections of the sublingual space are frequently bilateral. A patient with an abscess in the submandibular space has swelling that begins at the inferior border of the mandible and extends under the mandible and along the lateral surface of the superior portion of the neck to the midline. A sublingual abscess presents as a swelling under the tongue that raises the tongue and is limited by the midline or extends to the contralateral side.[13]

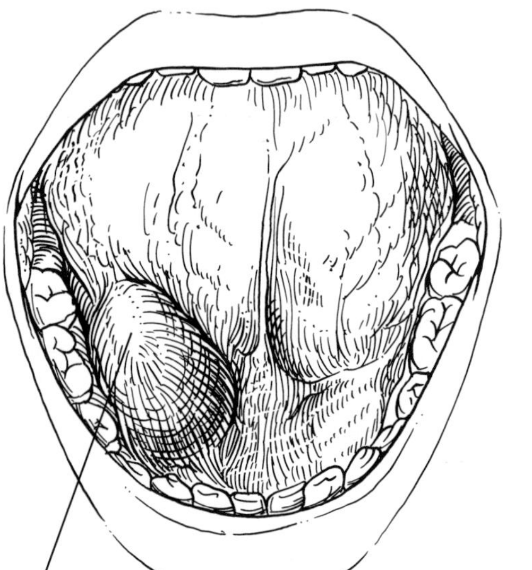

Figure 16–4. Sublingual space abscess. (Adapted from Archer WH. Oral & Maxillofacial surgery, vol., VI, 5th ed. Philadelphia, WB Saunders, 1975.)

Severe, rapidly occurring infections that involve the submandibular, sublingual, and submental spaces bilaterally and involve brawny edema of the anterior neck and submental areas along with elevation of the tongue and obstruction of the airway are referred to as Ludwig's angina and may be life threatening if they are not treated immediately. With current antibiotic therapy, Lugwig's angina is a rare occurrence.[14]

Infections involving the mandibular third molars frequently result in involvement of the *masseteric space*. This space lies between the lateral surface of the mandible and the masseter muscle. Buccal space infections can also spread into this space. Patients have large, tender, warm, hard swellings of the face over the angle of the mandible and above the inferior border of the mandible.[13]

The *pterygomandibular space* is located between the medial pterygoid muscle and the medial border of the ramus of the mandible. Infections in this space are a result of posterior spread of infection from the submandibular and sublingual spaces. A patient presents with little or no facial swelling but has severe trismus and pain.[13]

The *superficial temporal space* is separated from the deep temporal space by the temporalis muscle. These spaces are posterior and superior to the masseteric and pterygomandibular spaces. The deep temporal space is continuous with the infratemporal space. The superficial and deep temporal spaces become infected by extension of severe infections from the other spaces. A patient with a temporal space infection presents with a bulging temporalis muscle above the zygomatic arch. The associated cellulitis may involve the periorbital region and cause swelling and closure of the eyelids.[13]

Infections involving both the masseter and pterygomandibular spaces and sometimes the temporal spaces as well are known as *masticator space* infections.[13]

Priorities

A patient exhibiting systemic symptoms of an odontogenic infection should be placed on antibiotic therapy. A patient with coexisting conditions, such as insulin-dependent diabetes mellitus, immunosuppression, or renal failure, should also receive antibiotics. Penicillin is the antibiotic of choice for odontogenic infections. Metronidazole can be used in combination with penicillin if there is concern about gram-negative bacteria. Immediate drainage is important in the treatment of acute odontogenic infections. This includes the removal of the offending tooth or removal of the necrotic pulpal tissue of that tooth. Drainage of localized abscesses of dental origin can usually be accomplished intraorally at the site of dependence of the fluctuant area. Extraction of the offending tooth often serves to create adequate drainage of a localized odontogenic abscess.[12, 15]

The management of fascial space infections includes medical support of the patient, administration of appropriate antibiotics, early removal of the source of the infection, and surgical drainage of the infection, including placement of drains. Assessment and continued monitoring of the patient should be performed to ensure a patent airway. The patient should be provided with fluids, analgesics, and nutritional support. High-dose antibiotics should administered intravenously. Surgical management of an infection of the fascial space often requires incision, exploration, and placement of a drain. Locations of incisions into the various spaces can be seen in Figure 16–5. Making the incision in healthy skin or mucosa is important to prevent an unsightly scar. The incision should be placed, when possible, in an esthetically acceptable area such as in a natural skin crease or fold or under the inferior border of the mandible. A dependent location should be used so that gravity encourages drainage. Blunt dissection is carried out in the deeper tissues to explore the entire abscess cavity to be sure that any loculations of pus have been disrupted. The blunt dissection should be carried to the bone near the apex of the offending tooth or teeth. Drains should be placed in the wound and stabilized by being sutured to the skin. Drains should be removed as soon as possible after drainage has become minimal. The dressing should be changed daily and the wound cleaned of clots and dried purulence.[13, 16–18]

Serious complications may arise from space infections of odontogenic origin, including airway obstruction, mediastinitis, acute orbital cellulitis, intracranial infection, and necrotizing fasciitis.

Bilateral submandibular and submental space infections or Ludwig's angina result in acute respiratory obstruction if not treated aggressively (Fig. 16–6). Most cases of Ludwig's angina are caused by dental infections. Prior to the advent of antibiotics, more than a 50% mortality rate was associated with this disease, but antibiotics have reduced it to less than 5%. Early use of antibiotics for submandibular infections prevent many cases of Ludwig's angina. Infection can spread from the masticator space into the lateral pharyngeal space. This too can result in respiratory obstruction as well as septic thrombosis of the internal jugular vein and hemorrhage of the carotid artery.

Further extension of an infection in the lateral pharyngeal space can involve the pretracheal space, which descends into the anterior mediastinum, or the retropharyngeal space, which becomes the retrovisceral space and extends into the posterior mediastinum. The resulting mediastinitis is treated aggressively with antibiotics and surgical drainage using a transcervical approach. There is a 42% mortality rate associated with this kind of infection.[19]

In one reported study of acute orbital cellulitis, 10 of 190 cases (5%) resulted from odontogenic infection. A patient with acute orbital cellulitis presents with erythema and edema of the eyelids, chemosis, exophthalmos, and dull pain. Delayed treatment can result in cavernous sinus thrombosis, meningitis, subdural empyema, or brain abscess.[20]

Odontogenic infections, especially those originating in the maxillary teeth, can spread via the pterygoid plexus and emissary veins or via the angular veins and ophthalmic veins into the cavernous sinus and cause cavernous sinus thrombosis. This is associated with a high mortality rate. Aggressive antibiotic therapy and possible surgical drainage may be needed. Other neurologic complications resulting from odontogenic infection include meningitis, brain abscess, and subdural empyema.[21, 22]

Another serious and potentially fatal complication of odontogenic infection is necrotizing fasciitis. This is a rare infection in the maxillofacial region; it more commonly occurs in the abdomen and the extremities. The superficial

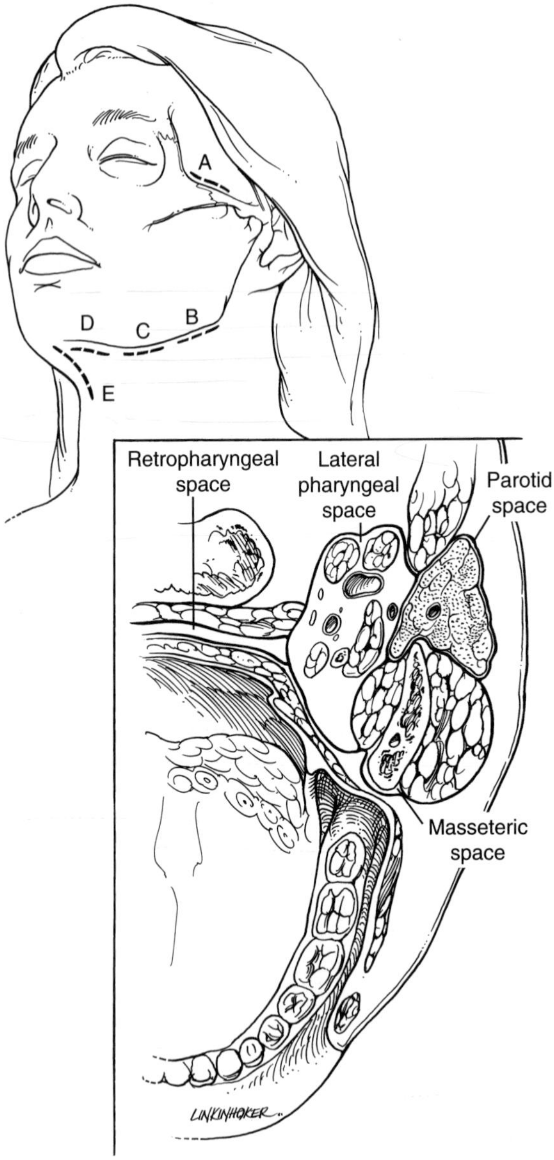

Figure 16–5. Location of incisions to drain space infections of the face. A: Temporal space. B: Submandibular and lateral pharyngeal space. C: Submandibular and sublingual space. D: Sublingual space. E: Bilateral submandibular and sublingual (Lugwig's) spaces.

fascia becomes infected, undermining the overlying soft tissues, and the infection progresses rapidly. The overlying tissues become dusky, showing small purple patches with ill-defined borders. Bullae measuring a few millimeters in diameter develop in the skin in the affected areas. Thrombosis of the vessels in the involved fascia causes the skin tissue beneath the bullae to become necrotic and cyanotic. A patient may have an associated condition such as diabetes mellitus, atherosclerotic coronary artery disease, peripheral vascular disease, or alcohol abuse. Early diagnosis is necessary to interrupt the progress of the disease. The diagnosis is made using computed tomography (CT), radiographs, and tissue biopsy with frozen section. A patient must be managed with aggressive antibiotic therapy, supportive care that includes management of concurrent debilitating diseases, fluid and electrolyte balance, and extensive surgical debridement of necrotic fascia and placement of surgical irrigating drains and antibiotic packings. The mortality rate for necrotizing fasciitis is about 30%.[23–25]

Outcomes

Recovery from odontogenic infections is usually uneventful. With adequate medical and surgical

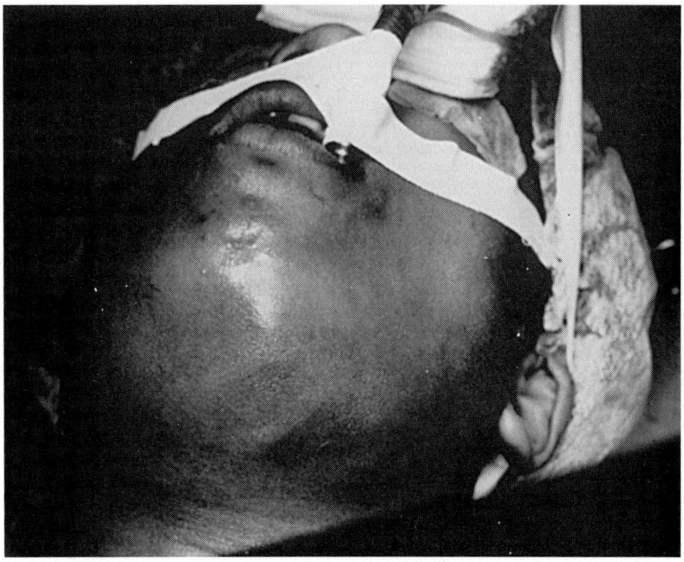

Figure 16–6. Ludwig's angina.

management, patients have few posttreatment problems. Drainage of space infections results in scarring of the operative site. Care is usually taken to keep these incisions in cosmetically appropriate locations, but scar revision is sometimes necessary.

ACUTE NECROTIZING ULCERATIVE GINGIVOSTOMATITIS

Acute necrotizing ulcerative gingivostomatitis is also known as Vincent's disease and more recently has been called necrotizing ulcerative periodontitis. The disease is most prevalent among teenage and young adult males. The disease is stress-related and also occurs under circumstances of poor oral hygiene. This explains the outbreak of the disease during World War I (when it was called trench mouth) and its frequent occurrence in college students during final examinations.[26, 27] More recently, very severe forms of this disease have been noted among patients who have the human immunodeficiency virus (HIV) and low CD4 counts. Ulcerations that invade the submucosal tissues, including muscle, and gingival ulcers that necrose bone have been documented in this population.[28, 29]

Presentation

This acute infection attacks the gingival margins of the teeth, especially the interproximal tissues. In the population without HIV, there are shallow ulcerations of the gingival margins and blunting of the interdental papillae, with formation of necrotic craters surrounded by marginal zones of erythema. The patient complains of severe pain, and recognizable halitosis is present. Rarely in the immune-competent population, but frequently in those with HIV, the ulcerations extend beyond the gingiva to the palate and buccal mucosa.[28]

Evaluation

The foul oral odor and necrosis of the interdental papillae are diagnostic of this disease. Microscopically, the associated bacteria, known as Vincent's organisms, are anaerobic fusiform and spirochetal bacteria (*Borrelia vincentii* and *Fusiformis fusiformis*).[14]

Priorities

The patient is treated with oral antibiotics for a week. Penicillin is the drug of choice. In addition, oral rinses with hydrogen peroxide solution or Peridex may be used. Early debridement by means of dental scaling and cleaning is also indicated.

Outcomes

Usually, the patient recovers rapidly after beginning antibiotic therapy. Instruction in oral hygiene is important to prevent recurrence.

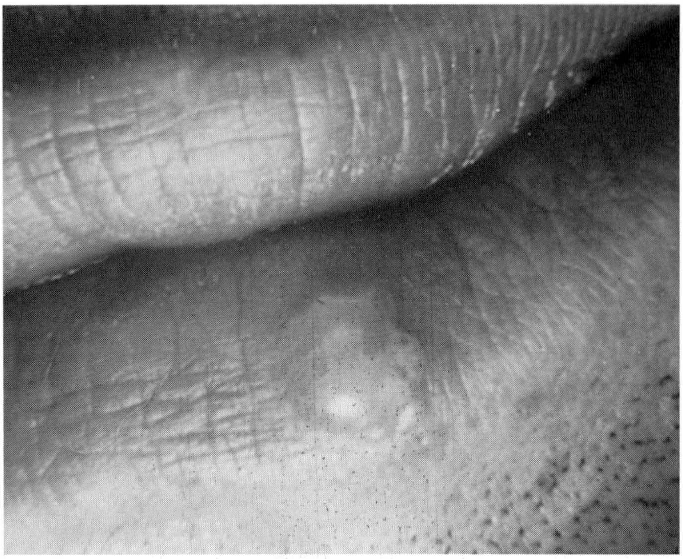

Figure 16–7. Herpetic vesicle of the lower lip.

PRIMARY HERPETIC STOMATITIS

Acute herpetic gingivostomatitis is the most common oral infection caused by the herpes simplex virus. This infection is actually systemic but has oral manifestations. The primary infection usually affects children under the age of 5. It is estimated that one third to one half the population of the United States experience recurrent herpetic lesions.[30]

Presentation

The virus invades the oral mucosa and after about 4 days' incubation presents initially as fever, cervical lymphadenitis, and oral pain. This is followed by vesicle formation on the tongue, buccal mucosa, and lips (Fig. 16–7). Occasionally, there are cutaneous lesions. The vesicles rupture to form ulcerations surrounded by erythematous halos. The gingivae become edematous, with bright red marginal erythema. The lesions last for 1 to 2 weeks.[31, 32]

Evaluation

The diagnosis of primary herpetic gingivostomatitis is usually based on the clinical findings. The virus can be isolated in animal or tissue culture. Tests used to assist in the diagnosis include immunologic and serologic tests. Intranuclear inclusion bodies can be seen on a smear. Viral antigens can be detected by immunofluorescence, and the virus can be typed with monoclonal antibodies and DNA hybridization techniques.[30, 33, 34]

Priorities

The disease is self-limiting, lasting 1 to 2 weeks. Supportive and symptomatic treatments are indicated. Of the antiviral drugs, only acyclovir is effective in treating severe cases and patients who are immunocompromised.

Outcomes

Most patients recover in 2 weeks. Many patients develop recurrent herpetic infections.

ORAL CAVITY HEMORRHAGE

Postsurgical hemorrhage after oral surgery may be immediate or delayed. Immediate hemorrhage is controlled at the time of surgery by the usual procedures of ligation of the bleeding vessel, electrocautery of the bleeding source, or packing and tamponade. Delayed bleeding may occur as early as the evening of the surgical procedure or as late as a week to 10 days later. The oral surgical procedures that most commonly result in postoperative bleeding are dental extractions (including wisdom teeth), biopsies, excisions, and orthognathic surgery. Serious postoperative bleeding has been reported with dental implant surgery as well.[35–39] A complete history should be obtained prior to the surgical procedure to identify any patient with a previous hemorrhagic episode or with a family history of a bleeding disorder. If the history is positive, appropriate laboratory studies should be obtained. A patient with a bleeding disorder should have a hematology consultation and preparation prior to surgery. In addition, a patient who is on a drug that may interfere with hemostasis, such as aspirin, anticoagulants, broad-spectrum antibiotics, alcohol, anticancer and cancer chemotherapeutic agents, may also have prolonged bleeding after surgery.

Postoperative bleeding is one of the most common complications of dentoalveolar surgery, but it is usually minor and self-limiting.

Bleeding complications appear to be more common with maxillary orthognathic surgery than with mandibular surgery. According to a review of the literature on mandibular surgery by Lanigan and colleagues, less than 1% of patients undergoing mandibular orthognathic surgery experience intraoperative or postoperative hemorrhage. Although no specific statistics are available, in 1986, in a survey reported by Lanigan's group of oral and maxillofacial surgeons about major vascular complications following orthognathic surgery, 800 surgeons out of 5,000 reported 39 cases of postoperative hemorrhage following maxillary surgery and 30 cases of intraoperative hemorrhage.[40, 41] In a small number of cases, the hemorrhage has been life threatening.

Presentation

A patient with postoperative hemorrhage resulting from a dentoalveolar procedure experiences welling of blood in the oral cavity if active bleeding is occurring. Postoperative oozing is normal and is often mistaken for postoperative bleeding. After maxillary osteotomy surgery, postoperative bleeding presents as brisk, bright-red bleeding from the nostrils and oral cavity. If the patient is in intermaxillary fixation, there should be concern about the airway. The vessels most commonly involved with hemorrhage after maxillary osteotomy are the internal maxillary artery, the posterior superior alveolar artery, and the greater palatine artery[42] (Fig. 16–8). If it

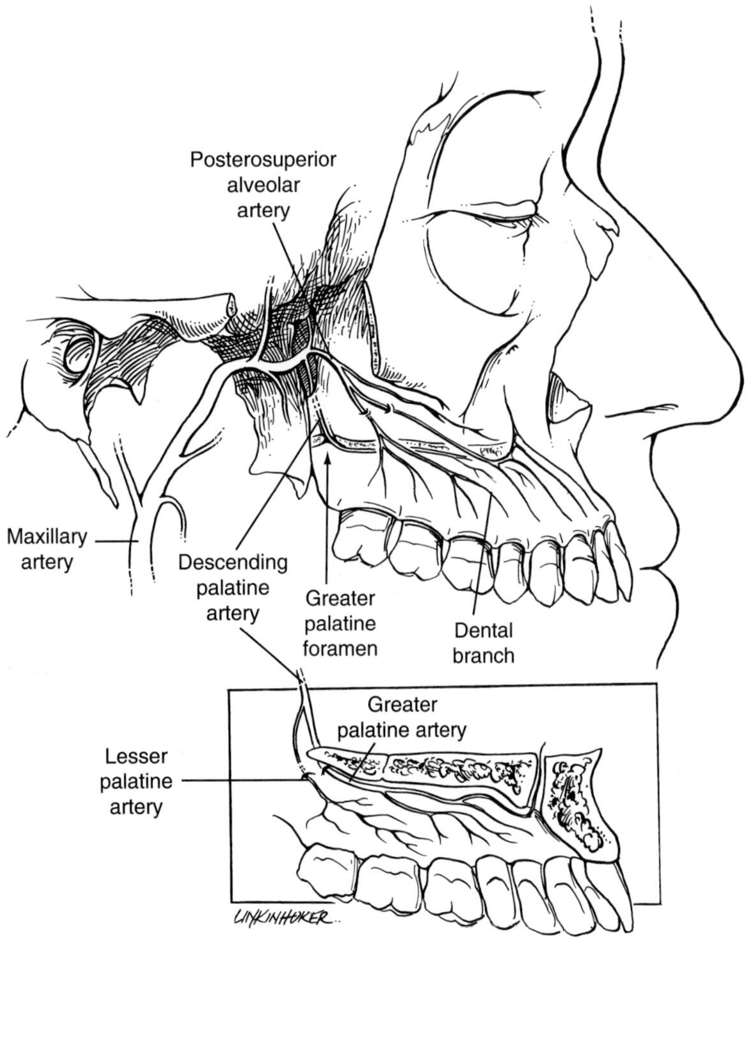

Figure 16–8. Blood vessels of the middle face.

becomes necessary to ligate or pack the bleeding vessels, it is, of course, necessary to take the patient back to the operating room to remove the internal rigid fixation. Although ligation of the external carotid artery may be considered in cases of extreme hemorrhage, because of collateral circulation, the procedure may not be as effective as desired. An angiogram and embolization of the bleeding vessel may also be considered. Postoperative hemorrhage after a mandibular osteotomy causes rapid swelling of the submandibular space, the buccal space, and the parapharyngeal spaces and potential airway embarrassment. The vessels most commonly involved in hemorrhage after mandibular osteotomy are the masseteric artery, the inferior alveolar artery, the posterior facial vein, and the anterior facial artery. External ligation can be accomplished on the last two arteries. Bleeding from the masseteric artery is usually controllable with packing. Reexploration of the surgical site is necessary to locate and ligate the inferior alveolar artery.

Evaluation

Good suction and an adequate light source are essential to evaluate a patient with bleeding that occurs after an oral or maxillofacial surgical procedure. The surgical site of the tooth extraction or biopsy should be clearly observed. Gauze packing may be used to put pressure on the site, which helps to identify the source of the bleeding. If the patient is immobilized, the intermaxillary fixation should be removed. The patient's physical status should be determined, and appropriate laboratory studies may be ordered—hematocrit or hemoglobin, prothrombin time, and partial thromboplastin time. If abnormal results are found, steps should be taken to correct these deficiencies, and hematology consultation should be obtained.[43]

Priorities

For postoperative bleeding after a dentoalveolar procedure, hemostatic agents such as oxidized cellulose, activated bovine collagen, or topical thrombin can be used to pack the wound and control the bleeding. Careful suturing of the surgical site to maintain the hemostatic packing is often needed.

For bleeding following maxillary surgery, vasoconstrictors can be used to decongest the nose and help in the evaluation of the bleeding. Local anesthetic injections in the nose and around the greater palatine foramen may also be helpful in controlling postoperative bleeding. Minor bleeding after maxillary surgery may sometimes be treated with only bed rest. Anterior and posterior nasal packing or even surgical exploration of the surgical site with direct ligation or packing of the bleeding source may be necessary. An angiogram can be used to identify the source of the bleeding and may include embolization of the specific vessel[44, 45] (Fig. 16–9). In extreme cases, ligation of the external carotid artery should be considered.

Bleeding after a mandibular procedure can be controlled by packing the medial or lateral mandible, by occluding the bleeding vessel with a clamp, ligature, or vascular staple, or by in-

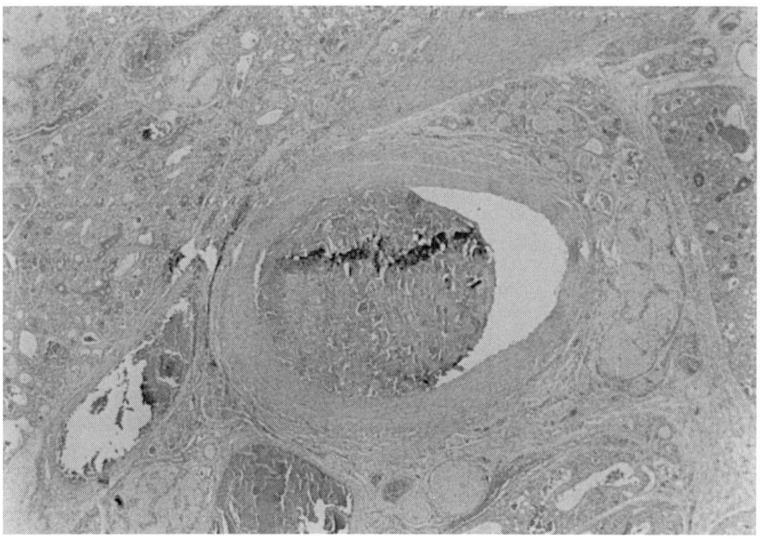

Figure 16–9. Photomicrograph of embolization of blood vessel with bead.

jecting local anesthetic with 1:100,000 epinephrine into the vessel wall. Extraoral dissection to isolate and control the bleeding is seldom necessary.

DENTOALVEOLAR INJURIES

Traumatic injuries to teeth and the dentoalveolar processes are very common and usually occur between the ages of 8 and 11. In the general population, there has been a reported 5.0% incidence of dentoalveolar injury in adults and a 1.3% incidence in children. The maxillary anterior dentition is most prone to injury at any age. Injuries include partial and complete avulsion of a tooth or teeth, fracture of the coronal portion of a tooth, fracture of the root portion of a tooth, and fracture of the alveolus containing a tooth or teeth.[46, 47] Most reports on the incidence of facial fractures conclude that children represent less than 5% of all cases, but Carroll and coworkers found that children represented 23% of all cases if dentoalveolar injuries were included.[48] In children, the most common causes are falls and accidents that occur during sports or play as compared to adults in whom assaults and motor vehicle accidents account for most injuries to the orofacial region. As a result of trauma involving primary dentition, 10% of cases involve crown or root fractures, and 75% of cases result in the avulsion of the primary teeth. In trauma involving adult dentition, 39% of cases involve fracture of the crown or root of the teeth.[49]

Presentation

In the case of a partially avulsed tooth, the patient may present with bleeding around the gingival collar and with mobility of a tooth. There is tenderness on palpation of the tooth. Periapical x-ray may show a widening of the space between the tooth and the bone, the periodontal ligament space. If there has been complete tooth avulsion, the tooth is missing from the socket. Inquiry should be made to determine whether the patient or a family member has recovered the tooth. When a tooth has been fractured, a portion of the crown of the tooth may be cracked or missing. Examination of the crown of the tooth may reveal that the underlying dentin is exposed. In this case, the tooth may be sensitive to cold. If the root of the tooth is fractured, the tooth may appear mobile and tender. Periapical x-ray may show a fracture line in the root. If there is an alveolar fracture, palpation of the teeth in the affected segment causes movement of the segment as a unit. There may be ecchymosis of the surrounding mucosa. The teeth may be displaced in such a way as to interfere with occlusion, so the patient cannot close the teeth completely. An x-ray may show a fracture in the bone surrounding the segment.

Evaluation

A careful history and physical evaluation should be carried out in any patient who has sustained maxillofacial injuries. Care should be taken to ensure that there are no associated occult injuries. Knowing the details of the accident that caused the injury makes it easier to predict and confirm the presence of a maxillofacial injury as well as the probability of an associated injury. If a tooth has been completely avulsed and not recovered, consideration should be given to the possibility of aspiration of the tooth and appropriate radiographic studies carried out.

A thorough examination of the oral cavity should be made. The tissues are inspected to determine the presence of lacerations, active bleeding, ecchymosis, or hematoma formation that might indicate the presence of a fracture of the underlying bone. The inspection should rule out the presence of foreign bodies in the oral cavity as well as in the nasal cavity and oropharynx. The ducts of the salivary glands should be evaluated for the presence of abrasions or lacerations. The examination of the teeth should note any missing or fractured teeth and the presence of mobility of individual teeth or segments of teeth. The positions of the teeth should be evaluated to be sure a tooth or group of teeth has not been displaced from its normal position in the dental arch. The patient's occlusion should be evaluated for changes from normal occlusion prior to the accident. This can be accomplished by simply asking if the patient's bite feels normal or changed. The teeth should be percussed with the end of an examining mirror. Tenderness of a tooth without other evidence of pathology may indicate an injury to the crown or root of the tooth. Panographic x-rays and periapical x-rays are the best means of evaluating the dentoalveolar structures radiographically.[50, 51]

Priorities

The management of dentoalveolar injuries follows the same principles as the management of other traumatic injuries. The maintenance of an adequate airway and the control of any hemorrhage are the immediate emergency measures that apply to every patient with a facial injury.

With respect to the dentition, the next important consideration should be teeth that have been completely avulsed and recovered. A parent or patient who calls the office or the emergency department and reports that a tooth has been avulsed should be told to carefully and gently rinse the tooth of gross contamination in water and immediately place the tooth into the socket of the alveolus. The general rule is that the longer the tooth is out of the mouth, the less likely the reimplantation is to be successful. The second best action is to place the tooth into a milk solution and bring the patient and the tooth immediately to the office or the emergency department. When the patient arrives, the tooth should be gently cleaned of gross contamination and quickly placed into the socket and stabilized with bonded wires or an acrylic splint. Teeth that have been allowed to dry out or that have been out of the mouth for more than 3 hours have a very poor prognosis for successful reimplantation.

Alveolar fractures and teeth that have been displaced from their normal positions in the dental arch are manually repositioned, under local anesthesia, to normal alignment based on the occlusion and stabilized with bonded wires, arch bars, or acrylic splints.[50] Teeth that have undergone crown fractures or root fractures must be treated by a dentist.[52]

MAXILLARY AND MANDIBULAR FRACTURES

The goal in the treatment of maxillary and mandibular fractures is to restore the function of the maxilla and mandible and the strength and contour of the bones. The functions of the maxilla and mandible include mastication and speech. These functions require both normal range of motion of the jaws and normal functional occlusion of the teeth. To achieve these goals, maxillary and mandibular fractures must be reduced, fixed, and immobilized.

Reduction of a fracture refers to the realignment of the proximal and distal fragments of the fractured mandible or maxilla to the preinjury state. This may be done under direct visualization, as in an open reduction, or may be accomplished indirectly by means of a closed reduction in which palpation of the fracture, manipulation of the fracture, and the reestablishment of occlusion are used to guide the reduction.

To obtain bony union at the site of a fracture, the site must be stabilized to avoid motion. Fixation of jaw fractures resists forces that might displace or move the fracture. Direct fixation of the fracture is performed during an open reduction using a nonrigid, semirigid, or rigid technique. The nonrigid technique utilizes interosseous wires to fixate the fracture. This technique is also dependent upon interdental wiring (intermaxillary fixation) to reestablish the patient's occlusion. A miniplate with unicortical or bicortical screws provides semirigid fixation of the fracture site as these plates are usually somewhat flexible. This technique is most often used with intermaxillary fixation as well. Rigid fixation is accomplished by using compression bone plates with bicortical screws or by using lag screws. It is most often used in the treatment of mandibular fractures. With this technique, long-term intermaxillary fixation is often unnecessary, although interdental wires are used to reestablish occlusion before the bone plates are secured with bone screws. When a fracture is treated using a closed reduction, fixation of the fracture is accomplished using intermaxillary fixation to prevent the movement of the proximal and distal fragments. Occasionally, external pins are used as a method of indirect fixation of a fracture.

Once reduction and fixation of a fracture have been accomplished, sufficient immobilization time must be allowed for the consolidation and healing of the fractured bone. In 80% of patients treated by using closed reduction, 4 weeks of intermaxillary fixation provide sufficient healing of the fracture site that the patient can begin to function again. This period of immobilization varies depending on the age and health of the patient, the patient's compliance, and the presence of local inflammatory factors such as periodontal disease, tooth infection, and wound infection.

Presentation

Maxillary and mandibular fractures occur as a result of motor vehicle accidents, sports injuries, social altercations, and work and home accidents. A patient usually presents to the emergency department, dentist's office, or physician's office with a history of trauma to the head and neck region. If a jaw fracture is present, there is usually the complaint that the bite is "off," that the teeth do not come together as they had prior to the accident, and that chewing food is difficult. There may be pain at the site of the injury or at a distant site in the maxilla or mandible. In the case of a mandibular fracture, there may be a complaint of numbness of the lip and chin on one side (or on both sides if there is a bilateral fracture). This is because of injury to the inferior alveolar nerve that is located within the body of the mandible. A patient with a maxillary fracture sometimes complains of numbness of the upper lip and nose, which occurs because of injury to the infraorbital nerve. A patient may present with swelling of the face along the lower jaw line, in front of the ear, or at the midface. There is usually a degree of trismus. There may be ecchymosis in the floor of the mouth and the buccal vestibule in the area of the fracture if it is located in the body or symphysis of the mandible. Ecchymosis or laceration of the palate is sometimes present if there is a partial maxillary fracture or if the maxilla is comminuted. If a body or symphysis fracture is displaced, a step is noted between the teeth on either side of the fracture line (Fig. 16–10). There may also be a laceration in the gingiva. Bimanual palpation of the mandible shows movement around the fracture site. Movement of the entire maxilla or of segments of the maxilla may be noted with palpation. Observation may reveal malocclusion.

A fracture of the condylar neck or condylar head may cause a laceration in the external auditory meatus and result in bleeding from the ear. A condylar fracture forced through the roof of the glenoid fossa into the middle cranial fossa may cause bleeding in the mastoid region and result in a positive Battle's sign, ecchymosis behind the ear. Bilateral fracture of the mandible in the body region can result in posterior displacement of the anterior mandible and airway obstruction.

Evaluation

Maxillary and mandibular fractures are classified according to the location of the fracture on the mandible, whether it is displaced or nondisplaced, whether it is compound, simple, or comminuted, and whether it is favorable or unfavorable; for example, a patient might have a displaced, compound fracture of the right angle of the mandible.

Mandibular fractures are located in the following regions, as defined by Kelly and Harrigan (Fig. 16–11). (1) A condylar process fracture extends from the sigmoid notch between the coronoid process and condyle to the posterior border of the ramus of the mandible. (2) A ramus fracture extends horizontally from the anterior to the posterior border of the ramus of the mandible or vertically from the sigmoid notch to the inferior border of the mandible. (3) An angle fracture is located posterior to the second molar tooth. It extends from a point along the curve that forms at the junction of the body and the ramus of the mandible in the retromolar area to a point along the curve that forms from the junction to the inferior border of the body of the mandible and the posterior border of the ramus of the mandible. (4) A body fracture occurs in the tooth-bearing portion of the mandible, extending from the cuspid area posterior to the second molar and from the

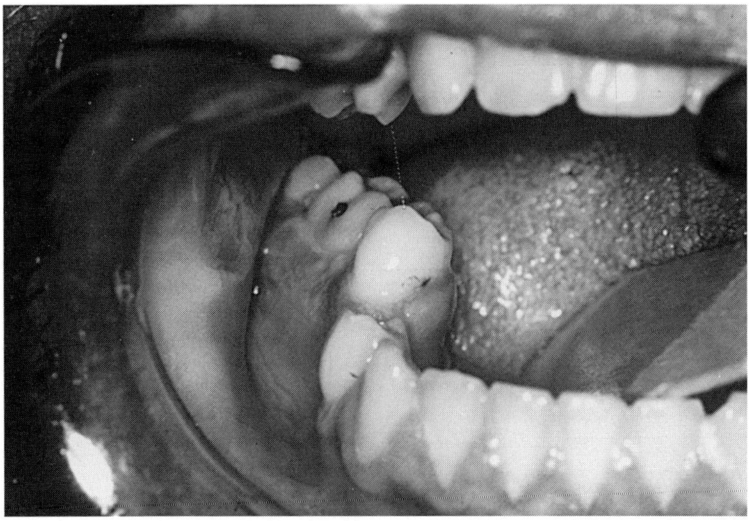

Figure 16–10. Mandibular body fracture with step deformity.

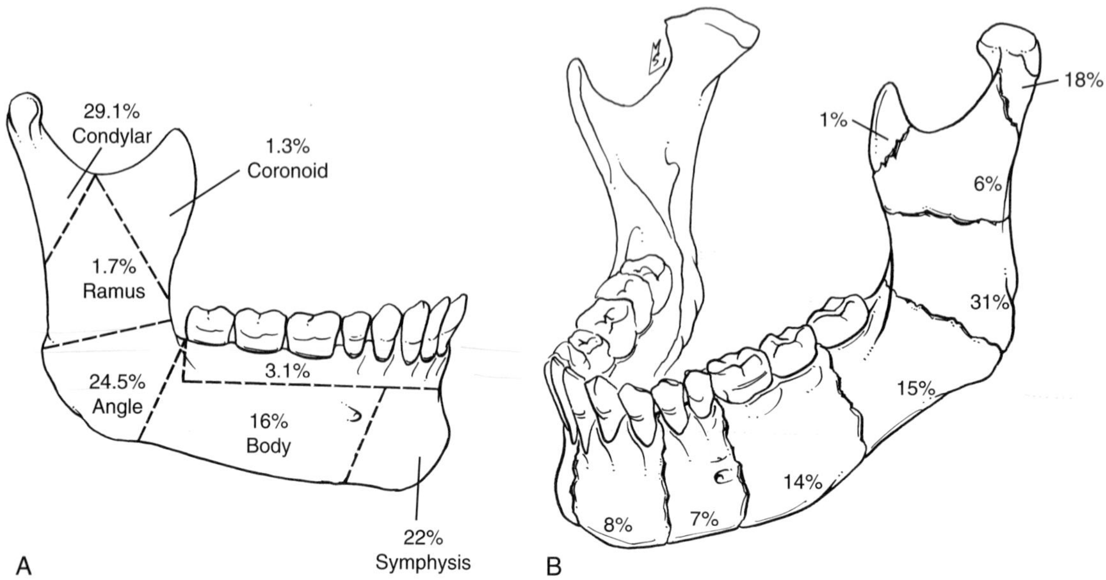

Figure 16–11A and B. The most common locations of mandibular fractures. (Adapted from Olson RA et al. J Oral Maxillofac Surg 1982; 40:23.)

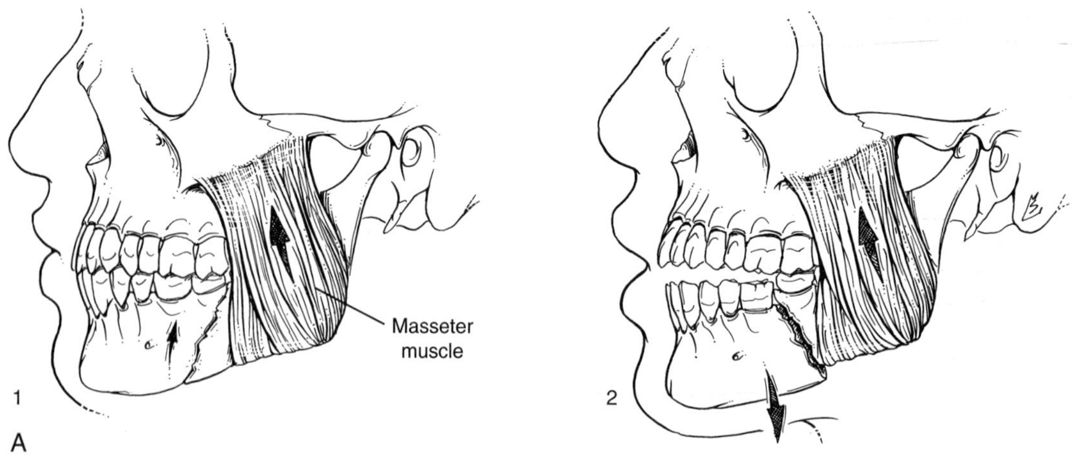

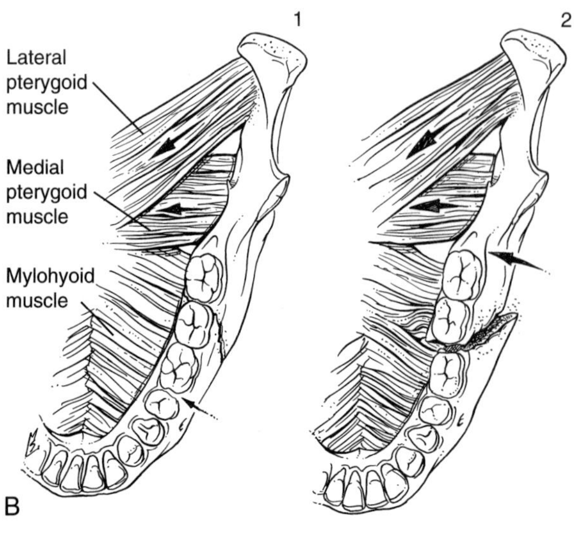

Figure 16–12A. Lateral view of a mandibular fracture. 1: A favorable fracture; the pull of the masseter muscle reduces the fracture. 2: An unfavorable fracture; the pull of the masseter muscle displaces the fracture.

Figure 16–12B. Axial view of a mandibular fracture. 1: A favorable fracture; the pull of the lateral pterygoid, medial pterygoid, and mylohyoid muscles reduces the fracture. 2: An unfavorable fracture; the pull of lateral pterygoid, medial pterygoid, and mylohyoid muscles displaces the fracture.

alveolar border to the inferior border of the mandible. (5) A symphysis fracture is located between the cuspids on either side, extending from the alveolar border to the inferior border of the mandible.

The most common location of a fracture of the mandible is the body, followed by the angle and the condylar neck. Fractures of the mandible represent approximately half of all facial fractures, and approximately 20% of patients with mandibular fractures have other, associated fractures of the facial skeleton. About 10% of patients with mandibular fractures have other injuries outside of the maxillofacial area.

A displaced fracture occurs when the continuity of the bone is disturbed and the proximal and distal fragments have moved out of alignment with each other. The fracture is defined as simple when there is no communication with the exterior, either the oral cavity or the skin surface. Condylar neck fractures, coronoid process fractures, and ramus fractures are usually simple fractures. All fractures that communicate with a laceration on the skin surface of the head and neck region are compound fractures. Because the teeth communicate with the oral cavity through the periodontal ligament space, a fracture of the body or symphysis of the mandible, where teeth are present, is a compound fracture. An angle fracture may or may not be compound, depending on the presence of a third molar and its relationship to the oral cavity. A comminuted fracture is one in which the fracture has created multiple fragments of bone at the fracture site.

Mandibular fractures are favorable when the line of the fracture and the pulling force of the attached muscles tend to reduce the fracture (Fig. 16–12*A* and *B*).

Bimanual palpation of the mandible usually helps to determine the presence and location of a mandibular fracture. The thumb of each gloved hand is placed on the occlusal surface of the teeth on either side of the suspected fracture site. The fingers of each hand are placed on the inferior border of the mandible. The mandible is then manipulated while the teeth are observed for movement. Independent movement between the teeth, along with pain, indicates the probable presence of a mandibular fracture. The best radiographic evaluation of a mandibular fracture can be obtained with a panographic x-ray, which generally shows the entire mandible in fine detail.[53] If a panograph is not available, right and left lateral oblique and posteroanterior views of the mandible provide most of the information needed to diagnose a mandibular fracture. A

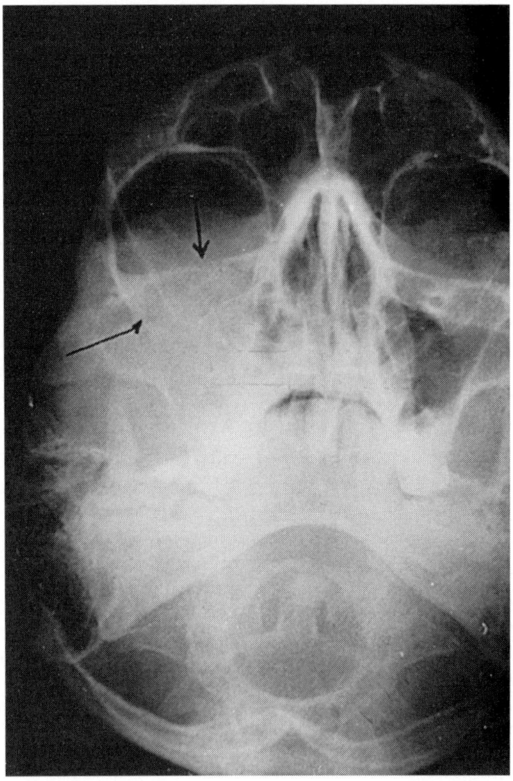

Figure 16–13. A Waters' view of a right zygoma fracture with maxillary sinus opacification.

modified Towne's view is helpful in determining the presence of a condylar neck or condylar head fracture. A CT scan is also useful in evaluating a mandibular fracture but can sometimes be confusing without three-dimensional reconstruction. The best method of imaging a maxillary fracture is a CT scan, as it can be difficult to diagnose based on conventional x-rays[54] (Fig. 16–13). Opacification of the maxillary sinus in a patient with midface trauma should raise suspicion of a maxillary fracture.

Priorities

Any patient presenting with trauma to the head and neck region must be completely evaluated. The provider of emergency care should not focus on the facial injury until other, more critical problems have been ruled out. Facial fractures are rarely fatal. According to the advanced trauma life support protocol, the first priority is the airway. Any obstruction of the airway must be immediately corrected and a patent airway maintained. Endotracheal intubation or tracheotomy should be performed if needed. Once an airway has been established, the vital signs should be obtained. Blood loss is the next consideration. Usually the sources of significant blood loss are injuries other than facial injuries. Critical injuries such as intracranial trauma, chest trauma, abdominal trauma, spinal trauma and other bone trauma must be identified so that treatment can be prioritized.[55–57]

Once the patient has been stabilized and more critical injuries have been attended to, the treatment of the maxillary or mandibular fracture should begin. The initial treatment should be aimed at controlling bleeding and obtaining temporary immobilization of the fracture until definitive treatment can be performed. Bleeding can be controlled by administering local anesthesia with a vasoconstrictor into the area of bleeding or by packing the wound with gauze or with a hemostatic agent such as activated collagen or oxidized cellulose. Temporary immobilization can be obtained by using a Barton-type bandage (Fig. 16–14), Ivy loop wires on the teeth (Fig. 16–15), or bone screws designed for temporary immobilization.[58, 59] Repair of lacerations of the mucosa and skin should be delayed until the jaw fracture

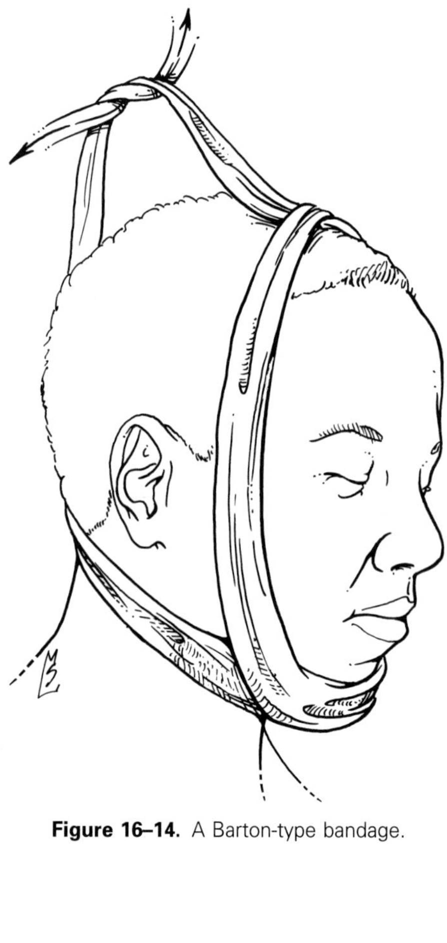

Figure 16–14. A Barton-type bandage.

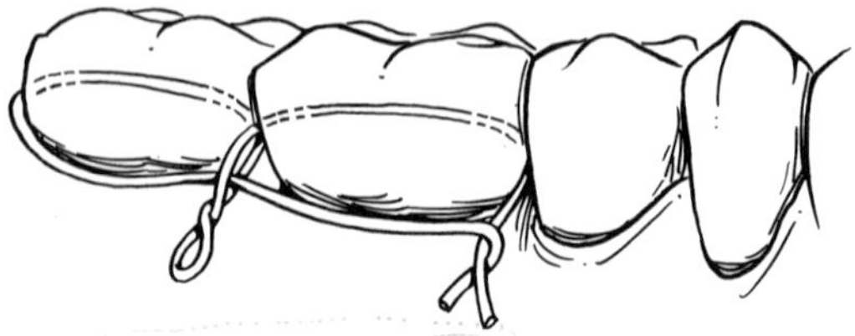

Figure 16–15. Ivy-loop wiring.

has been reduced, if the reduction is to be performed in the next few hours; otherwise, the wounds should be temporarily closed. Careful cosmetic closure of lacerations of the face prior to the reduction of a jaw fracture may result in disruption of the closure during the reduction of the fracture. Although early reduction of a fracture is recommended for patient comfort and reduction in the risk for postoperative infection, definitive treatment of a fracture can be delayed if other medical problems must be addressed first. Reduction of a maxillary or mandibular fracture can be delayed for 7 to 10 days without significantly complicating the surgery necessary to perform a successful reduction. The patient should be in some form of temporary immobilization during this delay.[60–62]

MANDIBULAR DISLOCATION

The mandibular condyle has two movements within the temporomandibular joint. First, the condyle rotates during the beginning of the opening movement. Second, the condyle translates along the articular eminence of the temporal bone in an anterior and inferior direction until it reaches the inferior aspect of the articular eminence.

Sometimes a patient exhibits hypermobility of the temporomandibular joint. Such hypermobility may be limited to hypertranslation whereby the condyle moves anteriorly and superiorly to the articular eminence or there may be subluxation or partial dislocation of the mandibular condyle out of the fossa, in which the condyle, during maximum opening, is anterior to the articular eminence, but the patient is able to close the mouth only after it has been caught open for a moment. In a subluxation, the patient is usually able to self-manipulate the jaw so it closes, reducing the joint spontaneously after it has been temporarily stuck in the open position. In a complete dislocation, the condyle is anterior to the articular eminence, and the patient is unable to reduce the joint and close the jaw. This is also referred to as an open lock.

Hypermobility is commonly found, and it accounts for the large number of cases of joint noise or joint symptoms. It is estimated that approximately 70% of the asymptomatic population have some form of hypermobility. The highest incidence occurs in females between the ages of 21 and 30. Complete dislocation of the joint is unusual.[63]

Presentation

In acute complete dislocation, it is important to obtain a careful history from the patient, including whether a causative event occurred such as mandibular trauma or a wide yawn. The duration of dislocation is an important prognostic factor. A patient whose jaw has been dislocated for many hours sometimes requires general anesthesia and open procedures to reduce the dislocation. A patient may have a neurologic or musculoskeletal disease such as a seizure disorder or a disorder of the basal ganglia that can cause acute and chronic dislocation of the mandible. Certain drugs that cause extrapyramidal reactions such as phenothiazines and some psychotropic drugs can be causative factors.

A patient with complete dislocation of the temporomandibular joint usually presents to the office or the emergency department in a great deal of pain and in an anxious state. This often prevents spontaneous reduction of the dislocation. Complete dislocation is caused by a combination of an overextension of the temporomandibular joint, as in yawning or wide opening, and an abnormal contraction of the protractor and elevator muscles of the mandible. The lateral pterygoid muscles, which protract the mandible, fail to relax when the condyle reaches the most anteroinferior location along the articular eminence. At the same time, the masseter, medial pterygoid, and temporalis muscles that elevate the mandible prematurely contract. This abnormal contraction of the muscles of mastication forces the mandibular condyle into the infratemporal fossa anterior to the articular eminence.

The resulting trauma to the capsule of the temporomandibular joint and to the ligaments supporting the joint results in severe pain. In bilateral dislocation, the patient is unable to voluntarily close the jaw completely and protrudes the jaw forward; occlusion occurs only on the posterior teeth. This is referred to as an open lock. Bilateral dislocation of the mandible is more common, but unilateral dislocations do occur. A patient with a unilateral dislocation presents with an anterior open lock, with the jaw deviated toward the contralateral side. The range of motion of the jaw is restricted and the patient may exhibit excessive salivation. There is a depression in the preauricular area anterior to the tragus. Palpation and radiographs show the condyle to be located anterior to the articular eminence, and the coronoid process is inferior to the zygomatic arch (Fig. 16–16).[64]

Priorities

Rapid recognition and early reduction of complete mandibular dislocations are important in order to prevent the need for complex surgical treatment of the dislocation and to avoid postreduction complications. An acute dislocation is treated by manually repositioning the condyle

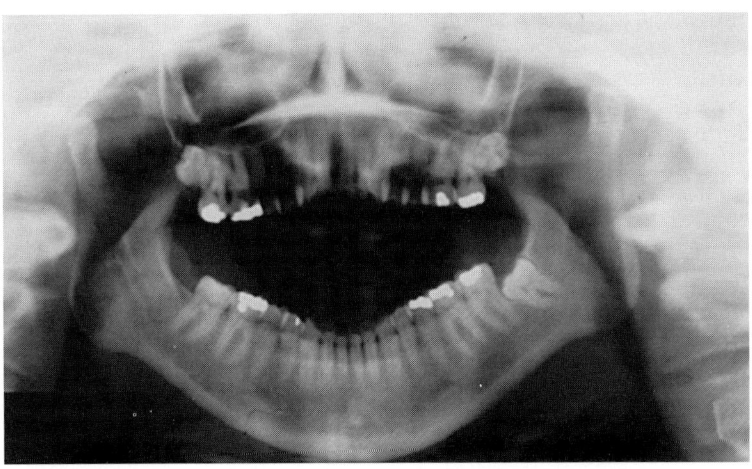

Figure 16–16. Panographic x-ray of bilateral mandibular dislocation.

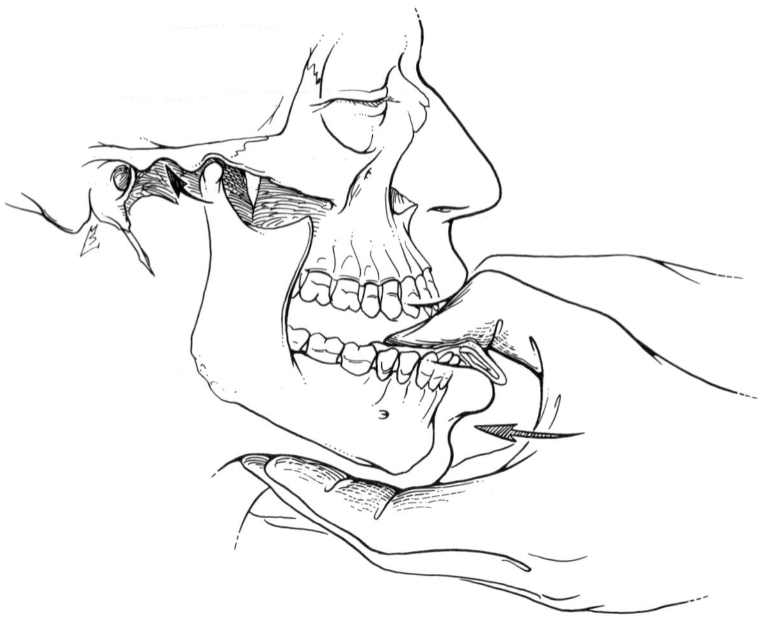

Figure 16–17. Bimanual reduction of mandibular dislocation.

into the glenoid fossa. Pain and the splinting of surrounding muscles can make this procedure difficult; sedation with medications such as benzodiazepams and local anesthetic injections may be necessary to relax the muscles.

Reduction is best accomplished with the patient sitting upright and the back supported. The surgeon is positioned in front of the patient. The surgeon places the thumbs lateral to the posterior molar teeth. The thumbs may be placed on the teeth, but care should be taken to protect the thumbs with gauze to prevent injury from accidental biting when the jaw reduces. The index and middle fingers are placed at the inferior border of the mandible anterior to the mandibular notch. The posterior mandible is depressed inferiorly with the thumbs as the chin is elevated anteriorly with the fingers. This moves the condyles inferior to the articular eminence and allows the surgeon to manipulate the condyles posteriorly into the glenoid fossas. It is usually easier to reduce one side at a time rather than attempt to reduce a bilateral dislocation simultaneously (Fig. 16–17).

If a dislocation has occurred more than a few hours earlier, it may not be possible to reduce the joints without the use of sedation and local anesthesia or even of general anesthesia in the operating room. Light sedation using 1 to 3 mg of midazolam or 5 to 10 mg of diazepam are slowly administered intravenously. Local anesthetic (2% lidocaine) is injected into the masseter and medial pterygoid muscles. The combination of the sedative drugs and the local anesthesia relaxes the muscles and allows the mandible to be reduced. If reduction cannot be accomplished with sedation and local anesthesia, general anesthesia in the operating room may be necessary. Rarely, an open surgical procedure is necessary to accomplish reduction.[65]

Outcomes

After the reduction of an acute dislocation of the mandible, a patient experiences pain in the muscles and the joints. Symptomatic treatment includes physical therapy, analgesia with nonsteroidal anti-inflammatory drugs, muscle relaxants, and sometimes intra-articular steroid injections. Recurrent dislocation of the mandible is common. A patient who develops chronic dislocation of the jaw may require surgical intervention to prevent additional episodes of dislocation.

REFERENCES

1. Kaldahl WB et al. Long-term evaluation of periodontal therapy. I: Response to four therapeutic modalities. J Periodontol 1996; 67:93–102.
2. Smith RG, Davies RM. Acute lateral periodontal abscesses. Br Dental J 1986; 161:176–178.
3. Leone SA et al. Correlation of acute pericoronitis and the position of the mandibular third molar. Oral Surg 1986; 62:245–250.
4. Mombelli A et al. Suspected periodontopathogens in erupting third molar sites of periodontally healthy individuals. J Clin Periodontol 1990; 17:48.
5. Blakey GH et al. Clinical/biological outcomes of treat-

ment for pericoronitis. J Oral Maxillofac Surg 1996; 54:1150–1160.
6. Ferrera PC et al. Uncommon complications of odontogenic infections [Review]. Am J Emerg Med 1996; 14:317–322.
7. Berge TI. Incidence of infections requiring hospitalization associated with partially erupted third molars. Acta Odontol Scand 1996; 54:309–313.
8. Ferrera PC, Busino LJ, Snyder HS. Uncommon complications of odontogenic infections. Am J Emerg Med 1996; 14:317–322.
9. Headley DB, Dolan KD. Infratemporal fossa abscess. Ann Otol Rhinol Laryngol 1991; 100:516–517.
10. Held JL et al. Cutaneous sinus of dental origin: a diagnosis requiring clinical and radiologic correlation. Cutis 1989; 43:22–24.
11. Topazian RG, Goldberg MH, eds. Oral and Maxillofacial Infections, 4th ed. Philadelphia, WB Saunders, 1987.
12. Sands T et al. Odontogenic infections. II: Microbiology, antibiotics and management. Oral Health, 1995; 85:11–23.
13. Sicher H, DuBrul EL, eds. Oral Anatomy, 5th ed. St. Louis, CV Mosby, 1970.
14. Regezi JA, Sciubba JJ. Oral Pathology: Clinical-Pathologic Correlations. Philadelphia, WB Saunders, 1989.
15. Comer RW et al. Dental emergencies: management by the primary care physician. Postgrad Med 1989; 85:63–77.
16. Heimdahl A, Nord CE. Treatment of orofacial infections of odontogenic origin. Scand J Infect Dis 1985; 45:101.
17. Gidley PW, Ghorayeb BY, Stiernberg CM. Contemporary management of deep neck space infections. Otolaryngol Head Neck Surg 1997; 116:16–22.
18. Peterson LJ et al. Contemporary Oral and Maxillofacial Surgery. St. Louis, CV Mosby, 1993.
19. Izumoto H et al. Successful utilization of the median sternotomy approach in the management of descending necrotizing mediastinitis: report of a case. Surg Today 1996; 26:286–288.
20. Thakar M, Thakar A. Odontogenic orbital cellulitis: report of a case and considerations on route of spread. Acta Ophthalmol Scand 1995; 73:470–471.
21. Rockoff, PR et al. Meningitis as a result of postextraction infection: report of a case. J Oral Surg 1972; 30:687–689.
22. Baddour HM, Durst NL, Tilson HB. Frontal lobe abscess of dental origin. Oral Surg 1979; 47:303–306.
23. Stamenkovic I, Lew PD. Early recognition of potentially fatal necrotizing fasciitis: the use of frozen-section biopsy. N Engl J Med 1984; 310:1689–1693.
24. Balcerak RJ, Sisto JM, Bosack RC. Cervicofacial necrotizing fasciitis: report of three cases and literature review. J Oral Maxillofac Surg 1988; 46:450–459.
25. Shindo ML, Nalbone VP, Dougherty WR. Necrotizing fasciitis of the face. Laryngoscope 1997; 107:107–109.
26. Haring JI. Case 1: acute necrotizing ulcerative gingivitis. RDH 1995; 15:13, 42.
27. Melnick SL et al. Epidemiology of acute necrotizing ulcerative gingivitis. Epidemiol Rev 1988; 10:191–211.
28. SanGiacomo TR et al. Progressive osseous destruction as a complication of HIV-periodontitis. Oral Surg 1990; 70:476–479.
29. Barr CE. Periodontal problems related to HIV-1 infection. Adv Dent Res 1995; 9:147–151.
30. Miller CS, Redding SW. Diagnosis and management of orofacial herpes simplex virus infections. Dent Clin North Am 1992; 36:879–895.
31. Kuzushima K et al. Clinical manifestations of primary herpes simplex virus type 1 infection in a closed community. Pediatrics 1991; 87:152–158.
32. Main DM. Acute herpetic stomatitis: referrals to Leeds Dental Hospital 1978–1987. Br Dent J 1989; 166:14–16.
33. Fox SF et al. Evaluation of a monoclonal antibody typing system for herpes simplex virus. Oral Surg 1987; 64:165–170.
34. Burns JC. Diagnostic methods for herpes simplex infection: a review. Oral Surg 1980; 50:346–349.
35. Engel JD, Supancic JS, Davis LF. Arteriovenous malformation of the mandible: life-threatening complications during tooth extraction. J Am Dent Assoc 1995; 126:237–242.
36. de Boer MP et al. Complications after mandibular third molar extraction. Quintessence Int 1995; 26:779–784.
37. Krepler K, Wedrich A, Schranz R. Intraocular hemorrhage associated with dental implant surgery. Am J Ophthalmol 1996; 122:745–746.
38. ten Bruggenkate CM et al. Hemorrhage of the floor of the mouth resulting from lingual perforation during implant placement: a clinical report. Int J Oral Maxillofac Implants 1993; 8:329–234.
39. Laboda G. Life-threatening hemorrhage after placement of an endosseous implant: report of three cases. J Am Dent Assoc 1990; 121:599–600.
40. Lanigan DT, Hey J, West RA. Major vascular complications of orthognathic surgery: hemorrhage associated with Le Fort I osteotomies. J Oral Maxillofac Surg 1990; 48:561–573.
41. Lanigan DT, Hey J, West RA. Hemorrhage following mandibular osteotomies: a report of 21 cases. J Oral Maxillofac Surg 1991; 49:713–724.
42. Tiner BD, van Sickels JE, Schmitz JP. Life-threatening, delayed hemorrhage after Le Fort I osteotomy requiring intervention: report of two cases. J Oral Maxillofac Surg 1997; 55:91–93.
43. Humphries JE, Baker RC. Occult hemophilia: prolonged bleeding follows extraction. J Am Dent Assoc 1992; 123:69–70.
44. Solomons NB, Blumgart R. Severe late-onset epistaxis following Le Fort I osteotomy: angiographic localization and embolization. J Laryngol Otol 1988; 102:260–263.
45. Lustbader DP et al. The use of percutaneous transcatheter embolization to control postoperative bleeding following Le Fort I osteotomy: report of three cases. J Oral Maxillofac Surg 1991; 49:426–431.
46. Luz JG, Di Mase F. Incidence of dentoalveolar injuries in hospital emergency room patients. Endodon Dent Traumatol 1994; 10:188–190.
47. Bader JD, Martin JA. Preliminary estimates of the incidence and consequences of tooth fracture. J Am Dent Assoc 1995; 126:1650–1654.
48. Carroll MJ, Hill CM, Mason DA. Facial fractures in children. Br Dent J 1987; 163:23–26.
49. Glendor U et al. Incidence of traumatic tooth injuries in children and adolescents in the county of Vastmanland, Sweden. Swed Dent J 1996; 20:15–28.
50. Stapleford RG. The management of dentoalveolar trauma—a review. J Can Dent Assoc 1990; 56:39–41.
51. Bakland LK, Milledge T. Treatment of crown fractures. J Calif Dent Assoc 1996; 24:45–50.
52. de Blanco LP. Treatment of crown fractures with pulp exposure. Oral Surg 1996; 82:564–568.
53. Chiles JL, Gores RJ. Anatomic interpretation of the orthopantomogram. Oral Surg 1973; 35:564–574.
54. Fox LA, et al. Diagnostic performance of CT, MPR

and 3DCT imaging in maxillofacial trauma. Comput Med Imaging Graph 1995; 19:385–395.
55. Comer RW et al. Oral trauma: emergency care of lacerations, fractures, and burns. Postgrad Med 1989; 85:34–41.
56. Peterson LJ, ed. Principles of Oral and Maxillofacial Surgery. Philadelphia, JB Lippincott, 1992.
57. Williams JL, ed. Rowe and Williams' Maxillofacial Injuries, 2nd ed. Edinburgh, Churchill Livingstone, 1994.
58. Divis BO. DIMAC wires: a new approach to interdental immobilization in the 1990s. J Otolaryngol 1992; 21:238–240.
59. Busch RF, Prunes F. Intermaxillary fixation with intraoral cortical bone screws. Laryngoscope 1991; 101:1336–1338.
60. Onishi K, Maruyama Y. Simple intermaxillary fixation for maxillomandibular osteosynthesis. J Craniofac Surg 1996; 7:170–172.
61. Oikarinen KS. Clinical management of injuries to the maxilla, mandible, and alveolus. Dent Clin North Am 1995; 39:113–131.
62. Siegert R, Weerda H. Immobilization of fractures of the facial skeleton: past and present. Facial Plast Surg 7:137–151.
63. Luz JGC, Oliveira NG. Incidence of temporomandibular disorders in patients seen at a hospital emergency room. J Oral Rehabil 1994; 21:349.
64. Nevakari K. Elapsiopraearticularis of the temporomandibular joint. Acta Odontol Scand. 1960; 18:123–170.
65. Merrill RG. Mandibular dislocation. In Keith DA, ed. Surgery of the Temporomandibular Joint. Boston, Blackwell Scientific, 1988.

CHAPTER 17

Nasal Emergencies

Michelle Marie Cullen, MD
Donald A. Leopold, MD

EPISTAXIS

Epistaxis, from the Greek word *epi*, meaning on, and *stazo*, to fall in drops, is defined as bleeding from the nose. The severity of epistaxis ranges from mild, anterior bleeding that resolves spontaneously to profuse, posterior bleeding with hypotension, anemia, and airway compromise that leads to death. An organized, systematic approach to and swift delivery of treatment contribute to the successful management of this condition.

Epistaxis is a common malady. Approximately 7% to 14% of the U.S. population experience at least one nosebleed. Of these, 90% originate from the anterior septum; the remainder originate from the lateral wall or the posterior septum.

All persons are at increased risk for developing epistaxis in the winter months because of lower humidity. The most commonly affected group during this time of year is males in the fifth decade of life. Certain medical conditions also pose increased risk for epistaxis (Table 17–1).

BOX 17–1

Conditions that Raise the Risk of Aspiration Due to Epistaxis

Neurologic disease (cerebral palsy, mental retardation, cranial nerve defects, etc.)
Pulmonary disease
Elderly patients
Immunocompromised patients

Some patients are at increased risk for aspiration of blood during an episode of epistaxis (Box 17–1). During history taking and physical examination, these conditions should be considered and appropriate airway precautions taken.

Presentation

The diagnosis of epistaxis is usually a simple one: the history of or finding of bleeding from the nose. In the case of anterior epistaxis, this is certainly true. However, posterior bleeding can occur insidiously and continue slowly for hours without the patient's knowledge. Significant blood loss can occur in this setting. These patients can present obtunded or in shock, or may die before receiving medical attention.

When treating any patient with epistaxis, it is of primary importance to evaluate and treat life-threatening conditions first. After stabilizing the patient's airway, breathing, circulation (ABCs), and bleeding, attention can be focused on the problem of epistaxis. Questions are usually asked while simultaneously obtaining hemostasis. Important information includes the amount, frequency, location, cause, and source (arterial or venous) of the bleeding. It is helpful to ask the patient to attempt to quantify how much bleeding has occurred with each episode (a teaspoon, tablespoon, cup, half gallon), how many episodes have occurred, how long the episodes last, and what measures stop the bleeding. Other important information to elicit includes factors that may be associated with the start of bleeding, the color of the blood (dark red or bright red), whether the blood runs out

Table 17–1. *Causes of Epistaxis*

Local Causes	Systemic Causes
Trauma • Dry air • Facial fracture • Nasal surgery • Digital trauma • Foreign body • Chemical and caustic agents • Cocaine Structural • Septal deviation • Septal perforation • Nasal mucosal adhesions Neoplasms • Polyps • Arteriovenous malformation, hemangioma • Juvenile nasopharyngeal angiofibroma • Encephalocele • Inverting papilloma • Papilloma • Nasopharyngeal carcinoma (World Health Organization types 1, 2, and 3) • Adenocarcinoma • Squamous cell carcinoma Inflammatory • Pyogenic granuloma • Granulomatous diseases (Wegener's granulomatosis, tuberculosis, sarcoidosis, syphilis, polymorphic reticulosis) • Sinusitis (acute and chronic; fungal, viral, bacterial, parasitic) • Rhinitis (allergic, atrophic) • Rheumatic fever • Diphtheria	Blood Dyscrasias • Platelet disorders (idiopathic thrombocytopenic purpura, von Willebrand's disease, Glanzmann's thrombasthenia) • Coagulation defects (hemophilia A and B) • Anticoagulant drugs (heparin, Coumadin, aspirin, nonsteroidal anti-inflammatory drugs) • Medical conditions that interfere with clotting mechanisms (liver disease, renal disease, polycythemia vera, leukemia, multiple myeloma, thrombocytopenia due to chemotherapy, vitamin A, D, E, K deficiencies) Hereditary • Hereditary hemorrhagic telangiectasia (Osler-Weber-Rendu disease) Other • Arteriosclerosis • Aging (atrophy of the nasal mucosa) • Vitamin C deficiency (poor wound healing) • Heavy metals (phosphorous, mercury, chromium) • Cardiovascular factors that increase venous pressure (congestive heart failure, mitral stenosis, coarctation of the aorta)

Note: Hypertension has *not* been shown to increase the incidence of epistaxis, but it is associated with prolonged bleeding and an increased amount of blood lost once bleeding begins.

of the nostrils or down the back of the throat, and if the bleeding occurs on the right or left side.

It is important to ask about the local, systemic, and related factors listed in Table 17–1. A thorough medical, surgical, social, family, and allergy history plus a medication list and a review of all systems produce these details.

The physical examination should focus initially on the ABCs, and the physician should continually reevaluate the stability of the patient. The general overall appearance of the patient can change from awake, alert, and stable to obtunded and in airway distress. Vital signs and a pulse oximetry check are important immediate steps to evaluate for hypertension, hypotension, tachycardia, and hypoxia.

Upon stabilizing the patient and the bleeding, a complete physical exam should be performed, with attention to the following details: sidedness of the bleeding (left or right); site of the bleeding (anterior, posterior, superior, or inferior); blood actively streaming down the posterior pharyngeal wall; or presence of nasal masses, septal spurs, septal perforation, nasal infection, nasal foreign body, or nasal granulomas. Other important physical details to survey include the presence of neck adenopathy, carotid bruits, jugulovenous distension, facial symmetry, facial tenderness, telangiectasias of the face and mucosal membranes, and signs of facial trauma or previous facial surgery. Attention should also be paid to evaluating the patient for the presence of hepatosplenomegaly, bruising of the extremities, overall neurologic status (including cranial nerves), the general ability of the patient to protect his or her airway, and the general cardiovascular and respiratory status of the patient (the ability to maintain oxygenation and tolerate a posterior nasal pack).

Evaluation

Initial laboratory evaluation should include a baseline hemoglobin and hematocrit (H&H) level, a platelet count, and a prothrombin time and partial thromboplastin time (PT/PTT). Even if a patient is not bleeding at the time of examination, it is helpful to have a baseline H& H against which to judge the amount of bleeding in past or future episodes. As previously stated, posterior bleeding can be insidious and a patient can lose a substantial amount of blood without realizing it. The patient's most recent H&H may have been done elsewhere and should be obtained and compared to the present result. It should also be noted that acute blood loss may not result in an immediate drop in hemoglobin, and that dehydration may result in a false-normal hemoglobin reading. In a situation involving moderate to severe bleeding, several additional blood tests are suggested (Box 17–2).

BOX 17-2

Suggested Blood Tests for Moderate to Severe Epistaxis

- Hemoglobin and hematocrit
- Type and cross or type and screen
- Prothrombin time and partial thromboplastin time
- Blood urea nitrogen and creatinine (to evaluate renal function and hydration)
- Liver function tests (to evaluate formation of clotting factors)
- Bleeding time (if a recurrent episode) or abnormal platelet count or prothrombin time and partial thromboplastin time
- Arterial blood gas and continuous pulse oximetry
- Electrocardiogram (if there is a history of heart disease, for baseline and to evaluate strain of hypoxia, hypotension, or hypertension and tachycardia on heart)

In general, the initial evaluation of epistaxis does not involve radiologic studies. A chest radiograph may be indicated if the patient is at risk for aspiration or has signs or symptoms of hypoxia. In special situations such as nasal masses and signs of infection, a facial computerized tomography (CT) scan may be indicated. In the case of juvenile nasopharyngeal angiofibroma, an angiogram and a magnetic resonance imaging (MRI) scan may be indicated as well. These tests are rarely necessary on an emergent basis and are performed after bleeding is under control and the patient stabilized. Lastly, a patient with a unilateral nasal mass should undergo a CT scan before biopsy unless a foreign body is clearly evident by history or physical exam. This is to avoid cerebrospinal fluid leakage or biopsy of herniated brain resulting from an unrecognized encephalocele.

Pathognomonic aspects of the history, physical examination, and workup in a case of epistaxis can indicate several rare conditions. Osler-Weber-Rendu disease presents as tiny, 1- to 3-mm, raised telangiectasias of the facial skin and mucosal membranes. The number and size of the telangiectasias worsen with age, and their presence in the gastrointestinal tract of these patients can cause life-threatening gastrointestinal bleeds. The severity of the bleeding in this condition is due to the lack of elastic tissue within the vessel walls of the telangiectasias.[1–3]

Encephalocele and mucocele can present as a widening of the nasal dorsum or periorbital bulge. Often juvenile nasopharyngeal angiofibroma has no signs or symptoms until the first severe posterior unilateral nosebleed, usually in a pubertal male. This condition can also be associated with fullness of the cheek or malar region, hypoesthesia of the second division of the trigeminal nerve, and infraorbital swelling. Cocaine abuse, although unfortunately not a rare condition, often presents as a septal perforation.

Priorities

The severity of epistaxis requiring intervention ranges from minor anterior bleeding, which resolves spontaneously, to profuse posterior bleeding with hypotension, anemia, and airway compromise leading to death. Swift delivery of treatment via an organized, systematic approach contributes to the successful management of this condition. Plans for initial emergency treatment of minor bleeding and of moderate to severe bleeding are outlined in Table 17–2.

An angiogram is indicated if rebleeding occurs following surgical treatment of epistaxis or previous embolization of epistaxis. It allows evaluation of the vessels that provide persistent flow to the bleeding site. Specialized hematology tests (for von Willebrand's factor, factor VIII, factor IX, platelet morphology, and a bone marrow biopsy) are appropriate if bleeding per-

Table 17–2. *Immediate Courses of Action for Epistaxis*

Minor Bleeding	Moderate or Severe Bleeding
• Stabilize airway, breathing, circulation • Heparin lock or IVF, send for CBC, PT/PTT • Equipment: head light, Frazier suction tube, Yankauer suction tube, tongue blades, bayonet forceps, 1 cm × 3 cm cotton neuropatties, nasal speculum, ½-inch × 72-in cotton ribbon, water soluble antibiotic gel, 10-mL Foley catheter, 0.5% phenylephrine, 1% lidocaine, 2% Pontocaine, or 4% cocaine, hemostat, Surgical, Gelfoam, or Avitene, silver nitrate sticks • Suction clots from nose or have patient blow nose; decongest nose with 0.5% phenylephrine • Anesthetize nose topically with 2% Pontocaine or 4% cocaine (spray, pledgets, or cotton) • Anesthetize nose locally with 1% to 2% lidocaine with 1:100,000 epinephrine to anterior nasal spine via sublabial injection or sphenopalatine vessels via greater palatine foramen or sphenopalatine foramen* • Identify site of bleeding (septum vs. lateral wall, anterior vs. posterior, superior vs. inferior) directly or with nasal endoscopy • Attempt to differentiate venous from arterial bleeding • Use chemical cautery; if it fails, use Avitene or anterior nasal packing • Control hypertension • Complete H&P, check labs • If bleed controlled, ambulate prior to D/C to check for rebleeding • May send patient home with anterior nasal pack; on oral antistaphylococcal antibiotics until packing is removed; stool softener and iron if necessary; no aspirin or NSAIDs; instructions for light activity, no nose blowing, no bending over, no straining; increase humidity; use normal saline drops in nose q 2 h • Follow-up in 2–5 days for nonabsorbable packing removal	• Stabilize airway, breathing, circulation • If bleeding is severe or patient cannot protect airway, consider intubation to protect airway • Suction airway, keep patient upright, place two largebore IVs and administer crystalloid • Continuous pulse oximetry and supplemental O_2 via nasal cannula in mouth • Control bleeding with posterior pack after suctioning nose • CBC, PT/PTT, LFTs, BUN/Cr, electrolytes, ABG, T&S, ECG, CXR if risk or suspicion of aspiration • Control hypertension • Complete H&P, check labs, correct abnormalities, transfuse if necessary • Monitor oxygen saturation and give all patients with posterior packing 40% supplemental oxygen • Admit; IVF, antistaphylococcal IV antibiotics, iron, continuous pulse oximetry, at least 4% O_2; monitor cardiac rhythm and oxygen saturation, baseline ECG; keep patient NPO; administer reversible narcotic if necessary • Repeat CBC in a.m.; recheck posterior pharyngeal wall for bleeding, check position of pack to avoid alar notching, soft palate and septal perforation • If no bleeding and H&H stable, advance to clear diet and remove or deflate pack on day 2–5 with aforementioned equipment bedside or take patient to treatment room • If patient rebleeds, repack and move on to surgical options, including cautery • If no bleeding after removal of posterior pack or surgical treatment, observe for at least 12 h, allow patient to ambulate • D/C home on 5–7 days of oral antistaphylococcal antibiotics, stool softener, and iron if necessary; no aspirin or NSAIDs; instructions for light activity, no nose blowing, no bending over, no straining; increase humidity; use normal saline drops in nose q 2 h

*Bleeding may cease due to injection of local anesthetic only.
ABG, arterial blood gas; BUN/Cr, blood urea nitrogen/creatinine levels; CBC, complete blood count; CXR, chest x-ray; ECG, electrocardiogram; LFTs, liver function tests; H&H, hemoglobin and hematocrit; H&P, history and physical examination; IV, intravenous; IVF, intravenous fluids; NPO, nothing by mouth; NSAIDs, nonsteroidal anti-inflammatory drugs; PT/PTT, prothrombin time/partial thromboplastin time; T&S, type and screen.

sists despite adequate therapy.[4] If examination of the nasal mucosa is suspicious for granulomatous disease, appropriate workup is indicated. Cardiac evaluation tests such as an echocardiogram may be indicated if jugulovenous distention, murmur, abnormal electrocardiogram, or carotid bruits are noted in order to investigate the cause of increased central venous pressure or the presence of atherosclerotic disease. The following consultation services may be appropriate in reference to the previously mentioned conditions associated with epistaxis or for the treatment of epistaxis: neuroradiology, hematology, oncology, internal medicine, rheumatology, or cardiology.

Following the immediate treatment and stabilization of a patient with epistaxis, (see Table 17–2), other therapeutic interventions may be necessary. These alternatives are indicated if initial treatment fails or is only partially successful or for long-term prevention of further episodes. Appropriate decisions regarding surgical or neuroradiologic treatment begin with a thorough understanding of the blood supply to the nose: how best to treat the nosebleed should be decided; then the other information gathered should be considered and a decision made as to whether that treatment is the best option for the patient). Therefore, a brief discussion of the blood supply to the nose and how it is involved in anterior and posterior epistaxis is presented and is followed by a list of nonoperative and operative interventions, in order of complexity.

ANTERIOR EPISTAXIS

Anterior epistaxis involves the nasal septum in 90% of cases. Because both the external carotid artery and the internal carotid artery supply the blood to the nose, it is important to decipher from where the bleeding originates. Superior bleeding originates from the anterior or posterior ethmoid arteries (the internal carotid artery). Anterior inferior bleeding originates from the septal branch of the facial artery, whereas posterior inferior bleeding originates from the sphenopalatine branch of the internal maxillary artery (the external carotid artery). It is imperative to make this distinction because the branches of the external carotid artery (the facial and internal maxillary arteries) can be safely embolized, but the branches of the internal carotid artery (the anterior and posterior ethmoid arteries) cannot be safely embolized because of the risk to the cerebral and ophthalmic circulation. Figure 17–1 demonstrates the blood supply to the septum; Figure 17–2 demonstrates the blood supply to the lateral nasal wall.

Embolization of the internal maxillary artery may be more appropriate for a patient not medically fit to undergo general anesthesia, for a patient not wishing to undergo general anesthesia, for a patient whose neurologic status must be monitored, and for a patient who has previously undergone failed surgical ligation.

Surgical ligation of the anterior or posterior ethmoid artery or the internal maxillary artery is appropriate for a patient with refractory bleeding who has failed conservative nonoperative measures and has no contraindications to general anesthesia. Ligation may also be attempted under local anesthesia with sedation after careful consideration of the patient, the nosebleed, and the general circumstances (for example, overall patient health, patient anxiety, airway control, amount of bleeding, patient condition, and surgical facilities).

Many nonoperative and operative interventions for anterior epistaxis exist. A brief discussion of those most often used is presented in order of complexity. The first nonoperative intervention for mild anterior epistaxis is usually chemical cautery. Silver nitrate is placed around the mucosa of the bleeding site as well as on it. Care is taken to avoid cauterizing the same area on the opposite septal mucosa so as to prevent a future septal perforation. Electrocautery may also be attempted in the office, utilizing the same principles. If cautery is unsuccessful or is impractical because of bleeding, anterior packing is usually the next nonoperative intervention. This can be performed with a variety of materials. Merocel ethmoid sponges or 1/2-inch gauze ribbon may be used[5] and should be coated with an antistaphylococcal water-soluble antibiotic such as Cleocin gel to decrease the risk of toxic shock syndrome and eliminate the risk of myospherulosis.[6] If anterior nasal packing is

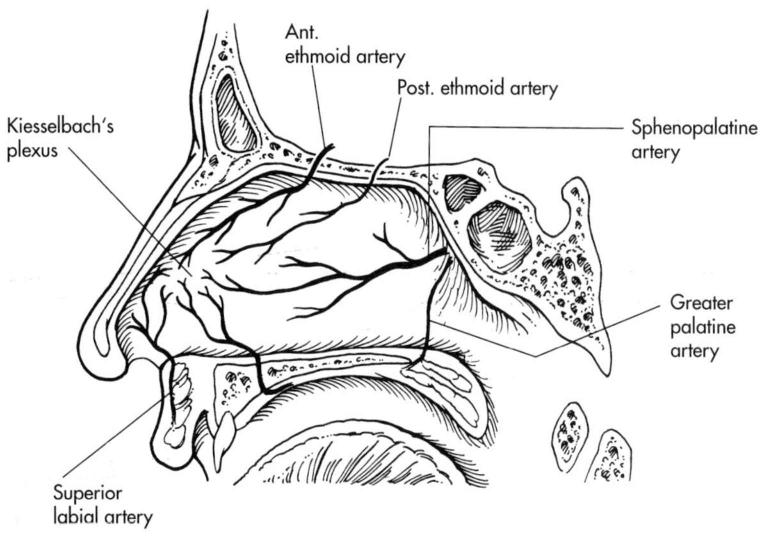

Figure 17–1. The blood supply of the nasal septum.

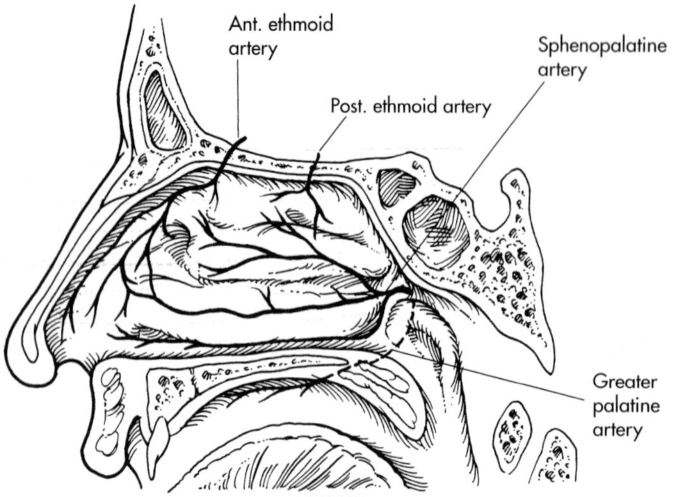

Figure 17–2. The blood supply to the lateral nasal wall.

used, the patient should also be placed on an oral antistaphylococcal antibiotic to further decrease the risk of toxic shock syndrome. Cases of toxic shock syndrome related to nasal packing are thought to occur when an endotoxin, produced by approximately one fifth of all strains of *Staphylococcus aureus*, is systemically absorbed.[7–9] The symptoms of toxic shock syndrome include fever, rash, hypotension, mucosal hyperemia, vomiting, diarrhea, multiorgan dysfunction, and desquamation during recovery. Death can occur if the condition is not recognized and swift treatment instituted, including removing and culturing the nasal packing, taking blood cultures, treating shock and organ failure, and giving intravenous antibiotic therapy.

Most nonabsorbable anterior nasal packs are removed in 3 to 5 days. Absorbable material with hemostatic properties, such as Surgicel, Gelfoam, and Avitene, are especially useful for anterior epistaxis in children and in patients with coagulopathies because the material need not be removed, and it assists with clotting. Surgicel wrapped around several long pieces of Gelfoam and coated with oxymetazoline is often an effective, comfortable, absorbable anterior nasal pack. Other nonoperative methods of controlling mild anterior epistaxis include local anesthetic block of the sphenopalatine artery either through the greater palatine foramen or directly into the region of the sphenopalatine artery, using a transnasal view.

If nonoperative intervention fails, operative alternatives include endoscopic electrocautery, cryotherapy, laser photocoagulation, septoplasty, anterior/posterior ethmoid artery ligation, internal maxillary artery (IMA) ligation using an endoscopic, a transantral, or a transpalatal approach, or embolization of the septal branch of the facial artery and the IMA.

POSTERIOR EPISTAXIS

As previously stated, the blood supply to the nose comes from both the external carotid and the internal carotid arteries, so it is very important to determine the source of the bleeding, as the branches of the internal carotid artery (the anterior and posterior ethmoid artery) cannot be safely embolized because of the risk to the cerebral and ophthalmic circulation. Another important issue to address when discussing the treatment of posterior epistaxis is the need for supplemental oxygen when utilizing a posterior pack; this is necessary because of the association of posterior nasal packing with hypoxemia.[10–13] At least 40% supplemental oxygen (preferably humidified oxygen) is recommended via face tent or orally positioned nasal cannula as soon as a posterior pack is placed not an hour or several hours later when the patient arrives on the ward. Furthermore, monitoring of cardiac and oxygen saturation is suggested while a posterior pack is in place to avoid apnea, hypoxia, or cardiac arrhythmia, all of which are postulated to be related to the nasopulmonary reflex that may be stimulated at any time when a posterior pack is in place.

Nonoperative interventions for the treatment of posterior epistaxis include chemical cautery, electrocautery, posterior packing (a classic gauze ribbon posterior pack, a double balloon "rhinorocket," a 10-mL Foley catheter placed posteriorly and filled with 5 to 10 mL of normal saline,[14] or gauze ribbon placed anteriorly), or local anesthetic block through the greater palatine foramen or directly into the region of the sphenopalatine artery via a transnasal view. Nonabsorbable nasal packing is usually left in place for 3 to 5 days and should be coated with antistaphylococcal antibiotic and water-soluble gel. Oral or intravenous antistaphylococcal antibiotics are also administered.

Operative interventions for the treatment of posterior epistaxis include endoscopic electrocautery,[15, 16] cryotherapy, laser photocoagulation, septoplasty, endoscopic sphenopalatine artery ligation,[17, 18] anterior/posterior ethmoid artery ligation, IMA ligation (via an endoscopic transantral,[19] external transantral, or transoral approach), embolization of the IMA and its branches or of the septal branch of the facial artery,[20, 21] or external carotid artery ligation.

Special mention must be made of the treatment of Osler-Weber-Rendu disease. A patient with this disease is prone to experience failure of standard therapies because of the regrowth and rebleeding of the small, fragile telangiectasias on the nasal mucosa.[1–3] If the standard treatments fail, several other options are available, including estrogen and progesterone treatments, CO_2 laser, argon laser,[22] Nd:YAG laser,[23] septodermoplasty, embolization, Young's procedure,[24] amniotic tissue graft of the nasal septum, cutaneous/myocutaneous grafts of the nasal septum, and vascularized free flaps such as the radial forearm flap. The argon and Nd:YAG lasers[23] have yielded particularly excellent results. Young's procedure is also successful, although it is a more drastic procedure and is used only as a last resort.[24]

Complications of nasal bleeding include hypoxia, hypotension or anemia leading to possible myocardial infarction or stroke, and aspiration pneumonia. Sequelae of anterior or posterior packing include myospherulosis, toxic shock syndrome, alar notching resulting from incorrectly placed packing,[25] septal or soft palate perforation caused by overinflated or incorrectly placed posterior packing,[26] acute or chronic sinusitis, and synechia. Oral antral fistula,[27] hypoesthesia, and hyperesthesia are all potential sequelae of IMA ligation. Complications of anterior or posterior ethmoid ligation include lacrimal duct injury, diplopia, enopthalmos, hypoesthesia, and blindness. Complications of embolization include hyper- or hypoesthesia, stroke, facial nerve paralysis, carotid artery injury, blindness, and headache.

In addition, there exists the risk of blindness resulting from injection of local anesthesia into the inferior turbinate. This is postulated to be caused by the embolization and subsequent infarction, or constriction, of the retinal artery as a result of its anastomosis with the arterial supply of the nasal mucosa.[28] It has classically been described as occurring with steroid injections with particle sizes greater than 7 μm.

Lastly, complications associated with the use of local and injectable anesthetics should be considered. Lidocaine is used commonly. Overdose of this local anesthetic is heralded by signs of central nervous system excitation followed by signs of central nervous system depression,[29] including excitement, disorientation, rambling speech, dizziness, twitching of facial muscles, shivering, tachycardia, hypertension, seizure, sweating, or vomiting; if overdose is not recognized, these signs and symptoms may be followed by hypotension, bradycardia, shock, apnea, coma, and death. At high doses, lidocaine decreases myocardial contractility and decreases peripheral vascular tone.

Outcomes

Almost all anterior epistaxis is effectively treated, probably because of the ease of accessibility and the small volume of bleeding involved. Unfortunately, the opposite is true of posterior epistaxis. This condition is usually more serious and more difficult to access. Recently, the two most common forms of second-line treatment for posterior epistaxis have been compared (complication and failure rates for IMA ligation vs. embolization). In general, although the rates vary from institution to institution according to the staff's skill, embolization of the IMA appears to have a slightly higher failure rate (20%) than ligation (12%). Major complication rates are nearly identical for both procedures (4% to 5%), although the types of major complications associated with IMA embolization are more serious (carotid artery injury, stroke). The risk of experiencing a minor complication, however, is much higher with IMA ligation than with embolization (26% vs. 14%). Long-term sequelae of epistaxis are identical to those mentioned above—hypoxia, hypotension, or anemia (leading to possible myocardial infarction or stroke) and aspiration pneumonia.[21, 30]

SEPTAL HEMATOMA

In a septal hematoma blood collects between the mucoperichondrium or mucoperiosteum of the nasal septum and the underlying septal cartilage or bone. It is an urgent situation because there is a risk of necrosis of the septal cartilage. The septal cartilage contains no blood vessels and relies on the overlying vasculature of the mucoperichondrium for viability. Blood collection between the mucoperichondrium and the septal cartilage results in diminution of the metabolic activity of the cartilage. A grace period of 1 to 3 days exists during which damage to the devascularized cartilage is reversible if the hematoma is evacuated. However, necrosis will be likely to occur if pressure and blood are not relieved within 72 hours. This results from the death of the chondrocytes in the cartilage matrix. The chondrocytes produce collagen, elastin, and matrix for the septal cartilage. Loss of viable chondrocytes because of an unevacuated septal hematoma can result in septal deformity, perforation, or infection.

Risk exists in any patient who has a condition that predisposes the nasal septum to bleeding, most commonly, septal surgery, septal trauma, nasal surgery, and nasal trauma. Other conditions include digital trauma that is self-inflicted (by those with mental retardation or other neurologic conditions that impair awareness of trauma to the self), platelet disorders (idiopathic thrombocytopenic purpura, von Willebrand's disease, Glanzmann's thrombasthenia), coagulation defects (hemophilia A and B), anticoagulant drugs (heparin, Coumadin, aspirin, nonsteroidal anti-inflammatory drugs), medical conditions that interfere with clotting mechanisms (liver disease, renal disease, polycythemia vera, leukemia, multiple myeloma, thrombocytopenia due to chemotherapy, deficiencies in vitamins A, D, E, or K, and hereditary hemorrhagic telangiectasia (Osler-Weber-Rendu disease).[31–33] Less common conditions that may be associated with septal bleeding and septal hematoma include granulomatous diseases,[34–37] chronic rhinosinusitis, arteriovenous malformations, hemangiomas, papillomas, and malignancy, the most common being squamous cell carcinoma.

Presentation

The history should be studied for any condition that predisposes a patient to a septal hematoma. The most common causes are nasal surgery and nasal trauma. Symptoms may be unilateral or bilateral and include nasal obstruction, pressure, and intense pain. Severe pain does not usually occur after septoplasty, so if it does occur, a septal hematoma should be suspected. Epistaxis may or may not be noted by the patient. If the hematoma has become infected, the patient may experience chills, a subjective feeling of temperature elevation, or purulent discharge.

The definitive diagnosis of a septal hematoma is clinical. Swelling of the upper lip and ecchymosis of the superior sublabial mucosa can occur with extravasation of blood into the surrounding tissues. An erythematous swelling on the anterior or posterior nasal septum, which is soft to palpation, is noted on nasal examination. The swelling can extend laterally to touch the inferior turbinates, and it is usually most pronounced in the middle inferior portion of the septum. If the hematoma remains undiagnosed and is not evacuated, the clot eventually undegoes liquefaction followed by fibrosis. This can result in a permanent thickening of the septum. If the hematoma becomes infected by means of a septal abscess or septal or nasal cellulitis, tenderness or erythema of the septum, nasal tip, nasal dorsum, and sublabial area may also be present.[38, 39] Fever, chills, and malaise may indicate serious infection and the possibility of bacteremia. Figure 17–3 shows the location of a septal hematoma developing between the septal cartilage and the septal mucoperichondrium.

Evaluation

In general, a septal hematoma is a localized process involving minimal blood loss. Recom-

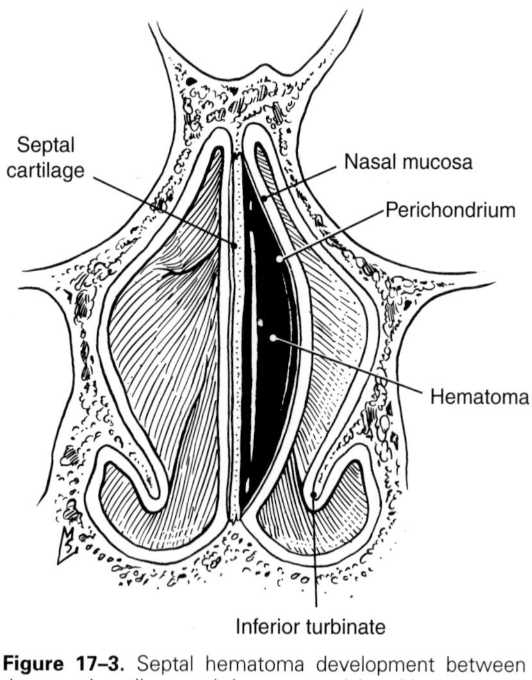

Figure 17–3. Septal hematoma development between the septal cartilage and the mucoperichondrium.

mended initial laboratory evaluation includes a complete blood count, including hemoglobin, hematocrit, platelet count, PT, and PTT. If a bleeding disorder is suspected from the history or from the initial laboratory workup, hematology consultation and bleeding time should be requested. If an infection or abscess is noted, a white blood cell count and differential should be obtained.

Radiologic studies are not necessary for diagnosis. However, because many patients with this disorder have been involved in multitrauma incidents, they often undergo radiologic studies of the head for other reasons. Blood can be seen on MRI or CT scans as a lucency between the mucoperiosteum or mucoperichondrium and the underlying cartilage and bone of the septum.

Pathognomonic aspects of the history and physical examination of a patient with an acute septal hematoma include a history of trauma or a bleeding disorder, increasing pain or nasal obstruction after nasal surgery or trauma, and a soft, tender unilateral or bilateral bulge in the nasal septum.

Priorities

True emergency evacuation of a septal hematoma should be performed in an infant younger than 1 year of age who is an obligate nasal breather. Bilateral septal hematomas in an infant could lead to life-threatening nasal airway obstruction. In this case, an oral airway should be placed and oxygen monitored until the condition is treated. If necessary, the child should be intubated. Following evacuation of the septal hematoma via a hemitransfixion incision and evacuation of the blood, a drain and septal splint or nasal packing should be placed to prevent the reaccumulation of blood. A young patient, who is an obligate nasal breather until approximately 1 year old, requires admission for airway observation while nasal packing or trumpets are in place. The evacuation of a septal hematoma should be made expeditiously but only after life-threatening abnormalities have been addressed and the patient has been stabilized. "The sooner the better" is a good axiom to apply to this situation. Evacuation of a septal hematoma within 72 hours of its formation has been associated with the best chance for survival of the chondrocytes within the cartilage. Septal abscess or infection of the hematoma requires immediate removal.

Although there are many variations, the basic therapeutic intervention for septal hematoma is presented here. First, ABC status must be assessed and addressed. Several key pieces of equipment are necessary: a nasal speculum, a Frazier suction tube, a head light, a no. 15 surgical blade, topical anesthetic (4% cocaine or 2% Pontocaine), topical decongestant, local anesthetic, culture swab, anterior nasal packing material (ribbon gauze or rolled Telfa or Merocel packing coated with a water-soluble antistaphylococcal antibiotic gel), a drain (sterile rubber band, small-bore flexible plastic tubing), a Cottle elevator, and 4-0 absorbable suture. One-dose intravenous antibiotics covering *Staphylococcus* species should be given for prophylaxis of toxic shock syndrome. The nasal cavity is decongested and anesthetized with topical agents. Local anesthesia is injected to the anterior septal region on the side of the hematoma. A sublabial injection into the anterior nasal spine is often helpful, and general anesthesia may be necessary for children, infants, or neurologically impaired patients.

If present, the previous hemitransfixion incision is utilized. If not present, a hemitransfixion incision is made on the side of the hematoma. If bilateral septal hematomas are diagnosed, stair-step incisions are made so as not to lie directly opposite one another. The hematoma is evacuated with suction.[38] If purulent, cultures of the material are sent for study. The wound is then evaluated for hemostasis, searching for any active bleeding sites. Usually, the site of bleeding has been tamponaded due to pressure from the hematoma formation, but bleeding may recur once pressure is removed. Next, the status of the septal cartilage is evaluated, and nonviable cartilage and bone are debrided. The pocket between the mucoperiosteum and septal cartilage and the bone is irrigated with normal saline and a drain (a sterile rubber band or small Penrose drain) is placed into it and secured with a nylon suture to the septum or to a septal splint. The incision is not tightly closed. Septal splints or running horizontal 4-0 chromic catgut sutures are placed to quilt the mucoperichondrial flaps against the septal cartilage.

If nasal packing is used, it is coated with antistaphylococcal, water-soluble antibiotic gel. Infants, the elderly, and patients with cardiac, pulmonary, or neurologic conditions affecting airway protection or awareness may require hospitalization, supplemental oxygen, and observation until the nasal packing is removed. In cases in which nasal breathing is preferred infants, the elderly, and those with pulmonary or cardiac disease), a nasal trumpet or trumpets may be used as nasal packing. Oral antibiotic therapy that covers *Staphylococcus* species is administered for 5 to 7 days in routine, noninfected cases.

If infection exists at the time of evacuation, the patient should be hospitalized for observation and administration of intravenous antibiotics to avoid the sequelae of progressive nasal infection which can include bacteremia, toxic shock, septic thrombophlebitis with brain abscess, meningitis, and cavernous sinus thrombosis.[39] The nasal packing and drain may be removed the following day and the septum inspected for reaccumulation of the hematoma. The nasal packing may be replaced for 3 to 5 days or left out. Needle aspiration of the hematoma is not recommended as the sole form of treatment because the hematoma may not be fully evacuated by this method.

Complications of septal hematoma can include septal perforation, significant loss of septal cartilage resulting in loss of nasal support and saddle-nose deformity, septal thickening resulting from the fibrosis of an unevacuated hematoma, and infection of the nasal septum or other nasal cartilage which can result in the sequelae mentioned earlier.

Sequelae of intervention can include undesirable, uneven cosmetic anterior septal incision, toxic shock syndrome, and bacteremia.

Outcome

Potential long-term sequelae of unevacuated septal hematoma include nasal airway obstruction from septal fibrosis and thickening, saddle-nose deformity, septal perforation, synechia to the lateral nasal wall, and epistaxis due to septal perforation.

NASAL FOREIGN BODY

A child often makes a game of placing an object into his or her nose or into the nose of another child. In most cases, the placement of an object into the nose does not constitute an emergency. However, there are several situations in which a foreign body in the nose does constitute an emergency. These foreign bodies include small batteries such as watch or hearing aid batteries, bilateral foreign bodies in the nose of an infant, and a food item lodged in the nasal cavity that may swell significantly if left in a moist environment, for example, a seed. A battery left in contact with the nasal mucosa can cause acute necrosis of the mucosa within several hours. Bilateral nasal foreign bodies can result in acute airway obstruction. Foods such as seeds or nuts can be difficult to remove and can cause more damage to the nasal mucosa when they are removed if the object has swollen.

In addition, certain patients are at increased risk for aspiration of nasal foreign bodies, including those with neurologic disease (for example, cerebral palsy, mental retardation, or cranial nerve defects) or pulmonary disease, institutionalized patients, elderly patients, immunocompromised patients, and infants and children. During history taking and physical examination, these conditions should be considered, and appropriate airway precautions should be taken prior to expeditious removal of the foreign body.

Children constitute the most common group of patients involved in foreign body placement in the nose. Institutionalized children and those with neurologic disease are also at risk for the presence of foreign bodies placed by other children. Immunocompromised patients are at increased risk for potential infectious complications resulting from foreign bodies in the nose and are at increased risk for infectious complications resulting from aspiration of foreign bodies. Also at risk for harboring nasal foreign bodies are patients who have undergone nasal surgical procedures and patients who have incurred trauma to the nose from any type of foreign material.

Presentation

A patient most at risk for having a foreign body in the nose, such as a child or an institutionalized person, is also the least likely to provide a history of having put an object into the nose in the first place. The symptoms that are commonly associated with the presence of a foreign body in the nose are listed in Box 17–3.

It is important to elicit information about how long the object may have been in the nose, the site of the symptoms, and precisely what the object might be. A representation of the foreign body is very helpful when selecting instruments for its removal. The size and shape of the object and the type of material it is made of are also helpful pieces of information.

The physical examination should include a complete head and neck examination and chest auscultation. The presence of one foreign body means there is a high risk of the presence of a second or third foreign body. A complete examination occasionally detects another for-

BOX 17-3

History of the Presence of a Foreign Body

Unilateral nasal discharge (particularly purulent or malodorous)
Foul odor from the nasal cavity
Unilateral or bilateral nasal pain
Recurrent rhinosinusitis
Intractable sneezing
Epistaxis
Headache
Nasal whistling
Cough
Postnasal drip
Nasal airway obstruction
Previous history of foreign body in the ear, nose, or throat

eign body. Pertinent aspects of the nasal examination include evaluation for edema, erythema, or ulceration of the nasal mucosa, granulation tissue (which may be confused with neoplasm or may completely encase the foreign body), septal perforation, and epistaxis. Classically, unilateral purulent discharge with or without sinusitis has been described as a sign that is highly likely to indicate the presence of a nasal foreign body; however, nasal obstruction or whistling and nasal crusting are common. If the foreign body has been present for a long time, it is possible to find a rhinolith, which is formed by the deposit of layers of calcium on the foreign body.

The remainder of the head and neck examination should be performed, keeping a high suspicion for the presence of other foreign bodies or complications secondary to the nasal foreign body. The ear is examined for serous otitis media and the presence of a foreign body and the nasopharynx is inspected for an impacted foreign body and choanal atresia (which can present with identical symptoms). The oral cavity is surveyed for the presence of a foreign body, indications include an ulceration of the soft or hard palate resulting from the longstanding presence of a foreign body and the presence of posterolateral oropharyngeal drainage.

It is imperative to inspect the larynx and chest in any patient with a suspected areodigestive tract foreign body. The consequences of missing a second object or a piece of the original object in these sites could be disastrous. Flexible fiberoptic examination of the larynx should be performed along with chest auscultation, paying special attention to the presence of unilateral wheezing, productive cough, or unilateral decrease or loss of breath sounds. A photograph of a nasal foreign body as seen on nasal endoscopy is shown in Figure 17–4.

Evaluation

No laboratory tests are necessary in a routine case of a nasal foreign body. Usually, an elevated white blood cell count is not present; however, an elevated white blood cell count may be noted with the presence of secondary sinusitis, facial cellulitis, parasitic or helminthic infestation, or other facial soft tissue infection.

Imaging studies of the nasopharynx and nose can be of value for identification of radiopaque foreign bodies such as metallic or calcified objects. Imaging studies might include fluoroscopy, lateral soft tissue films of the neck and nasopharynx, plain sinus films, and CT scans. Anatomic abnormalities related to the foreign body should be evaluated (sinusitis, perforation, soft tissue inflammation) as should disorders pertaining to differential diagnosis (choanal atresia, malignancy, benign tumor, nasal polyposis, encephalocele). If a clear view of the skull base cannot be seen or if there is no clear history or identification of a foreign body, a CT scan or MRI should be obtained to rule out the possibility of an encephalocele or meningoencephalocele. Figure 17–5 shows a CT scan of a nasal foreign body.

A chest radiograph that shows hyperinflation of a lobe or lung, atelectasis, pneumonia, or

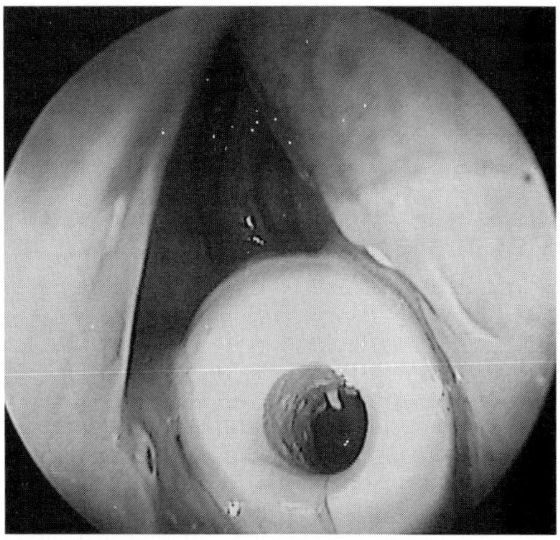

Figure 17–4. Photograph of an endoscopic view of a nasal foreign body.

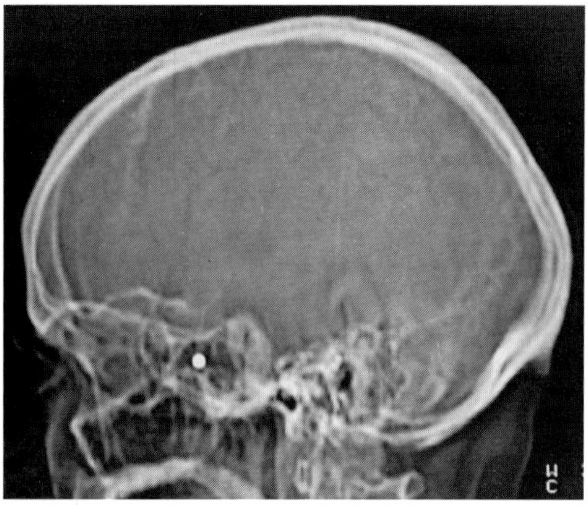

Figure 17–5. CT scan of a nasal foreign body.

opacity may indicate aspiration of a fragment of the foreign body or of another foreign body. Consideration should be given to performing bronchoscopy to rule out this possibility. A list of foreign bodies is presented in Table 17–3, but it cannot be complete, as any solid material can be placed into the nose.

A pathognomonic history and physical examination might include a unilateral malodorous or purulent nasal discharge and unilateral nasal obstruction.

Priorities

Several situations require expeditious removal of foreign bodies found in the nose: a small battery such as a watch or hearing aid battery, bilateral foreign bodies in the nose of an infant, and foods lodged in the nasal cavity that may swell significantly if left in a moist environment. A battery left in contact with the nasal mucosa can cause acute necrosis of nasal mucosa within several hours. Mucosal damage is caused by the continuous low current that is delivered directly to the tissues. Bilateral nasal foreign bodies can result in acute airway obstruction. Seeds and nuts can swell to two times their original size and can cause damage to the nasal mucosa on removal.

Certain groups of patients are particularly at risk for aspiration of nasal foreign bodies that are loose or are propelled backward from the nose into the nasopharynx and supraglottis. This can create an emergent situation of acute respiratory obstruction and possible death. Precautions must be taken to guard against aspiration of the object when any nasal foreign body is being manipulated. At greatest risk are patients with neurologic or pulmonary disease, institutionalized patients, elderly patients, immunocompromised patients, and infants and children. During history and physical examination, these conditions should be considered, and appropriate airway precautions should be taken prior to expeditious removal of any foreign body.

An immunocompromised patient is at increased risk for potential infectious complications resulting from a foreign body in the nose and from aspiration of the foreign body. Also at risk for harboring a nasal foreign body is a patient who has undergone nasal surgical procedure or who has incurred trauma to the nose from any type of foreign material.

The management of a foreign body in the nose is to remove it. The goal is to remove the foreign body without creating other problems, such as aspiration, epistaxis, pain, or impaction. The outline of a plan for the removal of a nasal foreign body is as follows.

First, the patient's ABCs are assessed and controlled; then a full history is taken and a head and neck examination is performed to look for other foreign bodies and for complications of the presence of a foreign body.

Table 17–3. *Foreign Bodies Found in the Nose*

Inanimate Foreign Bodies	Animate Foreign Bodies
• Objects left behind after trauma (e.g., bullets, motor vehicle parts) • Iatrogenic objects left behind after surgery or anesthesia • Food (e.g., seeds) • Rhinoliths (crystallized salts of calcium and magnesium around a small piece of organic or inorganic material) • Teeth, displaced bone • Any other object (the most common objects are beans, nuts, peas, chalk, erasers, crayons, marbles, cloth, meat, vegetables, fruit pits, jewelry, and pieces of plastic toys)	• Fungi (fungal balls, rhinosporidiosis) • Roundworms *(Ascaris lumbricoides)* • Screw worms **(Cochliomylia hominivorax, C. macellaris)* • Fly larvae *(Oestrus, Hypoderma, Dermatobia)* • Adult insects

The chest is auscultated and a chest radiograph is obtained.

Instruments necessary for removal of the object are gathered: a nasal speculum, an otoscope, bayonet forceps, alligator forceps (large and small), Hartmann forceps, blunt hook or nerve hook, a wire loop, a Fogarty catheter, a head light and excellent lighting, a flexible or rigid endoscope or both, a Frazier suction tube, topical anesthetic (4% cocaine or 2% Pontocaine), topical decongestant, local anesthetic, culture swabs, a procedure table, and the materials necessary for the treatment of anterior and posterior epistaxis. Strong consideration should be given to general anesthesia for a patient who has an increased risk for aspiration of the foreign body, a firmly impacted object, or a risk of bleeding.

It is helpful to have an idea of what the foreign body looks like. Ask the patient or a family member to draw a picture of the object or to bring you a representative object that is the same as or similar to the foreign body. This helps in the selection of the best instrument and method of removal for a particular object. It is also very helpful to fully explain the procedure to the child and the parent. Allowing the patient to see and feel the bluntness of the instruments used often significantly decreases the patient's anxiety and increases cooperation and patience. Restraints or a papoose may be necessary.

Next, topical anesthetic and decongestant are applied and, if warranted by the circumstances, local anesthesia. If foreign body manipulation is attempted in the office, placement of the procedure table in the Trendelenberg position can reduce the risk of aspiration. Good lighting and a head mirror or nasal endoscope are essential. Secretions are suctioned and any purulent material is cultured. Upon inspection, if no inanimate or animate object is seen, if the object is covered with granulation tissue, if there is no history of a foreign body, or if there is no clear distinction at the skull base, a CT scan or MRI should be performed prior to removal or biopsy to rule out an encephalocoele. The goal of treating the presence of a foreign body in the nose is to remove it, but before doing so, the physician's first goal is to be absolutely certain that the object in the nose is indeed a foreign body. Disastrous consequences can result from the attempted removal of an encephalocoele, carcinoma, or arteriovenous malformation.

Once the definitive diagnosis of a foreign body has been made, removal of rounded or smooth-surfaced foreign bodies is easily accomplished with a blunt hook. The blunt hook is slid past the foreign body, then turned 90 degrees and pulled gently toward the nostril. As removal is begun, the degree of impaction can be judged by the patient's discomfort. Hartmann or alligator forceps may be used if the foreign body has a part that can be grasped. If a large rhinolith or a large, partially degraded foreign body is present, it may break into smaller pieces that can be removed.[40–42]

Another useful piece of equipment is a Fogarty catheter. This small catheter may be inserted along the floor of the nose and past the object. The small balloon is then inflated and the catheter pulled forward, ideally pushing the foreign body in front of itself. A large or impacted foreign body may require general anesthesia, with or without a lateral rhinotomy, for removal. A trial of endoscopic visualization and instrumentation is suggested prior to resorting to a lateral rhinotomy.

Animate foreign bodies such as insects that are still moving at the time of attempted removal can be anesthetized or killed with the application of several drops of mineral oil. Once the foreign body has been removed, the nasal cavity, nasopharynx, supraglottis, and glottis are inspected for other foreign bodies and pieces of the removed foreign body.[43] The status of the nasal cavity is evaluated and mucous membrane ulceration, septal perforation, bleeding, or sinus infection are diagnosed and treated appropriately. Necrotic tissue and granulation tissue are debrided. For patients without infection, the use of saline mist for 10 to 14 days assists in removing static secretions and improves healing and mucociliary flow.

The foreign body is inspected for evidence of possible incomplete removal such as broken or missing pieces. It is appropriate to send the foreign body and any granulation tissue to pathology for documentation of removal and to rule out malignancy. The patient is seen in 2 to 4 weeks to survey for resolving sinusitis or other sequelae. Figures 17–6, 17–7, and 17–8 demonstrate the removal of a nasal foreign body with a Hartmann forceps, wire loop, and blunt hook.

Complications involving nasal foreign bodies can include aspiration, pneumonia, chronic bronchitis, or chronic cough. Rarely, irritation to the nasal mucosa can cause intractable sneezing. Serious complications such as acute airway obstruction, facial cellulitis, periorbital abscess, periorbital cellulitis, meningitis, encephalitis, brain abscess, or cavernous sinus thrombosis can occur. Less serious complications such as sinusitis, mucocele, mucopyocele, nasal polyps, septal abscess, acute or serous otitis media sec-

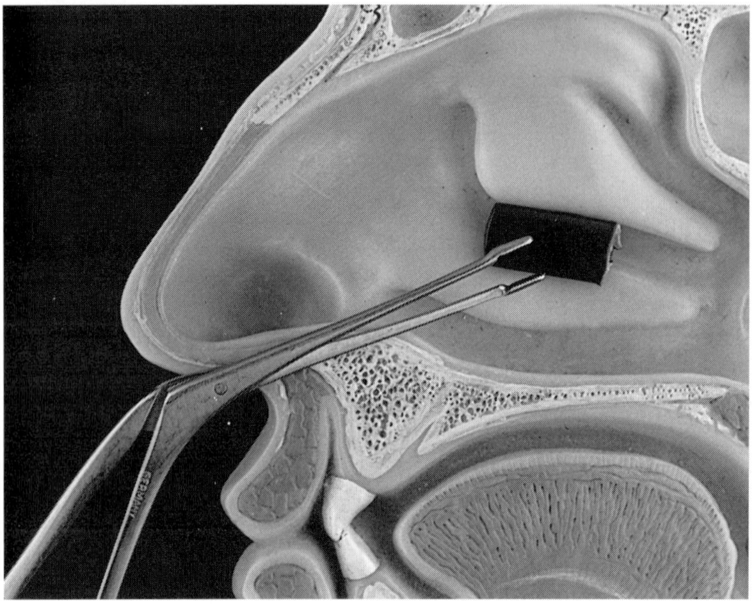

Figure 17–6. Removal of a nasal foreign body with Hartmann forceps.

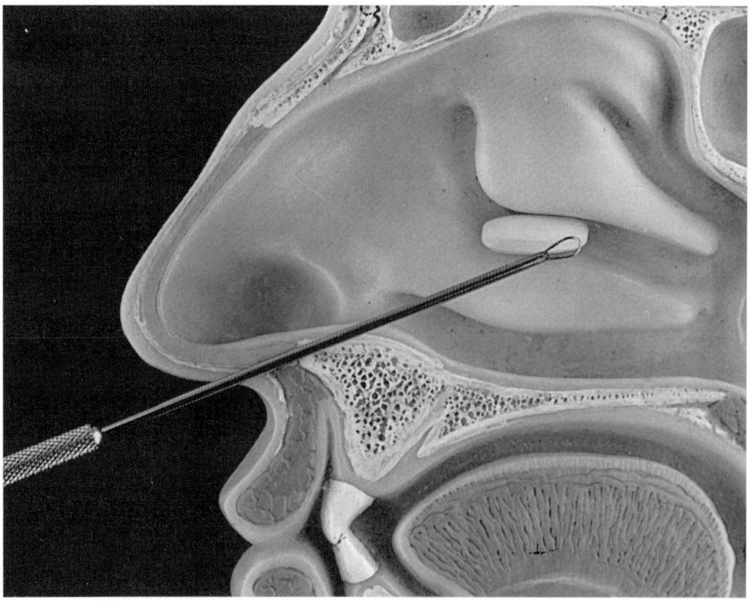

Figure 17–7. Removal of a nasal foreign body with a wire loop.

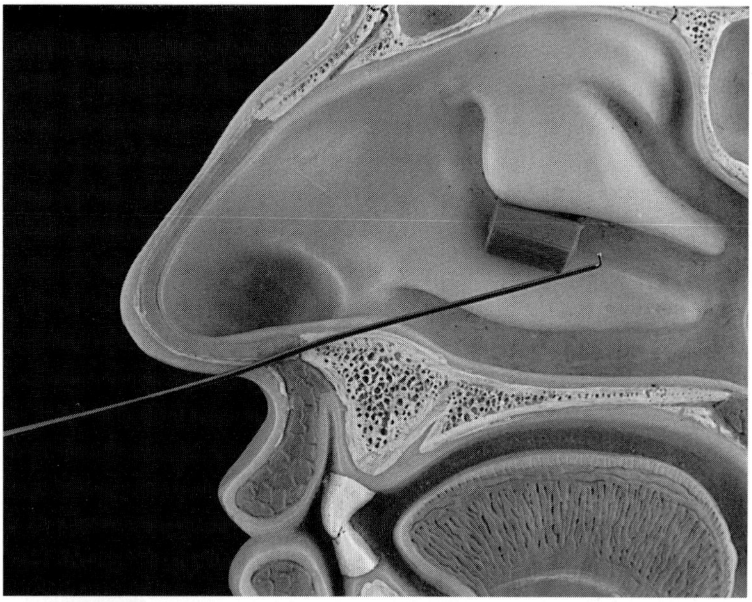

Figure 17–8. Removal of a nasal foreign body with a blunt hook.

ondary to eustachian tube inflammation can also occur.

Outcomes

Foreign bodies that remain present for long periods can result in septal perforation, soft palate perforation, hard palate perforation, anosmia, hyposmia, or ozena. Localized or cephalic tetanus and osteomyelitis have been reported to occur with the presence of long-standing nasal foreign bodies. Sequelae of intervention include aspiration of the foreign body or of pieces of the foreign body, epistaxis, nasal mucosal membrane synechia, and the possibility that a piece of the foreign body has been left in the nose or nasopharynx.

NASAL TRAUMA

The nasal bones are the most commonly fractured bones of the face. Of every 100 facial fractures in adults, 39 involve the nasal bones. A nasal fracture is not an acute emergency in itself. However, several conditions associated with nasal fractures are emergencies and as such must be evaluated before nonemergent follow-up treatment in 3 to 5 days. These conditions include cerebrospinal fluid leak, nasal soft tissue avulsion, septal hematoma, orbital injury, open nasal fracture, and brain injury. The diagnosis and management of all of these emergencies can be found elsewhere in this book. Only open nasal fractures and the presence of a displaced septum in a neonate are discussed here.

Open nasal fracture, a nasal fracture in which the nasal skin has been lacerated, exposing fractured bone and or cartilage beneath it, constitutes an emergency for three reasons. First, exposed cartilage requires timely (within 1 to 8 hours) coverage by soft tissue if it is to survive. Second, the thin dorsal skin involved in a nasal laceration requires prompt debridement, irrigation, and reapproximation for optimal cosmesis. Third, because the force required to produce an open nasal fracture is great, other serious, possibly life-threatening injuries may coexist in a patient with nasal trauma. Such injuries include cervical spine trauma,[44] cerebrospinal fluid leak, nasal soft tissue avulsion, septal hematoma, orbital injury, cervical spine injury, brain injury, epistaxis, septal hematoma, and other serious facial fractures.

Males are twice as likely as females to experience a nasal fracture; those in the 15- to 30-year age group have the highest incidence. There is a bimodal age distribution of nasal fractures in females, with increased incidence in the 15- to 25-year age group and in the over-60-year age group.

Activities that increase the risk of nasal fracture include interpersonal altercations, sports, falls, and motor vehicle accidents. Other causes include sharp trauma (knives and other sharp objects), gunshot wounds, and human and animal bites. (Treatment of bites is covered in Chapter 13.)

Because neonates and infants are obligate nasal breathers, septal deviation is a situation that can result in acute airway obstruction. Approximately 1% of newborn infants experience septal deviation during birth. There is an increased incidence of the condition in birth trauma during vaginal and forceps delivery. Neonatal septal deviation can also occur in utero because of crowding in cases of multiple births or because of the position of the fetus in the womb.

Presentation

A patient with an open nasal fracture presents with a history of trauma to the nose resulting from an interpersonal altercation, sports, a fall, or a motor vehicle accident. A significant amount of force—approximately 35 to 80 g—is required to produce a nasal fracture, so other facial fractures and head trauma can be present in a patient with nasal trauma. The physician should question the patient about the amount of time that has elapsed since injury. It is recommended that all open fractures be closed as soon as possible after injury—certainly within 12 to 24 hours—to avoid scarring and infection and to improve cosmetic closure. Knowing the approximate speed of the object that has struck the face and whether loss of consciousness occurred at the scene and noting the presence of other injuries gives the physician important knowledge about the risk of there being severe injury to other facial or craniofacial structures or to the cervical spine. A complete history is necessary, especially concerning previous nasal or facial surgery and the patient's preinjury olfactory status.[45, 46]

The age of a patient with a nasal fracture is important; it may help in determining the likelihood of upper and lower lateral cartilage dislocation. Younger patients are susceptible to dislocations of the nasal and septal cartilage whereas older patients are more prone to comminuted fractures of the nasal bones because they are likely to have brittle, osteoporotic bones. The majority of nasal fractures are lateral, the result of a laterally applied force.

The signs and symptoms of a nasal fracture include cosmetic deformity, pain in the nasal pyramid, epistaxis, nasal congestion, nasal airway obstruction, nasal edema, periobital ecchymosis, septal hematoma, crepitus, and tenderness. In an open nasal fracture, the skin of the nose has been lacerated, exposing fractured bone or cartilage. It is important to document and evaluate hypoesthesia of the nasal and surrounding skin, facial nerve function (nasal wrinkling), and olfactory function prior to the administration of a local or general anesthetic. It is also important to evaluate, document, and treat, if necessary a septal hematoma. Figure 17–9 demonstrates an open, displaced nasal fracture repaired with debridement, reduction, and primary closure.

A neonate with a displaced nasal septum can present shortly after delivery with acute airway obstruction and may also present with intermittent blood oxygen desaturations. Physical examination of the nose will reveal the problem. Subtle signs of septal deviation in a neonate include lateral deviation of the nose accompanied by angulation of the columella and loss of nasal tip support. Other subtle signs include flattening of the nostril on the side opposite the deviation and diminished movement of the ala on the side of deviation with nasal respiration.

Evaluation

An open nasal fracture can be a local process with minimal or significant blood loss. It is often associated with multitrauma and other injuries in which routine laboratory tests are ordered by emergency department physicians. In the case of an isolated open nasal fracture with moderate to significant blood loss, recommended initial laboratory evaluation includes a complete blood count, including hemoglobin, hematocrit, and platelet count, and PT/PTT. This allows estimation of the patient's actual blood loss and a baseline against which to judge possible future epistaxis or other bleeding. The platelet count and PT/PTT evaluate the patient's ability to form stable clots and screens for hemostatic disorders. If a bleeding disorder is suspected based on history or initial laboratory workup, hematology consultation and evaluation of bleeding time should be requested. If a delay in care has occurred and infection or abscess is noted, a white blood cell count and differential can be obtained. Radiologic studies are not necessary for diagnosis. However, because many patients with this disorder have been involved in multitrauma incidents, they commonly undergo radiologic studies of the head for other reasons. Displacement of the nasal bones and soft tissue can be seen on MRI, CT, and plain facial films. A head and facial CT scan is recommended in the case of an open nasal fracture caused by blunt trauma because

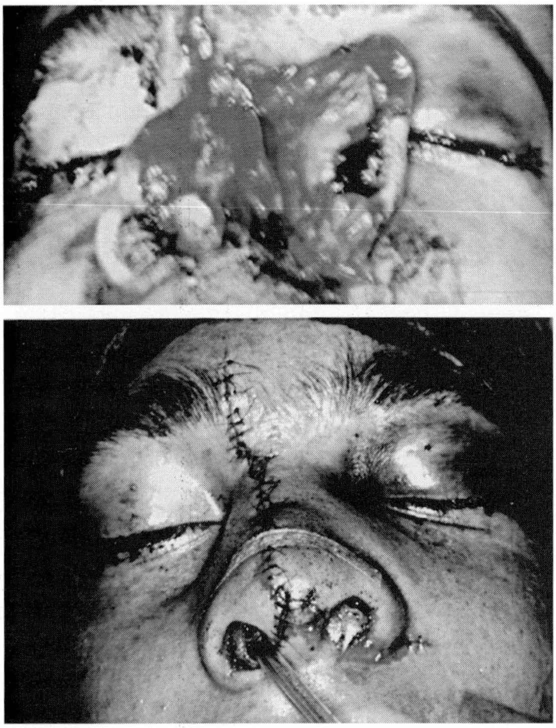

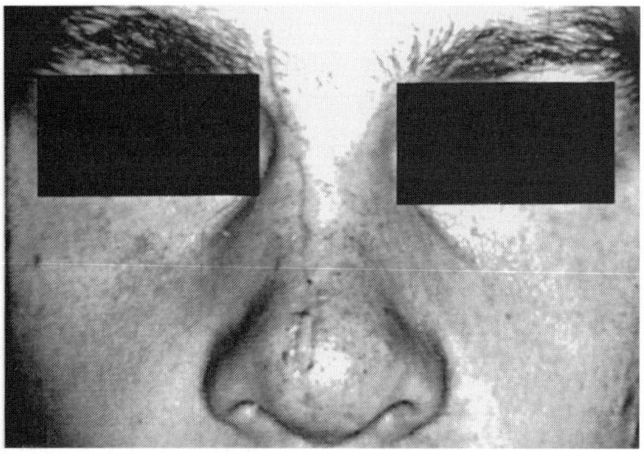

Figure 17–9. An open, displaced nasal fracture repaired with debridement, reduction, and primary closure.

the amount of force necessary to cause an open nasal fracture is enough to cause facial and brain injuries, which should be ruled out when evaluating the extent of nasal deviation, comminution, depression, or impaction. These injuries include frontal sinus fracture, skull base fracture, orbital apex and wall fractures, skull fracture, and brain injury. Figure 17–10 is a CT scan of a comminuted, displaced, depressed nasal fracture.

Priorities

When treating and evaluating an open nasal fracture, the ABCs and the cervical spine must be assessed and treated appropriately. Once these steps have been taken and a primary trauma survey of the patient has been made, attention can be turned to the nose. Pressure is applied to the nose if significant external nasal bleeding is present. Posterior epistaxis is treated

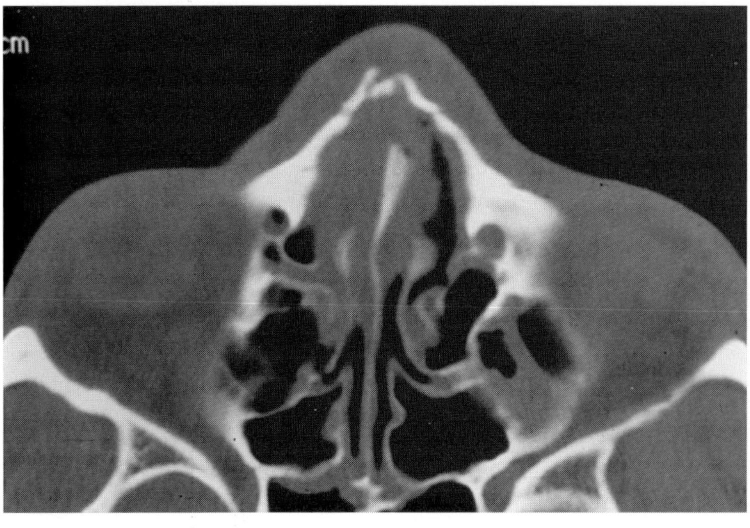

Figure 17–10. CT scan of a comminuted, nondisplaced nasal fracture.

if present. A secondary trauma survey is made and a thorough history is obtained. A complete head and neck examination is performed, including gentle examination of the wound. The nasal tissue is kept moist with saline-soaked gauze while radiologic studies are performed. A complete blood count and PT/PTT are performed if necessary, and the patient is administered a tetanus or rabies booster shot, if appropriate. Prior to manipulating an open nasal fracture, administration of an antistaphylococcal antibiotic is recommended.

General principles of surgery apply when repairing an open nasal fracture. The nose is anesthetized with local anesthesia (infraorbital, lateral nasal, or anterior septum), or closure can be performed under general anesthesia. The wound is irrigated and explored, taking care to evaluate for significant septal deviation, septal hematoma, skin loss, and upper and lower lateral cartilage dislocation. The wound is debrided of foreign bodies. Small pieces of loose cartilage and bone are removed and saved for possible use in reconstruction. Hemostasis is obtained and nasal bones are reduced, if necessary, prior to soft tissue closure. The internal nasal mucosae are reapproximated, as is the perichondrium of cartilage. The soft tissue edges are debrided sharply freshened, and reapproximated. Nasal packing, septal splints, and nasal splints are used as necessary, and local wound care is prescribed as is an antistaphylococcal antibiotic for 7 to 10 days. If necessary, closed or open reduction of the nasal fracture is performed 3 to 14 days after injury.

When treating septal deviation in a neonate, basic principles of medicine apply. The infant's ABCs are assessed and an oral airway, nasal trumpet, mask, or endotracheal tube is placed, if necessary. Once the airway has been stabilized, the physician may proceed with therapeutic intervention. This is usually a simple and quick maneuver. The septum is gently replaced into the maxillary crest with a superior and lateral movement, which may be accomplished by using a cotton swab, a Freer elevator, or digital pressure. Nasal packing is usually unnecessary. To reduce nasal edema, a topical nasal decongestant spray may be used for 3 to 5 days or topical ophthalmic Decadron 0.1% drops may be applied to the nasal cavity for 7 to 10 days.

Complications that can occur with an open nasal fracture include nasal scarring, septal deviation, airway and nasal obstruction, epistaxis, local infection of soft tissue, sinusitis, fibrosis, contracture of the nasal ala or nasal sill, and hypoesthesia of the nasal skin. Intractable sneezing, hyposmia, anosmia, synechia, septal hematoma, septal perforation, saddle nose, crooked nose, upper or lower lateral cartilage necrosis, or nasal collapse can also occur. Long-term complications that have been reported include trigeminal nerve branch neuroma, lacrimal duct obstruction with epiphora, and pseudohypotelorism. Complications of a severe fracture include frontal sinus fracture, meningitis, brain abscess, cavernous sinus thrombosis,[47] diplopia and visual impairment, and cerebrospinal fluid leakage. A high index of suspicion for other injuries must be employed when evaluating and treating nasal fractures, and follow-up is recommended to survey for long-term complications.

Outcomes

Possible sequelae of treatment of an open nasal fracture include secondary nasal deformity, cerebrospinal fluid leakage secondary to manipulation of nasal fragments, synechia of the nasal airway due to rough handling of internal mucosal membranes, hypoesthesia of nasal skin, chronic nasal pain, hyposmia, anosmia, suture or stitch abscess, and wound dehiscence.

Complications of septal deviation in a neonate include septal hematoma, septal abscess, facial cellulitis and its sequelae, acute nasal airway obstruction resulting in hypoxia or death, epistaxis, sinusitis and the sequelae associated with sinusitis, intractable sneezing, blunted midfacial growth, blunted sinus aeration and development, blunted nasal growth, hyposmia, and anosmia.

Sequelae of treatment of septal deviation in a neonate can include epistaxis, hyposmia, anosmia, septal hematoma, synechia of the nasal airway caused by rough handling of internal mucosal membranes, inadequate reduction of the septal deviation, and nasal edema.

NASAL MASS

A nasal mass is not an emergency in itself, but it must be managed so as to prevent the creation of an emergent situation. Performing a biopsy of a unilateral nasal mass that is then recognized as an encephalocele (herniation of the brain, dura, and cerebrospinal fluid through the skull base) can potentially result in very serious complications or in the death of the patient. The important point to be made here is that a unilateral nasal mass should never be biopsied prior to radiologic evaluation of the skull base. A corollary to this is that once the absence of a connection between the central nervous system and a unilateral or bilateral nasal mass has been confirmed, and a biopsy is performed, it is important to be prepared to deal with epistaxis at the time of the biopsy. A third point is that one should be highly suspicious for malignancy in evaluating any unilateral nasal mass.

An encephalocele may be congenital or may occur and develop secondary to trauma or surgery. Overall, caudal neural tube defects are more common than cephalic neural tube defects (lumbosacral spina bifida occurs five times more frequently than do cranial encephaloceles). The incidence of cranial encephaloceles is approximately 1 in every 35,000 live births in the United States, Europe, Australia, Japan, China, and India. There is a much higher incidence in southern Asia and Russia, where the occurrence is approximately 1 in every 6,000 births. The majority (75%) of cranial encephaloceles occur in the region of the occiput; the remainder are found in the parietal (15%) or nasofrontal area (10%). The majority of nasal encephaloceles are situated over the nasal dorsum (60%), with 30% occurring intranasally and 10% involving both regions. There is no sex predilection and there is an increased incidence in patients with Ehlers-Danlos syndrome, neurofibromatosis, cleft lip, cleft palate, or any other midline craniofacial fusion defects or syndromes that include such fusion defects.

Presentation

There are numerous causes of nasal masses. A differential diagnosis is made by performing a thorough history, physical examination, and radiologic evaluation. Biopsy is then usually necessary for definitive diagnosis. Again, biopsy of a nasal mass should be performed only after confirmation of the absence of a connection to the central nervous system by examination or radiologic study. An important piece of information to elicit when obtaining a history from a patient with a nasal mass is whether there has been a change in size with time or whether there is a change in size with crying or performing the Valsalva maneuver. Other important details are the presence of epistaxis, hypoesthesia, other cranial nerve deficits (especially changes in the sense of smell or in vision), pain, headaches, or epiphora. It is also helpful to know whether there has been a change in the appearance of the skin, a widening of the face, or any nasal obstruction and, if so, on which side and for how long. Furthermore, a history of the presence of a foreign body, nasal fluid leakage, a salty taste in the throat, headaches, the position in which leakage occurs, and the consistency of the nasal fluid are important details as are the presence of a purulent or malodorous discharge and a history of nasal trauma or surgery, meningitis, other congenital abnormalities, seizures, birth problems, or infection of the skin of the nasal dorsum.

When evaluating a nasal mass, it is important to note whether the mass is unilateral or bilateral and to look for the presence of external facial or cranial bulges, widening of the facial bones, telecanthus, skin discoloration, skin necrosis, or a small tuft of hair on the nasal dorsum, glabbella, or nasal tip. If an external bulge or hair tuft is present, the physician should note whether is it midline or off to one side. Other important signs include the presence of skin infection or discharge, rhinorrhea, abnormalities of cranial nerves I through XII (especially nerves I through VI), or other neurologic signs that may be indicative of increased cerebrospinal fluid pressure or tumor. It is important to perform a thorough nasal examination and flexible nasopharyngoscopy to determine the sidedness, color, size, consistency, and pulsation of the mass and to look for any evidence of leakage of cerebrospinal fluid at rest or with the Valsalva maneuver or crying and any signs of epistaxis or trauma. Erosion or pushing of surrounding structures, septal deviation, hypoesthesia of the nasal cavity, increase in the size of the mass with the Valsalva maneuver, bony defects of the nasal bones by palpation, or signs of infection are also important. Table 17–4 lists the most common nasal masses and their signs, symptoms, and distinguishing characteristics. Table 17–5 lists causes to consider in making a differential diagnosis of a nasal mass.

Evaluation

In evaluating a nasal mass, laboratory studies are usually not necessary. However, if leakage of cerebrospinal fluid is suspected, the presence of β_2-transferrin in the fluid or a glucose level higher than 50 mg/100 mL can be helpful in confirming that the fluid is indeed cerebrospinal fluid.[48, 49] For maximal results, fluid for β_2-transferrin analysis is best collected without using a sponge or tissue because the protein may settle or precipitate within these materials. Further-

Table 17–4. Common Types of Nasal Masses

Nasal Mass	Definition	Characteristics
Nasal dermoid	Subcutaneous collection of ectodermal and mesodermal elements Dermoid cyst remains superficial to nasal bones Dermoid sinus extends deep to nasal structures; 45% extend deep to nasal bones, 35% extend to cribriform	Tuft of hair noted on nasal dorsum or glabella Firm, noncompressible Nonpulsatile Occasionally lobulated May drain purulent material Majority are midline Usually diagnosed in children
Nasal glioma	Heterotopic remainder of neuroglial tissue	Overlying skin discoloration (reddish-blue) or telangiectasias Usually off midline Firm, noncompressible May appear polypoid intranasally Does not transilluminate More common in males; 60% are extranasal at the rhinion, 30% are intranasal, and 10% are a combination of intranasal and extranasal
Nasal cephalocele	Herniation of dura and cerebrospinal fluid White and gray matter not herniated or involved in sac	Usually present in infancy Pulsation of dura May or may not bulge with Valsalva maneuver Soft, compressible Bluish color Bulging nasal mass Transilluminates Associated with cerebrospinal fluid leak and meningitis
Nasal encephalocele	Herniation of dura, cerebrospinal fluid, and brain through bony defect in skull base Can occur in the following regions: nasoethmoid, nasoorbital, transethmoid, transsphenoid, sphenoethemoid, nasofrontal	Usually present in infancy Bulges with Valsalva maneuver Pulsation of dura Transilluminates Associated with cerebrospinal fluid leak and meningitis Soft, compressible Bluish color

more, the physician should be aware that optimal results may not be achieved in a patient with a low protein level in general (in the case of liver disease, for example) or if the analysis is performed more than 6 hours after specimen collection. If purulent nasal secretions and signs and symptoms of sinusitis are noted, a nasal culture and gram stain may be indicated.[50]

Radiographic evaluation is of utmost importance in evaluating a nasal mass. As stated previously, it is imperative to delineate the integrity of the skull base and the relationship between it and the mass in the workup of any nasal mass that cannot be clearly demarcated from the central nervous system by physical exam. A CT scan is an excellent study for evaluating the location, extent, and size of the mass as well as the status of the skull base, white matter, and size of the ventricles. An MRI scan should be obtained if the CT scan raises the possibility of an encephalocele. This will allow clear evaluation of the nasal soft tissue and the central nervous system. Also, because there is an increased incidence of ventricular dilation and corpus collosum agenesis with encephaloceles, an MRI scan is indicated if the CT scan shows definitive evidence of an encephalocele. Increased intracranial pressure may require treatment with medication or with a ventricular shunt prior to repair of the encephalocele. Failure to diagnose and treat increased intracranial pressure could result in leakage of cerebrospinal fluid or brain herniation after the repair of the encephalocele. Figure 17–11 shows the appearance of an encephalocele on a CT scan.

Priorities

A thorough history, physical examination, and radiologic workup and a high degree of suspicion prevent the complications involved in bi-

Table 17–5. *Differential Diagnosis of a Nasal Mass*

Differential Diagnosis	Comments
Lymphangioma	Soft, painless, compressible mass Usually continues to grow unless completely excised
Hemangioma	The most common head and neck neoplasm in children
Inverted papilloma	Usually occurs on the lateral nasal wall Has a 10% risk of malignant potential Is more common in males
Squamous papilloma	Usually occurs on the septum or ala or in the nasal vestibule
Squamous cell carcinoma	Most common paranasal sinus malignancy Associated with exposure to nickel In the nose, the most common sites are the anterior middle turbinate and the middle meatus
Olfactory neuroblastoma	Also known as esthesioneuroblastoma Arises from the olfactory neuroepithelium 20%–30% have regional or distant metastasis at presentation
Adenoid cystic carcinoma	Minor salivary gland malignancy May arise primarily or extend into the nasal cavity from a primary focus on the palate
Adenocarcinoma	Associated with woodworking In the nose, the most common sites are the anterior middle turbinate and the middle meatus
Chondrosarcoma	Rare tumor of the head and neck Most commonly presents at ages 30–40 years Treated with wide local excision and postoperative radiation therapy
Rhabdomyosarcoma	Most common soft tissue malignancy in children Most common site is the orbit with relatively rare occurrence in the paranasal sinus and nasal cavity; therefore, diagnosis of this malignancy in the nasal cavity should raise suspicion of extension from a primary orbital site
Melanoma	Dark, fleshy tumor that bleeds easily Most common head and neck sites are the oral cavity (50%), nasal cavity and sinuses (35%), and pharynx and larynx (15%)
Hemangiopericytoma	Slowly expanding asymptomatic mass Arises from the capillary pericyte of Zimmerman
Nasopharyngeal carcinoma (WHO types 1, 2, 3)	High incidence among the Chinese population Association of types 2 and 3 with Epstein-Barr virus Most common symptoms include neck mass, aural fullness, hearing loss, nasal airway obstruction, and epistaxis
Granulation tissue covering a foreign body	High index of suspicion in children and institutionalized patients
Superior or supreme turbinate	Normal anatomic structure Important not to mistake for a nasal mass
Large concha bullosa	Normal anatomic variant Important not to mistake for a nasal mass
Retroflexed uncinate process	Normal anatomic variant Important not to mistake for a nasal mass
Nasal polyposis	If found in any patient under 16 years of age, is suspicious for cystic fibrosis Unilateral nasal polyposis is suspicious for possible underlying malignancy
Lymphoma	Rarely found in nasal cavity Arises from lymphoid cells of bone marrow in the nasal bones or submucosal tissue
Fibrous dysplasia	Slow-growing tumor Mixture of fibrous and cancellous bone Most commonly occurs in the maxilla
Arteriovenous malformation	Growth is accelerated with hormonal changes
Mucosal changes secondary to granulomatous disease	Sarcoidosis, Wegener's granulomatosis, polymorphic reticulosis, etc.
Dacrocystitis	Symptoms include epiphora and pain Results from an obstruction of the upper nasolacrimal duct
Mucocele	Trapped mucus surrounded by inflamed sinonasal mucosa If infected, termed mucopyocele Can result in bone erosion or thickening that can mimic appearance of carcinoma on CT scan
Juvenile nasopharyngeal carcinoma	Occurs in pubescent males; usually a history of increasing nasal obstruction, severe epistaxis, and fullness of the cheek; CT or MRI scan shows characteristic bowing of the posterior wall of the maxillary sinus; embolization is usually performed prior to surgical excision; biopsy is not performed prior to resection because of the potential for severe epistaxis

WHO, World Health Organization.

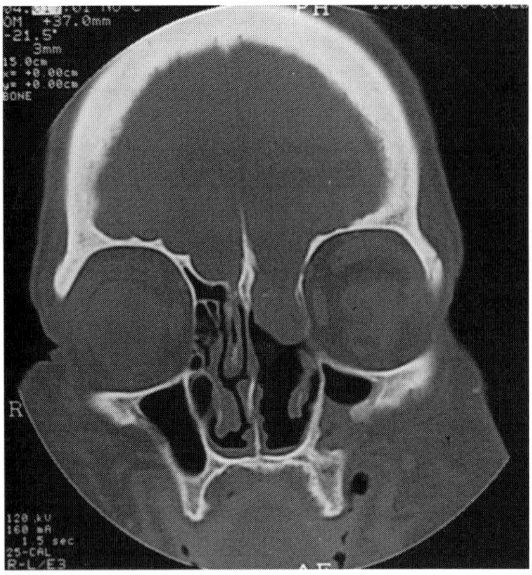

Figure 17–11. CT scan of a nasal encephalocele. (Courtesy of Douglas Mattox, M.D.)

opsying a nasal cephalocele. If the unfortunate circumstance arises in which complications occur, several immediate steps should be undertaken. First, the patient's ABCs and neurologic status must be evaluated. Hemostasis is obtained if bleeding is significant. A neurosurgery consultation is requested, and as soon as the patient has been stabilized, an emergent CT or MRI scan is performed. The physician should accompany the patient to, from, and during the radiologic study to deal with any sudden change in neurologic status until intracranial injury is ruled out. The nasal cavity should be evaluated and treated for active leakage of cerebrospinal fluid. If no leak is found and there are no acute radiologic findings, the patient should still be considered for inpatient neurologic observation overnight.

In a routine case, if central nervous system involvement is noted on radiology, neurosurgical consultation is appropriate. Genetics consultation may be indicated for a patient with craniofacial abnormalities or a suspicious family history.

The surgical treatment of a nasal cephalocele is performed on an elective basis after careful workup and surgical planning. The surgical approach to nasal dermoids, encephaloceles, and gliomas is discussed only briefly here, as treatment of nasal cephaloceles is not an emergency.

In general, encephaloceles, gliomas, and nasal dermoid sinuses with intracranial connections undergo primary surgical removal from above, with completion of the removal of the nasal portion secondarily. This can be done in a single- or a two-stage procedure. A transnasal endoscopic approach may be used alone in appropriate cases of small encephaloceles, gliomas, and dermoid sinuses.[51] The surgeon's endoscopic skill is an important factor when considering this approach. If a nasal mass is judged to be extracranial by imaging study but suspicious by examination for a nasal dermoid or glioma, it is wise to have a neurosurgeon available during excision of the mass in case a small tract is present and is found to extend intracranially. It is important to discuss this possibility with the patient preoperatively and obtain proper consent for all possibilities.

Extracranial external nasal masses can be removed through a variety of incisions, depending on the size and location of the mass. In general, nasal dermoids in the glabellar or rhinion region are excised through a vertical midline incision. An external rhinoplasty incision may be used, however, if a nasal dimple is present; it and its surrounding skin should be excised. Medial osteotomies are sometimes necessary to remove the sinus tract. Other approaches to excising a nasal mass are lateral rhinotomy incisions, closed rhinoplasty incisions, midfacial degloving, transconjunctival incisions, and bi- or hemicoronal incisions. These approaches can be combined with an endoscopic approach, or the endoscopic approach can be used alone in appropriate cases.

Outcomes

Complications in the presence of a cephalocele include meningitis, cerebrospinal fluid leakage, cosmetic deformity because of an expanding mass, anosmia, nasal airway obstruction, epistaxis, and erosion of the bones of the face. In addition, saddle-nose deformity, diplopia, telecanthus, stroke, seizure, increased intracranial pressure, sinusitis, septal deviation, and septal perforation can occur. Furthermore, there have been reports of facial scarring due to overlying skin change or necrosis, facial cellulitis, brain abscess, spontaneous pneumocephalus, intracranial bleeding, rhinorrhea secondary to nasal irritation, and interruption of parasympathetic nerve supply to the nasal mucosa. Eustachian tube dysfunction and velopharyngeal insufficiency can occur because of the effect of the mass on the nasopharynx.

Complications that can arise in biopsying an unrecognized mass in the central nervous system that is presenting as a nasal mass include meningitis, leakage of cerebrospinal fluid, anosmia, epistaxis, stroke, seizure, brain abscess, intracranial bleed, brain injury, pneumocephalus, orbital hemorrhage and injury, cranial nerve injury, and death.

REFERENCES

1. Bridger GP. Hereditary hemorrhagic telangiectasia. Arch Otolaryngol Head Neck Surg 1992; 118:992–993.
2. Guttmacher AE, Marchuk DA, White RI. Hereditary hemorrhagic telangiectasia. N Engl J Med 1995; 333:918–924.
3. Haitjema T et al. Screening family members of patients with hereditary hemorrhagic telangiectasia. Am J Med 1995; 99:519–524.
4. Lusher JM. Disease of coagulation: the fluid phase. In Nathan DG, Oski FA, eds. Hematology of Infancy and Childhood, 3rd ed. Philadelphia, WB Saunders, 1987, pp. 1293–1341.
5. Pringle MB, Beasley P, Brightwell AP. The use of Merocel nasal packs in the treatment of epistaxis. J Laryngol Otol 1996; 110:543–546.
6. Nissen RL. Myospherulosis: a review of etiology, diagnosis and treatment. Ear Nose Throat J 1984; 63:272–276.
7. Breda SD et al. Toxic shock syndrome in nasal surgery: a physiochemical and microbiologic evaluation of Merocel and Nu-Gauze nasal packing. Laryngoscope 1987; 97:1388.
8. Hull HF et al. Toxic shock syndrome related to nasal packing. Arch Otolaryngol Head Neck Surg 1983; 109:624.
9. Tag A et al. Toxic shock syndrome: otolaryngologic presentations. Laryngoscope 1982; 92:1070.
10. Cassisi NJ, Biller HF, Ogura JH. Changes in arterial oxygen tension and pulmonary mechanics with use of posterior packing in epistaxis. Laryngoscope 1971; 81:1261–1266.
11. Cook TA, Komorn RM. Statistical analysis of the alternative of blood gases produced by nasal packing. Laryngoscope 1972; 82:1802–1809.
12. Jacobs JR et al. Posterior packs and the nasopulmonary reflex. Laryngoscope 1981; 91:279–284.
13. Taasan V et al. The effect of nasal packing on sleep-disordered breathing and nocturnal oxygen desaturation. Laryngoscope 1981; 91:1163–1171.
14. Wurtele P. How I do it: emergency nasal packing using an umbilical cord clamp to secure a Foley catheter for posterior epistaxis. J Otolaryngol 1996; 25:46.
15. Wurman L et al. Selective endoscopic electrocautery for posterior epistaxis. Laryngoscope 1988; 98:1348–1349.
16. Pritkin JB, Calderelli DD, Panje NR. Endoscopic ligation if the internal maxillary artery for intractable posterior epistaxis. Ann Otol Rhinol Laryngol 1998; 107:85–91.
17. Winstead W. Sphenopalatine artery ligation: an alternative to internal maxillary artery ligation. Laryngoscope 1996; 106:667–669.
18. White PS. Endoscopic ligation of sphenopalatine artery (ELSA): a preliminary description. J Laryngol Otol 1996; 110:27–30.
19. Chandler JR, Serrins AJ. Transantral ligation of the internal maxillary artery for epistaxis. Laryngoscope 1965; 75:1151–1159.
20. Vikek JJ. Idiopathic intractable epistaxis: endovascular therapy. Head Neck Radiol 1991; 114:113–116.
21. Breda SO et al. Embolization for the treatment of epistaxis after the failure of internal maxillary ligation. Laryngoscope 1988; 99:809–813.
22. Lennox PA et al. A retrospective study of the role of the argon laser in the management of epistaxis secondary to hereditary hemorrhagic telangiectasia. J Laryngol Otol 1997; 11:34–37.
23. Velegrakis GA et al. Nd:YAG laser treatment of recurrent epistaxis in hereditary hemorrhagic telangiectasia. J Otolaryngol 1997; 26:384–386.
24. Lund VJ, Howard DJ. Closure of the nasal cavities in the therapy of refractive hereditary hemorrhagic telangiectasia. J Laryngol Otol 1997; 11:30–33.
25. Eliashar R, Sichel JY, Shah D. Preventing alar necrosis in using a Foley catheter for the control of posterior epistaxis. J Otolaryngol 1997; 26:166.
26. Streitmann MJ, Frable MA. Soft palate perforation: a complication of posterior nasal packing. Laryngoscope 1996; 114:806–807.
27. Morgan MK, Aldren CP. Oroantral fistula: a complication of transantral ligation of the internal maxillary artery for epistaxis. J Laryngol Otol 1997; 11:468–470.
28. Katz E. Intranasal steroid injection. J Otolaryngol 1985; 14:136–138.
29. DeJong RH, Ronfeld RA, DeRosa R. Cardiovascular effects of convulsant and supraconvulsant doses of amide local anesthetics. Anesth Analg 1982; 61:3.
30. Cullen MM, Tami TA. Comparison of internal maxillary artery ligation versus embolization for refractory epistaxis. Otolaryngol Head Neck Surg 1998; 118:630–642.
31. Lusher JM. Disease of coagulation: the fluid phase. In Nathan DG, Oski FA, eds. Hematology of Infancy and Childhood, 3rd ed. Philadelphia, WB Saunders, 1987, pp. 1293–1341.
32. Haitjema T et al. Screening family members of patients with hereditary hemorrhagic telangiectasia. Am J Med 1995; 99:519–524.
33. Guttmacher AE, Marchuk DA, White RI. Hereditary hemorrhagic telangectasia. N Engl J Med 1995; 333(14):918–924.
34. Krespi YP, Kuriloff, Aner M. Sarcoidosis of the sinonasal tract: a new staging system. Otolaryngol Head Neck Surg 1995; 112:221–227.
35. Sneller MC. Wegener's granulomatosis. JAMA 1997; 273:1288–1291.
36. Campbell SM, Montanaro A, Bardana EJ. Head and neck manifestations of autoimmune disease. Am J Otolaryngol 1983; 4:187–216.
37. Specks U, DeRemee RA. Granulomatous vasculitis. Rheumatol Dis Clin North Am 1990; 16:377–396.
38. Kastenbauer ER. Management of hematoma of the septum and abscesses of the nasal septum. Laryngo Rhino Otolaryngol 1997; 76:A1–A5.
39. Ginsberg CM, Leach JL. Infected nasal septal hematoma. Pediatr Infect Dis J 1995; 14:1012–1013.
40. Munoz A, Pedrosa I, Villafruela M. Eraseroma as a cause of rhinolith: CT and MRI in a child. Neuroradiology 1997; 39:824–826.
41. Ezsias A, Sugar AW. Rhinolith: an unusual case and an update. Ann Otol Rhinol Laryngol 1997; 106:135–138.
42. Celikkanat S et al. Rhinolithiasis. Rhinology 1997; 35:39–40.
43. Chaker AC et al. Bilateral rhinolithiasis. Ear Nose Throat J 1987; 57:50.
44. Ahmmed AU, Camilleri AE, Small M. Cavernous sinus thrombosis following the manipulation of fractured nasal bones. J Laryngol Otol 1996; 110:69–71.
45. Martin SH. Injury to the head and cervical spine. Otolaryngol Clin North Am 1976; 9:403–423.
46. Duvall AJ, Banovatz JD. Nasoethmoid fractures. Otolaryngol Clin North Am 1976; 9:507–515.
47. Hester TO, Camplbell JP. Diagnosis and management of nasal trauma for primary care physicians. J Ky Med Assoc 1997; 95:386–392.

48. Meurman EM et al. A new method for the detection of CSF leakage. Acta Otolaryngol 1979; 87:366–369.
49. Skedros PG, Chandler JR. Traumatic CSF leakage. Otolarygol Clin North Am 1983; 16:623–632.
50. Skedros PG et al. Sources of error in the use of beta-transferrin analysis for diagnosis of perilymphatic and CSF leaks. Otolaryngol Head Neck Surg 1993; 109:861–864.
51. Mattox DE, Kennedy DW. Endoscopic management of CSF leaks and cephaloceles. Laryngoscope 1990; 100:857–862.

SUGGESTED READING

Epistaxis

Abelson TI. Epistaxis. In Paperella et al., eds. Otolaryngology. Philadelphia, WB Saunders, 1991, pp. 1831–1841.

Culbertson MC, Manning SC. Epistaxis. In Bluestone CD, Stool SE, eds. Pediatric Otolaryngology. Philadelphia, WB Saunders, 1988, pp. 672–679.

Elwany S, Abdel-Fatah H. Endoscopic control of posterior epistaxis. J Laryngol Otol 1996; 110;432–434.

Leopore ML. Epistaxis. In Bailey BJ, ed. Head and Neck Surgery: Otolaryngology. Philadelphia, JB Lippincott, 1993, pp. 428–446.

Myer CM, Cotton RT. Epistaxis. In A practical approach to pediatric otolaryngology. Chicago, Year Book, 1988, pp. 122–133.

Petruson B. Epistaxis: a clinical study with special reference to fibrinolysis. Acta Otolaryngol Suppl 1974; 317:3.

Raczkowksi VF et al. Cocaine acts in the central nervous system to inhibit sympathetic neural activity. J Pharmacol Exp Ther 1991; 257:511–519.

Rood SR et al. The management of epistaxis: self-instructional packet. Alexandria, VA, American Academy of Otolaryngology—Head and Neck Surgery.

Verlander JM, Johns ME. The clinical use of cocaine. Otolaryngol Clin North Am 1981; 14:521–531.

Wurman LH. Epistaxis. In Gates GA, ed. Current Therapy in Otolaryngology-Head and Neck Surgery, 5th ed. St. Louis, Mosby, 1994, pp. 354–358.

Septal Hematoma

Macrei DR. Epistaxis and nasal trauma. In Cummings CW, ed. Otolaryngology: Head and Neck Surgery, St. Louis, Mosby, 1992, pp. 734–735.

Marlowe FI. Injuries of the nose, facial bones and paranasal sinuses. In Bluestone CD, Stool SE, eds. Pediatric Otolaryngology. Philadelphia, WB Saunders, 1988, p. 769.

Myer CM, Cotton RT. Facial trauma. In A practical approach to pediatric otolaryngology. Chicago, Year Book, 1988, p. 222.

Rabuzzi DD, Hengerer AS. Complications of nasal and sinus infections. In Bluestone CD, Stool SE, eds. Pediatric Otolaryngology. Philadelphia, WB Saunders, 1988, pp. 745–746.

Wood RP, Jafek BW, Eberhard R. Nasal obstruction. In Bailey BJ, ed. Head and Neck Surgery: Otolaryngology. Philadelphia, JB Lippincott, 1993, p. 311.

Nasal Foreign Body

Macrei DR. Epistaxis and nasal trauma. In Cummings CW, ed. Otolaryngology: Head and Neck Surgery, St. Louis, Mosby, 1992, pp. 723–725.

Myer CM, Cotton RT. Nasal obstruction. In A Practical Approach to Pediatric Otolaryngology. Chicago, Year Book, 1988, pp. 93–95.

Shapiro RS. Foreign bodies of the nose. In Bluestone CD, Stool SE, eds. Pediatric Otolaryngology. Philadelphia, WB Saunders, 1988, pp. 752–759.

Wood RP, Jafek BW, Eberhard R. Nasal obstruction. In Bailey BJ, ed. Head and neck surgery: Otolaryngology, Philadelphia, JB Lippincott, 1993, pp. 302–323.

Nasal Trauma

Arden RL, Mathog RH. Nasal fractures. In Cummings CW, ed. Otolaryngology: Head and Neck Surgery. St. Louis, Mosby, 1993, pp. 737–753.

Bailey BJ. Nasal fractures. In Bailey BJ, ed. Head and Neck Surgery: Otolaryngology. Philadelphia, JB Lippincott, 1993, pp. 991–1007.

Boekhus GJ. Nasal fracture. In Paperella MM, et al., eds. Otolaryngology. Philadelphia, WB Saunders, 1991, pp. 1823–1830.

Marlowe FI: Injuries of the nose, facial bones and paranasal sinuses. In Bluestone CD, Stool SE, eds. Pediatric Otolaryngology. Philadelphia, WB Saunders, 1988, pp. 767–769.

Myer CM, Cotton RT. Nasal fracture. In A Practical Approach to Pediatric Otolaryngology. Chicago, Year Book, 1988, pp. 222–223.

Ridenour BD. Nasal fracture. In Gates GA, ed. Current Therapy in Otolaryngology: Head and Neck Surgery 5th ed. St. Louis, Mosby, 1994, pp. 132–138.

Encephalocele

DeSanto LW. Neoplasms. In Cummings CW, ed. Otolaryngology: Head and Neck Surgery. St. Louis, Mosby, 1993, pp. 754–763.

Hao SP, Wang HS, Lui TN. Transnasal endoscopic management of basal encephalocele-craniotomy is no longer necessary. Am J Otolaryngol 1995; 16:196–199.

Hengerer AS, Newburg JA. Congenital malformations of the nose and sinuses. In Bluestone CD, Stool SE, eds. Pediatric Otolaryngology. Philadelphia, WB Saunders, 1988, pp. 718–728.

Kennedy EM et al. Transpalatal approach for the extracranial surgical repair of transsphenoidal cephaloceles in children. J Neurosurg 1997; 87;677–681.

Khan MA, Salahuddin I. Intranasal meningoencephalocele and the use of fibrin glue. Ear Nose Throat J 1997; 76:464–467.

Knudsen SJ, Bailey BJ. Midline nasal masses. In Bailey BJ, ed. Head and Neck Surgery: Otolaryngology. Philadelphia, JB Lippincott, 1993, pp. 329–341.

McDonald WS, Zagzag D, Thorne CH. Frontonasal encephalocele and associated congenital brain tumor. J Craniofac Surg 1995; 6:386–389.

Myer CM, Cotton RT. Nasal obstruction. In A practical approach to pediatric otolaryngology. Chicago, Year Book, 1988, pp. 91–93.

Newboune JP et al. Frontal sinus cephalocele associated with hydrocephalus. J Comput Assist Tomogr 1997; 21:840–841.

Pashley NR. Congenital anomalies of the nose. In Cummings CW, ed. Otolaryngology: Head and Neck Surgery. St. Louis, Mosby, 1993, pp. 702–712.

Sessions RB, Hudkins C. Congenital anomalies of the nose. In Bailey BJ, ed. Head and Neck Surgery: Otolaryngology. Philadelphia, JB Lippincott, 1993, pp. 793–801.

Stanievich JF, Lore JM. Tumors of the nose, paranasal sinuses and nasopharynx. In Bluestone CD, Stool SE, eds. Pediatric Otolaryngology. Philadelphia, WB Saunders, 1988, p. 780–792.

Turgut M et al. Congenital nasal encephalocele: a review of 35 cases. J Craniomaxillofac Surg 1995; 23:1–5.

CHAPTER 18

Paranasal Sinus Emergencies

Bert W. O'Malley, Jr., MD

INVASIVE FUNGAL RHINOSINUSITIS

Invasive fungal rhinosinusitis is characterized by mucosal infiltration by mycotic organisms and angiocentric invasion into paranasal sinus soft tissue and bone as well as into orbital and intracranial structures. The primary risk factor for invasive fungal rhinosinusitis is an immunocompromised state. High-risk patients are those with hematologic neoplasms requiring high-dose chemotherapy bone marrow transplantation, those who test positive for the human immunodeficiency virus (HIV) and who have acquired immunodeficiency syndrome (AIDS), insulin-dependent diabetics, patients with underlying primary hematologic deficiencies, and patients who require heavy steroid therapy for autoimmune diseases.[1, 2] Invasive fungal rhinosinusitis is, in most cases, a surgical emergency that continues to be lethal in 50% to 80% of cases.[3]

Presentation

A patient's history reveals one or more underlying disease processes, such as those mentioned earlier, that cause immunocompromise. On initial presentation, a patient's symptoms, physical examination, and radiographic findings are the same as those of classic acute sinusitis, and many have already been treated with steroids and intravenous broad-spectrum antibiotics for 7 to 21 days. Up to 80% of patients with invasive fungal rhinosinusitis have a history of a regimen of more than three antibiotics.

The most common presenting symptoms included fever and facial and periorbital pain and swelling as well as nasal congestion, rhinorrhea, and headache.[4] Less common at presentation are ophthalmologic complaints such as decreased visual acuity or ophthalmoplegia. Many patients present with two or more of these symptoms.

Evaluation

All patients with the history and symptoms noted earlier should receive rigid nasal endoscopy and biopsy of tissue suspicious because of visible mucosal abnormalities, including erythema with edema, granulation, and pale, white, or black discoloration. Also ulcerated tissue, mucosal sites that do not bleed when manipulated, and areas that have decreased sensation upon manipulation should raise the suspicion of invasive fungal disease. Tissue biopsy identifies the presence of fungal hyphae in the submucosa and angiocentric invasion and provides the definitive diagnosis.

The two most common invasive fungal infections are mucormycosis and aspergillosis. Mucormycosis is a general term used to describe invasive disease caused by organisms belonging to the class Phycomycetes (also called Zygomycetes). The most common genera are *Rhizopus*, *Mucor*, and *Absidia*. Patients with poorly controlled diabetes and patients in ketoacidosis are at high risk, as the fungi appear to favor an environment of high glucose and acidity. Microscopic examination demonstrates tissue necrosis and vascular invasion with nonseptate, branching hyphae (Fig. 18–1). Organisms of the genus *Aspergillus* are the most commonly identi-

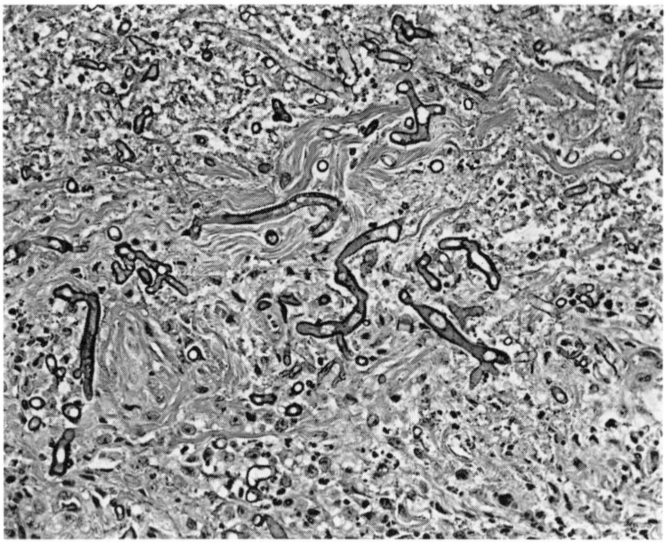

Figure 18–1. Photomicrograph of early invasion of *Mucor* species into the subcutaneous tissues of the maxillary sinus mucosa. Note the nonseptated hyphae.

fied organisms in the fungal infections of invasive rhinosinusitis in nondiabetic, immunocompromised patients. The most prevalent species are *A. fumigatus*, *A. flavus*, and *A. niger.* Histologic characteristics of involved paranasal tissue include necrosis and vascular invasion with septated fungal forms that have acute (45-degree angle) branching (Fig. 18–2).

In early and potentially curable invasive fungal rhinosinusitis, the middle turbinate is the most common site of involvement, followed by the ethmoid and maxillary sinuses and then the nasal septum and the inferior turbinate (Fig. 18–3).[4] Mucosal discoloration is an inconsistent finding and should not be a criterion for definitive diagnosis nor should one decide against biopsy of even mildly inflamed tissues.

Hematologic derangements are common at the time of diagnosis and should be used to heighten awareness of the possibility of invasive fungal disease. Neutropenia (a white blood count lower than 500), thrombocytopenia (a platelet count lower than 60,000), and anemia (a hematocrit level less than 30%) are common findings in these patients. HIV-positive patients with AIDS may have CD4 counts lower than 50.

All patients should have computed tomography (CT) scans of the paranasal sinuses, and magnetic resonance imaging (MRI) scans may also be obtained for patients with evidence or suspicion of intracranial or central nervous system (CNS) involvement on history and physical examination (Fig. 18–4). Evidence of invasion such as erosion of bone within or beyond the confines of the sinonasal region is highly suggestive of invasive fungal disease; however, when no erosion or abscess is found, patients

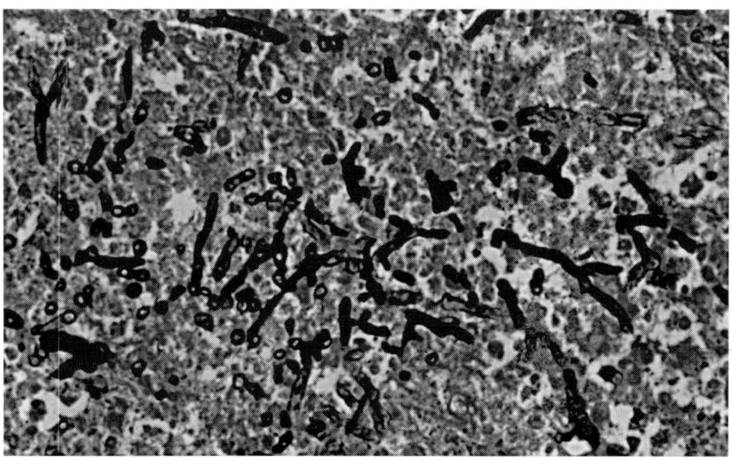

Figure 18–2. Photomicrograph of extensive *Aspergillus fumigatus* invasion and necrosis of the maxillary sinus mucosa. Note the classic acute (45-degree) angled branches and septated hyphae.

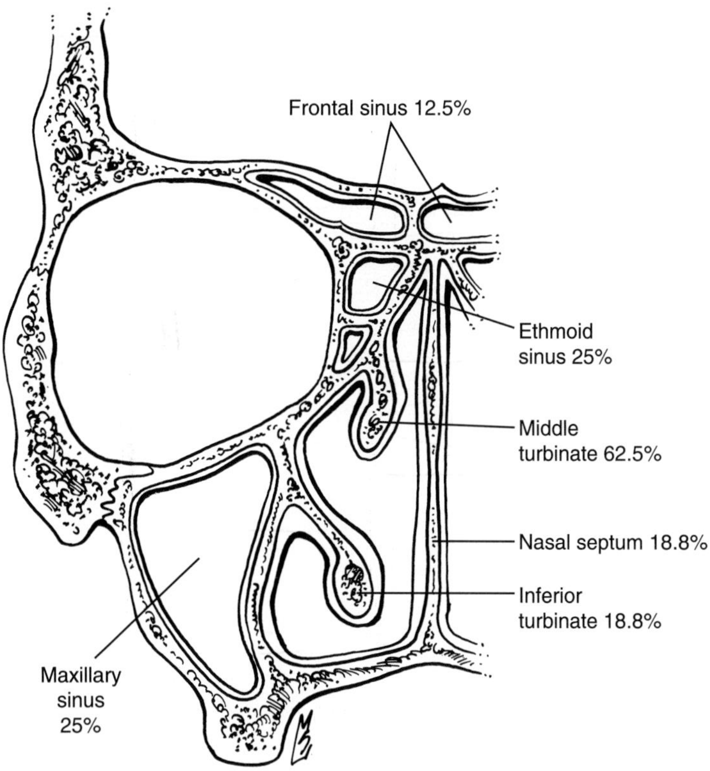

Figure 18–3. The most common sites of early fungal invasion shown for the right nose and paranasal sinus cavities. The middle turbinate has the highest incidence of fungal invasion, and it may serve as a useful site for early biopsy to rule out fungal invasion.

may still have significant invasive disease with involvement of the CNS (Fig. 18–5).

Priorities

Nasal biopsy and surgery should be preceded by correction of thrombocytopenia to higher than 60,000 and replacement of any needed coagulation factors. Treatment is initiated as soon as the diagnosis is made from tissue biopsy and should not be delayed while waiting for analysis of cultures taken at the time of the nasal sinus examination. Amphotericin B is the choice of antifungal chemotherapy, with dosing up to 1 mg/kg/day or higher. A full course of amphotericin B involves a total dose of 2 grams or more.[5] Granulocyte colony stimulating factor may also be used in an attempt to stimulate an increase in the white blood cell count, although this therapy requires further investigation to prove its efficacy or benefit.

In general, surgical resection of involved structures is recommended.[4,6] Although the resolution of neutropenia is critical for survival, surgical debridement eradicates or slows the progression of the invasive disease and allows time for bone marrow recovery. The scope of surgical resection varies with the extent of disease. For limited disease, transnasal endoscopic surgery, external ethmoidectomy, or the Caldwell-Luc operation is appropriate. For more extensive or invasive disease, radical surgical resection may be required, including medial maxillectomy, total maxillectomy with orbital exenteration, or craniofacial resection. Multiple or repeat surgical procedures may be required to control even limited disease. The goal of surgery is to obtain complete resection of the diseased tissue. Demonstration of viable, bleeding tissue margins intraoperatively is a good clinical indicator of adequate resection, but whenever possible, biopsies of margins or residual tissue should be evaluated with frozen sections. Blood, platelet, and coagulation factor replacement may be required for even minor surgical procedures in these patients and should be available as needed before, during, and after the surgery.

Outcomes

In a recently reported series, the survival rate for patients with invasive fungal rhinosinusitis was 40%.[4] Of the survivors, 90% had complete surgical resection that was documented by a combination of frozen-section analyses of surgical margins and clinical documentation of viable

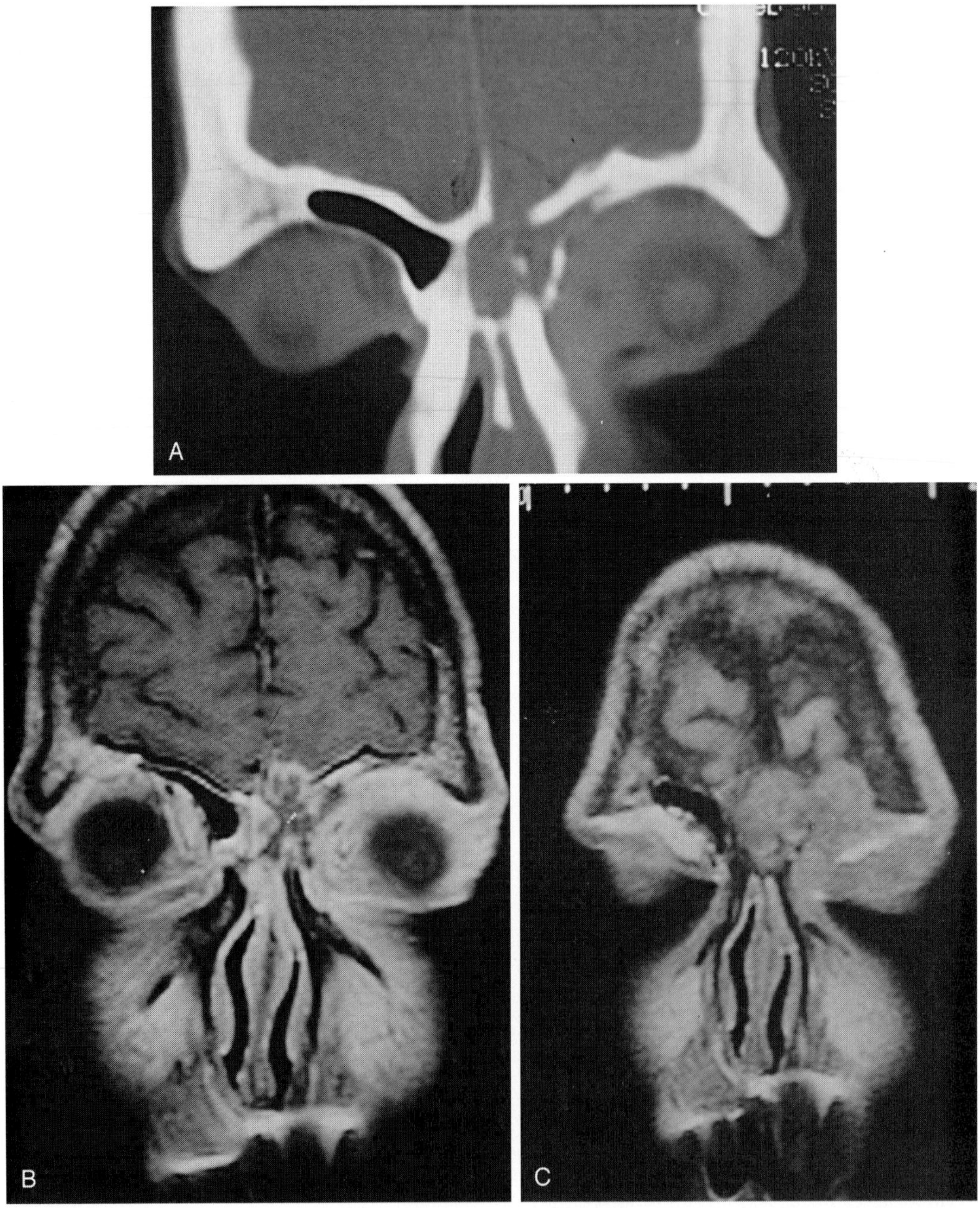

Figure 18–4. A: Coronal CT image showing left frontal sinusitis with a defect in the bony roof. B: Coronal MRI with contrast, demonstrating the frontal sinus infection and intracranial extension. C: Coronal MRI depicting extensive intracranial invasion and involvement of the frontal lobe by invasive *Aspergillus* species fungal sinusitis in an HIV+ patient.

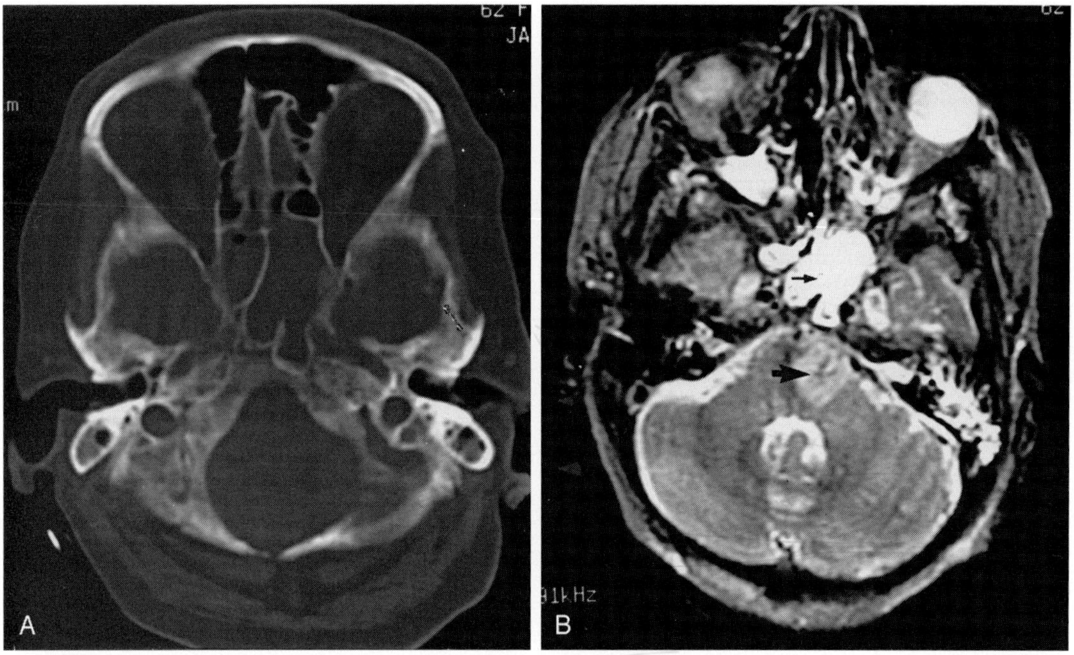

Figure 18–5. A: Axial CT image showing ethmoid and sphenoid sinusitis in an immunocompromised patient. There is no evidence of bony erosion. B: Axial MRI with contrast of the same patient (performed on the same day as the CT scan), demonstrating extension of the infectious process into the brain stem (large arrowhead) and corresponding sphenoid sinusitis (small arrow). Sphenoid sinus mucosal biopsy and necrotic bone in the clivus confirmed the presence of invasive *Aspergillus fumigatus.*

bleeding tissue. In the same series, the mortality rate was 90% for patients who had residual disease after surgical intervention. These patients typically had invasive disease that extended beyond the paranasal sinuses into deep soft tissues or to the skull base at the time of diagnosis. Therefore, the need for radical surgical resection portends a poor prognosis.

The overall mortality rate in invasive fungal rhinosinusitis remains 50% to 80% by some estimates.[3] Although surgery and amphotericin B are important, long-term survival ultimately depends on bone marrow recovery and reversal of the hematologic derangements. For patients who respond to intervention, close follow-up with frequent rigid nasal endoscopy is necessary so that disease relapse or progression can be identified and treated early.

PERIORBITAL AND ORBITAL INFECTION CAUSED BY SINUSITIS

Orbital and periorbital infections usually arise as a complication of sinusitis and require immediate intervention.[7] The incidence of such complications is not well documented but published series have reported ranges of 0.5% to 3.9%.[8] Orbital infections occur more frequently in pediatric and adolescent patients, and orbital cellulitis is the most common cause of proptosis in children. The ethmoid sinus is the predominant site of origin of orbital sequelae, but the sites vary with the patient's age. In infants, both maxillary and ethmoid sinus infections contribute to the development of orbital complications. In school-age children, ethmoid sinusitis is the major origin; in adolescents and adults, ethmoid sinusitis followed by frontal sinusitis are the common sources of orbital infections. The pediatric population is at higher risk for orbital sequelae of sinusitis for a number of reasons. Children and adolescents have a higher frequency of upper respiratory tract infections, and anatomically they have greater bony vascularity, thinner paranasal sinus bones, and smaller sinus ostia than adults.[9]

The levels of orbital involvement range from periorbital or preseptal cellulitis to subperiosteal abscess, to direct orbital cellulitis or abscess. Periorbital or preseptal cellulitis is by far the most common of these and is found in 80% to 95% of cases of orbital extension of sinusitis.[7, 10] Direct orbital involvement is less common because the orbital septum (a continuation of the frontal periosteum) is a significant natural barrier to the spread of sinus infection.

Presentation

Periorbital cellulitis presents concurrently with sinusitis and its associated symptoms. The predominant findings on physical examination are eyelid edema and erythema. The eye is painful and tender to palpation, but there is no proptosis, chemosis, or ocular dysmotility. Visual acuity is normal in these cases as is the fundoscopic examination.

A subperiosteal abscess results from direct extension of ethmoid sinusitis or, less commonly, of frontal sinusitis or mucopyocele. A discrete collection of pus is found between the lamina papyracea, or superior bony orbit, and the periorbita (orbital septum). Along with the physical findings and symptoms of periorbital cellulitis, subperiosteal abscess may cause proptosis with either lateral or downward displacement of the globe.

Orbital cellulitis occurs when infection courses through the orbital septum to create an acute inflammatory reaction within the orbital fat, muscles, and nerves and the globe itself. Proptosis results from edema and distension of inflamed intraorbital vessels. Conjunctival lymphatics become obstructed by the inflammatory process and cause chemosis, which is readily apparent on physical examination. Ulcerations indicate direct involvement of the globe.

An orbital abscess arises from direct erosion of a subperiosteal abscess through the periorbita or from coalescence of orbital cellulitis. A single collection or multiple collections of pus may be present in both the extraconal and intraconal compartments of the eye. Physical findings include severe proptosis, chemosis, and pain, with partial or complete ophthalmoplegia, optic neuritis, and vascular ischemia. Irreversible optic nerve damage and blindness are common presenting findings and sequelae.

Evaluation

Although the physical findings provide important clues to the diagnosis of periorbital or orbital infections resulting from sinusitis, radiographic examination is critical in delineating the extent of orbital involvement. A CT scan with intravenous contrast provides the definitive diagnosis and differentiates a more common periorbital cellulitis from a less common subperiosteal abscess (Fig. 18–6). An MRI scan may be used alone or in conjunction with a CT scan to localize abscesses or define the extent of an intraorbital inflammatory process. Imaging studies reveal thickened sinus mucosa or evidence of acute sinusitis in the primary paranasal sinus source. A CT scan may reveal the thinning of bony walls or loss of bony definition between the sinus and orbit. Orbital complications of acute sinusitis do not commonly demonstrate frank bone erosion on a CT scan. A mucopyocele of the frontal sinus, however, often demonstrates bone erosion or dehiscence in the presence of orbital extension. An MRI scan may provide better differentiation between a subperiosteal or orbital abscess and orbital cellulitis.

Sinus cultures or direct cultures of abscess contents may prove helpful in directing appropriate antibiotic therapy. The most common organism identified in the pediatric population with periorbital cellulitis is *Hemophilus influenzae*, especially in children under 3 years of age.[7] Cultures of the contents of subperiosteal or orbital abscesses, however, reveal *Staphylococcus aureus* and *Streptococcus pneumoniae* in the majority of cases. Less common in abscesses are mixed cultures or anaerobic organisms such as *Bacteroides*. No organisms may be identified in 30% to 50% of cases because of antibiotic therapy administered prior to the time cultures are obtained.

Priorities

All potential periorbital or orbital infections should be evaluated and followed by an ophthalmologist. For patients with periorbital or preseptal cellulitis, hospitalization and prompt administration of intravenous antibiotics proves sufficient treatment and should stop the progression to more serious orbital or even intracranial complications. Topical nasal decongestants as well as oral decongestants are typically administered in conjunction with antibiotic therapy. Because of its efficacy against *H. influenzae*, ampicillin can be given intravenously in divided doses up to 200 mg/kg/day. The combination of ampicillin with sulbactam (Unasyn) may be chosen for its benefit against β-lactamase–producing bacteria. Combination therapy with the addition of chloramphenicol may also be chosen as may alternative antibiotics such as cefuroxime. For adolescents or adults and in cases of periorbital or orbital abscesses, high-dose penicillins with β-lactamase–protecting agents are usually sufficient. Nafcillin

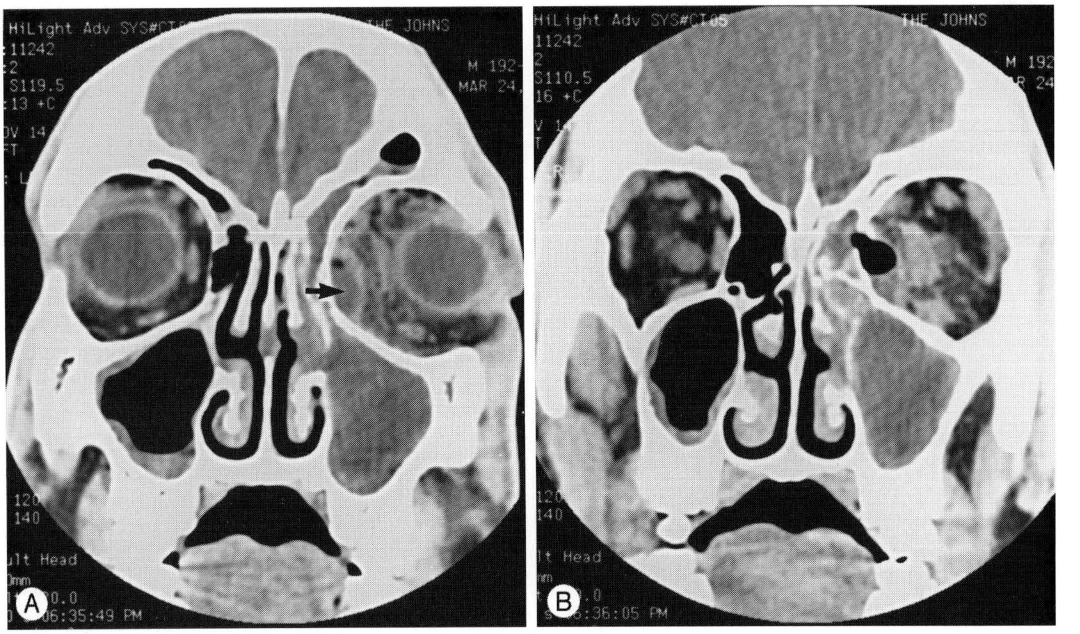

Figure 18–6. A: Coronal CT image demonstrating a subperiosteal abscess *(arrow)*. B: CT image of the same patient showing a defect in the lamina papyracea and intraorbital air.

may also be chosen, especially when penicillinase-producing organisms are suspected or identified. Steroids are not typically used in the face of uncontrolled infection and are generally not recommended for orbital complications of sinusitis.

Subperiosteal and orbital abscesses require prompt institution of intravenous antibiotics as well as surgical intervention after abscess diagnosis and localization by radiographic imaging studies. The external ethmoid approach to incision and drainage with ethmoidectomy and placement of Penrose drains is the classic choice for surgical intervention. However, endoscopic ethmoidectomy, removal of lamina papyracea, and intranasal drainage of the abscess is a possible alternative approach. The periobita should not be incised in cases of isolated subperiosteal abscess. Other paranasal sinus cavities should be opened and drained according to their potential role in causing the orbital infection.

In cases of orbital cellulitis, medical management is usually sufficient to treat the acute process; surgery is reserved for cases in which there is persistent or progressive infection. High-dose intravenous antibiotics and careful and frequent clinical examination in conjunction with ophthalmologic examination are used to assess the progression of the disease. An increase in intraorbital pressure caused by the cellulitis may induce central retinal artery compression and lead to decreased retinal perfusion. Medical treatment for this complication includes administration of acetazolamide, mannitol, or timolol. In these cases, lateral canthotomy and inferior cantholysis may be performed to reduce pressure-related injury to the optic nerve. Loss of or decrease in visual acuity or ocular motility, progression of erythema, edema, and chemosis, or persistence of or increase in fever or pain over 48 to 72 hours warrants repeat radiographic imaging studies followed by surgical intervention. External ethmoidectomy with sphenoidotomy or frontal sinusotomy or an endoscopic approach to sinus drainage and orbital decompression may be chosen, depending on the severity and origin of the disease.[11, 12]

Outcomes

Visual loss and other, associated morbidities are uncommon with periorbital or preseptal cellulitis that is treated with prompt intravenous antibiotic therapy. In cases of subperiosteal abscess, antibiotics and surgical intervention provide adequate therapy with minimal associated morbidity. Orbital cellulitis and orbital abscess, depending on the severity or progression of the disease, may result in diffuse loss of orbital contents and loss of vision, even with appropriate medical and surgical interventions. Intraorbital surgery in cases of orbital abscess may also result in injury to extraocular muscles or orbital cranial nerves, including the optic nerve. CNS involvement and cranial nerve neuropathies may occur, especially in cases of orbital cellulitis and abscess. The most devastating of CNS complications is cavernous sinus thrombosis which may be lethal in 70% to 80% of cases. Fortunately, cavernous sinus thrombosis occurs in only an estimated 1% of all cases of orbital infections and complications of sinusitis.[7, 9] A more detailed discussion of CNS complications and emergencies as a result of bacterial sinusitis is found in the following section.

INTRACRANIAL INFECTION RESULTING FROM SINUSITIS

Intracranial infections may occur after acute or chronic sinusitis; their incidence among patients requiring hospitalization for sinusitis is reported as being 3.7%.[13] For those patients who require hospitalization and treatment for intracranial infection, sinusitis has been the cause in a reported 5.9% of patients and has surpassed otologic disease as the most common cause of brain abscess.[14] Frontal sinusitis is the cause of intracranial involvement in the majority of cases, followed in descending order of frequency by sinusitis of the ethmoid, the sphenoid and, rarely, the maxillary sinuses.[15] The population that is most susceptible and that has the highest incidence is adolescents and young adults. This incidence corresponds with the period of frontal sinus development, which occurs between the ages of 10 and 20.

Frontal lobe cerebral abscess followed by meningitis are the most common intracranial infections that result from sinusitis. Sinusitis is also the most common cause of cerebral abscess.[16] The other, less common intracranial complications of sinusitis are epidural abscess, subdural abscess, and cavernous sinus thrombosis. Infection can enter the intracranial cavity by a variety of pathways. Infections may spread from the frontal sinus as a thrombophlebitis that tracks along the veins of Breschet, which are valveless diploic veins that directly connect the mucosa of the frontal sinus and the dural veins. Also, intracranial infection may result from thrombophlebitis along the small veins passing through the cribriform plate or along the ethmoidal veins that drain into the cavern-

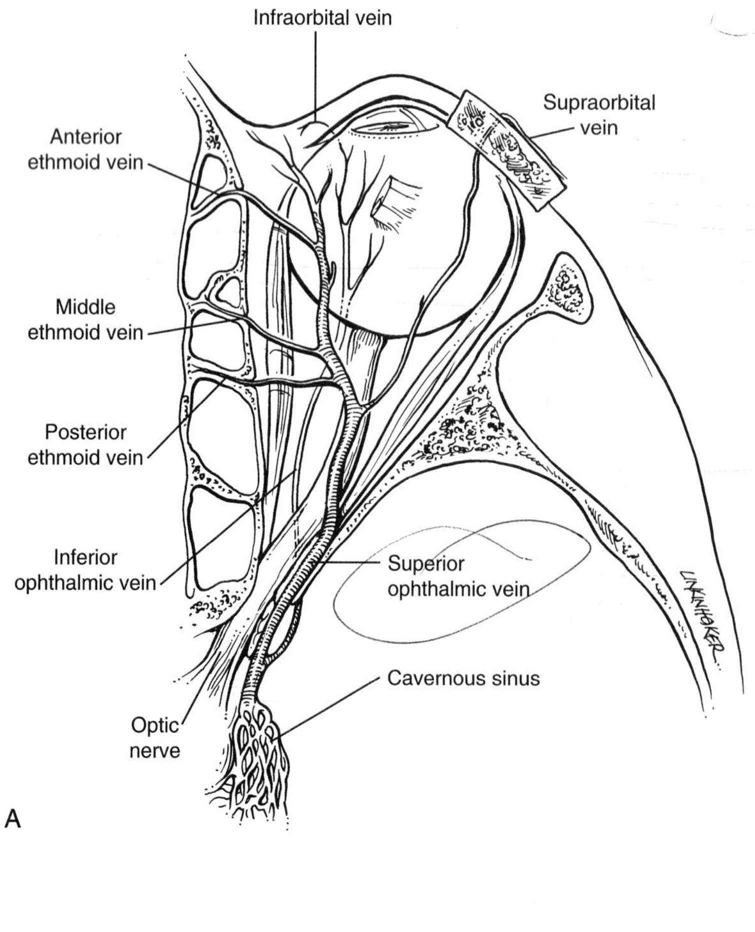

Figure 18–7. A: The ethmoid and orbital veins through which paranasal, periorbital, and orbital infections may travel to the cavernous sinus.

ous sinus via the ophthalmic vein (Fig. 18–7A). Facial veins and veins from the paranasal sinuses and temporal bone may also serve as conduits for the spread of infection intracranially and into the cavernous sinus (Fig. 18–7B). Intracranial infection may also result from direct extension through congenital or acquired bony dehiscence. Other avenues include the tracking of infection along perineural sheaths or a result of mucocele extension or osteomyelitis.

Presentation

Aside from the general symptoms of sinusitis, a patient may complain of persistent fever and headaches over a prolonged course of acute or chronic sinusitis. In a patient with meningitis, physical examination may reveal nuchal rigidity, or a patient may present later in the course of infection with depressed consciousness or focal neurologic defects. Neurologic symptoms may not be present in a patient with early epidural or cerebral abscess, and suspicion should be high in the face of persistent headache and spiking fevers. The patient's history is therefore very important in making a diagnosis before life-threatening complications occur. A patient typically describes a significant or prolonged episode of sinusitis followed in the later stage by a headache and agitation that may be the result of a focal or diffuse area of cerebritis. There may be a subsequent quiescent period during which the patient is totally asymptomatic while the abscess coalesces. When the abscess expands, headache and agitation return and pro-

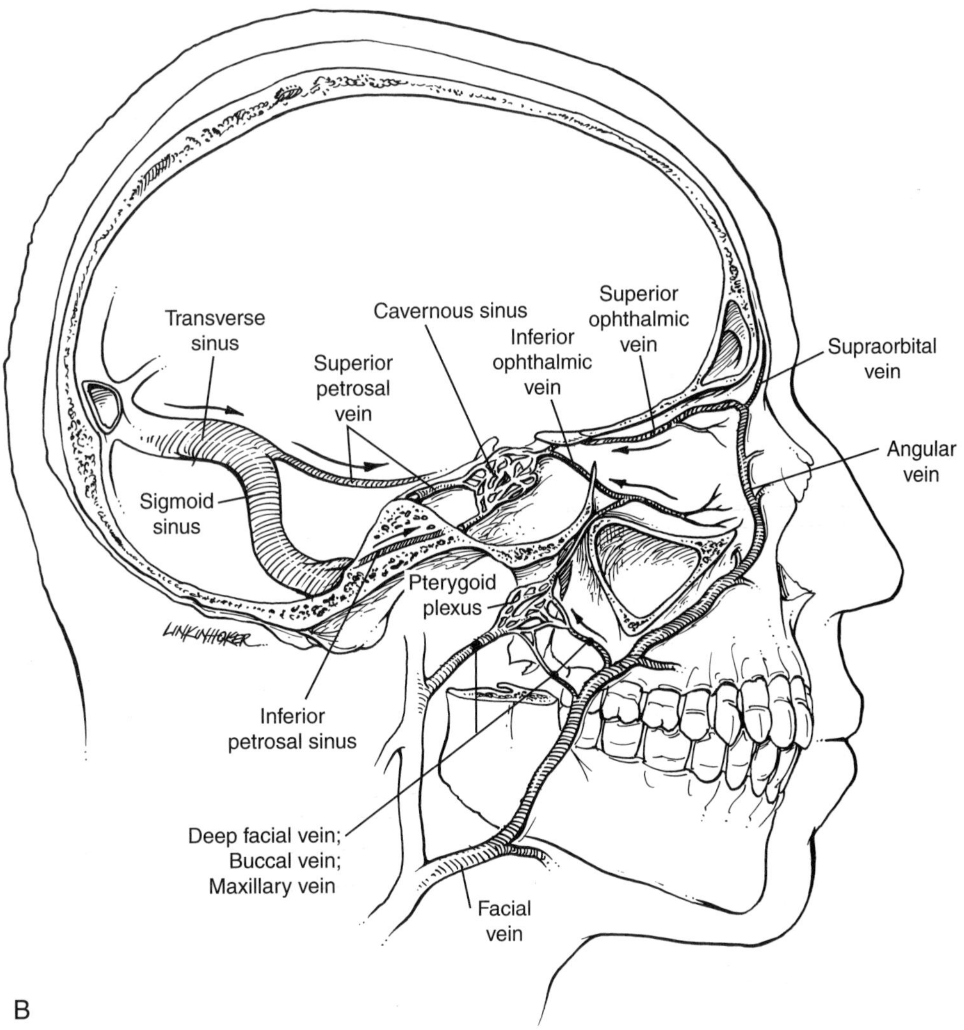

Figure 18–7 *Continued.* B: The facial vein, paranasal sinus veins, and intracranial veins that drain into the cavernous sinus and that may serve as routes for intracranial spread of infection.

gress, followed by the onset of lethargy. Large abscesses present with motor or sensory deficits, seizures, or mental status changes. Ruptured abscesses may present with severe deficits and are commonly fatal. The signs and symptoms of a subdural abscess are more pronounced than those of an early epidural or cerebral abscess and include severe headache and high fevers with meningeal signs that quickly progress to changes in mental status; neurologic deficits may be present, too.

The ethmoid and sphenoid sinuses are the most common sites of origin of cavernous sinus thrombophlebitis. *Staphylococcus aureus* is the offending organism in the majority of cases, and it gains access to the cavernous sinus via retrograde thrombophlebitis from the ophthalmic veins.[13] The classic presentation is that of the orbital apex syndrome with proptosis, ophthalmoplegia, decreased visual acuity, and anesthesia in the V_1 and V_2 distribution. A patient typically presents with high, spiking ("picket fence") fever patterns similar to those of lateral sinus thrombosis of otologic origin.

Evaluation

Radiographic imaging studies confirm intracranial infection and differentiate meningitis from abscess.[16] Imaging studies also identify the sinus cavity of origin and the overall extent of sinus disease. Axial and coronal CT scans using contrast or MRI scans using gadolinium are the modalities of choice for making the diagnosis (Fig. 18–8). Both axial and coronal fine-cut imaging may demonstrate bone erosion or areas of dehiscence or frank abscess. When osteomyelitis of primarily the frontal sinus is suspected, a bone scan using either technetium-99m-pertechnetate or gallium-67-citrate may confirm the diagnosis.[17]

Lumbar puncture does not play a major role in the diagnosis or evaluation of intracranial infections resulting from sinusitis except in cases of meningitis when it may confirm the diagnosis and provide a source for cultures. Caution should be exercised in performing a lumbar puncture when the diagnosis is unclear. A patient with an intracranial abscess may experience brain herniation through the foramen magnum after a lumbar puncture, and a CT or MRI scan should be performed to rule out abscess before performing this procedure.

Priorities

Prompt diagnosis and therapeutic intervention using a multispecialty approach (infectious disease, otolaryngology–head and neck surgery, neurosurgery) ensures the greatest chance of effective treatment. Upon clinical and radiographic diagnosis, intravenous antibiotics with broad coverage for both gram-positive and anaerobic organisms should be administered. When cultures and sensitivities of organisms can be obtained from sinus cavities, lumbar fluid, or an abscess, antibiotic regimens are tailored based on the results. Anticonvulsant therapy may be considered for severe cases of intracranial infection or abscess, as the incidence of seizures is as high as 86% in these cases.[18] Sys-

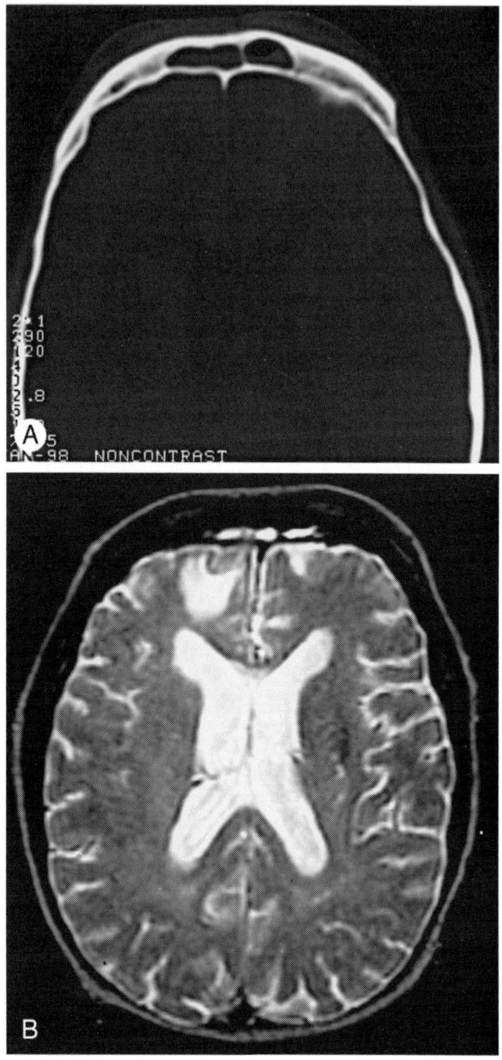

Figure 18–8. A: Axial CT image demonstrating infection in the right frontal sinus and an intact posterior bony wall. B: MRI of the same patient demonstrating a frontal lobe abscess that most likely arose from direct extension of the infection through the veins of Breschet, which allow communication between the sinus mucosa and the dural veins.

temic steroids may be administered to reduce intracranial pressure in cases in which significant cerebral edema exists, but there is no definitive proof of their benefit in cases of intracranial infection.

For meningitis related to sinusitis, intravenous antibiotics are administered. Surgery of the infected sinuses is reserved for disease that is refractory or persistent despite medical intervention. In general, surgical intervention is indicated in all cases of intracranial abscess or significant osteomyelitis or mucopyocele.[13] The surgical approach is determined by the extent and site of the abscess. Surgical options include formal craniotomy, site-directed burr holes, osteoplastic flap drainage and cranialization of the frontal sinus, and frontal sinus trephination and drainage through the posterior table. The less aggressive frontal sinus trephination or even endoscopic approach to the drainage of an epidural abscess may not definitively address underlying sinus pathology and may result in recurrent infection. Also, bony defects resulting from the infection or the surgical drainage procedure remain, so direct dural contact with the sinus and mucosa is an issue to be considered.

For cavernous sinus thrombosis, intravenous antibiotics and close systemic and neurologic monitoring is the primary intervention. Upon stabilization of the patient, surgical drainage of the sinus of origin is recommended. The use of anticoagulant therapy is controversial. It is thought by some that anticoagulation may prevent the thrombus from propagating and help to stimulate recanalization of the venous channels. Others theorize that the cavernous sinus may contain or act as a trap for the septic thrombus or clot, and anticoagulation may actually promote clot fragmentation with resultant formation of smaller septic emboli capable of escaping the sinus.

Outcomes

Prompt diagnosis and intervention are the best means of reducing both morbidity and mortality resulting from intracranial infections.[14] Overall neurologic sequelae occur in 25% of patients with sinogenic intracranial infection. For subdural and cerebral abscesses as well as for cavernous sinus thrombophlebitis, mortality rates are reported in the range of 10% to 30%. These three infections also have higher incidences of long-term morbidity caused by the focal neurologic deficits, seizure disorders, and multiple cranial neuropathies that occur in up to 50% of patients.[19]

NASOORBITOETHMOID TRAUMA

Nasoorbitoethmoid (NOE) fractures usually occur as a result of severe trauma to the anterior facial skeleton, most commonly caused by motor vehicle accidents. With the introduction of seat belts with shoulder belts, the incidence of these fractures has been greatly reduced. Regardless of the mechanism of trauma, the principles of injury remain the same in that the force of the impact fractures the nasal bones and drives them posteriorly and superiorly into the ethmoid complex.[20] The ascending process of the maxilla, the lamina papyracea, and the lacrimal bone are typically fractured. The anterior wall of the frontal sinus may also be fractured and displaced posteriorly. The most critical structures that may be injured in NOE fractures are the eye and the brain. Approximately 10% to 30% of patients with NOE fractures have corresponding ocular injuries, including vitreous hemorrhage, detached retina, dislocated lens, and rupture of the globe.[21] Concurrent intracranial trauma is not uncommon with these fractures and up to 40% of patients may demonstrate cerebrospinal fluid (CSF) leaks.[21] (The evaluation and management of intracranial and ocular emergencies after facial trauma are presented in detail in Chapters 24 and 25.) After thorough initial evaluation and stabilization of the patient (see Chapter 1), including airway and bleeding control, surgical reconstruction should be undertaken. Given the complexity of the anatomy at the junction of the frontal, nasal, ethmoid, and orbital regions, these fractures are considered the most difficult to manage with respect to both functional and cosmetic outcome.[20]

Presentation and Evaluation

As mentioned, a patient with an NOE fracture has a history of acute isolated traumas or multiple trauma to the head. Complaints include midfacial pain and nasal obstruction, and a patient may have epiphora and diplopia, depending on injury to the lacrimal system and the involvement or entrapment of the extraocular muscles. Usually, a patient presents with epistaxis or provides a history of significant epistaxis. A clear ring around a central spot of blood on a pillow or sheet may be a halo sign

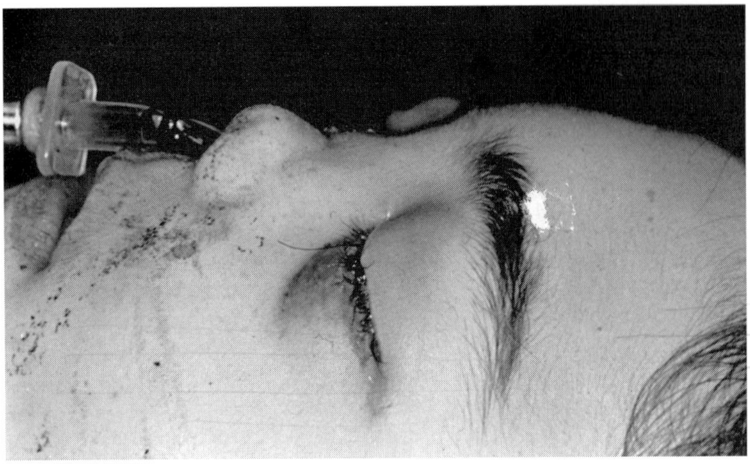

Figure 18–9. A patient who sustained a nasoorbitoethmoid fracture in a high-speed motor vehicle accident. Note the classic "pigsnout" deformity.

and indicate the presence of a CSF leak. On physical examination, there is a distinct facial deformity characteristic of NOE fractures that is termed a "pigsnout" deformity (Fig. 18–9). It occurs as a result of the loss of the nasal tip and dorsal projection, with exaggerated upward rotation of the tip. In classic NOE fractures, one or both medial canthal tendons may be lacerated or disrupted as a result of the traumatic episode.[21, 22] Along with the flattening of the nasal dorsum, the disruption of the medial canthal tendon causes an increased intercanthal distance that is readily recognized on physical examination as telecanthus (Fig. 18–10). The average normal intercanthal distances for women and men range from 25 to 38 mm. Another common physical finding is the absence of the "bow string sign" in which a taut medial canthus is not palpated upon lateral gaze. Coupled with these obvious physical findings, a CT scan confirms the diagnosis of an NOE fracture. The CT scan readily depicts the prolapse of the nasal bones into the ethmoid sinuses and the resulting telescoping of the ethmoid sinuses laterally (Fig. 18–11). A CT scan also identifies other injuries to the orbital bones or skull base.

Priorities

Once a patient has been stabilized and the management of the eye and intracranial injuries has been begun or completed, prompt surgical intervention is required to achieve the greatest success. Delay in surgical intervention allows fibrosis to occur and that makes the bony reduction and reconstruction very difficult, especially with respect to the repair of the medial canthal tendon. Although surgical reduction of the fracture may be achieved under general anesthesia using simply an Asch forceps, external ethmoidectomy incisions with bilateral bony hook reduction are usually required. For increased exposure to the nasofrontal area, a bicoronal incision with elevation of the frontal scalp and

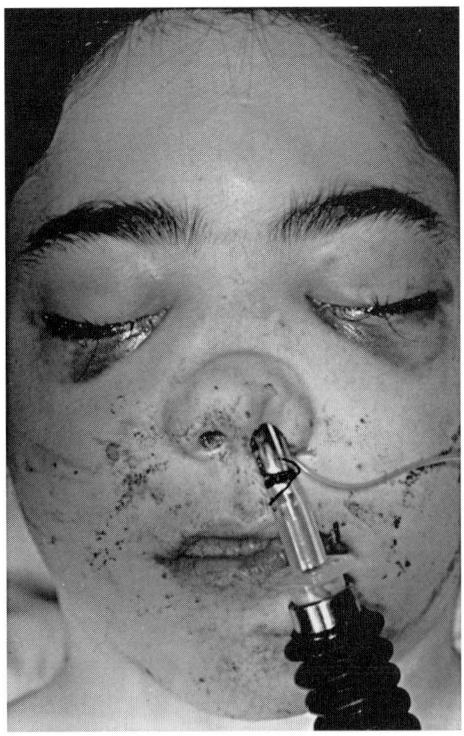

Figure 18–10. The patient with the nasoorbitoethmoid fracture showing telecanthus resulting from bilateral disruption of the medial canthal tendon.

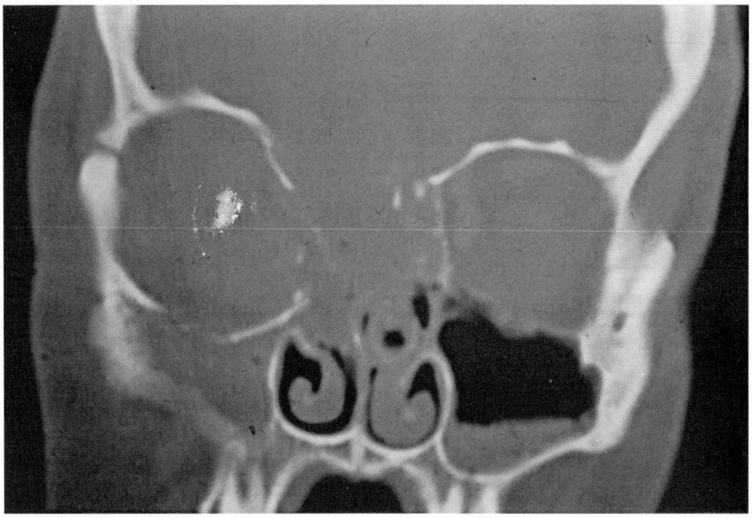

Figure 18–11. Coronal CT image showing comminuted ethmoid sinuses and telescoping of the bony ethmoid laterally, with disruption of the cribiform plate and skull base. A CSF leak was present initially but resolved spontaneously after surgical reduction of the bony ethmoid cavity.

pericranium may be utilized. Upon completing the initial bony exposure to the nasoorbitoethmoid region, the periorbita is elevated from the ethmoid labyrinth to the level of the posterior ethmoid artery. The bone hooks are then placed bilaterally just anterior to the posterior ethmoid artery, and a downward and anterior pull is performed. After reducing the fracture, miniplate or microplate rigid fixation is used to stabilize the fractures and recreate the anatomy. Following reduction and rigid fixation, repair of the medial canthal tendons at the site of anatomic insertion is performed. The medial canthal tendon may be wired to remaining bony fragments of the lacrimal crest or attached to the miniplates used for fracture fixation. The tendon may even have to be wired to the opposite lateral nasal bone. Repair is more difficult in cases of bilateral disruption of the medial canthal tendons and bilateral comminuted nasal and lacrimal bone fractures.[23] Silastic buttons may be placed in the medial canthal region and secured by wires or suture to further reduce and support the medial canthus.[24] An initial slight overcorrection of the medial canthi is the optimal reconstructive goal. The lacrimal apparatus may require repair and stenting with small Silastic tubing for 4 to 8 weeks to reconstitute a patent lacrimal conduit.

Outcomes

Despite prompt surgical intervention, residual cosmetic and function deformities are common after an NOE fracture. Nasal depression may persist as may a widened intercanthus. Diplopia may persist or may occur as a later sequela of direct injury, entrapment, or scarring around the extraocular muscles. Also, epiphora may result from unrecognized lacrimal apparatus trauma or ineffective repair.

FRONTAL SINUS FRACTURE WITH POSTERIOR WALL DISRUPTION

A frontal sinus fracture that disrupts the posterior wall is considered an emergency and requires immediate complete evaluation and prompt surgical management. Although an isolated anterior wall fracture may require surgical intervention, it does not carry the same risk of intracranial complications and usually does not require emergent surgical intervention. There are varying opinions regarding the management of small linear or nondisplaced posterior frontal sinus fractures. The general management concept is that if the posterior frontal sinus fracture results in any degree of bony displacement, the patient is at risk for subsequent intracranial infection, including brain abscess, mucocele, mucopyocele, or meningitis, so prompt surgery is required. In the case of a small linear fracture, this risk is greatly diminished and some advocate frequent clinical evaluation and follow-up with CT scans. Unfortunately, even fine-cut CT scanning may not provide conclusive differentiation between a linear and a mildly displaced posterior wall fracture. In general, the physician should have a low threshold for recommending surgical exploration and definitive treatment of most fractures involving the posterior wall of the frontal sinus.

Presentation and Evaluation

In most cases, a patient with a frontal sinus fracture is a victim of an unrestrained motor vehicle accident, but occasionally blunt or penetrating trauma to the forehead is encountered. As with NOE fractures, the use of shoulder belts has greatly diminished the incidence of frontal sinus fractures. The force required to fracture the frontal sinus is greater than that required to fracture any other facial bone, including the mandible; an estimated 800 to 1,200 foot-pounds are needed to cause a frontal sinus fracture.[25]

The complaint of frontal headache is uncommon, but the patient may have anesthesia in the distribution of the supraorbital nerve. A patient typically has nasal bleeding, and the possibility of a CSF leak should be ruled out. Massive hemorrhage is not common except in the case of an anterior or posterior compound fracture; it occurs as a result of sagittal or dural sinus tears. On physical exam, a patient typically has a laceration over the forehead and displays a bony and soft tissue depression at the site of injury. Any patient with suspected frontal sinus injury (as with suspected intracranial injury) should undergo a fine-cut (1- to 2-mm) CT scan with axial and coronal cuts after being stabilized in the emergency room (Fig. 18–12). The extent of the frontal sinus fracture determines the method of surgical treatment.[26]

A patient with substantial disruption of the posterior wall or a major frontal sinus fracture may also have concurrent pneumocephalus, CSF leakage, hemorrhage, or other intracranial trauma. These issues should be evaluated and resolved upon patient presentation. (See Chapter 24 for a more detailed discussion of the evaluation and management of intracranial trauma.) A severely comminuted anterior or posterior frontal sinus fracture is most likely to be found in a patient with a history of multiple trauma such as from major motor vehicle accident or a work-related fall.

Priorities

After stabilizing a patient and managing any acute neurologic trauma, prompt surgical intervention is the treatment of choice for a posterior frontal sinus fracture. The surgical approach may vary with the location and extent of the posterior wall fracture. Approaching the frontal sinus via a bicoronal incision is the most common choice, but using an existing laceration or even a deep brow crease may be acceptable. The frontal sinus is then exposed using either an osteoplastic flap or a frontal craniotomy approach. Fractures or bone defects of less than 25% of the frontal sinus may be treated with an osteoplastic flap procedure. Prior to performing an osteoplastic flap procedure, a 1:1 or 6-foot Caldwell x-ray view of the frontal sinus is taken

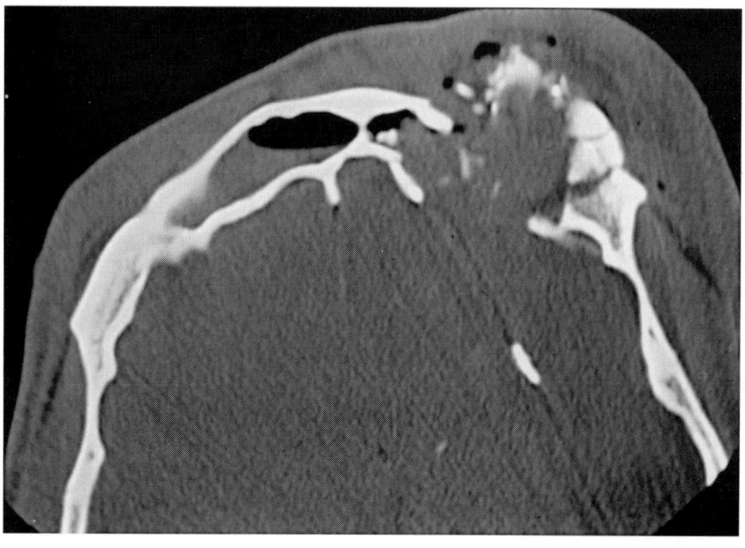

Figure 18–12. Axial CT image demonstrating a severely comminuted frontal sinus fracture with large anterior and posterior wall defects.

for use as a template to outline the extent of the frontal sinus. Comminuted fractures and those with bone defects of 25% or more are better addressed through a frontal craniotomy.

When using an osteoplastic flap approach for more limited fractures, the fracture site is identified and debrided of loose bony fragments. Any dural tears are repaired primarily and a pericranium or temporalis patch graft may be used to supplement this closure. The frontal sinus mucosa is dissected free from the remaining bone and approximately 1 to 2 mm of sinus wall are drilled away with a combination of cutting and diamond burrs to ensure complete removal of all sinus mucosa. Microscopic visualization aids in identifying small remnants of mucosa. The frontonasal duct is packed with free temporalis muscle or fascia graft to prevent upward migration of frontal recess or ethmoid sinus mucosa. The frontal sinus is then obliterated with a free-fat graft, cancellous bone chips, or commercially available hydroxyapatite bone cement.[27]

For larger or comminuted frontal sinus fractures, a formal frontal craniotomy and frontal sinus cranialization is performed. After removing the craniotomy bone flap, frontal sinus bone fragments are debrided and the posterior wall completely removed using rongeurs and drills with cutting and diamond burrs. Dural defects are repaired and reinforced as needed. The frontal sinus mucosa is removed and the frontonasal duct is packed with free graft. A pericranial flap is raised, placed into the frontal sinus, and reflected onto the floor of the anterior cranial fossa to obliterate the dead space and reduce regrowth of mucosa.[28] If a comminuted frontal table fracture also exists, these bone fragments are debrided of mucosa and reattached to the frontal bone or craniotomy bone flap with rigid plate fixation.

Outcomes

Frontal sinus obliteration procedures are generally very effective in reducing the morbidity of posterior frontal sinus fractures. When promptly and appropriately managed, the incidence of complications resulting from frontal sinus fractures, such as persistent CSF leakage, meningitis, brain abscess, and mucocele formation, is low. However, the risk of these complications increases with the severity of the fracture. Major complications have been reported to be 10% in a series of 72 patients with predominantly combined anterior and posterior table frontal sinus fractures.[29] Meningitis occurred in 6%, and mucoceles developed in 6% of the patients reported on in this series.[29]

REFERENCES

1. Denning DW, Stevens DA. Antifungal and surgical treatment of invasive aspergillosis: review of 2121 published cases. Rev Infect Dis 1990; 12:1147–1201.
2. Drakos PE et al. Invasive fungal sinusitis in patients undergoing bone marrow transplantation. Bone Marrow Transplant 1993; 12:203–208.
3. Waitzman AA, Birt BD. Fungal sinusitis. J Otolaryngol 1994; 23:244–249.
4. Gillespie MB, O'Malley BW Jr, Francis HW. New concepts in invasive fungal rhinosinusitis. Arch Otolaryngol Head Neck Surg 1998; 124:1–7.
5. Rhame FS. Lessons from the Roswell Park bone marrow transplant aspergillosis outbreak. Infect Control 1985; 6:345–346.
6. Kennedy CA et al. Impact of surgical treatment on paranasal fungal infections in bone marrow transplant patients. Otolaryngol Head Neck Surg 1997; 116:610–616.
7. Schramm VL, Curtin HD, Kennerdell JS. Evaluation of orbital cellulitis and results of treatment. Laryngoscope 1982; 92:732–738.
8. Arjomand EM, Lusk RP, Muntz HR. Pediatric sinusitis and subperiosteal abscess formation: diagnosis and treatment. Otolaryngol Head Neck Surg 1993; 109:886–894.
9. Fearon B, Edmonds B, Bird R. Orbital-facial complications of sinusitis in children. Laryngoscope 1979; 89:947.
10. Goodwin WJ, Winshall M, Chandler JR. The role of high-resolution computerized tomography and standard ultrasound in the evaluation of orbital cellulitis. Laryngoscope 1982; 92:728–731.
11. Mann W, Amedee RG, Maurer J. Orbital complications of pediatric sinusitis: treatment of periorbital abscess. Am J Rhinol 1997; 11:149–153.
12. Manning SC. Endoscopic management of medial subperiosteal orbital abscess. Arch Otolaryngol Head Neck Surg 1993; 119:789–791.
13. Clayman GL et al. Intracranial complications of paranasal sinusitis: a combined institutional review. Laryngoscope 1991; 101:234–239.
14. Giannoni CM, Stewart MG, Alford EL. Intracranial complications of sinusitis. Laryngoscope 1997; 107:863–867.
15. Fairbanks D, Vanderveen T, Bordley J. Intracranial complications of sinusitis. In English G, ed. Otolaryngology, vol. II. New York, Harper & Row, 1983, pp. 1–28.
16. Maniglia et al. Intracranial abscesses secondary to nasal, sinus and orbital infections in adults and children. Arch Otolaryngol Head Neck Surg 1989; 115:1424–1429.
17. Gardiner LJ. Complications of frontal sinusitis: evaluation and management. Otolaryngol Head Neck Surg 1986; 95:333–343.
18. Wald ER et al. Sinusitis and its complications in the pediatric patient. Pediatr Clin North Am 1981; 28:777–796.
19. Karlin RJ, Robinson WA. Septic cavernous sinus thrombosis. Ann Emerg Med 1984; 13:449–455.
20. Donald PJ. Frontal and ethmoid complex fractures. In Donald PJ, Gluckman JL, Rice DH, eds. The Sinuses. New York, Raven, 1995, pp. 401–419.

21. Cruse CW, Blevins PK, Luce EA. Naso-ethmoid-orbital fractures. J Trauma 1980; 20:551–556.
22. Stranc MF. The pattern of lacrimal injuries in naso-ethmoid fractures. Br J Plast Surg 1970; 23:339–346.
23. Converse JM, Hogan VM. Open-sky approach for reduction of naso-orbital fractures. Plast Reconstr Surg 1970; 46:396.
24. Duvall AJ, Banovetz JD. Nasoethmoidal fractures. Otolaryngol Clin North Am 1976; 9:507–514.
25. Nahum AM. The biomechanics of maxillofacial trauma. Clin Plast Surg 1975; 2:59.
26. Olson EM et al. Frontal sinus fractures: evaluation of CT scans in 132 patients. Am J Neuroradiol 1992; 13:897–902.
27. Rohrich RJ, Mickel TJ. Frontal sinus obliteration: in search of the ideal autogenous material. Plast Reconstr Surg 1995; 95:590–585.
28. Thaller SR, Donald PJ. The use of pericranial flaps in frontal sinus fractures. Ann Plast Surg 1994; 32:284–287.
29. Wallis A, Donald PJ. Frontal sinus fractures: a review of 72 cases. Laryngoscope 1988; 98:593–598.

CHAPTER 19

Neck Emergencies

Shelly J. McQuone, MD

A variety of life-threatening processes can affect the numerous, closely related vital structures located within the neck. Compression of the airway by abscess or hematoma, severe hemorrhage from a major blood vessel, and fulminant infection with the potential for spread to adjacent mediastinal structures are some of these emergencies. This chapter addresses such infectious emergencies of the neck as deep-space neck infections, acute sialadenitis, and craniocervical necrotizing fasciitis, as well as vascular emergencies of the neck including intraoperative vascular injury, postoperative hematoma, and postoperative exposure or rupture of the carotid artery. Penetrating trauma to the neck (Chapter 12), trauma to the larynx (Chapter 11), and isolated airway emergencies (Chapter 9) are discussed elsewhere.

INFECTIOUS EMERGENCIES OF THE NECK

Deep-Space Neck Infections

Deep-space neck infections remain relatively common despite significant advances in antibiotic therapy. Although the morbidity and mortality previously associated with these infections have been dramatically reduced, they continue to pose challenging and occasionally life-threatening problems. Well-defined fascial planes make up the boundaries of a number of potential spaces in the neck. An abscess collection can occur within any of these spaces. Thorough knowledge of the anatomy of the fascial layers of the neck is critical to understanding the clinical implications and pathways of spread of deep-space neck infections (Fig. 19–1).

The two primary fascial layers in the neck are the superficial and the deep cervical fasciae. Enveloping the platysma and the muscles of facial expression, the superficial cervical fascia does not play a significant role in the pathogenesis of deep-space neck infections. The deep cervical fascia is further divided into three separate layers known as the superficial, middle, and deep layers. The superficial layer of the deep cervical fascia surrounds the trapezius and sternocleidomastoid muscles, the muscles of mastication, and the parotid and submandibular glands. The middle layer of the deep cervical fascia, or visceral layer, invests the pharynx, larynx, trachea, esophagus, thyroid gland, and parathyroid glands. Posteriorly, the middle layer forms the buccopharyngeal fascia, creating the midline raphe adherent to the prevertebral fascia. The deep layer of the deep cervical fascia envelops the vertebrae and paraspinous muscles, and divides again into the alar layer and the prevertebral layer. The alar layer is anterior, extending from the skull base to the mediastinum; the prevertebral layer is posterior, extending from the skull base to the coccyx. All three layers of the deep cervical fascia contribute to the carotid sheath.

These fascial layers form the boundaries of the potential spaces in the neck; the close anatomic relationships among these spaces direct their paths of infectious spread. The *submandibular* space is located inferior to the floor of the mouth and superior to the digastric muscle (Fig. 19–2). Its anterior border consists of the mylohyoid muscle and the anterior belly of the digastric muscle; the posterior belly of the digastric muscle forms its posterior border. This space rests medial to the platysma muscle and the

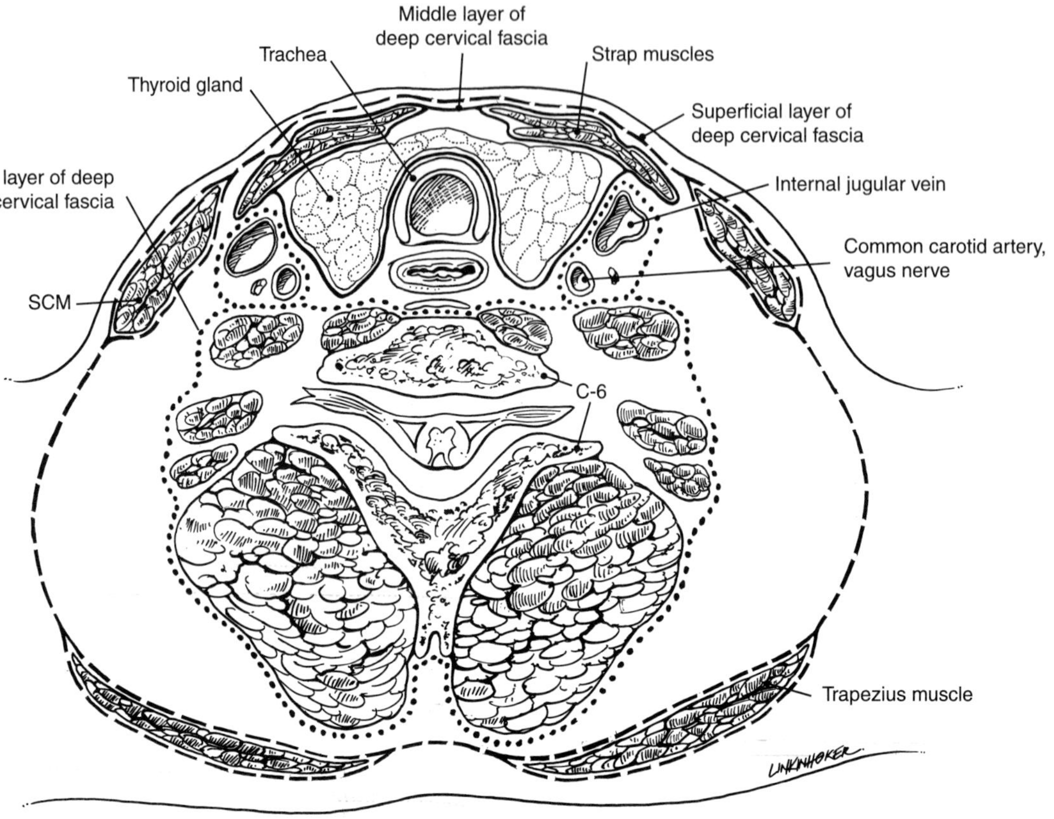

Figure 19–1. Cross-sectional drawing of the neck, depicting layers of the superficial and deep cervical fasciae at the level of the 6th cervical vertebra. SCM = sternocleidomastoid muscle.

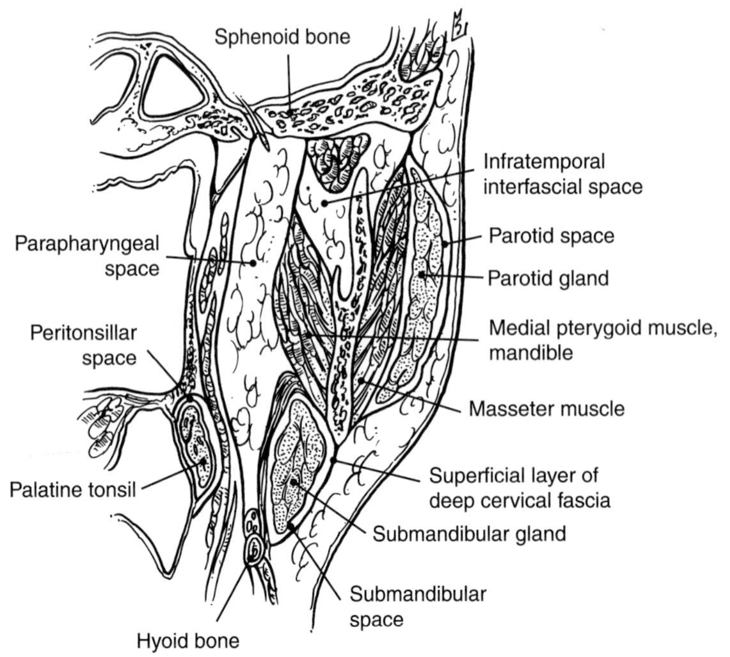

Figure 19–2. Coronal drawing of the left lateral neck, demonstrating the peritonsillar, parapharyngeal, submandibular, and parotid spaces.

mandible, and lateral to the hyoglossus and mylohyoid muscles. The *sublingual* space is the supramylohyoid aspect of the submandibular space.

The *parapharyngeal*, or *lateral pharyngeal*, space forms an inverted conical space whose superior boundary is the base of the skull. Its apex and inferior border is the hyoid bone. The parapharyngeal space lies lateral to the superior constrictor muscle and medial to the parotid gland, mandible, and lateral pterygoid muscle. Anteriorly, this space extends to the pterygomandibular raphe, and posteriorly, to the prevertebral fascia (see Fig. 19–2).

The *visceral* space extends from the hyoid bone to the mediastinum. Anteriorly, this space is limited by the superficial layer of the deep cervical fascia. Posteriorly, it is continuous with the retropharyngeal and prevertebral spaces, and laterally, it communicates with the parapharyngeal and carotid sheath spaces. The *carotid sheath* is lateral to the visceral space, anterior to the prevertebral space, and medial to the sternocleidomastoid muscle (see Fig. 19–1).

The *retropharyngeal* space lies between the skull base and the tracheal bifurcation in the superior mediastinum, approximately at the level of the 4th thoracic vertebra. This space is posterior to the pharynx and esophagus but anterior to the alar fascia. The *prevertebral* space extends from the skull base to the coccyx, posterior to the prevertebral fascia and anterior to the vertebral bodies. The loose areolar tissue between the two divisions of the deep layer of the deep cervical fascia is called the *danger space* since infection may rapidly traverse this area, spreading directly to the posterior mediastinum.

The peritonsillar space occupies the area between the fascial capsule of the tonsil and the superior constrictor muscle and is not a genuine deep neck space (see Fig. 19–2). Infections of the *peritonsillar* space, however, are grouped with infections of the deep spaces of the neck because of similar presentations and potential complications.

The great majority of infections involving the submandibular, sublingual, and parapharyngeal spaces are odontogenic, resulting from bacterial erosion through the pulp of a tooth into the deeper soft tissues of the neck. An odontogenic infection may involve the sublingual or the submandibular space, or both, depending on the relationship between the offending tooth root and the mylohyoid line. The sublingual space becomes infected if the tooth root lies superior to this line, generally including the premolars or the first molar. An infected tooth whose root lies inferior to this line, like the third molar, preferentially involves the submandibular space. The root of the second molar usually rests at the mylohyoid line and therefore can involve either space (Fig. 19–3).

Virtually all odontogenic abscesses are polymicrobial, composed of various combinations of the aerobic and anaerobic organisms normally found in the oral flora. The predominant aerobic species in the mouth is *Streptococcus;* the most common anaerobic species are *Bacteroides*, *Fusobacterium*, and *Peptostreptococcus.* Not surprisingly, these species are also the most common isolates from odontogenic infections. Approximately half of odontogenic infections are a mixture of aerobic and anaerobic organisms; the other half are purely anaerobic at the time of culture. Very rarely (5%), cultures from an abscess reveal solely aerobic organisms. An odontogenic abscess typically starts as a streptococcal cellulitis. As the infection progresses, the tissues become increasingly hypoxic, allowing anaerobic species to predominate.[1]

In addition, there are a number of nonodontogenic causes of deep-space neck infections. Peritonsillar abscesses, for example, are not odontogenic but originate from infection of the pharynx and tonsils. Direct extension from an adjacent space is another nonodontogenic cause of deep-space neck infection. Carotid sheath infections, visceral space infections, and prevertebral space infections often result from the spread of an infection of the parapharyngeal or submandibular space. Visceral space infections can also arise following traumatic injury to the larynx or esophagus, following surgical proce-

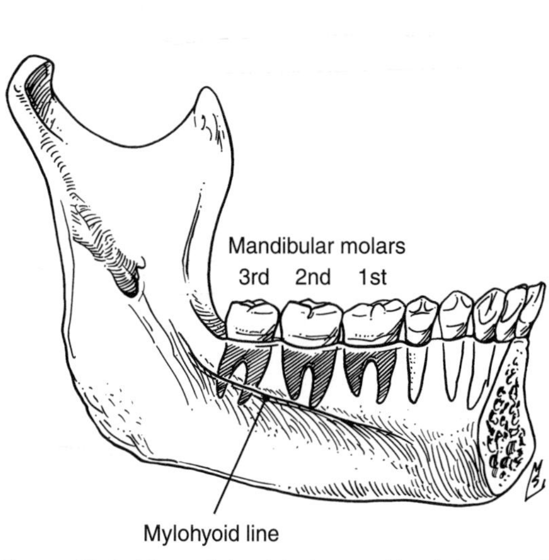

Figure 19–3. View of the right inner table of the mandible, demonstrating the relationship between the mylohyoid line and the roots of the mandibular molars.

dures performed on the neck, and following acute thyroiditis. Infections of the prevertebral space classically arose from tuberculosis of the spine. Formation of a Pott's abscess was relatively common prior to modern antitubercular therapy. Penetrating trauma is an another cause of prevertebral space infection.[2]

In the population of intravenous drug abusers, a common source of deep-space neck infection is a retained foreign body. Attempted intravenous access through deep cervical injection can result in needles breaking within or near the carotid sheath space and causing subsequent abscess formation.[3, 4]

PRESENTATION

A patient with a deep-space neck infection typically presents with both systemic and localized symptoms and signs. Systemic complaints include fever, chills, malaise, and loss of appetite. Localized symptoms include trismus, dysphagia, odynophagia, hoarseness or other change in voice, otalgia, and dyspnea. Localized signs include intraoral or external neck swelling, drooling, and temperature elevation. Understanding the particular patterns of these signs and symptoms facilitates clinical differentiation of the potential spaces involved. Clinical presentation can also predict the location of an abscess if one is present (Table 19–1).

A patient with a *peritonsillar* abscess generally presents with dysphagia and odynophagia, ipsilateral otalgia, and a "hot-potato voice," described as such because of its muffled quality. Trismus is less pronounced. Physical examination classically reveals a unilateral soft palatal bulge, often with uvular deviation away from the abscess. Exudative tonsillitis may or may not be evident (Fig. 19–4). Peritonsillar abscesses require urgent management because of their potential to spread to the lateral pharyngeal space.

An isolated *sublingual space* abscess presents as a bulging fullness in the floor of the mouth. A patient generally complains of pain, with or without dysphagia. In an isolated abscess of the *submandibular space*, a patient complains of dysphagia and mild trismus. On physical examination, unilateral submandibular fluctuance and tenderness are apparent.

Because the submandibular and sublingual spaces are contiguous posterior to the mylohyoid muscle, infection can easily involve both

Table 19–1. *Signs and Symptoms of Deep-Space Neck Infections*

Space	Trismus	Dysphagia	Source	Edema	Unique Sign/Symptom
Peritonsillar	Minimal	Yes	Tonsil	Soft palate	Uvular deviation, hot-potato voice, otalgia
Submandibular (Ludwig's angina)	Marked	Yes	2nd and 3rd mandibular molars	Diffuse, collar	Brawny edema, firm floor of mouth
Parapharyngeal (lateral pharyngeal)	Severe	Yes	Teeth (odontogenic)	Tonsil, lateral pharyngeal wall, ± soft tissue neck	
Carotid sheath	Variable	Variable	Direct extension IVDA, trauma	SCM	Pitting edema over SCM, torticollis
Retropharyngeal	Yes	Yes	URI, nasopharynx, sinuses	Unilateral bulge, posterior pharyngeal wall	± Drooling, cervical rigidity, hot-potato voice
Prevertebral	Variable	Variable	Direct extension trauma, TB	Midline bulge, posterior pharyngeal wall	± Drooling, cervical rigidity, hot-potato voice (TB may be chronic)
Pterygopalatine	Severe	No	Maxillary molars	Gingiva, face, or eye	
Masticator	Extreme	No	3rd mandibular molar	Posterior mandibular ramus	External swelling minimal compared to trismus
Visceral	Variable	Yes	Direct extension trauma	Variable	± Hoarseness, dyspnea, cutaneous emphysema

IVDA, intravenous drug abuse; URI, upper respiratory infection; TB, tuberculosis; SCM, sternocleidomastoid muscle.

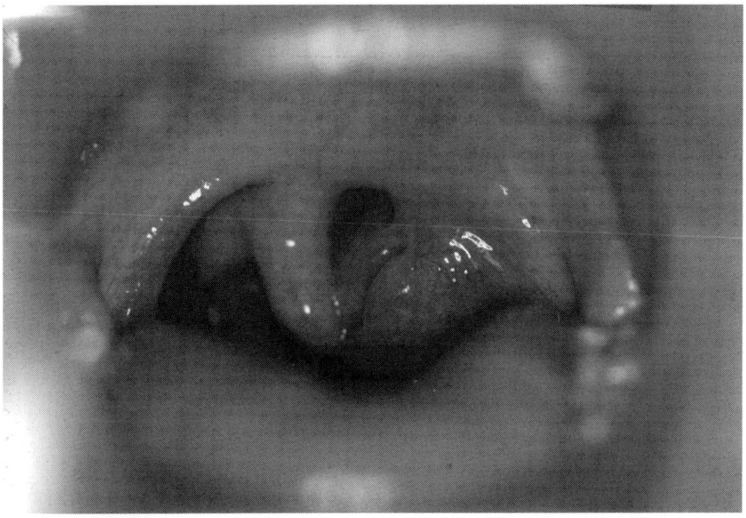

Figure 19–4. A patient with a left peritonsillar abscess. Note the unilateral bulge of the soft palate and associated erythema.

spaces. *Ludwig's angina* is a rapidly spreading, gangrenous cellulitis of both compartments that appears as diffuse, brawny edema of the neck without discrete fluctuance. The floor of the mouth becomes firm and elevated, displacing the tongue posteriorly. Trismus becomes pronounced, and airway compromise may quickly progress to asphyxiation (Fig. 19–5).

The hallmarks of a *parapharyngeal, or lateral pharyngeal, space* abscess are severe dysphagia, odynophagia, and marked trismus. In contrast to a peritonsillar abscess, no exudate is seen over the tonsils, but a unilateral fullness of the tonsil or lateral pharyngeal wall can be seen intraorally. Occasionally, external soft tissue swelling may be appreciated.

Infection of the *visceral space* presents with severe dysphagia and odynophagia and with minimal trismus. Dyspnea and hoarseness may occur, and crepitus may be palpable. Pitting edema over the sternocleidomastoid muscle and torticollis are virtually pathognomonic for *carotid sheath space* involvement. *Retropharyngeal* abscesses generally occur in the pediatric population; thorough discussion of this process can be found in Chapter 21.

Infections of the *prevertebral space* display a more indolent clinical course than their anterior counterparts because of the compact and relatively contained nature of this compartment. Physical findings are few, but if the abscess is located in the superior cervical aspect of this space, a midline bulge may be seen intraorally. Signs and symptoms are determined by the vertical location of the abscess, as this space extends from the base of skull to the coccyx.

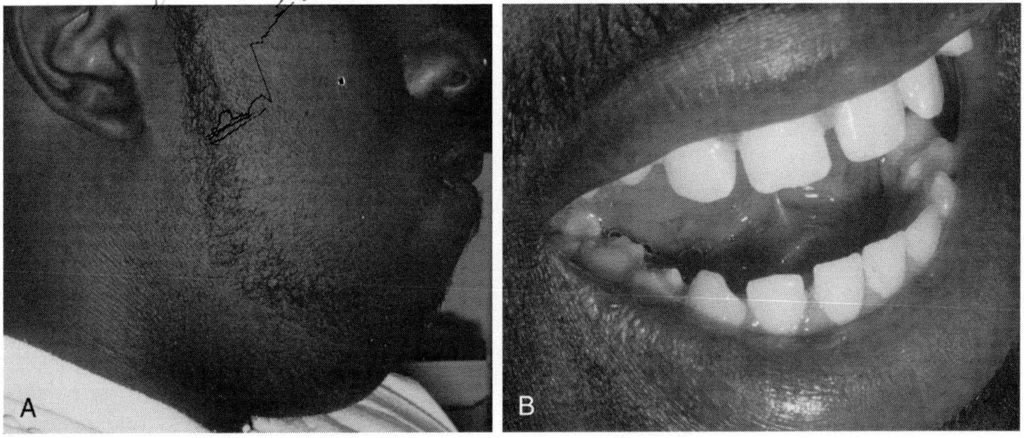

Figure 19–5. A patient with Ludwig's angina. A: External view demonstrating submental swelling. B: Intraoral view demonstrating brawny edema of the floor of the mouth.

EVALUATION

The presence of a deep-space neck abscess is suggested by the clinical presentation. An elevated white blood cell count may be useful in clinically subtle cases, but laboratory tests are otherwise uninformative. Most cases are confirmed with computed tomography (CT) imaging to document the presence and location of an abscess (Fig. 19–6), but there are several important exceptions. Advanced processes, such as Ludwig's angina and large abscesses acutely compressing the airway, require urgent airway control without benefit of imaging studies. A *peritonsillar abscess* is a purely clinical diagnosis that does not require imaging studies unless there is suspicion of its extension to adjacent spaces (Fig. 19–7).

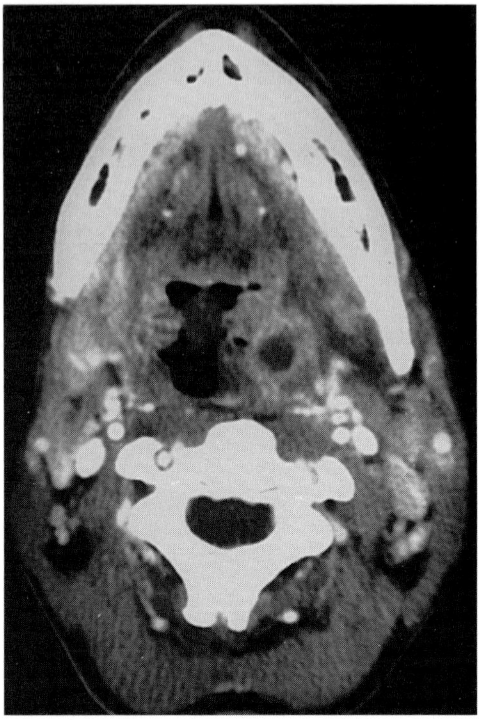

Figure 19–7. Axial CT image demonstrating a left peritonsillar abscess. The imaging study was obtained to rule out extension into the lateral pharyngeal space.

PRIORITIES

The first priority in managing deep-space neck infections is to secure the airway. The airway may be obstructed by posterior displacement of the tongue, as in Ludwig's angina, or may be directly compressed by a large abscess collection. Evaluation of the upper airway with a flexible fiberoptic laryngoscope is extremely useful if the patient's clinical condition permits. If the clinician deems the airway significantly impaired on visual inspection, it should be secured by intubation performed urgently in the operating room. Nasotracheal fiberoptic intubation is generally the preferred technique of airway control in these patients, as orotracheal intubation is usually not feasible secondary to trismus or edema. Preparations for tracheostomy should be made in all cases, because distortion of landmarks and associated edema may mandate a surgical airway.

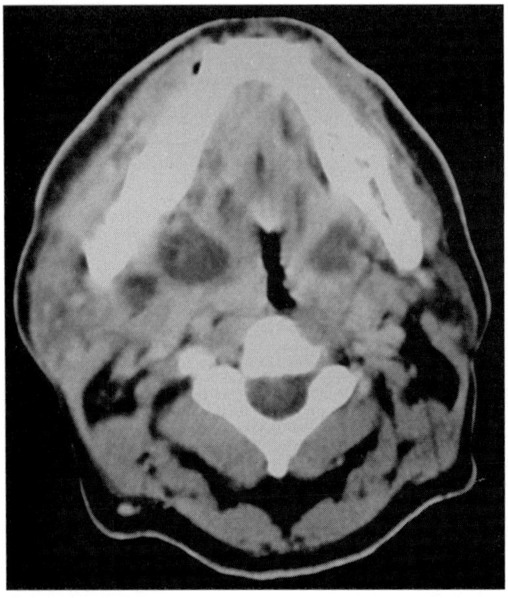

Figure 19–6. Axial CT image of a deep-space neck abscess involving the parapharyngeal spaces bilaterally.

In many cases, the patient is asymptomatic with respect to the airway, and early fiberoptic laryngoscopic evaluation demonstrates an uncompromised airway. In these instances, time is available for imaging studies, but the patient should be carefully monitored throughout the evaluation.

If the patient's condition is tenuous or deteriorating, fiberoptic evaluation of the airway may not be possible. Symptoms such as worsening stridor, shortness of breath, and decreasing level of consciousness and signs such as inability to maintain oxygen saturation, cyanosis, and increasing use of accessory respiratory musculature are associated with significant deterioration of the patient's condition. Emergency tracheotomy or cricothyroidotomy must be performed for immediate airway control under these circumstances. (See Chapter 9 for a comprehensive review of these techniques.)

Following assessment and control of the airway, the second priority in the management of deep-space neck infections is drainage of the abscess. If the airway is stable, CT imaging can be performed to determine the precise location of an abscess collection. The treatment of a neck abscess is surgical drainage. All submandibular, lateral pharyngeal, visceral space, and carotid sheath abscesses should be drained transcervically for adequate visualization and protection of major vessels (Fig. 19–8). A submandibular, anterior sternocleidomastoid, or submental incision is selected, depending on the location of the abscess. Finger exploration of the abscess cavity should be avoided, especially in an intravenous drug abuser, whose neck may harbor an unidentified needle.

There are few exceptions to the recommendation of external drainage. Among them are peritonsillar abscesses, which may be approached transorally in the office setting or the emergency department. In select cases of small or questionable peritonsillar abscesses, needle aspiration may prove useful diagnostically and therapeutically,[5] but transoral incision and drainage remain the standard treatment.[6] In addition, some retropharyngeal and high cervical prevertebral abscesses may be approached transorally (see Chapter 21). Small abscesses isolated in the sublingual space may be safely drained transorally as well.

The management of deep-space neck infections involves prompt initiation of appropriate intravenous antibiotic therapy. Oral antibiotics are employed only in an early infection that has not yet progressed to abscess formation. The choice of antibiotic is guided by the microbiology of the infection. Traditionally, high-dose penicillin was selected because it covers both aerobic and anaerobic organisms, penetrates into infected tissues, and is relatively inexpensive. The emergence of β-lactamase–producing organisms in deep-space neck infections, which have been reported in up to 46% of isolates from neck abscesses,[7] mandates the addition of a β-lactamase inhibitor such as clavulanic acid or metronidazole to an empiric penicillin regimen.

Clindamycin is an effective alternative agent but, like penicillin, resistance to this drug argues against its use as single-agent therapy. The combination of a second-generation cephalosporin such as cefoxitin or cefuroxime with clindamycin is an effective therapeutic regimen in the treatment of deep-space neck infections.[8] Cultures should be obtained from all drained abscesses, and the final selection of antibiotics is based on sensitivity results.

OUTCOMES

A deep-space neck infection that is not recognized and promptly treated can be fatal. Progressive airway obstruction can result in asphyxiation. Untreated or inadequately treated abscesses of the deep neck spaces spread along fascial planes to contiguous spaces, increasing the rate of complications.

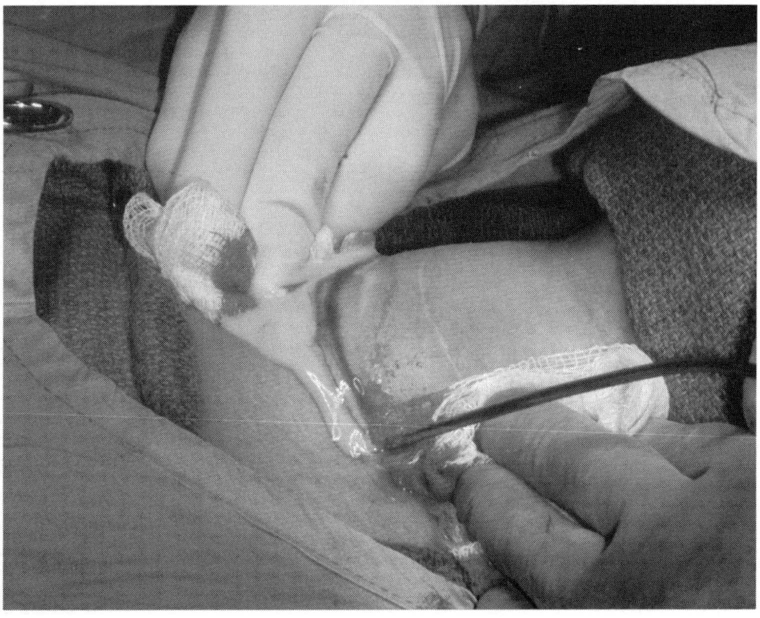

Figure 19–8. Transcervical drainage of a visceral-space abscess in a patient status post-thyroidectomy.

The most common infectious complication of a deep-space neck infection is septic thrombosis of the internal jugular vein, also known as Lemierre's syndrome (Fig. 19–9).[9] The thrombosis may extend proximally to the lateral or cavernous sinus systems or may embolize distally to the pulmonary system. As a result, metastatic abscesses of the brain and lungs can occur. Septic thrombosis of the internal jugular vein is managed with long-term intravenous antibiotic therapy.[10] Ligation of the vein has no proven benefit, and anticoagulation therapy remains controversial.[11, 12] Those advocating systemic anticoagulation believe extension of thrombus is minimized and risk for pulmonary embolism is decreased.[12]

One of the most feared complications of a deep-space neck infection is carotid arterial erosion, which is fatal in 20% to 40% of cases.[13] A sentinel oral or pharyngeal bleed may herald this ominous event. Onset of shock and the accumulation of a hematoma in the neck may be associated with arterial erosion. An unexplained palsy of cranial nerves IX, X, XI, or XII or the development of Horner's syndrome can also signal carotid arterial involvement.[14] The management of carotid rupture is discussed in a later section of this chapter.

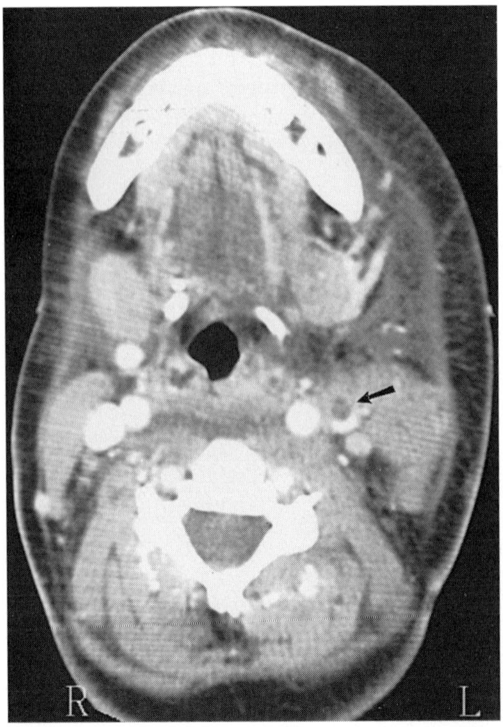

Figure 19–9. Axial CT image of a patient with septic thrombosis of the left internal jugular vein (Lemierre's syndrome) indicated by the arrow. The patient presented initially with a peritonsillar abscess.

Spread of infection outside the confines of the neck is another hazardous consequence of inadequate treatment of a neck abscess. Inferior extension of infection may result in mediastinitis, a life-threatening condition discussed in Chapter 20. Hematogenous extension may lead to sepsis and ultimately to multiorgan system failure (see Chapter 3). In addition, an untreated abscess can spontaneously rupture into the airway, causing acute airway compromise or the subsequent development of aspiration pneumonia.

The extended management of deep-space neck infections includes careful postoperative monitoring of the airway to direct the timing of extubation or tracheotomy decannulation. Extractions of involved teeth in odontogenic infections should be expedited to permit resolution and to prevent recurrence of infection. Additionally, a patient who has a recurrent peritonsillar abscess is a candidate for tonsillectomy after the resolution of the acute process.

Fortunately, with proper airway management, timely surgical drainage, and appropriate antibiotic therapy, most deep-space neck infections resolve without adverse sequelae.

Acute Sialadenitis

Although severe bacterial infection can arise from any of the major salivary glands, the majority involve the parotid gland. The gland is located within the parotid space, which contains the parotid gland, facial nerve, external carotid artery, and retromandibular vein (see Fig. 19–2). Considered one of the deep neck spaces, the parotid space communicates directly with the parapharyngeal space. Acute suppurative parotitis is a life-threatening infection that is distinguished from nonemergent parotid inflammation by its bacterial nature, affinity for debilitated patients, and alarmingly high mortality rate. Common in weakened, elderly patients recovering from surgical procedures, acute suppurative parotitis is also known as surgical parotitis and postoperative parotitis. In addition to postoperative dehydration, patients with chronic, debilitating medical conditions and those with compromised immune function appear to be at increased risk for the development of acute parotitis, which affects men and women equally.

The mechanism believed responsible for this infection is stasis of salivary flow and retrograde migration of bacteria from the oral cavity to the parotid parenchyma. The most commonly cultured organism is penicillin-resistant *Staphylococcus aureus*, but streptococcal species, anerobic species and, rarely, gram-negative organisms have also been recognized as causes of this infection.[15]

Salivary stasis can be caused by dehydration, which is exacerbated by a variety of factors. Postoperative patients are susceptible to dehydration because of the uncompensated-for losses of blood and body fluids associated with many surgical procedures. Patients in their 6th and 7th decades of life often have comorbidities such as congestive heart failure and renal insufficiency that limit aggressive fluid resuscitation. For the majority of upper and lower aerodigestive tract procedures, patients are routinely maintained without oral intake postoperatively and consequently are without regular salivary stimulation.

Salivary secretion is further reduced by medications that have anticholinergic or diuretic side effects. Stasis of salivary flow can also result from sialolithiasis, although this condition is generally associated with chronic, recurrent salivary gland infections rather than with an acute suppurative process.

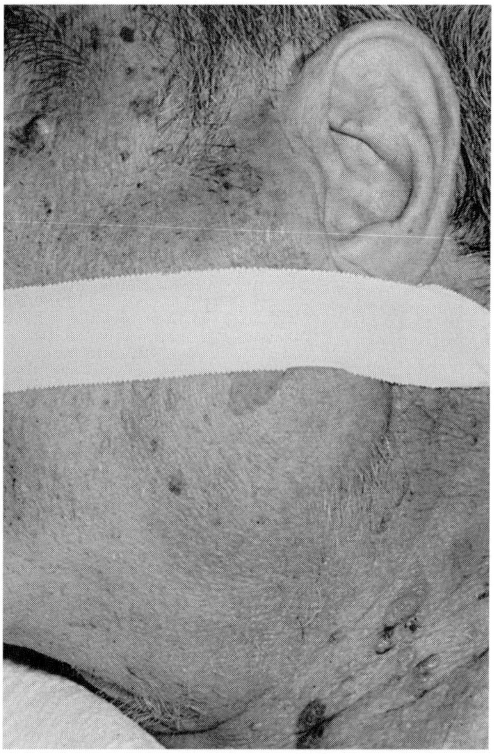

Figure 19–10. An intubated patient with acute suppurative parotitis.

PRESENTATION

A patient with acute suppurative parotitis demonstrates both systemic and localized symptoms. Bacterial parotitis manifests itself as the sudden onset of induration, erythema, edema, and extreme tenderness over the cheek and angle of the mandible (Fig. 19–10). Parotitis most commonly appears within 2 weeks after surgery; its peak occurrence falls between postoperative days 5 and 7.[16] Although primarily unilateral, bilateral involvement has been reported in up to 25% of cases.[17] Systemically, a patient usually appears toxic, displaying high fever, profound dehydration, and even delirium. A patient may be overtly septic or may display signs of multiorgan system failure.

EVALUATION

Acute suppurative parotitis is a clinical diagnosis. Awareness of conditions that predispose to this infection and recognition of the findings described above secure the diagnosis. Review of a patient's intake and output as well as assessment of skin turgor can help to confirm dehydration. The mucous membranes of the oral cavity appear dry and sometimes crusted, indicating reduced salivary flow. Stensen's duct may appear erythematous or inflamed, and massage of the parotid gland may express pus from the ductal orifice. In cases of early parotitis or complete ductal obstruction, however, purulence may not be visualized. Fluctuance is rarely palpable externally because of the dense, fibrous nature of the parotid fascia. The infection is often restricted to diffuse parenchymal involvement of the gland rather than organized into a discrete abscess. If, however, an abscess is suspected based on physical findings, needle aspiration can be employed diagnostically. Cultures should be obtained if purulent fluid is found.

The white blood cell count is markedly elevated, but additional laboratory testing is rarely contributory. Imaging studies are not recommended initially, but if the infection proves refractory to several days of aggressive, standard therapy, a CT or ultrasound scan is performed to exclude the possibility of abscess collection (Fig. 19–11).

PRIORITIES

Acute suppurative parotitis requires urgent, aggressive therapy to prevent local as well as sys-

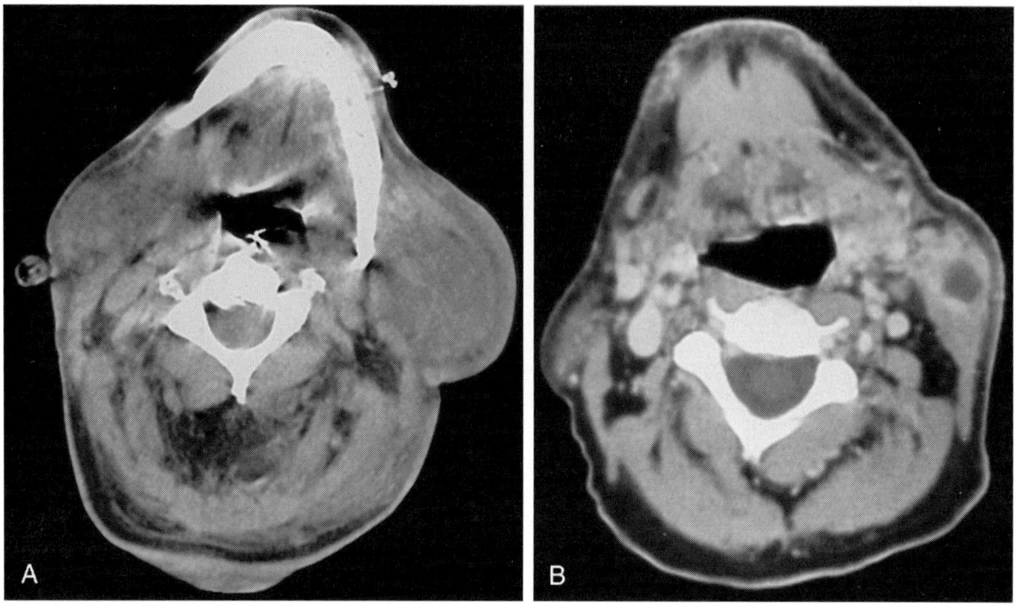

Figure 19–11. A: Axial CT image of a patient with acute suppurative parotitis of the left parotid gland. B: Axial CT image of a patient with acute suppurative parotitis that has progressed to form a left intraparotid abscess.

temic complications. The initial management of acute suppurative parotitis is nonsurgical and emphasizes correction of dehydration and underlying medical conditions whenever possible. Every attempt must be made to reverse salivary stasis and stimulate salivary flow. Application of warm compresses, maximization of oral hygiene and mouth irrigations, and administration of sialogogues such as lemon drops or orange juice promote salivary flow. External massage of the parotid gland or bimanual massage of the gland intraorally as well as externally should be employed if the patient can tolerate these measures. When neither saliva nor pus can be expressed from Stensen's duct, cannulation of the duct with lacrimal probes can establish ductal patency. A patent duct is essential, as therapy is directed at improving salivary flow.

Intravenous antibiotic therapy is the primary treatment of acute suppurative parotitis. Broad-spectrum coverage for *Staphylococcus aureus*, *Streptococcal* species, and anaerobes is required. If cultures were obtained from Stensen's duct or by needle aspiration, these results are used to further direct specific antibiotic therapy.

Failure to improve after 48 hours of aggressive nonsurgical therapy is an indication that an imaging study should be performed to exclude abscess formation (see Fig. 19–11). If a discrete abscess is identified, surgical drainage is undertaken using a standard parotidectomy incision. More commonly, however, the gland is diffusely inflamed. A small population of patients who are without discrete abscesses and who are refractory to nonoperative interventions may be candidates for surgical exploration if their medical conditions permit. The gland is approached with a standard, anteriorly based facial flap, and multiple superficial, radial incisions are created in the parotid fascia parallel to the facial nerve branches (Fig. 19–12). The wound is loosely approximated over a drain. The central aspect of the wound is often allowed to heal by secondary intention.

OUTCOMES

The prognosis of acute suppurative parotitis is variable and is related primarily to the medical condition of the affected patient. Classically, this infection has been a predictor of poor prognosis in a postoperative patient and is associated with a 20% to 40% mortality rate.[16, 17] Because of the underlying debilitation of most patients afflicted with bacterial parotitis, the most ominous consequences of this infection are systemic. Acute parotitis can rapidly lead to systemic sepsis although, conversely, a septic state often predates the parotitis. Complications of sepsis, such as shock and multiorgan failure, are discussed in Chapter 3.

Communication between the parotid space and the parapharyngeal space accounts for the potential extension of an infection into the deep

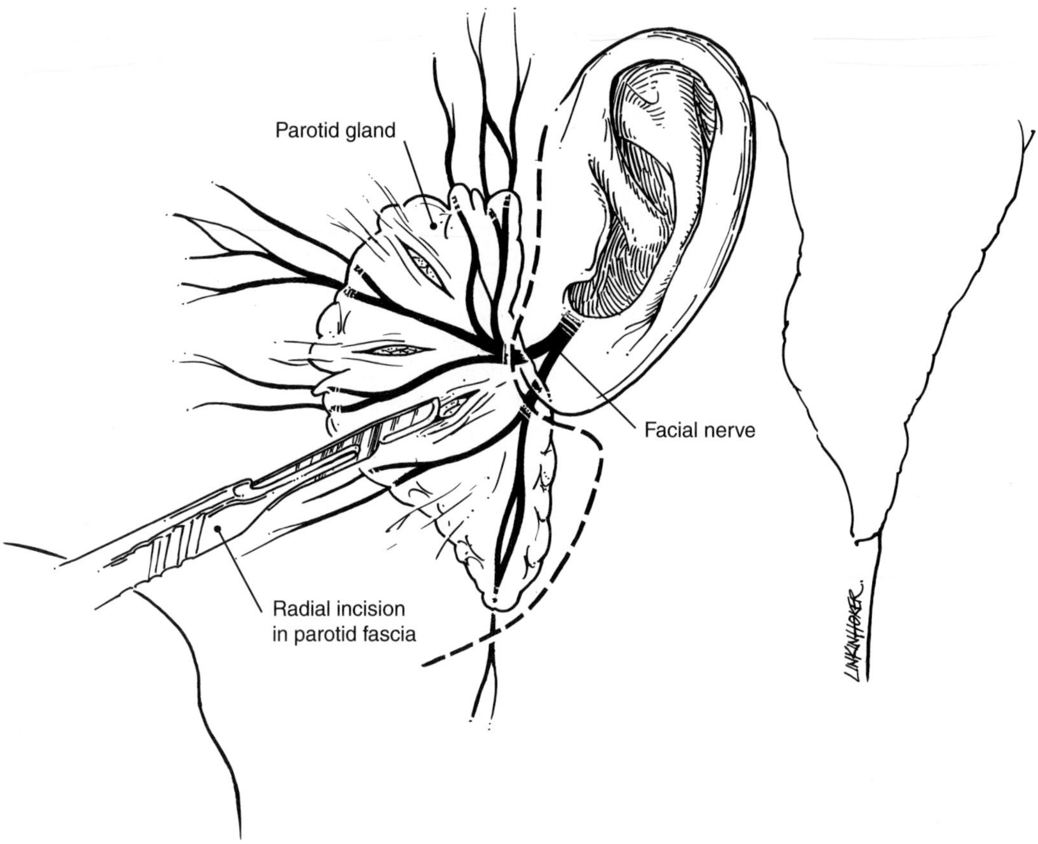

Figure 19–12. Surgical approach to drainage of acute suppurative parotitis refractory to medical management.

spaces of the neck. Any of the complications of a neck abscess may ensue, including mediastinitis, internal jugular vein thrombosis, and carotid arterial erosion. Proximal extension of a thrombosis of the retromandibular vein can also cause jugular venous thrombosis. Rarely, acute parotitis causes dysfunction of one or more branches of the facial nerve. Gradual onset of facial weakness over a period of several days may herald the presence of an abscess, and surgical exploration is often undertaken in this setting. Adequate treatment of the parotitis usually leads to resolution of the facial weakness.[18]

Early recognition and timely initiation of therapeutic interventions often lead to complete resolution of infection. The majority of patients who survive an episode of surgical parotitis do not develop adverse sequelae. A small number of patients, however, suffer from chronic recurrent parotitis, probably secondary to ductal stenosis sustained during the initial infection. These cases require formal parotidectomy, ideally performed at a time when inflammation and infection are minimal.

Necrotizing Fasciitis

Described as "hospital gangrene" in 1871 by Joseph Jones, a Confederate army surgeon, necrotizing fasciitis is predominantly a disease of the abdominal wall, perineum, and lower extremities. Involvement of the head and neck is rare and has been termed craniocervical necrotizing fasciitis (CCNF), a severe, rapidly progressive necrotizing process of the cervical fascia that is classically associated with high mortality rates. CCNF involves primarily the superficial layer of the cervical fascia, but the infection can spread to the deep cervical fascial layers as well. (The anatomy of the cervical fascial layers is reviewed earlier in this chapter [see Fig. 19–1].)

Typically, CCNF occurs in adult patients, and there is equal distribution among males and females. Approximately 50% of the time, this infection occurs in patients with predisposing comorbid conditions, typically diabetes mellitus, atherosclerotic vascular disease, alcoholism, or cirrhosis.[19, 20]

Craniocervical necrotizing fasciitis is most commonly odontogenic in origin, but additional causes include blunt and penetrating traumas (especially those involving the mandible) and direct extension of a tonsillar or cutaneous infection. CCNF is a polymicrobial infection composed of aerobic organisms with or without a synergistic facultative anaerobe. The most common aerobic organisms are group A β-hemolytic *Streptococcus* species and *Staphylococcus aureus;* the most common anaerobic organisms are *Bacteroides*, *Peptostreptococci*, and *Fusobacterium* species.[21]

PRESENTATION

Necrotizing fasciitis presents with both local and systemic findings. The affected area of the neck or scalp is edematous, warm, and tender to palpation. Underlying soft tissue necrosis produces a variety of changes in skin color. The skin may appear red or purplish prior to the development of frank gangrene. Bullae may form over the cervical skin as well. These local changes are caused by thrombosis of the nutrient blood vessels supplying the skin and subcutaneous tissues of the neck.

Systemically, patients are critically ill and may appear toxic. Confusion, weakness, malaise, and dehydration are all systemic symptoms associated with CCNF. Jaundice secondary to overwhelming sepsis is occasionally seen with this entity as well.

EVALUATION

Physical examination of patients with necrotizing fasciitis reveals the findings discussed above in addition to fever, which may initially be low-grade. Assessment of the vital signs may reveal hypotension or tachycardia as well.

Laboratory evaluation includes a complete blood count, blood chemistries and electrolytes, and blood cultures. Anemia, hyponatremia, hypoproteinemia, and hypocalcemia may all be associated with CCNF secondary to sequestration of extracellular fluids in the inflamed areas. Leukocytosis occurs in immune-competent patients. Cultures should be obtained of the fluid within the cutaneous bullae, if present, as well as of the blood. Needle aspiration of the neck seldom provides useful information in this diffuse process.

The classic radiographic appearance of CCNF on plain films or CT imaging reveals extensive subcutaneous emphysema. This finding is helpful in evaluating the initial extent of disease and in assessing disease progression during treatment.

PRIORITIES

Craniocervical necrotizing fasciitis can spread rapidly through the superficial and then through the deep cervical fascia and commonly extends to the anterior chest wall and mediastinum. The first priority in managing this aggressive infection is to secure the airway. Tracheostomy may be necessary if normal anatomic landmarks are distorted. In addition, early tracheostomy may be advantageous in these tenuous patients who generally require postoperative ventilatory support and multiple surgical procedures.

The most important therapeutic measure in the treatment of CCNF is aggressive, radical surgical debridement. Exploration of the neck and resection of all necrotic fascia are critical for control of this rapidly progressive infection. Often, necrosis extends into the chest, and general or thoracic surgical consultation is indicated in these instances. Debridement of necrotic tissue must extend until healthy tissue is encountered at all surrounding margins. A substantial degree of cutaneous involvement inevitably results in a large wound, which should be packed open with a well-moistened gauze dressing at the completion of the operation. The infected tooth of origin should be extracted during the procedure, as well.

Broad-spectrum intravenous antibiotic therapy should be implemented as soon as a diagnosis of necrotizing fasciitis is suspected. Initial coverage should include a penicillinase-resistant penicillin, clindamycin, and often an aminoglycoside for the rare gram-negative organism. The antibiotic regimen may be modified when culture results are available.

In the immediate postoperative period, patients with CCNF generally require an intensive care unit for monitoring and ventilatory support. Any associated metabolic and electrolyte disturbances should be addressed promptly, and treatment of predisposing medical conditions should be maximized.

OUTCOMES

A rapidly progressive craniocervical necrotizing fasciitis can involve the deep cervical fascia. If the infection extends in this direction, any of the complications of a deep-space neck infection can occur, including airway obstruction, jugular venous thrombosis, and arterial erosion. Pharyngocutaneous fistulas have also occurred in this setting. CCNF has a great propensity to spread along the superficial fascial layers into the anterior chest wall. Deeper involvement in the chest may lead to mediastinitis, thoracic empyema, pneumonia, pericardial effusion, or pleural effusion. Systemically, this infection produces bacteremia, and circulating endotoxins lead to multisystem organ failure. The kidney is especially sensitive to this insult; renal failure may be the first manifestation of multiple organ failure.

Following initial intervention, serial chest radiographs or CT scans are often helpful to exclude continued progression or extension of disease. Multiple surgical debridements may be necessary to control this infection. The use of supplemental hyperbaric oxygen therapy has been shown to reduce both mortality and the number of operations required.[22]

Craniocervical necrotizing fasciitis remains a difficult problem that has a mortality rate ranging from 20% to 70%.[19–21] The highest mortality rates are seen in patients with predisposing conditions such as diabetes.[19] In patients who survive CCNF, skin grafts can eventually be placed over the granulating neck wound to facilitate recovery.

VASCULAR EMERGENCIES OF THE NECK

Blood vessels of vital importance traverse the neck, linking the heart and the brain. The carotid arteries, the jugular veins, and their branches constitute large, high-flow vascular structures whose unplanned disruption demands immediate attention. Vascular emergencies of the neck can occur in the operating room or in the postoperative period. Rarely, nonoperated patients with cancer or severe infections are at risk for a vascular emergency. Penetrating trauma to the neck, another important cause of major vascular disruption, is discussed in Chapter 12.

Most surgical procedures of the neck place major vascular structures at risk. The controlled ligation of the internal jugular veins or of branches of the external carotid or jugular venous systems is common in numerous neck surgical procedures. Inadvertent disruption of the common or internal carotid artery, the internal jugular vein, one of the subclavian vessels, the vertebral arteries, or the innominate artery, however, constitutes a vascular emergency for the head and neck surgeon (Fig. 19–13).

Intraoperative Injury

PRESENTATION

Signaled by the rapid accumulation of a substantial amount of blood within the operative field, violation of a major vascular structure is not subtle. The source vessel of the hemorrhage is usually suggested by the anatomic location of the dissection. Bright red, pulsatile bleeding connotes an arterial source, whereas dark, nonpulsatile bleeding suggests a venous injury.

The potential for a major vascular emergency exists in any operation involving exposure or dissection of these vessels, but several procedures and preoperative diagnoses carry recognized predilections for vascular complications. When a patient is judged to be at high risk for intraoperative vascular injury, appropriate precautions should be taken preoperatively. Specific examples follow.

A patient with bulky, malignant cervical disease is at risk for vascular invasion of the major vessels by tumor. A CT scan with intravenous contrast can evaluate the relationship between the vessels and the tumor. If suspicion of carotid invasion is raised, a standard angiogram or magnetic resonance angiogram (MRA) may further delineate vascular encasement by tumor. Knowledge of this situation allows for appropriate operative planning. The surgeon may obtain a preoperative balloon occlusion study to assess the neurologic risk of carotid artery ligation or may consult with a vascular surgeon regarding bypass grafting. Unequivocal carotid arterial involvement carries an exceedingly grim prognosis that is not improved by surgical intervention.[23] In this instance, many surgeons would deem the tumor unresectable and spare the patient an unnecessary surgical procedure.

A patient with bilateral neck disease may demonstrate radiographic evidence of bilateral jugular venous invasion by tumor. The surgeon may elect to perform the neck dissection in two separate stages to avoid the risks associated with simultaneous resection of the bilateral internal jugular veins such as upper airway obstruction, massive facial or intracranial edema, blindness, and even death. Alternatively, simultaneous bilateral internal jugular vein ligation may be undertaken with improved safety if the external or anterior jugular venous systems are spared. Concomitant tracheostomy is often prudent in these cases to avoid the airway compromise associated with lack of venous outflow if collateral circulation is insufficient.

A patient with a carotid body tumor, or para-

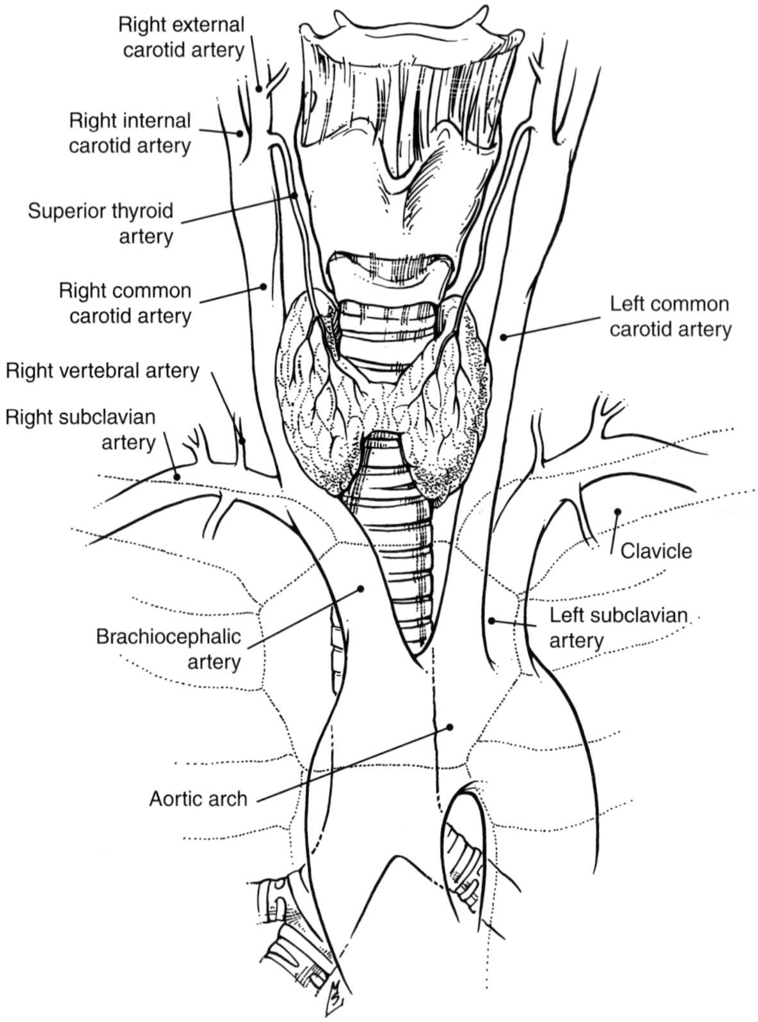

Figure 19–13. Major arteries of the neck.

ganglioma, is also at increased risk for vascular injury. Carotid body tumors arise from a small conglomerate of cells intimately related to the bifurcation of the common carotid artery. Many surgeons advocate the use of preoperative angiography with selective embolization of vessels supplying the tumor to reduce the significant vascularity of these lesions.[24] Preoperative vascular surgical consultation should be obtained in all cases in anticipation of arterial injury or inability to separate the tumor from the artery.

EVALUATION AND PRIORITIES

Significant intraoperative hemorrhage is instantly apparent and presents an immediate threat of considerable blood loss. Regardless of the source of the bleed, the application of direct pressure is the first measure taken to control it. The anesthesiologist should be informed of the potential for substantial blood loss and should adjust fluid volume support accordingly. If a current type and cross match is not confirmed by the blood bank, a blood sample should be sent promptly in the event that blood transfusion is necessary.

Although bleeding from the internal jugular vein is generally less feared than disruption of the carotid artery, it can be extremely problematic. If the injury is small and accessible, it is amenable to simple closure with a silk tie or primary repair with an 8-0 or 9-0 monofilament suture. If the venotomy is large but the contralateral internal jugular vein is intact, the vein can be resected by double ligation at the skull base and the inferior neck. If, however, the contralateral vein has been resected during the procedure, every attempt should be made to maintain flow through the injured vein by repairing it. Vein interposition grafts have been placed in an attempt to maintain flow in a single remaining vessel, but assessment of this technique has not been addressed objectively.

Simultaneous sacrifice of the bilateral internal jugular veins has been associated with marked facial edema, upper airway obstruction, increased intracranial pressure, blindness, and even death.[25] If tumor involvement of the bilateral veins is unexpectedly encountered, preservation of the anterior or external jugular venous system reduces the risk of complications. Postoperatively, elevation of the head of the patient's bed and intravenous steroids may be of benefit. Tracheostomy may be necessary to protect the airway in the event of significant venous outflow obstruction and resultant airway edema.

Hemorrhage from the internal jugular vein at the base of the skull can prove difficult to manage. Pressure applied against the bony skull base provides temporary control while the surgeon attempts to circumferentially free the vessel from surrounding tissue. Care must be taken to avoid clamping tissue hastily and without good visualization because cranial nerves X, XI, and XII are at risk for injury in this area. Various methods of tamponading the flow of blood while isolating the vessel have been employed. A Fogarty balloon catheter can be placed intraluminally during repair of the vessel (Fig. 19–14). Whenever possible, the vessel should be isolated and ligated. If controlled ligation cannot be accomplished, the injured vein can be packed at the skull base with muscle, fat, or a biologic hemostatic agent such as Avitene or Surgicel. Local tissue can be closed over the opening to maintain proper positioning of the packing. The vein should be properly ligated inferiorly in these instances.

The inferior limit of the neck dissection is another area where inadvertent vascular injury commonly occurs, often due to limited exposure. The subclavian and innominate vessels are at risk in this location (see Fig. 19–13), and application of direct pressure is difficult because access is restricted by the clavicle. A sponge on a clamp may facilitate immediate control of bleeding. In the case of a venous bleed, a clamp may be placed over the injury on the vessel and gently twisted while elevating the vessel into the operative field. This maneuver serves to stop the bleeding temporarily, providing time for visualization and repair. Care must be taken not to extend the injury with this method.

Injury to the subclavian artery is unusual but requires urgent vascular or thoracic surgical consultation. Sternotomy or thoracotomy may be necessary for adequate exposure of the vessel.

An especially precarious situation is entry into the innominate artery, which can occur during tracheostomy when exposure is limited. Occasionally, this vessel overlies the anterior tracheal wall, and extreme care must be taken during inferior dissection, especially if a tracheostomy is placed below the 4th tracheal ring. Although tracheostomy is regarded as a simple and routine procedure, this complication can be fatal.[26] Similarly, the innominate artery is at risk during thyroidectomy. Injury to this vessel may require sternotomy for access during repair.[27]

Apart from blood loss and associated hypovolemia, a significant venous bleed also creates a risk for air embolism. With disruption of the internal jugular or subclavian veins, air enters the venous circulation and returns to the heart, where it can subsequently embolize to the lungs. A large amount of embolized air may

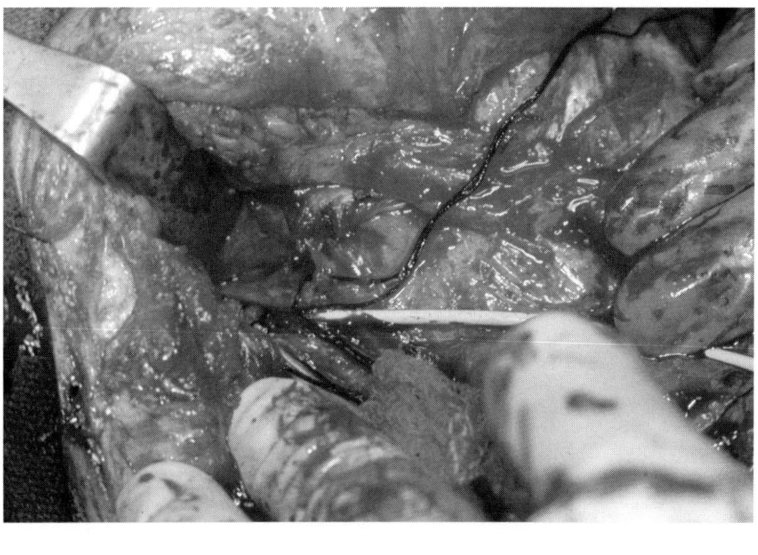

Figure 19–14. Placement of a Fogarty catheter into an injured internal jugular vein near the skull base for temporary vascular control during repair of the injured vessel.

cause hypotension and, ultimately, circulatory compromise. A churning sound heard over the precordium heralds this ominous event. Temporary control of the hemorrhage with pressure or packing should be implemented while the patient is placed in the head-down, left-lateral decubitus position. This position traps air in the right side of the heart, minimizing embolization to the lungs, and is maintained until the patient is hemodynamically stable. Sometimes needle aspiration of the air from the right ventricle is necessary to achieve stability.[27]

Intraoperative injury of the carotid artery is among the most dramatic complications of head and neck surgery, and it is greatly feared because it can rapidly lead to significant neurologic impairment or death. Immediate and temporary control of the hemorrhage with direct digitial pressure or a vascular clamp facilitates assessment of the extent of arterial damage. Dissection of the vessel superior and inferior to the rent should be performed, and vascular loops placed circumferentially around the artery for proximal and distal control. Tension on these loops can be applied to tamponade bleeding during primary repair of the vessel with a 5-0 or 6-0 monofilament suture. If the tissue is not amenable to simple repair, alternatives include bypass grafting or patch grafting. Intraoperative consultation with a vascular surgeon is indicated to aid in the vascular reconstruction. If grafting is not deemed feasible due to irreparable tissue damage, inability of the vessel to support an anastomosis, or lack of access to a surgeon skilled in arterial revascularization, arterial ligation is the remaining option.

Some surgeons advocate the intraoperative measurement of distal arterial stump pressure to determine the patient's tolerance for carotid artery ligation. A 22-gauge needle attached to a pressure transducer is inserted into the artery distal to a clamp temporarily occluding blood flow. If stump pressures exceed 70 mm Hg, collateral circulation is considered adequate for ligation without reconstruction. For stump pressures between 55 and 70 mm Hg, a conservative recommendation is resection with reconstruction. Stump pressures below 55 mm Hg require that reconstruction be undertaken in conjunction with a temporary intraoperative shunt.[28]

OUTCOMES

Intraoperative disruption of a major cervical vessel can lead to the patient's demise. Timely control of the hemorrhage and subsequent maintenance of hemodynamic stability allows many patients to recover without adverse effects. Unanticipated resection of bilateral internal jugular veins, however, is an unusual situation that requires close postoperative monitoring for signs of increased intracranial pressure, airway obstruction secondary to edema, or visual compromise.

Unplanned injury to, or ligation of, the carotid artery may also lead to serious postoperative sequelae. Unanticipated ligation of the carotid artery is associated with a mortality rate that ranges from 10% to 50% and with a 25% to 50% risk of a cerebrovascular event.[29, 30] The degree of neurologic impairment varies in severity and longevity, ranging from transient ischemia to permanent incapacitation. Neurologic impairment may be immediately apparent upon the patient's awakening or may manifest itself as a late event, presumably due to extension of thrombus from the distal stump or repaired segment. If carotid arterial ligation is unavoidable, the artery should be resected as near to the skull base as possible to prevent the formation of a pouch harboring a thrombus. In addition, some surgeons advocate the use of subcutaneous heparin postoperatively for prevention of delayed neurologic sequelae,[31] but its benefit in this situation remains controversial.

Hematoma

Hematoma formation is a potential complication of any surgical procedure. An open blood vessel may be unrecognized intraoperatively because of temporary vessel spasm. Postoperative relaxation of a previously spasmodic vessel and technical error related to inadequate vessel ligation are among the mechanisms that contribute to hematoma formation. An undrained collection of blood under the surface of the skin in the neck poses the additional risk of airway compromise.

PRESENTATION

A hematoma usually appears as a distended area, initially soft but later firm to palpation (Fig. 19–15). With time, the area becomes ecchymotic. If closed suction drains are in place, they may reveal brisk, bright-red output. Alternatively, clotted blood may render drains nonfunctional. Blood may visibly ooze from the suture line or drain sites.

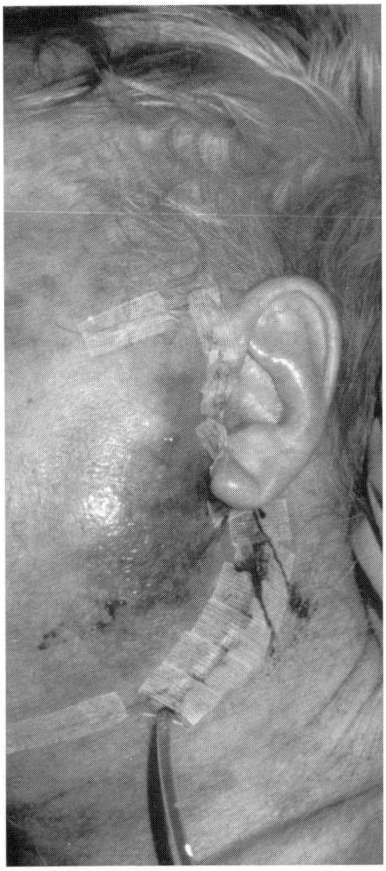

Figure 19–15. Hematoma after parotidectomy.

EVALUATION

Postoperative hematoma is diagnosed solely on the basis of the physical examination during which the above findings are recognized. The hematoma may present immediately, even prior to extubation in the operating room, or may manifest itself hours after the procedure. The stripping of a functioning drain and the application of direct pressure may evacuate blood from the wound and prevent reaccumulation if it has been detected early, but generally, a return to the operating room is required.

PRIORITIES

As an expanding cervical mass, a hematoma can create pressure on the airway. If the patient shows signs of respiratory compromise, such as stridor or poor oxygen saturation, airway control by intubation is warranted, and return to the operating room should be expedited. Evacuation of a hematoma at the bedside is undertaken if the airway cannot be secured and the patient is progressively deteriorating.

The wound is reopened and the clot evacuated, preferably in the operating room. After copious irrigation, the wound is carefully examined for the source of the bleeding. Adequate hemostasis is achieved, and fresh suction drains are placed.

OUTCOMES

Prompt recognition and evacuation of a hematoma usually results in complete recovery without adverse sequelae. These collections can, however, create pressure necrosis in the cervical flaps, and an unrecognized hematoma can be a source for wound infection. Hematomas are occasionally associated with significant blood loss, but this situation is rare in the head and neck where potential spaces for unrecognized accumulation of a substantial blood volume are limited.

Postoperative Carotid Arterial Exposure or Rupture

Carotid rupture, or "blowout," is perhaps the most devastating complication of head and neck surgery and is highly stressful for both the patient and the health care team. Impending rupture of the carotid artery can be quite subtle. Exposure of the artery after wound dehiscence places a patient at great risk for eventual arterial rupture.

The majority of patients at risk for exposure or rupture of the carotid artery are those previously treated for squamous cell carcinoma of the head and neck. A history of radical neck surgery is the primary risk factor for subsequent carotid exposure, and many of these patients have undergone resections involving dissection of tumor off the carotid artery. This type of dissection may sacrifice the adventitia of the vessel and compromise the blood supply of the arterial wall, weakening the vessel and placing it at risk for future rupture. Carotid arterial blowout has been reported as occurring from 1 week to nearly 3 months postoperatively, with a mean time of occurrence of just over 2 weeks after surgical resection.

Postoperative wound complications constitute another notable risk factor for carotid arterial damage. Between 60% and 80% of patients suffering carotid exposure and eventual rupture have active wound infections; most commonly, they are associated with a pharyngocutaneous or orocutaneous fistula. In addition, the majority of patients suffering carotid blowouts demonstrate flap necrosis.[29, 30, 32] Radiation therapy, administered either pre- or postoperatively, is another significant risk factor for carotid rupture. Radiation therapy obliterates the vasa vasorum, encourages early atherosclerosis, and promotes adventitial fibrosis, further weakening the arterial wall. Finally, persistence or recurrence of tumor poses a substantial risk to the integrity of the carotid artery. Tumor invasion of the vessel wall can lead directly to vascular breakdown.

PRESENTATION

An exposed carotid artery is not always apparent in a neck wound or fistula. Even if the vessel cannot be visualized, a sentinel bleed may herald its impending rupture. One or more episodes of brisk red bleeding from the neck or oral cavity often signal carotid blowout. Sentinel bleeding usually stops spontaneously or with minimal manipulation and is attributed to a periodically leaking pseudoaneurysm of the carotid artery.

An acute arterial rupture presents dramatically and cannot be mistaken for bleeding from a lesser vessel. It is a traumatic experience for patients, family members, and health care workers alike.

EVALUATION AND PRIORITIES: EXPOSED CAROTID ARTERY

Early recognition of an exposed vessel is paramount to the prevention of a catastrophic carotid rupture. Carotid precautions, implemented as soon as arterial exposure is identified, include the availability of a current blood sample in the blood bank and the maintenance of adequatedly sized intravenous catheters.

To prevent rupture, the vessel must be kept moist at all times, and meticulous care must be given to the wound. Intravenous antibiotic therapy is initiated to minimize underlying infection and promote the formation of granulation tissue. Hyperbaric oxygen therapy is occasionally employed to enhance oxygenation and tissue recovery. In the presence of a pharyngocutaneous fistula, saliva must be diverted away from the exposed artery. The exposed vessel should be resurfaced as soon as the wound is healthy. Pedicled myocutaneous flaps are commonly used for this purpose, as are split-thickness skin grafts in the presence of adequate granulation tissue.

A frank discussion with the patient and his or her family members is imperative once the risk of carotid rupture has been established. The prognosis of the underlying disease and the mortality rate inherent in emergent carotid ligation should be presented to patients and their families. One study demonstrated survival periods of less than 18 months following successful carotid ligation, even in patients without evidence of recurrent disease.[30] A clear plan must be in place regarding the level of resuscitation to be pursued in the event of rupture. In patients with recurrent or persistent disease, the choice of supportive care is a reasonable alternative to surgical intervention.

An episode of sentinel bleeding should be treated as an impending carotid blowout. After a decision in favor of maximal resuscitation has been reached, the patient should undergo testing for tolerability of carotid resection. The morbidity and mortality rates involved in carotid artery ligation are much lower in elective procedures than in unplanned ligations. A variety of tests are currently available to predict the neurologic safety of carotid resection.

Pressure measurements can be obtained from the distal carotid artery after temporary proximal occlusion of the vessel. High "stump pressure" readings correlate loosely with successful ligation, but this method is highly unreliable as it offers no information regarding cerebral blood flow or neurologic impairment. The analogous technique of direct stump pressure measurements can be valuable in an emergent intraoperative setting, as previously discussed. Ocular pneumoplethysmography is another technique used to predict carotid artery resectability; it reflects retinal artery filling pressures, which can be correlated with distal arterial flow. Unfortunately, these values do not correlate with flow in the anterior and middle cerebral arterial systems supplying the brain.[33]

The most commonly employed test of carotid resectability is the temporary balloon occlusion (TBO) test. This method involves cannulation of the carotid artery by a catheter that is inserted into the femoral artery. Balloon occlusion of the artery is undertaken with simulataneous assessment of neurologic function by electroencephalogram monitoring, clinical examination, or both. If neurologic compromise occurs within a somewhat arbitrarily designated time period (usually about 15 minutes), the patient is considered a high risk for stroke. If elective ligation is undertaken under these circumstances, arterial bypass grafting and temporary intraoperative shunting are necessary.[33]

Unfortunately, a patient who passes a TBO study remains at fairly high risk for neurologic impairment. Some centers use a xenon-enhanced CT (Xe-CT) image of cerebral blood flow to further assess such a patient.[33] This study is a high-resolution image that is the only direct measure of cerebral blood flow currently available. Following the TBO study, the arterial catheter remains in place, and the patient is taken to the CT scanner. The patient breathes a mixture containing xenon, a radiodense gas that rapidly saturates tissues. CT images are obtained with and without the balloon's being reinflated, and the difference in cerebral blood flow before and after occlusion is calculated. If a patient passes both the TBO test and the Xe-CT image of cerebral blood flow, carotid ligation is considered quite safe. If a patient passes the TBO test but fails the Xe-CT scan, cartoid ligation with bypass grafting is recommended. Although the Xe-CT scan increases the sensitivity of TBO testing, it is not universally available. Opponents of this method consider it an unnecessary increase in time, patient risk, and cost.

A patient deemed a candidate for elective arterial resection as a result of passing both the TBO test and the Xe-CT scan or the TBO test alone often has an alternative to surgical ligation. Endovascular therapeutic occlusion with detachable balloon embolization is now widely offered to patients with impending carotid rupture. Performed under intravenous sedation, this technique offers the advantage of precise localization of the leak or aneurysm in the artery. Success rates are comparable to those achieved with surgical ligation, and the procedure carries the identical risks of acute or delayed neurologic impairment.[35] Embolization can immediately follow a balloon occlusion study, without the need to transport the patient or remove the catheter. If detachable balloon occlusion is not available for a patient considered a candidate for carotid resection, surgical ligation of the vessel is performed.

EVALUATION AND PRIORITIES: ACUTE CAROTID RUPTURE

In the event of a carotid blowout, direct and immediate pressure must be applied to the vessel by the first person to arrive on the scene. Digital pressure should not be removed for any reason until definitive therapy is initiated, and no attempt should be made to clamp or ligate the vessel at the bedside because of the risk of exsanguination. If bleeding emanates from the oral cavity or oropharynx, direct external pressure may require supplementation with pharyngeal packing. In this instance, the airway must be secured prior to the placement of packing.

Volume resuscitation with Ringer's lactate solution, normal saline, or whole blood should be started immediately. Large-bore intravenous catheters are inserted, and arterial lines are placed for monitoring. Maintenance of an adequate blood pressure to ensure cerebral blood flow is the single most critical aspect in the management of acute carotid rupture. Hypotension, either preoperatively or intraoperatively, is the most reliable predictor of poor outcome in acute arterial rupture.

If the patient can be hemodynamically stabilized, endovascular therapeutic occlusion with detachable balloon embolization may be an option in the acute setting, provided that the equipment and personnel are readily available. Studies report an 80% to 100% survival rate for patients undergoing balloon embolization for acute carotid arterial rupture.[32, 33] If the patient cannot be hemodynamically stabilized, arrangements are made for immediate and direct transport to the operating room for surgical ligation. Constant digital pressure is held en route and during surgical preparation. Pressure is not released until the vessel is adequately exposed and controlled with clamps or vessel loops (Fig. 19–16). The artery is ligated away from any areas suspicious for tumor invasion with a 0 silk tie and suture ligature. In addition, oversewing the ligated vessel with monofilament suture further buttresses the closure.

OUTCOMES

Morbidity and mortality rates for both emergent and elective carotid arterial ligation are high. Mortality rates after acute carotid arterial rupture range from 40% to 80%,[29–33] whereas mortality rates after elective arterial ligation are much lower—less than 10%.[33, 34] The rate of neurologic impairment in emergent ligation has been cited as being 25% to 80%, depending on the series.[29–33] Morbidity relates to both acute and delayed neurologic sequelae. To reduce the occurrence of late stroke, many surgeons advocate the use of subcutaneous heparin sulfate, administered at 5,000 U every 12 hours, in patients who have undergone carotid ligation or embolization.[31]

Morbidity and mortality rates appear overall to be somewhat lower in patients who receive elective detachable balloon embolization therapy for impending carotid rupture than in those who undergo elective surgical ligation of the artery.[34, 35] Even in patients who withstand an

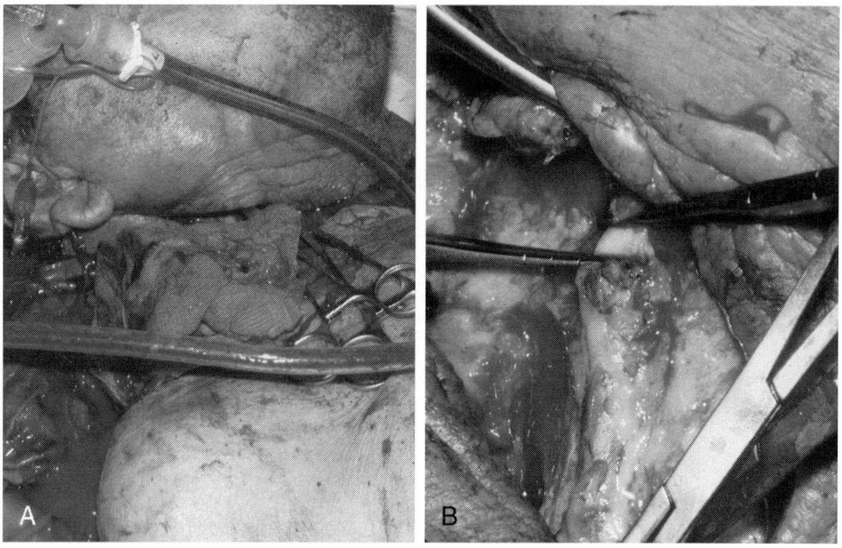

Figure 19–16. A: Emergency control of a ruptured right carotid artery. B: The site of arterial erosion in the same patient after control of the vessel.

acute arterial rupture, long-term survival may be substantially diminished. In all cases, prevention of carotid blowout provides the best chance for survival.

REFERENCES

1. Peterson LJ. Odontogenic infections. In Cummings CW et al., eds. Otolaryngology: Head and Neck Surgery. St. Louis, Mosby–Year Book, 1993, pp. 1199–1215.
2. Marra S, Hotaling AJ. Deep neck infections. Am J Otolaryngol 1996;17:287–298.
3. Williams MF, Eisele DW, Wyatt SH. Neck needle foreign bodies in intravenous drug abusers. Laryngoscope 1993;103:59–63.
4. Tom MB, Rice DH. Presentation and management of neck abscess: a retrospective analysis. Laryngoscope 1988;98:877–881.
5. Spires JR et al. Treatment of peritonsillar abscess: a prospective study of aspiration vs. incision and drainage. Arch Otolaryngol 1987;113:984–986.
6. Wolf M, Even-Chen I, Kronenberg J. Peritonsillar abscess: repeated needle aspiration versus incision and drainage. Ann Otol Rhinol Laryngol 1994;103:554–557.
7. Brook I. Diagnosis and management of anaerobic infections of the head and neck. Ann Otol Rhinol Laryngol 1992;101:9–15.
8. Gidley PW, Ghorayeb BY, Stiernberg CM. Contemporary management of deep neck space infections. Otolaryngol Head Neck Surg 1997;116:16–22.
9. Vandenberg SJ, Hartig GK. Lemierre's syndrome. Otolaryngol Head Neck Surg 1998;119:516–518.
10. Yau PC, Norante JD. Thrombophlebitis of the internal jugular vein secondary to pharyngitis. Arch Otolaryngol 1980;106:507–508.
11. Cohen JP, Persky MS, Reede DI. Internal jugular vein thrombosis. Laryngoscope 1985;95:1478–1482.
12. Tovi F, Fliss DM, Noyek AM. Septic internal jugular vein thrombosis. J Otolaryngol 1993;22:415–420.
13. Alexander DW, Leonard JR, Trail ML. Vascular complications of deep neck abscesses. Laryngoscope 1968;78:361–370.
14. Langenbrunner DJ, Dajani S. Pharyngomaxillary space abscess with carotid artery erosion. Arch Otolaryngol 1971;94:447–457.
15. Brook I. Diagnosis and management of parotitis. Arch Otolaryngol Head Neck Surg 1992;118:469–471.
16. Yonkers AJ, Krous HF, Yarington CT. Surgical parotitis. Laryngoscope 1972;82:1239–1247.
17. Lary B. Postoperative surgical parotitis. Arch Surg 1963;89:653.
18. Andrews JC et al. Parotitis and facial nerve dysfunction. Arch Otolaryngol Head Neck Surg 1989;115:240–242.
19. Gallia LJ, Johnson JT. Cervical necrotizing fasciitis. Otolaryngol Head Neck Surg 1981;89:935–937.
20. Kantu S, Har-El G. Cervical necrotizing fasciitis. Ann Otol Rhinol Laryngol 1997;106:965–970.
21. Spankus EM et al. Craniocervical necrotizing fasciitis. Otolaryngol Head Neck Surg 1984;92:261–265.
22. Riseman JA et al. Hyperbaric oxygen therapy for necrotizing fasciitis reduces mortality and the need for debridements. Surgery 1990;108:847–850.
23. Brennan JA, Jafek BW. Elective carotid artery resection for advanced squamous cell carcinoma of the neck. Laryngoscope 1994;104:259–263.
24. Ward PH et al. Embolization: an adjunctive measure for removal of carotid body tumors. Laryngoscope 1988;98:1287–1291.
25. Ahn C, Sindelar WF. Bilateral radical neck dissection: report of results in 55 patients. J Surg Oncol 1989;40:252–255.
26. Biller HF, Ebert PA. Innominate artery hemorrhage complicating tracheotomy. Ann Otol Rhinol Laryngol 1970;79:301–306.
27. Longnecker CG. Venous air embolism during operation on the head and neck. Plast Reconstr Surg 1965;36:619–621.
28. Ehrenfeld WK, Stoney RJ, Wylie RJ. Relation of carotid stump pressure to safety of carotid artery ligation. Surgery 1983;93:299–305.
29. Hillerman BL, Kennedy TL. Carotid rupture and tissue coverage. Laryngoscope 1982;92:985–988.

30. Baxter WF. Survival after unplanned carotid rupture. Laryngoscope 1979;89:385–392.
31. Leikensohn J, Milko D, Cotton R. Carotid artery rupture: management and prevention of delayed neurologic sequelae with low-dose heparin. Arch Otolaryngol 1978;104:307–310.
32. Citardi MJ et al. Management of carotid artery rupture by monitored endovascular therapeutic occlusion (1988–1994). Laryngoscope 1995;105:1086–1092.
33. Morrissey DD et al. Endovascular management of hemorrhage in patients with head and neck cancer. Arch Otolaryngol Head Neck Surg 1997;123:15–19.
34. de Vries EJ et al. A new method to predict safe resection of the internal carotid artery. Laryngoscope 1990;100:85–88.
35. Zimmerman MC et al. Treatment of impending carotid rupture with detachable balloon embolization. Arch Otolaryngol Head Neck Surg 1987;113:1169–1175.

CHAPTER 20

Thoracic Emergencies

Richard F. Heitmiller, MD
Stephen C. Yang, MD

There is anatomic and physiologic overlap between cervical and thoracic structures. Management of disease processes in the cervicothoracic region requires an understanding of chest anatomy and surgical principles. Many thoracic surgical emergencies are immediate, life-threatening problems that require prompt recognition, diagnosis, and management.

ESOPHAGEAL PERFORATION

Esophageal perforation is a surgical emergency; it commonly occurs unexpectedly, is frequently iatrogenic, and is invariably associated with high rates of morbidity and mortality. Its potential impact on postinjury swallowing, and therefore on quality of life, can be great, depending on the timing of repair and the nature of any underlying esophageal disease. Esophageal perforation is a significant injury because it results in leakage of the highly virulent oral bacteria into a well-vascularized mediastinum or pleural space where there is rapid bacterial absorption and early sepsis.

Jones and Ginsberg reported that the causes of esophageal perforation were instrumentation in 43%, trauma in 19%, spontaneous occurrence in 16%, foreign bodies in 7%, operative injuries in 8%, tumor in 5%, and miscellaneous causes in the remaining 3% (Fig. 20–1).[1] Iatrogenic injury (instrumentation plus operative injury) therefore accounts for over half of the cases of perforation. In their series, 40% of patients who developed perforation had no underlying esophageal disease. Ferguson has shown that the likelihood of developing postinstrumentation esophageal perforation is 47% for patients with benign disease and 88% for patients with malignant esophageal tumors.[2]

Trauma and instrumentation are the most common causes of perforation. Traumatic esophageal perforation accounts for 19% of cases and invariably follows penetrating injury. The cervical esophagus is most commonly involved. Reported perforation rates related to instrumentation vary depending on whether the data are viewed prospectively or retrospectively.

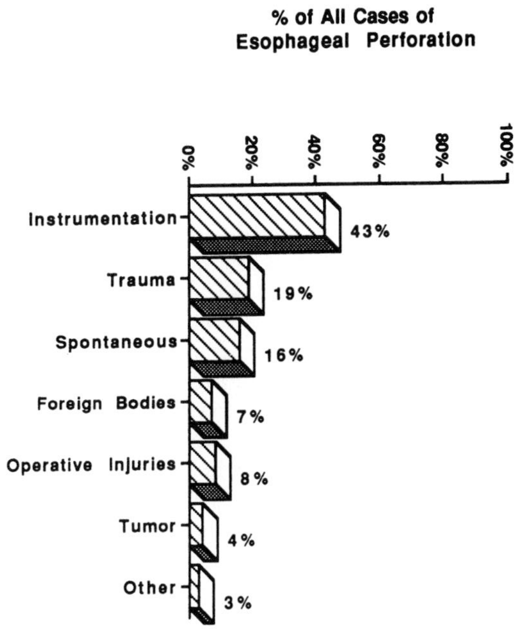

Figure 20–1. Etiology of esophageal perforation. (Reprinted with permission from the Society of Thoracic Surgeons [The Annals of Thoracic Surgery 1992, 53, pages 534–543].)

Prospectively, perforation following esophagoscopy is uncommon, occurring with a frequency of 0.03% and 1.00% for flexible and rigid esophagoscopy, respectively. Perforation rates following esophageal dilation are similar, regardless of the technique used—0.04% to 0.09% for mercury-filled dilators, 0.06% for metal olive dilators, and 0.3% for balloon dilators.[3] Considering patients with esophageal cancer specifically, insertion of a plastic stent carries a 6% risk of perforation, whereas wire-guided stents have approximately a 1% incidence of perforation.[2] Retrospectively, Jones and Ginsberg reported the type of instrumental perforation to be esophagoscopy in 35%, pneumatic dilation in 25%, bougienage in 20%, sclerotherapy in 2%, and miscellaneous procedures in the remainder, 18%.[1] Stent placement accounts for 40% of perforations in patients with esophageal cancer.[2]

Presentation and Evaluation

The diagnosis of perforation must be suspected in order to be established. A higher level of suspicion should be present for patients who have recently undergone esophageal instrumentation, who have known esophageal pathology, and who have sustained penetrating trauma, but in some patients, it occurs spontaneously. The objectives of the diagnostic workup are to determine whether a leak is present, whether it is cervical, thoracic, or abdominal, whether it is free or contained, and whether there is any associated esophageal pathology.

Clinically, patients with esophageal perforation present with constant, severe pain arising from the perforation site. They may also complain of pain on swallowing (odynophagia), worsening dysphagia, and dyspnea. Physical findings include fever, cervical subcutaneous emphysema, changes in voice, and dullness to chest percussion, suggesting effusion.

Plain films of the chest may reveal pneumomediastinum, pneumothorax, pleural effusion, or subcutaneous emphysema. On rare occasions, pneumoperitoneum is identified. Lateral neck films may be helpful in detecting small amounts of air in the prevertebral space.

By far the most effective means of achieving the diagnostic goals is to use contrast esophagography (Fig. 20–2). A water-soluble agent, Gastrografin, is administered first unless there is perceived risk of aspiration. If further detail is needed, or if no leak is identified, then dilute barium is used. Although false negative rates as high as 10% are reported, we have found this test to be invaluable because it fulfills all of the diagnostic objectives. A small red rubber catheter or nasogastric tube can be inserted into the cervical esophagus so that contrast can be directly infused in patients who are unable to swallow. Video esophagographic techniques increase the sensitivity of these studies.

Computed tomography (CT) scans of the chest and upper abdomen are useful to assess the extent of the leak, to help determine whether it is contained or free, and to evaluate the esophagus with respect to associated pathology. If a contrast swallow has demonstrated that a patient has a free perforation, it is not routine to add CT scanning to the diagnostic workup.

Theoretically, esophageal perforation can be diagnosed endoscopically. However, both rigid and flexible esophagoscopy risk extending the injury, the former by mechanical means and the latter by means of air insufflation. In addition, the sensitivity of endoscopy is less than that of contrast radiography, and it cannot differentiate between free and contained leaks.

Priorities

Prompt diagnosis and early surgical intervention are the keys to successful outcome. Once the diagnosis has been established, all oral intake is stopped, and the patient is treated with intravenous hydration, broad-spectrum antibiotics to cover oral flora, and H_2 blockers to reduce gastric acid secretions. Early surgical exploration—within the first 24 hours—and primary repair of the leak site yield the best results. This is not always possible because of delay in diagnosis, the extent of the injury, or associated esophageal pathology. Associated pathology is synchronously repaired only if it does not jeopardize closure of the leak. Specific treatment options vary depending on whether the leak is free or contained, on the site of the leak, and on the presence or absence of esophageal pathology.

CONTAINED PERFORATION

Occasionally, a contained esophageal perforation is encountered. It may be managed nonoperatively by ceasing oral intake and providing intravenous fluids, alimentation, and antibiotics. Nasogastric drainage does not appear to be necessary in the successful management of such a patient. Cameron and associates established the criteria for managing a patient nonoperatively:

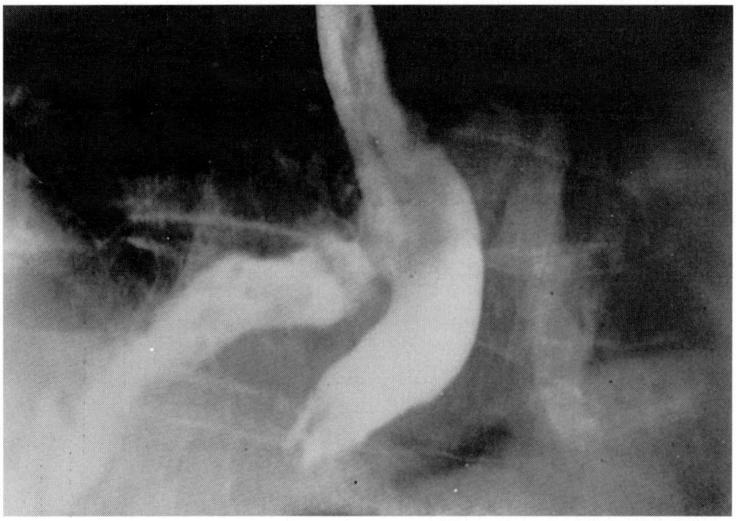

Figure 20–2. A film from a contrast esophagogram showing free distal esophageal perforation draining into the right pleural space.

(1) the esophageal leak is contained within the mediastinum; (2) the contained cavity drains back into the esophagus; (3) the patient has few symptoms; and (4) there is no evidence of clinical sepsis.[4] The surgeon must be willing to proceed operatively if a patient's status deteriorates during conservative therapy.

FREE CERVICAL PERFORATION

In the case of a patient with a free cervical perforation treatment options include primary repair and drainage. Primary repair is preferred whenever it is possible. The cervical esophagus is exposed and the leak site debrided. Closure is performed using two layers of sutures. The inner layer closes and inverts the mucosa, and the outer layer closes the esophageal musculature. This technique is illustrated in Figure 20–3. It is important to visualize the extent of the mucosal opening prior to repair. Extending the muscular injury to visualize the underlying mucosa may be necessary. The incision is then closed in layers. If, on cervical exploration, it is felt that the leak cannot be safely closed because of the extent of injury, the presence of friable tissue, or concerns about mediastinitis, the cervical incision should be packed and left widely open. Dry dressings are used until the salivary drainage stops, and then wet-to-dry normal saline dressings are employed until the wound closes by secondary intention.

FREE THORACIC OR ABDOMINAL PERFORATION

The options available for treating a free thoracic or abdominal performation include primary repair, diversion and drainage, primary resection, and observation. Primary repair is the preferred approach whenever it is possible.[5] A thoracotomy is recommended to visualize both thoracic and abdominal perforation sites. Lower-third esophageal perforations are approached through a left thoracotomy, whereas more proximal intrathoracic esophageal injuries are approached through the right chest. The leak site is closed using the same suture technique described earlier (see Fig. 20–3). Secondary reinforcement of

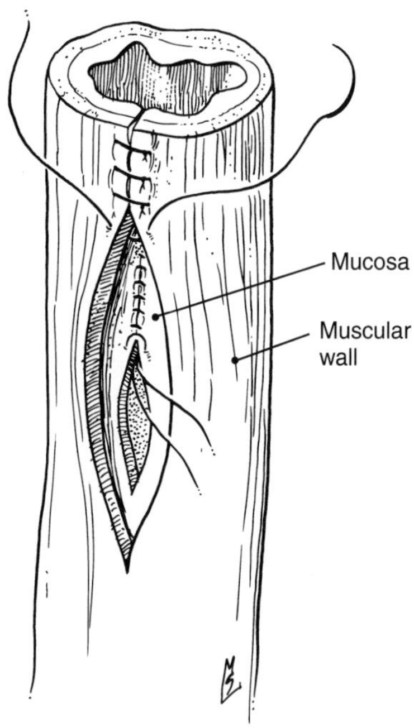

Figure 20–3. The technique of primary esophageal surgical repair is demonstrated.

the suture line with local vascularized soft tissue flaps (parietal pleura, pericardial fat, or intercostal muscle) is recommended. Adequate chest drainage is mandatory, and nasogastric drainage is commonly used for 3 to 5 days to protect the suture line.

If a patient is not a candidate for primary repair because thoracotomy carries increased risk because of the presence of comorbidities, sepsis, friable tissue or the extent of the esophageal injury, then diversion and drainage are performed. The virulence of an esophageal rupture results from the leakage of saliva into the chest. Complete salivary diversion by means of cervical esophagostomy, as shown in Figure 20–4, stops the source of sepsis and permits spontaneous healing of the distal leak site.[6] A gastrostomy for gastric drainage, a jejunostomy for enteral alimentation, and adequate chest tube drainage are routinely added. Once the sepsis has resolved and the leak site sealed, the esophagus is repaired by cervical esophagoesophagostomy or esophageal replacement with stomach or colon tissue.

Sometimes a patient presents with perforation in the setting of esophageal cancer or irreparable benign esophageal disease. If the diagnosis is made promptly and the patient is fit, one-stage esophagectomy, gastric pull-up, and cervical esophagogastric anastomosis may be considered.[7]

Chest drainage and observation of free perforations in the chest or abdomen have been advocated by some, but most studies show this tactic to be associated with an extremely high likelihood of mortality. Therefore, observation is not recommended if a patient is a candidate for other therapeutic options.

Outcomes

Bladergroen and colleagues reported a 21% overall mortality rate after esophageal perforation.[8] They stressed the importance of early diagnosis. Excluding nonoperative intervention, all forms of therapy demonstrated improved survival if treatment was instituted within 24 hours of the injury. Primary closure within 24 hours resulted in a 92% survival rate.

Jones and Ginsberg identified five factors that affect survival after esophageal perforation: etiology, location, delay in diagnosis (defined as more than 24 hours), associated esophageal disease, and treatment selection.[1] Mortality rates, based on cause of perforation, were 9% for trauma, 19% for iatrogenic/instrumentation, and 39% for spontaneous perforation. Perfora-

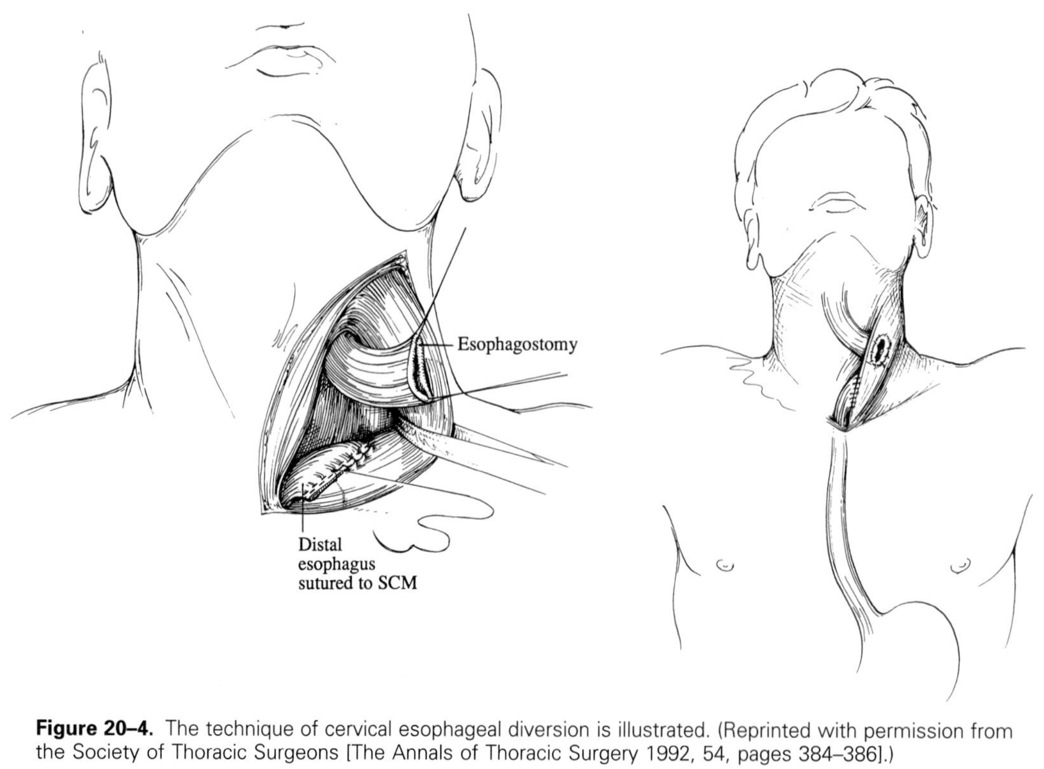

Figure 20–4. The technique of cervical esophageal diversion is illustrated. (Reprinted with permission from the Society of Thoracic Surgeons [The Annals of Thoracic Surgery 1992, 54, pages 384–386].)

tion in a cervical location resulted in a lower mortality rate (6%) than perforation in an intrathoracic location (34%). Survival rates improved with early diagnosis and treatment (79% to 87%) compared to cases in which there was delay in treatment (55% to 67%). Patients with esophageal cancer have a higher mortality rate than patients with benign disease or no disease. Primary repair results in the highest likelihood of survival.

Reeder and associates have demonstrated a trend toward improved survival rates after esophageal rupture.[9] In their series, overall mortality was 19%: diagnosis during the first 24 hours, 9%, and diagnosis after 24 hours, 29%.

CAUSTIC INGESTION

Caustic ingestion, either accidental or intentional, occurs in 5,000 to 15,000 cases per year in the United States.[10] Caustic ingestion is a devastating injury with a high mortality rate, serious morbidity, and significant adverse effects on esophageal function and, therefore, on quality of life. More recently, there has been a change in management principles from nonoperative to early surgical intervention for patients with significant esophageal injuries.

The list of reported ingested caustic agents is long and includes lye, bleach, sulfuric acid, hydrochloric acid, nitric acid, ammonia, iodine, and other. Lye ingestion, by far the most common agent, accounted for 60% of cases in Postlethwaite's extensive review.[11] It is clinically relevant to know the causative agent. Lye or alkaline ingestion results in a deeply penetrating injury to the pharyngeal and esophageal wall. In contrast, acid ingestion causes a mucosal surface coagulation necrosis that prevents deep penetrating pharyngeal and esophageal injury, yet results in a more extensive gastric injury.

The clinical course of a lye ingestion injury may be divided into five phases. Phase one is the acute phase in which there is edema and bowel wall necrosis. The concentration and volume of lye swallowed determine the depth of the injury. Phase two is the onset of inflammation that begins at 24 to 48 hours. Phase three is the period of necrotic eschar slough that occurs at 7 days. Phase four begins at 2 weeks and involves the onset of fibrosis. Phase five is notable for esophageal stricturing that begins at week 3 or 4.

Presentation

Symptoms vary depending on the concentration, the volume, and the nature of the ingested agent, for example, its acidity. With lye ingestion, patients complain of oral, pharyngeal, cervical, and thoracic pain, dysphagia, cough, tachypnea, and wheezing. Mild gastrointestinal symptoms predominate in minor injuries. As the extent of injury increases, respiratory symptoms become more prominent. Severe injuries are associated with profound respiratory distress and shock. Acid ingestion may result in greater gastric than esophageal symptoms.

Evaluation

Contrast esophagograms and CT scans are not routinely used in the acute evaluation of a patient after caustic ingestion unless there is suspicion of bowel wall perforation. Contrast swallowing studies may be used to follow the progression of later stricture formation.

The value of early diagnostic esophagoscopy is uniformly accepted. The endoscope is advanced to the proximal extent of the injury in order to assess the degree of damage. Further endoscopic advancement, which risks iatrogenic perforation, is avoided. Numerous grading systems, similar to the clinical grading of epidermal skin burn depth, have been devised based on endoscopic findings.

Priorities

In the past, treatment plans included the use of steroids, antibiotics, fluid resuscitation, and observation; they were based largely on the experimental work of Johnson[12] and Haller and Bachman.[13] If a stricture developed, it was managed with serial dilations or esophageal resection and replacement. Early surgery was reserved for patients with bowel perforation. More recently, the trend has been toward early surgery for patients with higher-grade injuries, even without perforation.[14–16] Based on their extensive experience, Andreoni and coworkers[17] currently use the following treatment plan: (1) nonoperative therapy for mild to moderate injuries, (2) early surgery (within 24 to 36 hours) for more serious injuries, and (3) emergency surgery for bowel perforation.

Outcomes

The mortality rate in cases of caustic ingestion, even with therapy, ranges from zero to 8.6%, but the rate varies with the extent of injury.

Survival rates after therapy continue to improve. Andreoni and colleagues, using the treatment algorithm described, reported an overall treatment mortality rate of 6.8%.[17] Three of the four deaths in this series occurred in the patients who had sustained the most severe injuries. The reported frequency of stricture, mediastinitis, and esophageal perforation are 18%, 20%, and 15%, respectively, for the three grades of injury.[11]

ESOPHAGEAL FOREIGN BODY

A patient of any age can ingest a foreign body that lodges in the esophagus, but the majority of cases involve patients under the age of 2 years. An enormous array of ingested objects has been reported. An impacted foreign body may result in few symptoms and may simply be extracted, or it may produce severe symptoms, become impacted, and lead to fatal complications. Foreign bodies lodge in the hypopharynx or just below the cricopharynx in 73% of cases, in the middle of the esophagus in 15% of cases, and in the lower esophagus in 12% of cases.[18]

Presentation and Evaluation

A foreign body in the esophagus results in gastrointestinal symptoms (pain, dysphagia, regurgitation, and excessive salivation), and respiratory symptoms (stidor, dyspnea, and cough). The degree of seriousness of the symptoms is determined by the size, nature, and location of the foreign body; 10% of patients are asymptomatic.

Radiopaque objects are easily identified on plain chest film (Fig. 20–5). Radiolucent objects are identified by administering a barium swallow during which time the object is coated with contrast. Perforation is identified in a contrast esophagogram or a CT scan.

Priorities

The vast majority of esophageal foreign bodies can be successfully removed endoscopically, using either rigid or flexible esophagoscopy. Details concerning the techniques available to the endoscopist are described in Chapter 10. On rare occasions, a foreign body has to be extracted surgically by means of an esophagotomy or an esophagectomy. Management of perforation has already been covered above.

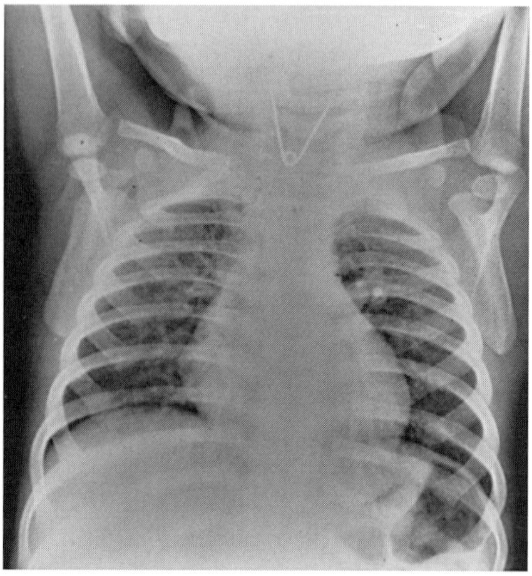

Figure 20–5. A plain radiograph depicting an ingested safety pin in a child.

Outcomes

The reported mortality rate among patients with esophageal foreign bodies is 0.27% to 0.46%. Hemorrhage and sepsis are the two most common causes of death. The frequency of perforation is 2.5%.[18]

ACQUIRED TRACHEOESOPHAGEAL FISTULA

The tracheoesophageal fistula (TEF) is part of a spectrum of esophagorespiratory fistulas that share similar symptoms and complications. The reported distribution of fistulas is tracheobronchial in 65% of cases and bronchoesophageal in 30% of cases; in 5% of cases, the fistula connects the esophagus to a small bronchus or lung periphery.[19] A TEF bypasses the normal cascade of defensive safeguards that separate the airway and esophagus and may cause few symptoms or acute respiratory failure, depending on its size, location, and associated pathology. Acquired TEFs are uncommon. In the United States, 5% of patients with esophageal cancer develop a TEF.[19] They are reported to occur in 2.4% and 0.1% of patients after tracheal resection[20] and trachestomy,[21] respectively. The most common are airway and esophageal malignancies, trauma (including iatrogenic trauma), and infection. Approximately half of acquired TEFs are of malignant origin, and 70% of all nonmalignant fistulas are caused by intubation injury.

Presentation

Symptoms vary according to the volume and direction of flow through the fistula. In most patients, the direction of flow is from the esophagus into the airway, which results in increased tracheal secretions and cough. These symptoms characteristically worsen with oral intake. Repeated tracheobronchitis and pneumonia are common. These infections may be severe and difficult to resolve completely. Patients who are intubated on positive-pressure ventilation present with acute respiratory distress because the mechanically delivered breath is vented across the fistula into the esophagus. Signs of developing TEF in a ventilated patient include (1) the need for progressive increase in cuff pressure to obtain a seal, (2) the inability to maintain pressure support, (3) the incomplete return of the complete volume of a delivered breath during expiration, and (4) increasing tracheal secretions.

Evaluation

Contrast esophagography is effective in identifying fistulas, particularly those that reach into distal airway or lung parenchyma (Fig. 20–6). Water-soluble agents should be employed because of the obvious risk of aspiration. Video esophagography techniques increase the accuracy of this test.

The fistula may be identified endoscopically using either esophagoscopy or bronchoscopy. Bronchoscopy is more sensitive if the fistula is in the lobar or more proximal airway.

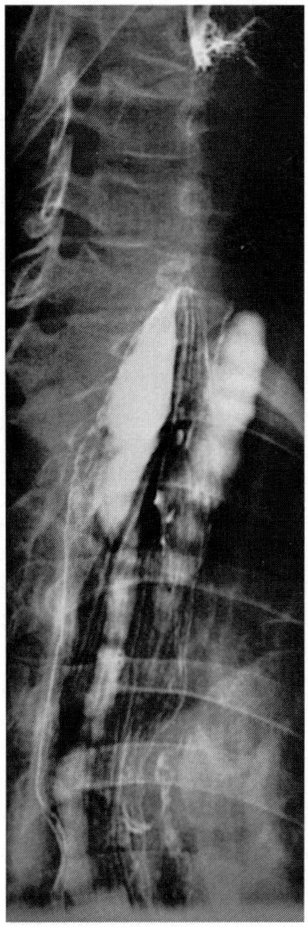

Figure 20–6. Contrast esophagography demonstrating an esophageal fistula into the distal trachea.

Priorities

Prompt diagnosis and management of TEFs are essential to prevent potentially life-threatening respiratory complications. Acute management principles are airway protection and reduction of gastrointestinal secretions. In a nonintubated patient, airway protection involves suctioning and antibiotics. In an intubated patient, the endotracheal or tracheostomy tube is advanced so that the cuff is below the fistula, the cuff is reinflated, and the tube is secured. This is not always possible in a patient with a distal tracheal or bronchial fistula. In such a patient, options include manipulation of the ventilator settings to higher rates with lower pressures and volumes, frequent airway suctioning, placement of a double-lumen endotracheal tube, and selective main-stem intubation. The patient may be positioned on his or her side with the dominant lung up. Reduction of gastrointestinal secretions includes cessation of oral intake, institution of gastric drainage (preferably by gastrostomy), and administration of H_2 blockers to reduce gastric secretions.

Definitive repair involves surgical interruption of the fistula and separate primary closure of the trachea and esophagus. The surgical approach is determined by the level of the fistula: above the thoracic inlet, a transverse cervical incision usually provides adequate exposure although sometimes a partial vertical sternal split through the manubrium is necessary for lower lesions; intrathoracic fistula are best approached via a right thoracotomy, unless the distal left main-stem bronchus is involved, in which case, a left thoracotomy is appropriate. In all cases, well-vascularized soft tissue (neck strap muscle, pectoralis muscle, intercostal muscle, parietal pleura, or pericardium) should be interposed between the two suture lines to prevent recurrence.

Outcomes

Short- and long-term results depend on the preoperative condition of the patient. The reported operative mortality rate using this technique is 5.0% to 7.1%, usually because of suture line recurrence or dehiscence, or mediastinal sepsis.

MEDIASTINITIS

A number of clinical and perioperative factors contribute to the development of mediastinitis. Three major categories of mediastinitis are acute bacterial, granulomatous, and sclerosing. The acute infections, however, are the most commonly encountered and must be addressed emergently. If unrecognized or left untreated, acute mediastinitis can lead to rapid sepsis and, therefore, be a life-threatening problem.

The causes of acute bacterial mediastinitis are listed in Table 20-1. The majority of such infections are secondary to surgical procedures, including median sternotomy for cardiac procedures and mediastinoscopy or mediastinotomy for mediastinal surgery.[22] Complications that arise from these procedures include superficial or deep tissue infection and sternal dehiscence or osteomyelitis. Superficial wound infections occur in approximately 4% of patients after median sternotomy, with 1% to 2% involving the deeper tissues and mediastinum. Factors that increase the risk for postoperative wound complications include cardiopulmonary bypass, reexploration for postoperative bleeding, postoperative cardiogenic shock, external chest compression, diabetes, obesity, and use of bilateral internal mammary arteries for coronary artery bypass.

Table 20–1. *Causes of Acute Bacterial Mediastinitis*

Postoperative Causes
Median sternotomy
Mediastinoscopy
Mediastinotomy
Tracheostomy
Neck dissections
Esophageal Perforation and Leakage
Instrumentation
Spontaneous
Surgery
Oral and Cervical Infections
Other Causes
Subdiaphragmatic infection
Pneumonia
Lung abscess
Pleural empyema

A more fatal form of acute mediastinitis is associated with bacterial contamination spread by instrumental or spontaneous disruption of the esophagus,[23] and it accounts for more than 90% of cases not associated with postoperative complications. Irrespective of the cause of the perforation, fatal septicemia is inevitable without prompt recognition and therapy. Acute mediastinitis can arise after esophageal surgery such as esophagectomy, diverticulectomy, or myotomy. Other, less common causes that should be considered include pneumonia, lung abscess, and pleural empyema due to direct extension. These have become rare because of the availability and effectiveness of present-day antibiotics.

Acute descending, necrotizing mediastinitis is an unusual form of mediastinitis, that results from virulent oral pathogens that cause an oropharyngeal infection or abscess in the cervical region despite the use of antibiotics. This kind of abscess is commonly the result of the progressive spread of odontogenic infections (of the second or third molar), peritonsillar or retropharyngeal abscesses, Ludwig's angina, epiglottitis, or traumatic pharyngeal perforations that might occur during endotracheal intubations. These are usually mixed infections of both aerobic and anaerobic organisms. β-hemolytic streptococcus is often the only organism present, but other organisms that have been isolated include *Fusobacterium*, *Bacteroides*, *Peptostreptococcus* species, *Staphylococcus aureus*, and other anaerobic streptococci. If unrecognized or uncontrolled, these infections dissect along the pretracheal or retrovisceral spaces or along the carotid sheaths to involve the anterior and visceral compartment of the mediastinum. (See Chapter 19 for a complete discussion of deep-space neck infections.)

Presentation and Evaluation

Classic signs and symptoms of acute bacterial mediastinitis are infrequently encountered and are determined by the cause and anatomic level of involvement. Manifestations common to all causes include fever, tachycardia, leukocytosis, and pain localized to the neck, back, or chest. The presentation of mediastinitis associated with esophageal pathology has already been covered.

Mediastinitis associated with a surgical procedure can present as early as 3 days after the operation but usually presents within 3 weeks. Clinical findings include wound pain or chest pain, fever, wound erythema or discharge, and sternal instability. Laboratory evaluation reveals leukocytosis. Chest roentgenograms are rarely helpful in the early diagnosis of mediastinitis. However, disruption of or configuration changes in the sternal wires may indicate sternal separation. Chest CT scans may show abnormal fluid or air collections and may help to plan surgical management.

Mediastinitis caused by descending, necrotizing infections usually occurs in a patient receiving antibiotic therapy for a deep cervical infection. Symptoms develop within 48 hours of the infection, but signs of initial involvement of the upper mediastinum are nonspecific, which makes early diagnosis quite difficult. As sepsis develops, the neck and upper chest may demonstrate diffuse brawny induration, pitting edema, and crepitance. Other symptoms include substernal chest pain, dysphagia, cough, fever, and dyspnea. The findings of friction rubs and effusions indicate involvement of the pleura and pericardium. Pneumomediastinum may produce a characteristic crunching sound that is audible over the pericardium and is known as Hamman's sign. As the infection progresses into the abdomen via the esophageal hiatus, the retroperitoneal space and free peritoneum may become involved. Chest radiographs may demonstrate a widening of the retrocervical space with or without an air-fluid level, anterior displacement of the tracheal air column, mediastinal emphysema, and loss of the normal lordosis of the cervical spine. In the latter phases, there may be evidence of pleural or pericardial involvement (Fig. 20–7). A CT scan, however, better delineates the extent of disease and is useful in identifying the extent of the mediastinitis so proper drainage can be planned. In addition to the abnormal findings on plain radiographs, a CT scan may demonstrate loss of normal fat planes, formation of abscesses, lymphadenopathy, and the presence of gas bubbles.

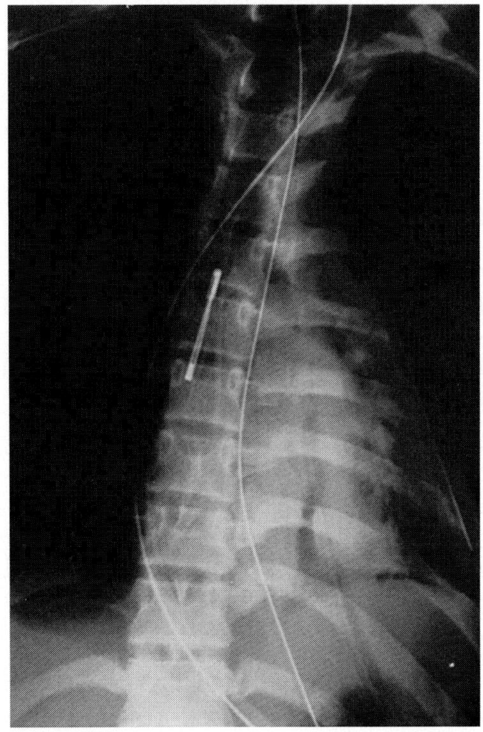

Figure 20–7. A chest x-ray demonstrating pneumomediastinum caused by mediastinitis.

Priorities

Proper management for all types of mediastinitis includes early diagnosis, correction of the inciting cause, fluid resuscitation, appropriate antibiotics, complete surgical drainage and, on occasion, tracheostomy. For postoperative mediastinitis, operative intervention includes adequate tissue debridement of the soft tissues, bone, and cartilage, wound drainage, and sternal rewiring. Myocutaneous flap coverage is required for larger defects.[24]

Acute mediastinal infections contained above the level of the carina may be drained via an anterior cervical mediastinotomy, leaving soft rubber drains in place. Below this level, thoracotomy is required in addition to cervical drainage in order to attain wide drainage of the mediastinum. Subxiphoid drainage may be necessary for processes that involve the anterior mediastinum. Depending upon the severity of involvement, large-bore drainage tubes can be left in place around the infected tissue bed which is continuously irrigated (3 L/day) with antibiotics or diluted povidone-iodine for 7 to 14 days postoperatively.[25] Tracheostomy is advocated when the possibility of major hemorrhage is present and to ensure access to the airway.[26] If, however, elective tracheostomy is required after median sternotomy, it should be delayed for 2 weeks after the primary procedure to avoid complications of descending mediastinitis.

Outcomes

Treatment of sterile sternal dehiscence involves simple rewiring of the sternum and is associated with excellent short- and long-term results. With the routine use of muscle and omental flaps for postoperative mediastinitis, the mortality rate has been reduced to 2%.[27, 28] Mortality associated with acute descending mediastinitis is as high as 40%.

Death related to any type of mediastinitis is usually associated with the development of postoperative complications—sepsis, blood vessel erosion resulting in exsanguination, aspiration, metastatic intracranial infection, empyema, and pericardial tamponade. Early recognition and prompt treatment remain the keys to keeping mortality rates down.

TENSION PNEUMOTHORAX

Leakage of air from the lung parenchyma becomes valvular when it moves freely into the pleural space during inspiration but is prevented from escaping the pleural space during expiration. A tension pneumothorax develops as pressure in the pleural space becomes greater than the atmospheric pressure, and it is further aggravated when the airway pressure is increased by coughing or straining. With increasing positive intrapleural pressure, the lung collapses further, and the mediastinum shifts to the opposite side. An emergency situation develops, causing impairment of venous return, decreased cardiac output, tachycardia, and shock. This process can occur rapidly, so a tension pneumothorax is an immediately life-threatening complication.

The causes of a tension pneumothorax are similar to those of a simple pneumothorax. Obstructive and restrictive pulmonary diseases associated with the development of a spontaneous pneumothorax include congenital subpleural blebs, bullae from chronic obstructive pulmonary disease, cystic fibrosis, pneumocystis pneumonia, metastatic cancer, eosinophilic granuloma, asthma with mucous plugging, and lung abscess. Several conditions enhance the valvular effect after a spontaneous pneumothorax. Airway factors include inflammation, granulation tissue, blood clots, and mucous plugging. Parenchymal factors include interstitial pneumonitis, fibrosis, and pneumonia associated with *Pneumocystis carinii*. Although infrequent, sometimes a tension pneumothorax may be an early manifestation of spontaneous rupture or perforation of the esophagus that occurs before systemic symptoms appear.

Iatrogenic causes are most commonly associated with the insertion of central venous or pacemaker lines (subclavian or internal jugular)

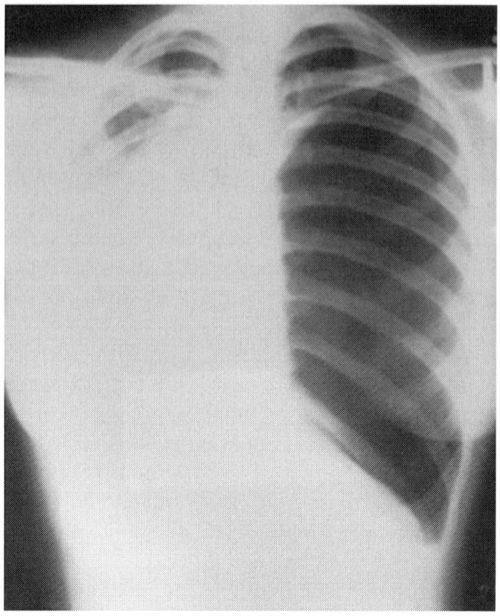

Figure 20–8. A plain radiograph showing the effects of a left tension pneumothorax.

and with complications after surgery, specifically, bronchoscopy with biopsies, surgical dissection around the cervical region, laparoscopic surgery, mediastinal surgery and, especially, with dissection around the pleura and trachea. A pneumothorax epidemic has been noted in the drug-addicted population. Injection of drugs into a neck, subclavian, or chest vein can inadvertently puncture the pleural space. Chronic intravenous drug abuse is also associated with injection of inert particles that embolize to the lung, resulting in restrictive interstitial disease. Repeated cocaine inhalation can lead to obstructive pulmonary disease. Other acquired causes include blunt or penetrating trauma, cardiopulmonary resuscitation, and positive-pressure ventilation.

Presentation and Evaluation

In the early clinical stages, a patient shows signs and symptoms of increasing respiratory distress, anxiety, sweating, dyspnea, and pain. A patient in extremis may present with hypotension, cyanosis, jugular venous distention, contralateral tracheal deviation, decreased breath sounds, tympany to percussion, and subcutaneous emphysema which eventually lead to cardiopulmonary arrest in the absence of immediate intervention. Although classic teaching states that the diagnosis is made only by physical examination and that there is no need for confirmation by chest radiograph, the features that can be seen on chest films include radiolucency of the affected side, contralateral shift of the mediastinum, and ipsilateral depression of the diaphragm (Fig. 20–8). Tension pneumothorax should also be suspected in a patient with chest trauma (especially rib fractures) undergoing general anesthesia who suddenly experiences cardiopulmonary deterioration and a simultaneous increase in ventilatory pressures.

Priorities

Immediate treatment is imperative to avoid total circulatory collapse. A large-bore needle is inserted through the second intercostal space anteriorly (Fig. 20–9). If the diagnosis is correct, a rush of air is heard, or the barrel of a glass syringe is pushed upward. After immediate decompression of the pleural space, tube thoracostomy can be performed in a controlled situation.

Outcomes

A review of the literature suggests that delayed pneumothorax has an incidence of approximately 0.4% in all central venous access attempts, and it results in tension pneumothorax in 22.0% of these cases.[29] It is much more common after subclavian than internal jugular approaches, especially in difficult or multiple attempts. After correction of tension pneumothorax by tube thoracostomy, most cases are given conservative management with good results. Although the overall mortality rate of patients who have experienced tension pneumothorax is unknown, the event is uniformly fatal if left undiagnosed.

MASSIVE HEMOPTYSIS

Massive, life-threatening bleeding into the tracheobronchial tree is an uncommon event, but it poses an imminent threat to life as a result of aspiration and asphyxiation rather than of exsanguination. Massive hemoptysis has been arbitrarily defined as the expectoration of more than 600 mL of blood in a 24-hour period. Exsanguinating hemorrhage occurs when the volume exceeds 150 mL/h.

The frequency of occurrence of the various causes of hemoptysis has changed over the past few decades as disease epidemiology has

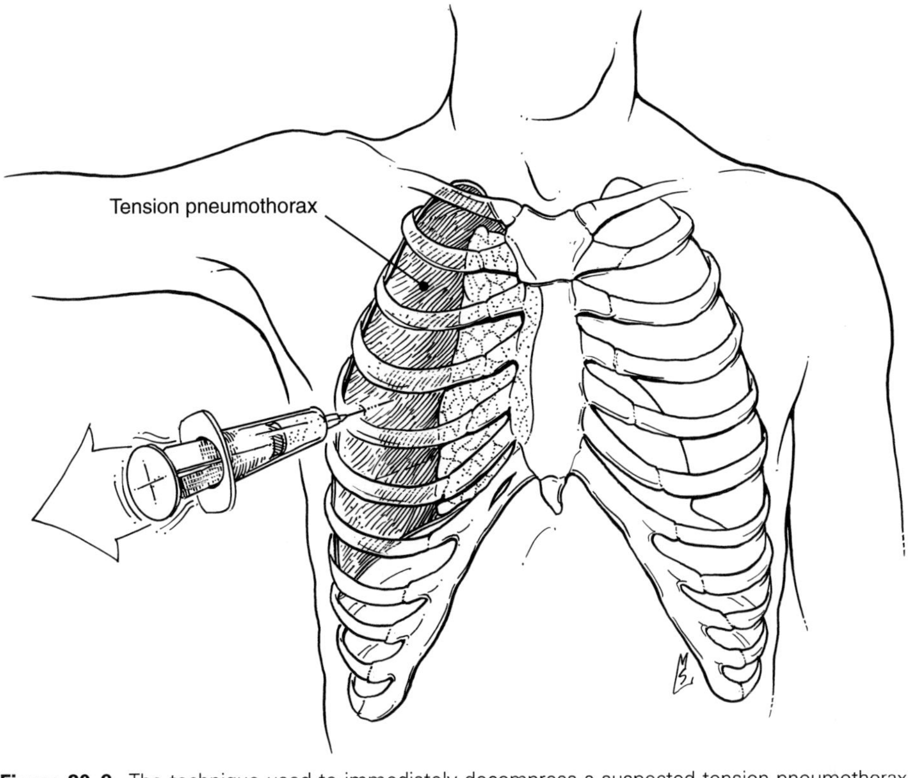

Figure 20–9. The technique used to immediately decompress a suspected tension pneumothorax.

changed. In the 1930s, hemoptysis was pathognomonic of tuberculosis. Although the incidence of tuberculosis has decreased, it remains the most common cause of massive hemoptysis, followed by bronchiectasis, chronic bronchitis, bronchogenic carcinoma, mitral stenosis, and arterial fistulization.

There are many causes of massive hemoptysis (Table 20–2); 95% of cases originate in the bronchial arterial system and inflammatory diseases account for the majority of those cases, with tuberculosis alone accounting for 70% of cases, followed by aspergillosis (especially in an old tuberculosis cavity), histoplasmosis, bronchiectasis, broncholithiasis, lung abscess, and sarcoidosis. The origin of bleeding in almost all cases is the rich bronchial arterial supply to these cavities. Neoplasms are rarely a cause of massive hemoptysis, but when they are, they are usually located in the truncus anterior of the right or left upper lobe of the lung and present with intermittent hemoptysis. Massive terminal hemoptysis has been found to occur in 3.3% of patients with lung cancer and is more commonly associated with cavitated squamous cell carcinoma.[30] After pulmonary embolism from a distal source, tissue infarction is followed by a rapid influx of bronchial arterial circulation, and the resulting hemoptysis is worsened by systemic heparinization.

Approximately 5% of bleeding originates in the pulmonary circulation. Sources include iatrogenic injuries such as those caused by catheter tip perforation or overinflation of the balloon of a Swan-Ganz catheter. Pulmonary arteriovenous fistulas are associated with hereditary hemorrhagic telangiectasis (Osler-Weber-Rendu disease) in 60% of cases. These fistulas result in a left-to-right shunt to the pulmonary arterial and venous structures. As this angiodysplastic disorder progresses, the vascular wall thins out and becomes prone to rupture.

The remaining 1% of cases arise from nonbronchial systemic arteries and are caused by trauma, tracheoinnominate fistulas, and thoracic aortic aneurysms that communicate with the bronchial system.

Table 20–2. *Causes of Hemoptysis*

Inflammatory
Tuberculosis
Aspergillosis
Bronchiectasis
Necrotizing pneumonitis
Cystic fibrosis
Lung abscess
Neoplastic
Bronchogenic carcinoma
Bronchial adenoma
Primary tracheal tumors
Vascular
Pulmonary embolism/infarction
Arteriovenous fistula
Traumatic
Lung contusion or laceration
Bronchial rupture
Foreign body
Iatrogenic
Invasive monitoring (Swan-Ganz catheter)
Bronchoscopy
Cardiac
Mitral stenosis
Acute pulmonary edema
Coagulation disorders

Presentation and Evaluation

It is important to localize the site of bleeding quickly. The patient's history often helps to establish the cause of the hemoptysis. It is important to verify that the blood is coming from the lungs and not from a lesion in the mouth, nose, or pharynx. Special attention should be paid to (1) the appearance and amount of the blood or clot, (2) the duration of bleeding, (3) any associated chest pain, (4) the relationship of bleeding to activity, (5) the presence of wheezing or the bubbling of secretions, (6) a previous history of heart or lung disease, and (7) a history of smoking.

Evaluation should start with a good chest radiograph, which may reveal the location by the presence of a cavity, mass, cavitation, or localized pulmonary infiltrate or atelectasis. However, massive hemoptysis may still occur in an area that appears normal by chest radiography. In appropriate situations, other studies that may be helpful include CT scans, ventilation-perfusion scans, pulmonary angiograms, and selective bronchial artery angiograms. However, in acute situations that involve massive life-threatening hemoptysis, stabilization of the patient's condition and use of life-saving maneuvers preclude a complete radiologic workup.

Although a good history and physical examination and radiologic studies may suggest the diagnosis, bronchoscopy is invariably required to determine the cause, to localize the lesion and more important, to clear the tracheobronchial tree of blood in order to maintain adequate ventilation. It is useful in localizing the site of disease, particularly if a patient has bilateral pathology. Although rigid bronchoscopy is useful in providing a wide conduit for suctioning blood and clots while allowing ventilation and good visualization, flexible bronchoscopy has the advantages of being more readily available and easier to perform.

Priorities

MEDICAL THERAPY

The management of a patient with massive hemoptysis has five main goals: (1) to maintain a patent airway to prevent asphyxiation; (2) to localize the site of bleeding; (3) to determine the cause of bleeding; (4) to arrest the hemorrhage; and (5) to direct treatment toward the underlying cause.[31] Although the initial management of massive hemoptysis remains conservative, the timing of surgical intervention is difficult to determine. Of paramount importance are the maintenance of a patent airway and support of the patient's vital signs. If the bleeding site is known, it is best to place that side in a dependent position to minimize aspiration of blood and to preserve ventilation in the nonbleeding lung. Oxygen supplementation is indicated in the presence of hypoxemia and, if possible, intubation with a double-lumen endotracheal tube is performed to reduce blood contamination of an uninvolved lung. Suction devices should be readily available at the bedside. Venous access should be established with a large-bore cannula, along with monitoring of oxygen saturation by an indwelling arterial line. Blood should be typed and crossmatched with several units available for use.

As soon as the patient is stable, bronchoscopy should be performed to identify the site of the bleeding. Intravenous sedation and an antitussive (codeine) may be used to help suppress excessive or violent coughing. If the bleeding is massive and unmanageable with the fiberoptic technique, rigid bronchoscopy may be required. In addition to the wide aperture that allows for ventilation and the suctioning of blood and clots, the rigid scope allows passage of suction cannulas, balloon catheters, and cold-infusion solutions. Should bronchoscopy fail to identify the source or control the bleeding, bronchial arteriography should be performed. With the development of arterial embolization, the need for surgical intervention has been reduced. Once the airway has been protected and the patient stabilized, bronchial arteriography is performed to identify the bleeding site. The appropriate vessel is embolized, usually with Gelfoam. Methods of control are outlined in Table 20–3.

Table 20–3. *Methods of Controlling Massive Hemoptysis*

Medical Management
Avoid intubation
Use the semi-Fowler's position
Suppress the cough reflex
Control hypertension
Provide appropriate monitoring
Perform early bronchoscopy
Administer broad-spectrum antibiotics
Methods of Control
Endobronchial Methods
Perform iced saline lavage
Employ balloon tamponade
Intubate with a double-lumen tube
Use bronchial blockers
Place endobronchial packing
Administer vasoconstrictors
Use an external tube to drain a bleeding cavity
Institute positive end-expiratory pressure
Provide radiation treatment

SURGICAL THERAPY

Surgery is advocated when more than 600 mL of blood have been lost in a period of 24 hours or less.[32] Other circumstances requiring urgent resection (24 to 48 hours after control of hemorrhage) include the presence of a fungal mass, lung abscess, persistent radiodense lesion, or irretrievable endoluminal obstructing clot (Table 20–4). Pulmonary resection remains the most effective method of controlling and preventing massive hemoptysis, but it is associated with a high mortality rate under emergent conditions.

The initial management of a patient undergoing emergent surgical therapy is similar to the initial steps taken in the management of a patient undergoing medical therapy: maintenance of a patent airway, hemodynamic stabilization, identification and localization of the bleeding source, avoidance of contralateral lung soilage, and attempt to control hemorrhage. In

Table 20–4. *Operative Indications for Massive Hemoptysis*

Immediate
Persistent massive hemoptysis:
> 600 mL/24 h or > 200 mL/h
Tracheoinnominate fistula
Aortobronchial fistula
Chest trauma
Urgent (delayed 24–48 h)
Fungus ball
Lung abscess
Persistent radiodense lesion
Irretrievable endoluminal obstructing clot

a nonemergent situation, preoperative knowledge of the patient's pulmonary function along with the absence of medical contraindications, distant metastasis, and cardiac valvular disease help to predict a more favorable outcome.

The principles of surgical excision include maximal resection of disease combined with optimal sparing of normal lung tissue. Intraoperative maneuvers include early division of the appropriate bronchus and extrapleural dissection, with surgical procedures including pulmonary resection, thoracoplasty, cavernostomy, and massive ligation of the hilum. Intrapericardial control of the pulmonary artery may be required in certain instances.

Outcomes

Factors that correlate directly with morbidity and mortality resulting from massive airway bleeding include (1) the rate of bleeding, (2) the amount of bleeding, (3) contamination of the dependent lung, (4) underlying pulmonary function, (5) the presence of anticoagulation, (6) the antecedent disease state, and (7) the mechanism of bleeding. Mortality rates range from 10% to 25%, irrespective of medical or surgical management and the type of surgical procedure involved.

Massive hemoptysis due to primary pulmonary disease can be managed with medical therapy alone in 90% of cases. When required, arterial embolization is successful in more than 75% of patients. Rebleeding occurs in 25%; however, in the presence of a mycetoma or residual pulmonary disease, the rebleeding rate is over 40%. Thus, it is suggested that successful embolization be followed by elective surgical intervention if the patient's overall condition, underlying disease, and pulmonary function are amenable to resection. With this combined approach, operative mortality is reduced to 8%.[39] In a patient who has an unresectable lesion, the mortality rate is higher than 50%.

When resection is performed as an emergency procedure, the mortality rate is significantly higher; it is dependent upon the extent of resection. Pneumonectomy, especially when combined with an extrapleural dissection, has an associated mortality rate on the order of 40%. Lobectomy and lesser resections are associated with mortality rates of 30% and 4%, respectively. Despite the morbidity following pulmonary resection, major complications generally occur in less than 15% of cases with a disease-free survival of up to 90% at 5 years among patients undergoing successful initial operations.[40]

Postoperative complications can occur in up to 60% of patients.[40] Pleural empyema is the most common complication, followed by respiratory failure, pneumonia, bronchopleural fistula, and pulmonary edema.

TRACHEOINNOMINATE FISTULA

Airway hemorrhage usually presents as a complication, commonly of tracheostomy. A tracheoinnominate fistula (TIF) is a unique situation that requires specific initial management and surgical treatment. This type of vascular emergency is likely to present itself to head and neck surgeons. The incidence of TIFs after tracheostomies ranges from zero to 1.0%, averaging 0.3%.[33] Postoperative hemorrhage occurs in approximately 3% of all tracheostomies, with TIF accounting for approximately 10% of these cases. A TIF can occur as early as 2 days postoperatively, but the peak incidence is at 1 to 2 weeks, and 72% of all cases occur within 3 weeks after tracheostomy.[34] A TIF can also occur as a complication of tracheal surgery, stenting, or resection; the rate is less than 1%.[35]

Two thirds of all cases of TIFs are a result of pressure necrosis—caused by the tracheostomy tube tip or by a high-pressure cuff—of the wall of the trachea, with subsequent ulceration and fistulization into the innominate artery.[34] These types of erosions have decreased because of the use of high-volume, low-pressure cuffs. Although rare, an erosion of the artery can occur at the inferior margin of a low-placed tracheostomy stoma as the inner curve of the tracheostomy tube erodes its way into the artery.[36] The innominate artery is the vessel most commonly involved in airway fistulization after tracheal surgery, but other vessels in close proximity that can cause a similar presentation include the innominate vein, common carotid artery, inferior thyroid artery, thyroid ima artery, and aortic arch.[37] A TIF following tracheal resection or surgery is usually a result of necrosis or excessive tension at the suture line, in the absence of tissue separation from the adjacent artery. Irrespective of the mechanism of fistulization, factors that increase the risk of a TIF include prior radiation, diabetes mellitus, steroid therapy, sepsis, hypotension, prolonged ventilation, and stomal infection.

Presentation and Evaluation

The differential diagnosis of a TIF includes bleeding stomal or tracheal granulation tissue and tracheitis. Although any hemorrhage from a tracheostomy site deserves further investigation, a TIF usually manifests itself as a sentinel bleed followed by a brief period of quiescence. Fiberoptic tracheoscopy and bronchoscopy can be performed via the tube itself to clear the airway and to inspect the distal tracheobronchial tree for pathology. If no active bleeding source is found, the balloon is deflated slowly and the tracheostomy tube is gently pulled back over the bronchoscope. The proximal and anterior tracheal wall is inspected for ulceration. If hemorrhage should continue or recur, the tube should be replaced rapidly, the balloon overinflated, and the tube tilted backward to tamponade the fistula site.

Priorities

Prevention of TIF is the key. A tracheostomy should be performed under proper circumstances, but though it is often considered a minor procedure, it must be performed with meticulous attention to detail, particularly anatomic placement and the correct positioning of the tube postoperatively.

When massive hemorrhage begins, management strategy includes control of the airway, immediate arterial compression, and subsequent treatment of the injured artery. Bedside control of hemorrhage by means of cuff overinflation or digital arterial compression can be lifesaving. If this fails to control the hemorrhage, the airway should be secured orally and the tracheostomy tube removed. A finger should be inserted through the tracheostomy stoma, and control of the innominate artery fistula gained by digital compression of the artery anteriorly against the posterior shelf of the sternum or right sternoclavicular joint.[38] In some cases, the innominate artery must be bluntly dissected from the trachea through this same exposure in order to gain control.

Immediate surgical exploration is mandatory to control the proximal and distal innominate artery. Often, an upper, partial sternal split through the manubrium rather than a full sternotomy can be employed for exposure.[37] In most cases, the artery is simply ligated because of the presence of a large defect. Oversewing or patch repair of the bleeding site (such as with pericardium) may be employed for a smaller defect. However, interpositioning repair with synthetic grafts should be avoided, as it invariably results in infectious complications. In any case, a flap of viable tissue (such as muscle or pericardium) should be interposed between the artery and the trachea to avoid fistula recurrence at the suture line.

Outcomes

Mortality following TIF repair is approximately 75%, with most patients dying as a result of underlying disease or associated morbidity.[41] Neurologic injury and arm ischemia are unusual. In one series, of 70 reported survivors, only 40 lived more than 2 months postoperatively.[37] Recurrent bleeding and death are significantly lower with arterial ligation than with attempted repair.[42]

SUMMARY

The thoracic surgical emergencies described in this chapter are rare complications associated with head and neck surgery or head and neck diseases. A patient who is experiencing any of

Table 20–5. *Summary of Thoracic Surgical Emergencies*

Emergency	Diagnostic Tests	Intervention
Esophageal perforation	Contrast esophagography Chest and abdominal CT scans	NPO, IV hydration, and antibiotics Contained: supportive care Free: primary surgical repair or esophageal diversion
Caustic ingestion	Esophagoscopy	Based on injury grade: supportive care vs. surgery
Esophageal foreign body	Chest x-ray Contrast esophagography	Endoscopic removal
Acquired tracheo-esophageal fistula	Contrast esophagography Esophagoscopy/ bronchoscopy	Airway protection Reduce GI secretions Surgical repair
Mediastinitis	Neck and chest CT scan Contrast esophagography	Surgical debridement and drainage
Tension pneumo-thorax	History and physical exam Chest x-ray	Needle decompression Tube thoracostomy
Hemoptysis	Bronchoscopy	Airway protection Arterial embolization Surgical resection
Tracheo-innominate fistula	Bronchoscopy Arteriography	Airway protection Arterial tamponade Surgical repair

these emergencies may present to a head and neck surgeon initially because the signs and symptoms are in proximity to the cervicothoracic region or because the signs and symptoms mimic many disease processes of the head and neck. These emergent problems are summarized in Table 20–5. Regardless of its cause, each problem deserves early evaluation and prompt, aggressive intervention.

REFERENCES

1. Jones WG, Ginsberg R.J. Esophageal perforation: a continuing challenge. Ann Thorac Surg 1992; 53:534–543.
2. Ferguson MK. Esophageal perforation and caustic injury: management of perforated esophageal cancer. Dis Esophagus 1997; 10:90–94.
3. Handy JR Jr, Reed CE. Esophageal injury. In Baue AE et al., eds. Glenn's Thoracic and Cardiovascular Surgery, 6th ed. Stamford, CT, Appleton & Lange, 1996, pp. 747–759.
4. Cameron JL et al. Selective nonoperative management of contained intrathoracic esophageal disruptions. Ann Thorac Surg 1979; 27:404–408.
5. Whyte RI, Iannettoni MD, Orringer MB. Intrathoracic esophageal perforation: the merit of primary repair. J Thorac Cardiovasc Surg 1995; 109:140–144.
6. Fraser CD, Heitmiller RF. Cervical esophago-esophageal anastomosis. Ann Thorac Surg 1992; 54:384–386.
7. Yeo CJ et al. Treatment of instrumental perforation of esophageal malignancy by transhiatal esophagectomy. Arch Surg 1988; 123:1016–1018.
8. Bladergroen MR, Lowe JE, Postlethwaite RW. Diagnosis and recommended management of esophageal perforation and rupture. Ann Thorac Surg 1986; 42:235–239.
9. Reeder LB, DeFilippi VJ, Ferguson MK. Current results of therapy for esophageal perforation. Am J Surg 1995; 169:615–617.
10. Goldman LP, Weigert JM. Corrosive susbstance ingestion: a review. Am J Gastroenterol 1984; 79:85–90.
11. Postlethwaite RW. Chemical burns of the esophagus. In Postlethwaite RW, ed. Surgery of the Esophagus, 2nd ed., Norwalk, CT, Appleton-Century-Crofts, 1986, pp. 317–344.
12. Johnson EE. A study of corrosive esophagitis. Laryngoscope 1963; 73:1651.
13. Haller JA Jr, Bachman K. The comparative effect of current therapy on experimental caustic burns of the esophagus. Pediatrics 1964; 34:236.
14. Hawkins DB, Demeter MJ, Barnett TE. Caustic ingestion: controversies in management: a review of 214 cases. Laryngoscope 1980; 90:98–109.
15. Estrera A, et al. Corrosive burns of the esophagus and stomach: a recommendation for an aggressive surgical approach. Ann Thorac Surg 1986; 41:276–283.
16. Gossot D, Sarfati E. Early blunt esophagectomy in severe caustic burns of the upper digestive tract. J Thorac Cardiovasc Surg 1987; 94:188–191.
17. Andreoni B et al. Esophageal perforation and caustic injury: emergency management of caustic ingestion. Dis Esophagus 1997; 10:95–100.
18. Postlethwaite RW. Foreign body. In Postlethwaite RW, ed. Surgery of the Esophagus, 2nd ed., Norwalk, CT, Appleton-Century-Crofts, 1986, pp. 201–210.
19. Conlan AA. The malignant tracheoesophageal or bronchoesophageal fistula. In Delarue NC, Wilkins EW Jr, Wong J, eds. International Trends in General Thoracic Surgery, vol. 4. St. Louis, Mosby, 1988, pp. 388–395.
20. Hilgenberg AD, Grillo HC. Acquired non-malignant tracheo-esophageal fistula. J Thorac Cardiovasc Surg 1983; 85:492–498.
21. Thomas AN. The diagnosis and treatment of tracheo-esophageal fistula caused by cuffed tracheal tubes. J Thorac Cardiovasc Surg 1973; 65:612–619.
22. El Oakley RM, Wright JE. Postoperative mediastinitis: classification and management. Ann Thor Surg 1996; 61:1030–1036.
23. Burnett CM, Rosemurgy AS, Pfeiffer EA. Life-threatening acute posterior mediastinitis due to esophageal perforation. Ann Thor Surg 1990; 49:979.
24. Bryan AJ et al. Median sternotomy wound dehiscence: a retrospective case control study of risk factors and outcome. J R Coll Surg Edinb 1992; 37:305–308.
25. Bryant LR, Spencer FC, Trinkle JK. Treatment of median sternotomy infection by mediastinal irrigation with an antibiotic solution. Ann Surg 1969; 169:914.
26. Wheatley MJ et al. Descending necrotizing mediastinitis: transcervical drainage is not enough. Ann Thorac Surg 1990; 49:780–784.
27. Jurkiewicz MJ et al. Infected median sternotomy wound: successful treatment by muscle flaps. Ann Surgery 1980; 191:738.
28. Nahai F et al. Primary treatment of the infected sternotomy wound with muscle flaps: a review of 211 consecutive cases. Plast Reconstr Surg 1989; 84:434–441.
29. Plewa MC, Ledrick D, Sferra JJ. Delayed tension pneumothorax complicating central venous catheterization and positive pressure ventilation. Am J Emerg Med 1995; 13:532.
30. Miller RR, McGregor DH. Hemorrhage from carcinoma of the lung. Cancer 1980; 46:200.
31. Jones DK, Davies RJ. Massive haemoptysis: medical management will usually arrest the bleeding. Br Med J 1990; 300:889.
32. Gourin A, Garzon AA. Operative treatment of massive hemoptysis. Ann Thorac Surg 1974; 18:52.
33. Dyer RK, Fisher SR. Tracheal-innominate and tracheal-esophageal fistula. In Wolfe WG, ed. Complications in Thoracic Surgery: Recognition and Management. St. Louis, Mosby-Year Book, 1992, p. 294.
34. Jones JW et al. Tracheo-innominate artery erosion: successful surgical management of a devastating complication. Ann Surg 1976; 184:194.
35. Grillo HC et al. Postintubation tracheal stenosis: treatment and results. J Thorac Cardiovasc Surg 1995; 10:486.
36. Deslauriers J et al. Innominate artery rupture: a major complication of tracheal surgery. Ann Thor Surg 1975; 20:671.
37. Wright CD. Management of tracheoinnominate artery fistula. Chest Surg Clinic N Am 1996; 6:865.
38. Cooper JD. Trachea-innominate artery fistula: successful management of 3 consecutive patients. Ann Thorac Surg 1977; 24:439–447.
39. Uflacker R et al. Management of massive hemoptysis by bronchial artery embolization. Radiology 1983; 146:627.
40. Guimaraes CA. Massive hemoptysis. In Pearson FG et al., eds. Thoracic Surgery. New York, Churchill Livingston, 1995, pp. 581–596.
41. Grillo HC, Mathisen DJ. Cervical exenteration. Ann Thorac Surg 1990; 49:401.
42. Dyer et al. Tracheo-innominate artery fistula. J Am Coll Surg 1994; 179:626.

CHAPTER 21

Pediatric Head and Neck Emergencies

David E. Tunkel, MD
John P. Little, MD

Children can experience a variety of head and neck disorders that require urgent evaluation and emergent treatment. These disorders include obstruction of the upper airway, complications of common head and neck infections (neck space infections and abscesses, intracranial and orbital complications of sinusitis, and intracranial and intratemporal complications of otitis media), bleeding from the nose or pharynx, maxillofacial trauma, and secondary effects of pediatric malignancies.

The scope of pediatric head and neck emergencies is far too broad for complete discussion in this chapter. We illustrate general management principles by presenting several types of pediatric head and neck emergencies. Some of the more common ear, nose, and throat emergencies outlined in other chapters of this textbook affect children primarily. See Chapter 10 for discussion of airway foreign body management, and see Chapters 18 and 23 for treatment of complications of sinusitis and otitis media.

AIRWAY EMERGENCIES

Airway compromise is the most feared pediatric head and neck emergency, producing anxiety in the child, the parent, and the clinician. A wide variety of disease processes can cause upper airway obstruction in a child. The hallmark symptom of obstruction of the large airways in a child is stridor. The small cross-sectional diameter of the pediatric subglottis is easily compromised, and in an infant, one millimeter of airway edema can reduce the cross-sectional area of the subglottic airway by 60%.[1] A small child also has limited pulmonary reserve, so impaired ventilation can rapidly cause hypoxemia and hypercarbia.

Symptoms of airway obstruction can occur because of obstructing anatomic lesions located anywhere between the nose and the carina. A child with signs of upper airway obstruction may have fixed anatomic lesions in the airway that are causing impaired ventilation, such as subglottic stenosis, aspirated foreign bodies, or mass lesions. A child might also have impaired airway patency caused by dynamic processes during active respiration, such as obstructive sleep apnea, vocal cord paralysis, laryngomalacia, or tracheomalacia. The site of obstruction in the upper airway can usually be determined by a thorough history and physical examination; verification of the level of obstruction and identification of the cause of airway compromise involve the use of radiographic studies and airway endoscopy.

The pace of the diagnostic evaluation of a young child or infant with stridor is influenced by the clinical setting and the presence or absence of signs of airway compromise. An infant with inspiratory stridor that has been present for weeks to several months without signs of respiratory compromise should be given an orderly evaluation that includes a thorough history and physical examination, neck and chest radiographs, and awake flexible fiberoptic laryngoscopy. Additional testing is based on the findings of the initial workup.[2] An infant or young child who has experienced rapid onset of stridor and shows signs of respiratory compromise such as worsening stridor, chest retractions, tachypnea, or cyanosis should have his or her airway secured rapidly at the time of the diagnostic workup. This may require evaluation in the operating room under anesthesia, using direct laryngoscopy and rigid bronchoscopy to locate the anatomic lesion. The airway is secured simultaneously with endotracheal intubation, rigid bronchoscopy, or even tracheotomy when necessary.

Safe management of pediatric airway emergencies requires a coordinated team approach in order to make an appropriately rapid response. This team should include pediatric otolaryngologists, pediatric anesthesiologists, pediatric intensivists, and pediatric emergency physicians working in concert to quickly evaluate the severity of the airway obstruction and outline the best diagnostic and therapeutic maneuvers to prevent airway catastrophe. Access to specialized equipment is essential. Operative laryngoscopes, rigid ventilating bronchoscopes, and foreign body extraction equipment must be available in age-appropriate sizes, and tracheotomy equipment should be prepared (Fig. 21–1). Anesthesia tools include all equipment necessary for induction of general anesthesia as well as endotracheal tubes (including tubes smaller than thought necessary for the given age and size), laryngeal mask airways, nasopharyngeal and oral airways, and masks for bag-mask ventilation. Inhalation of helium-oxygen mixtures may be helpful to temporarily improve ventilation in children with airway obstruction.[3]

BILATERAL VOCAL CORD PARALYSIS

Vocal cord paralysis is the second most common cause of stridor in infants, and bilateral vocal cord paralysis is the most common cause of stridor with severe respiratory distress occurring at birth.[4] Some children may have a history of birth trauma or chest surgery, but bilateral vocal cord paralysis is most commonly associated with abnormalities of the central nervous system.

Presentation

Bilateral vocal cord paralysis presents with inspiratory or biphasic stridor associated with varying degrees of respiratory distress. Respiratory compromise may worsen with agitation or crying, and aspiration of feedings may be seen in some infants. With bilateral vocal cord paralysis, the quality of the cry is often quite normal, unlike the hoarse, breathy cry associated with unilateral impairment of vocal cord motion. In cases of airway obstruction resulting from bilateral vocal cord paralysis, the vocal cords are usually found in a paramedian position. Neonates with central nervous system abnormalities, notably the Arnold-Chiari malformation, are most likely to have bilateral vocal cord paralysis. Such paralysis can also be seen in children with hydrocephalus before increased intracranial pressure is treated or when a ventriculoperitoneal shunt has ceased to function.

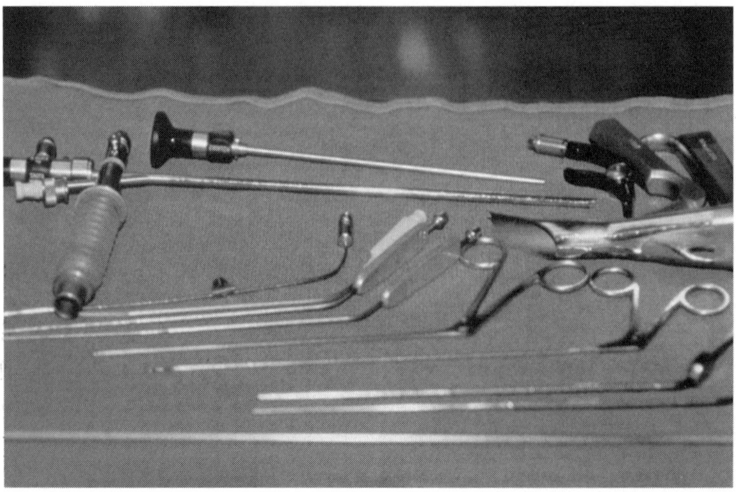

Figure 21–1. Equipment for an airway endoscopy in a young child includes a variety of operative laryngoscopes, ventilating bronchoscopes, and suction tubes.

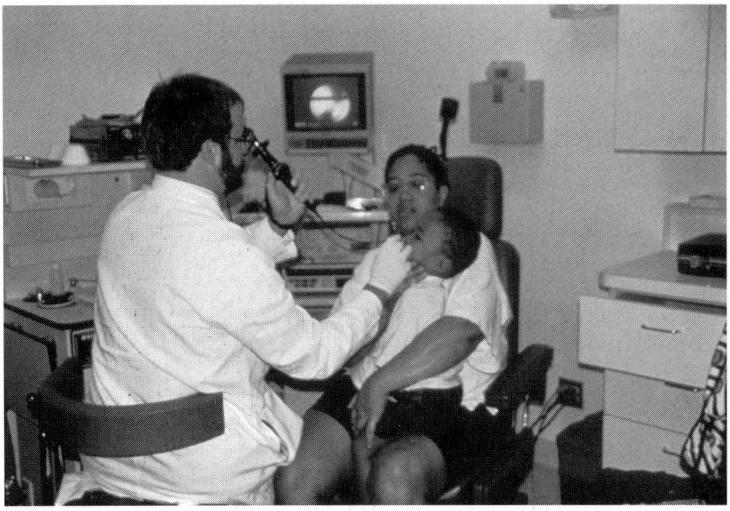

Figure 21–2. Fiberoptic laryngoscopy in an awake, upright child allows assessment of laryngeal dynamics, including vocal cord motion.

Evaluation

Transnasal fiberoptic laryngoscopy is the best tool for diagnosis of vocal cord motion abnormalities in children. This examination is best done when children are awake and upright which allows full appreciation of glottic and supraglottic dynamics during all phases of respiration (Fig. 21–2). In neonates who have required intubation for airway obstruction and in whom vocal cord paralysis is suspected, extubation is performed in a controlled setting (an intensive care unit or operating room) and fiberoptic laryngoscopy is performed. If bilateral vocal cord paralysis is confirmed and respiratory distress is present, these neonates are reintubated and long-term airway control by means of tracheotomy should be considered. Although laryngeal electromyography is a useful prognostic tool for adults with vocal cord paralysis, the use of this test in young children has been limited.[5]

The differential diagnosis of bilateral vocal cord paralysis includes a wide variety of congenital and acquired laryngotracheal disorders. In young infants with stridor, laryngomalacia is the most common diagnosis. Laryngomalacia rarely causes severe respiratory distress, does not affect the quality of the cry, and can be distinguished by the findings of inspiratory supraglottic tissue collapse on fiberoptic laryngoscopy (Fig. 21–3). Subglottic stenosis can also cause respiratory distress in neonates and is diagnosed by characteristic radiographic and endoscopic findings that display narrowing of the subglottic lumen (Fig. 21–4).

Priorities

As with all forms of neonatal airway compromise, stabilization of the airway is the foremost

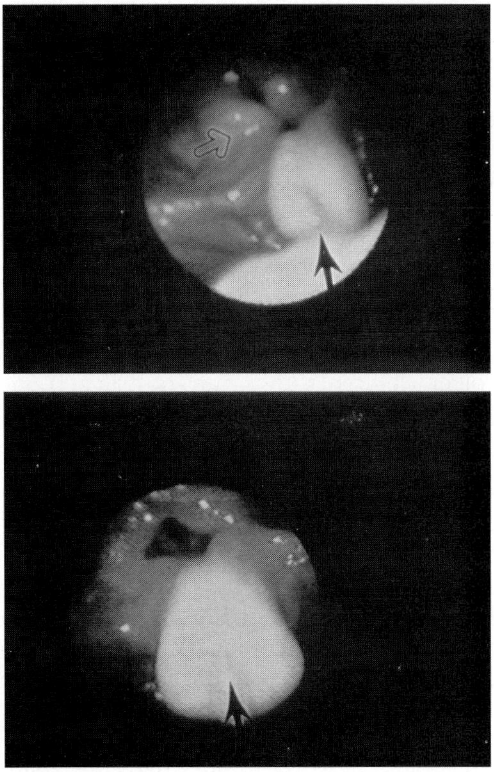

Figure 21–3. These endoscopic images of the larynx of an infant with laryngomalacia show the folding of the epiglottis *(solid arrow)* and the prolapse of the aryepiglottic folds *(open arrow)* into the laryngeal inlet during inspiration.

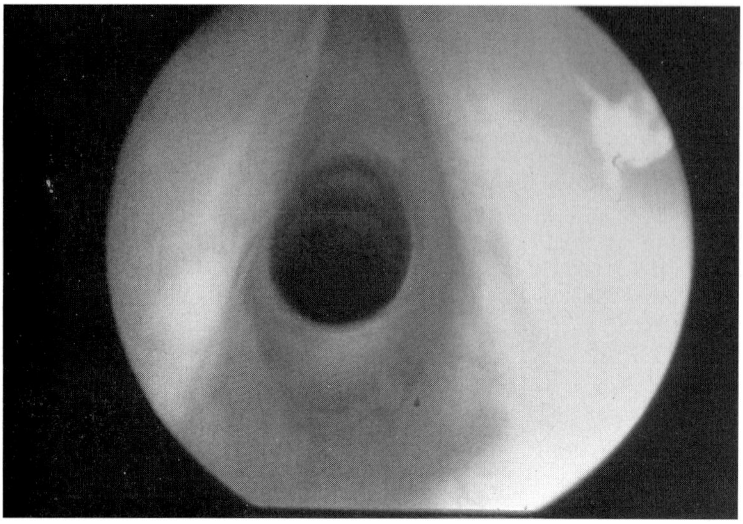

Figure 21–4. Direct laryngoscopy and bronchoscopy under general anesthesia showing circumferential subglottic stenosis.

priority in infants with respiratory embarrassment caused by bilateral vocal cord paralysis. Clinical assessment of ventilation and oxygenation should address the need for endotracheal intubation. Vocal cord paralysis does not limit the ability to pass an age-appropriate endotracheal tube; if a tube cannot be passed, an additional or different airway lesion is likely, for example, subglottic stenosis. After the airway has been stabilized with intubation, assessment focuses on possible associated abnormalities of the central nervous system that would affect prognosis. If airway compromise appears to be a long-term issue, tracheotomy is recommended. If vocal cord paralysis does not resolve, vocal cord lateralization techniques, arytenoidectomy, or posterior vocal cord transection can be attempted to allow decannulation of older children with airway obstruction and irreversible vocal cord paralysis.[4, 6, 7]

Outcomes

Tracheotomy is usually recommended for infants with severe respiratory difficulties resulting from bilateral vocal cord paralysis so as to stabilize the airway until vocal cord motion returns or surgery is performed to improve the glottic airway. Recent literature suggests that some children with stridor caused by bilateral vocal cord paralysis but without signs of respiratory distress can be observed without tracheotomy.[8, 9] This approach requires close monitoring of the respiratory and swallowing functions and serial evaluations of symptoms, growth, and so on. In our experience, the majority of children born with bilateral vocal cord paralysis without initial respiratory distress or associated central nervous system abnormalities can be observed cautiously without tracheotomy and have excellent chances for spontaneous recovery of vocal cord function.[9]

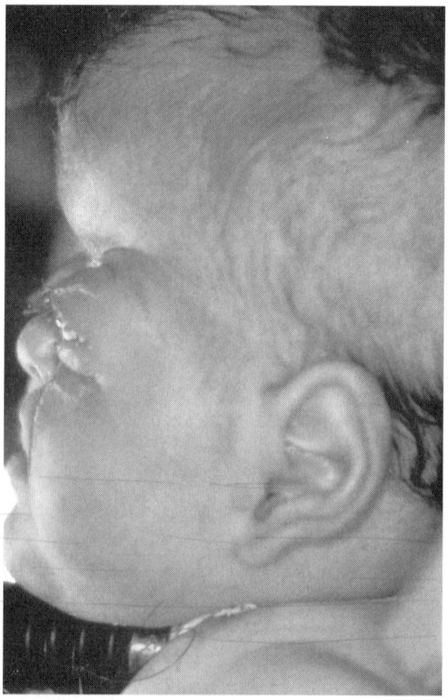

Figure 21–5. This infant with Apert syndrome required a tracheotomy because of severe airway compromise caused by midfacial and mandibular hypoplasia.

CRANIOFACIAL ABNORMALITIES AND AIRWAY OBSTRUCTION

Infants with craniofacial abnormalities may experience life-threatening airway obstruction in the neonatal period. A wide variety of syndromic and nonsyndromic craniofacial disorders commonly involve hypoplasia of the midface and the mandible and small nasal or nasopharyngeal airways (Fig. 21–5). The Pierre Robin sequence, a triad of signs including a wide U-shaped cleft of the secondary palate, glossoptosis, and micrognathia, is marked by varying degrees of upper airway obstruction and feeding difficulties that are usually noted during the first 24 hours of life.[10] The incidence of this triad is between 1 in 30,000 and 1 in 50,000 live births, and more than 80% of affected children have the triad as part of another specific syndrome.[11] Mandibular hypoplasia is associated with deficiency of supraglottic and pharyngeal airway support, retrodisplacement of the tongue, and collapse of supraglottic tissues (Fig. 21–6A and B).

Craniofacial structural abnormalities can be associated with neuromotor disorders and pharyngeal hypotonia that leads to additional airway compromise. Craniofacial abnormalities may include choanal atresia with airway obstruction at the nasopharyngeal level. Laryngotracheal abnormalities can occur in association with craniofacial abnormalities in some syndromic children, causing obstruction at several different areas of the upper airway.[12] For example, children with mucopolysaccharidoses such as Hunter's or Hurler's syndrome often have severe obstructive sleep apnea syndrome because of abnormal craniofacial anatomy. These patients can develop laryngotracheal obstruction caused by intramural deposits in the larynx and trachea. Similarly, infants with Down's syndrome have characteristic craniofacial features that include macroglossia, maxillary hypoplasia, narrow nasopharynx and skull base, and small nasal passages. A small subset of these children may also have laryngotracheal lesions such as laryngeal stenosis, tracheomalacia, or tracheal stenosis.[13]

Presentation

Craniofacial disorders usually obstruct the airway at the pharyngeal level, and such obstruc-

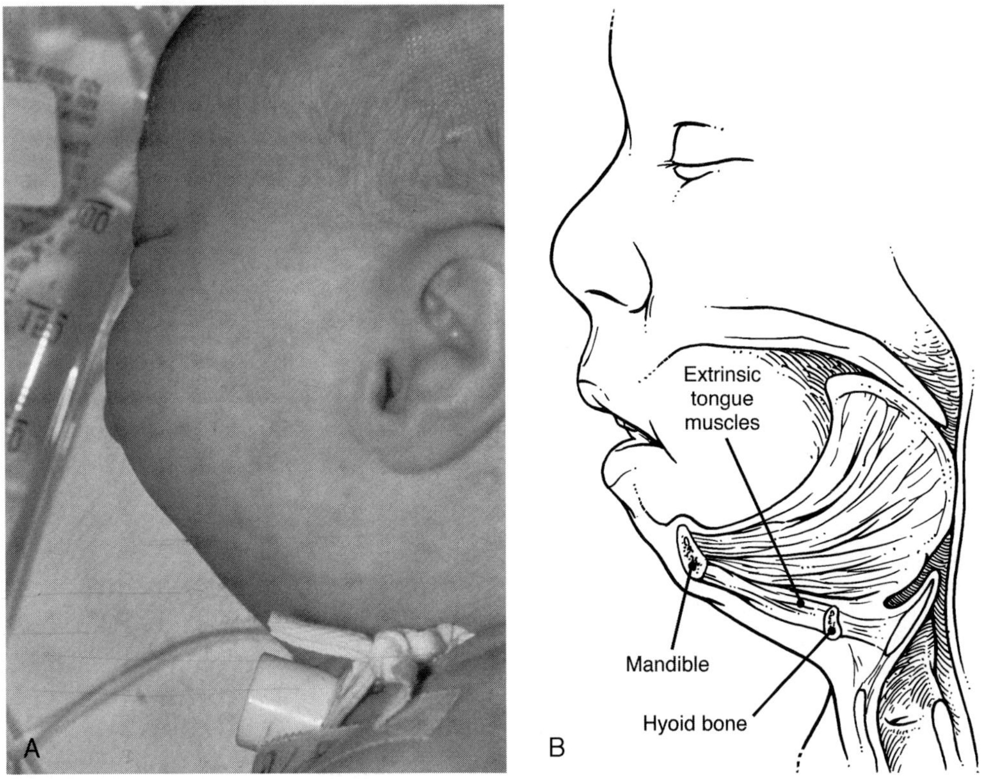

Figure 21–6. A: This infant had severe micrognathia as part of Pierre Robin triad. B: Micrognathia impairs airway function, with loss of support of the tongue and the suprahyoid muscles.

tion worsens when pharyngeal tone decreases during sleep. These neonates may have apneic periods during sleep that include arterial oxygen desaturation and hypercapnia. Feeding problems may occur because of respiratory difficulties or because of mechanical problems caused by cleft palate, tongue size and shape, or other malformations. Stridor, stertor, and loud, irregular snoring can be seen in these patients.

Evaluation

When airway obstruction is not life threatening, these children should undergo full evaluation, including head and neck examinations that emphasize facial skeletal structure and nasal patency. Fiberoptic nasopharyngoscopy is performed to assess pharyngeal and laryngeal anatomy. Radiographic imaging, including computerized tomography (CT) scans, can display two- and three-dimensional skull and bony facial anatomy (Fig. 21–7). Many of these infants have airway obstruction that worsens during sleep, so polysomnography may be useful to assess the severity of breathing abnormalities related to sleep disorders.[14] If airway obstruction is severe, airway support precedes any further diagnostic measures.

Priorities

Initial management of these infants includes positioning them to optimize respiratory function during sleep and feeding.[10] The prone position is usually discouraged because of the association of this position with sudden infant death syndrome,[15] but a prone or side position may decrease airway obstruction when craniofacial anomalies are present. This positioning allows the tongue to move forward, opening the hypopharyngeal airway. If positioning does not improve respiratory function, nasopharyngeal airways may be placed to bypass pharyngeal obstruction. Endotracheal intubation may be necessary if respiratory distress is severe. Infants born with the Pierre Robin triad are more likely to require airway intervention if they also have other abnormalities caused by unique or named syndromes.[16]

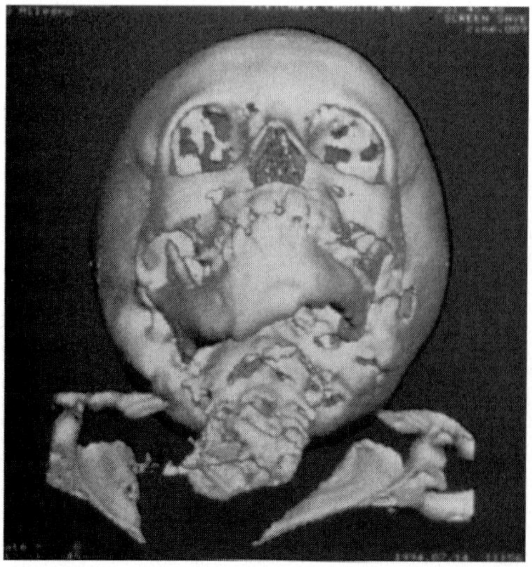

Figure 21–7. A three-dimensional CT image of a child with hemifacial microsomia shows asymmetric mandibular and facial anatomy.

Infants with small mandibles and glossoptosis can prove extremely difficult to intubate, which complicates efforts to stabilize the airway in neonates with respiratory distress. Exposure of the larynx by means of conventional direct laryngoscopy may prove difficult, and alternative methods may be necessary to accomplish intubation. An anterior commissure laryngoscope inserted into the lingual gutter, approaching the supraglottis from the side and moving toward the midline, may allow exposure of the larynx for successful endotracheal intubation.[17] A rigid bronchoscope combined with optical telescopes that have 0-degree and 30-degree angles of visualization may facilitate intubation. The laryngeal mask airway may prove to be life saving in infants in whom the larynx cannot be visualized, as it bypasses the supraglottic/hypopharyngeal obstruction and supports the airway until tracheotomy or intubation has been achieved.[18] "Blind" (nonvisualization) methods of intubation using light wands may be helpful in intubating infants with craniofacial anomalies, but experience with such techniques in infants is limited.[19] On rare occasions, tracheotomy is performed in an unsecured airway because intubation proves impossible.

If long-term airway management is necessary, tracheotomy is performed. Some authors have advocated the use of nasopharyngeal airways for weeks or months to secure the airway until sufficient craniofacial growth or neuromotor development has occurred to allow improvement of upper airway obstruction, but this approach is not universally accepted.[12, 16] A tracheotomy is maintained until mandibular growth and improvement of airway support and function are noted on examination, endoscopy, and ancillary tests such as polysomnography.[20] New methods of midfacial advancement and mandibular lengthening using bone grafting and distraction osteogenesis may expedite tracheotomy removal in some children with craniofacial abnormalities.[21–23]

Outcomes

Infants with craniofacial abnormalities are at high risk for airway obstruction, which may present as stridor and impaired ventilation, obstructive sleep apnea, or difficulties with intubation during induction of anesthesia. Using the preparations and strategies for airway management discussed here, the sequelae of sleep apnea and airway obstruction can be avoided. Children with isolated Pierre Robin triad are usually managed with positioning or nasopharyngeal airways, which may be necessary for the first 1 to 6 months of life.[12] Children with more complex craniofacial problems, such as midfacial and mandibular hypoplasia and additional lower airway anomalies, may be tracheotomy-dependent for several years until craniofacial growth occurs or corrective surgery is completed.

CHOANAL ATRESIA

Choanal atresia, congenital occlusion of the junction between the posterior nasal cavity and the nasopharynx, occurs in 1 in 7,000 live births. Bilateral choanal atresia occurs half as frequently as unilateral choanal atresia.[24] Bilateral choanal atresia can present as an emergency in the neonatal period when severe respiratory difficulty is commonly associated with feeding.

Presentation

Bilateral choanal atresia, when present, is commonly identified soon after infants are delivered, but unilateral choanal atresia may not be diagnosed for months to several years, as the symptoms of unilateral nasal obstruction and rhinorrhea may be mistaken for sinusitis or other, more common conditions.[25] Bilateral choanal atresia causes airway compromise in neonates because young infants are obligate nasal breathers. The respiratory difficulty caused by bilateral choanal atresia may improve with crying, as mouth breathing occurs then, but when at rest and when feeding, impressive respiratory distress can be observed.

Evaluation

Bilateral choanal atresia must be differentiated from other causes of neonatal airway obstruction. This diagnosis is suggested by inability to pass a 6-French catheter through either side of the nasal cavity and is confirmed by fiberoptic nasal examination with rigid and flexible telescopes or by performing an axial CT scan of the midface (Fig. 21–8A and B). Bony atresia has been considered to be nine times more common than membranous atresia, but the use of noncontrast CT scans suggests that most patients with choanal atresia have some combination of bony and membranous abnormalities.[24] Approximately 50% of infants with choanal atresia have other congenital anomalies, the most common being the abnormalities seen in the CHARGE association, which includes a group of congenital anomalies: *c*oloboma (iris defects), *h*eart defects, choanal *a*tresia, growth *r*etardation, *g*enitourinary abnormalities, and *e*ar defects.[26]

Priorities

Stabilization of the airway is the foremost priority in children with respiratory embarrassment

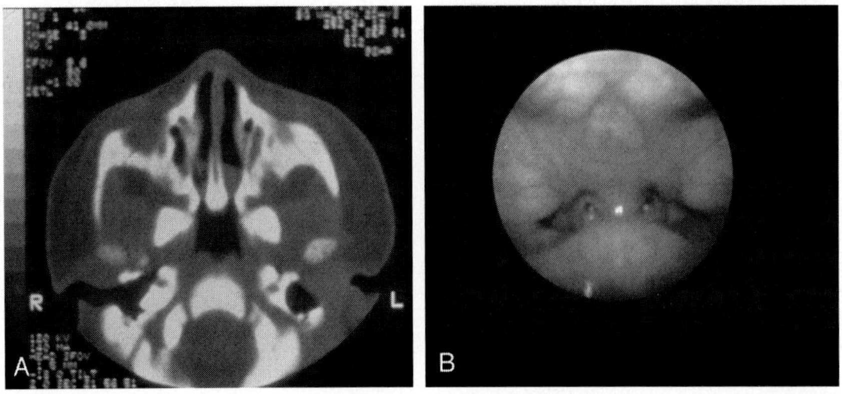

Figure 21–8. A: An axial CT image of the midface shows bilateral choanal atresia. B: An endoscopic photograph of bilateral choanal atresia viewed from the nasopharyngeal side, using a 120-degree telescope.

resulting from bilateral choanal atresia. Oral airways, mouth props, and special nipples have been used to allow respiration through the mouth by these infants who are obligate nasal breathers. Orogastric tube feeding may be necessary to provide nutrition and hydration until the respiratory pattern has been stabilized. Children who have associated craniofacial or neuromotor disorders in addition to bilateral choanal atresia may require endotracheal intubation to relieve marked respiratory distress.

After initial stabilization of the airway, a complete evaluation is performed to determine the anatomy of the choanal atresia plate and the midface. In syndromic children, other airway lesions must be excluded. Isolated choanal atresia can be repaired through a transnasal or a transpalatal approach, even in the neonatal period.[27] New methods of visualization through endoscopes and the use of powered instrumentation to remove the atresia plates have improved results with transnasal approaches.[28–30] Revision surgery or dilation may be necessary later in childhood regardless of the surgical approach and technique used.

Outcomes

Children with isolated bilateral choanal atresia can expect restoration of nasal and nasopharyngeal airway patency with current surgical techniques, although revision surgery may be needed. Syndromic children with choanal atresia may require long-term airway management by means of tracheotomy, as craniofacial anatomy and neuromotor issues may compromise upper airway function even with restoration of patent choanal openings.

POSTTONSILLECTOMY HEMORRHAGE

Tonsillectomy with or without adenoidectomy remains one of the most common surgical procedures performed on children. Its most serious complication not related to anesthesia is hemorrhage. The prevalence of bleeding after adenotonsillar surgery has been reported to be between 0.1% and 9.3%.[31, 32] Hemorrhage after adenotonsillectomy has been divided into primary hemorrhage, bleeding that occurs in the first 24 hours after surgery, and secondary hemorrhage, bleeding that occurs later than 24 hours after surgery.

Primary hemorrhage is less common than secondary hemorrhage, occurring in 0.14% to 2.7% of patients after adenotonsillectomy.[33] Early posttonsillectomy bleeding is more likely to be serious than is secondary bleeding, and it often requires operative intervention because of the brisk bleeding and the impaired airway-protection reflexes present during the postoperative period.[34] Primary hemorrhage is usually caused by the reopening of small vessels in the surgical wound.[35]

Secondary hemorrhage occurs most commonly between postoperative days 5 and 10 and is believed to be caused by the sloughing of the eschar in the tonsillar fossa or, local infection or because of local trauma due to inappropriate diet.[35] Secondary hemorrhage rates reported in the literature range from 0.5% to 9.3%.[32]

The rate for blood transfusion after adenotonsillectomy has been reported to be 0.04%.[31] Mortality after tonsillectomy was not a rare event early in the 20th century, but modern surgical and anesthetic techniques have reduced mortality rates after adenotonsillar surgery to between 1 in 16,000 and 1 in 35,000.[31, 35]

Although bleeding episodes usually are self-limited and affect a minority of patients, the physician must be skilled in handling these emergencies, given the large number of patients who undergo adenotonsillectomy.

Presentation

Children with posttonsillectomy bleeding can present dramatically, with massive oral bleeding and even airway compromise. More often, parents notice bloody stains on bed linen or blood on lips or tongue caused by brief self-limited episodes of bleeding from the tonsillar fossa.

Evaluation

All reports of bleeding after adenotonsillectomy merit evaluation. A complete history of the bleeding episode or episodes should be obtained, including estimates of the amount of blood lost and notation of associated symptoms. Cooperative children without active bleeding should be examined for the presence of fresh blood or clotting in the tonsillar fossa. Clinicians should note the site of the clot or blood; this information helps to direct treatment should bleeding recur. If a clot is present, most pediatric otolaryngologists attempt clot removal to assess for active bleeding within the fossa.[36] Some favor leaving clots undisturbed in uncooperative children to avoid restarting active hemorrhage that would require operative intervention.

Young children with active bleeding are likely to require evaluation in the operating room under anesthesia, establishment of a safe airway, and control of the bleeding with cautery, ligature, or packing.

Routine laboratory assessment of coagulation status (prothrombin time, activated partial thromboplastin time, platelet count, and bleeding time) does not predict the risk of posttonsillectomy hemorrhage.[35, 37, 38] Histories of bleeding disorders in patients or in family members should prompt formal evaluation of coagulation prior to surgery. These laboratory tests are not obtained routinely in patients before adenotonsillectomy, but we obtain such tests when patients present with bleeding after surgery, particularly in patients with primary hemorrhage or repeated secondary hemorrhages. Any history of drug use that would affect clotting (aspirin, ibuprofen, or ketorolac) is obviously significant.

Priorities

Postoperative hemorrhage after adenotonsillectomy creates two major issues: airway compromise caused by aspiration of blood and the physiologic effects of blood loss. Preoperative assessment of bleeding risk by taking a thorough history and performing laboratory tests when indicated is key to reducing the risk of postoperative bleeding.

Intraoperative assessment of blood loss is also necessary during tonsillectomy, especially when operating on young children who have small volumes of circulating blood. The maximal allowable blood loss during surgery before transfusion is considered is calculated by using the following formula:

Maximal Allowable Blood Loss =

EBV × (Starting Hct − Lowest Allowable Final Hct)/Starting Hct

where the estimated blood volume (EBV) is 70 mL/kg for most children, and the lowest allowable final hematocrit (Hct) is usually 25%.[31, 33] The use of electrocautery for tonsillar dissection has reduced intraoperative blood loss, and this technique may reduce the rate of postoperative bleeding as well.[39] Meticulous hemostasis should reduce the risk of primary hemorrhage. The use of ketorolac, a nonsteroidal anti-inflammatory agent, has been associated with an increased risk of hemorrhage after tonsillectomy, and this drug should be avoided.[40, 41]

The parents and caretakers of children who undergo adenotonsillectomy should be instructed to avoid hard foods that may abrade the tonsillar fossa and to avoid the use of aspirin-containing analgesic products. Most important, they must understand that bleeding from the mouth after surgery is not normal and that evaluation is required should this occur.

When bleeding is reported after tonsillectomy, clinicians must assess their patients for signs of continued bleeding, airway compromise, and/or hypovolemia. Decisions concerning children with bleeding after adenotonsillar surgery are influenced by their ages and levels of cooperation and by the presence of active bleeding.[36] In one retrospective review of secondary hemorrhage after adenotonsillectomy in children, 13% of children required major intervention, including operation or blood transfusions.[32] All of these interventions were necessary within 24 hours of readmission for observation after reported hemorrhage. We have a low threshold for admission to observe children after report of oral bleeding or hematemesis after adenotonsillectomy. These children are discharged after 24 hours of observation if bleeding does not recur.

If active bleeding is present, attention is given to careful maintenance of the airway, using a head-up position and suction to aid in clearing bloody secretions from the pharynx. Intravenous access is established, and crystalloid is given to replace intravascular losses. The hematocrit should be measured, but this may underestimate blood loss in the acute period. In older, cooperative children with pharyngeal bleeding, packing with tonsil sponges followed by application of hemostatic agents (Avitene, phenylephrine, tannic acid, bismuth subgallate, etc.) or cautery to the bleeding site may be possible. In most children, when bleeding is brisk, evaluation and management are performed after rapid transport to the operating room.

Induction of general anesthesia during active pharyngeal bleeding requires preparation to suction the pharynx during laryngoscopy and intubation. Rapid-sequence induction with cricoid pressure is usually performed because these patients may have blood and food in the stomach. The surgeon should be prepared to use operative laryngoscopes to accomplish intubation or to even perform tracheotomy in the rare event that intubation is unsuccessful. After intubation, the pharynx is examined, and the actively bleeding tonsillar fossa is packed with a tonsil sponge. Any bleeding site is controlled with cautery or with ligation. Hemorrhage from the nasopharynx after adenoidectomy is unusual and is usually early bleeding associated with retained adenoid tissue or inadequate surgical hemostasis. Removal of residual adenoid tissue and hemostasis with electrocautery is effective in controlling bleeding from the adenoid bed. An orogastric tube should be placed to empty the stomach of bloody secretions and intravenous fluid given to restore intravascular volume. Preparations for transfusion are made if bleeding is severe and recurrent and if hematocrit is very low (generally less than 20% to 25%).

In the rare instance in which massive bleeding cannot be controlled by local surgical measures in the pharynx, ligation of the external carotid artery has been described, as it reduces flow to the tonsil, which is supplied by branches of the external carotid artery, including the internal maxillary artery, ascending pharyngeal artery, facial artery, and lingual artery (Fig. 21–9).[31] In patients with unusual patterns of recurrent or massive bleeding, angiography has been used to identify injuries to branches of the external carotid artery and to the internal carotid artery itself.[31, 42, 43] Aneurysms of the external carotid artery branches have been treated by interventional radiologists who use embolization techniques.

Outcomes

Post-tonsillectomy hemorrhage is an emergency that is seen by virtually every surgeon who performs this procedure, given the number of procedures performed and the frequency of this event. Most bleeding is self-limited, either stopping spontaneously or responding to local measures. Unfortunately, death after adenotonsillectomy is still reported, and mortality that occurs after the immediate postoperative period almost always involves hemorrhage in some way. Appropriate preoperative workup, careful hemostasis during surgery, and attention to any signs of bleeding in the postoperative period minimize the potential for serious morbidity or death caused by post-tonsillectomy hemorrhage.

RETROPHARYNGEAL ABSCESS

Retropharyngeal abscess is an infrequent but serious problem that occurs because of the suppuration of lymph nodes in the retropharyngeal space. A review of deep-space head and neck infections in children found retropharyngeal abscesses to be second in frequency to peritonsillar abscesses.[44] Recent series have reported increasing numbers of retropharyngeal abscesses in adults[45] and in older children,[46] but this disease remains most common in infants and young children.[47] Although the exact incidence of the

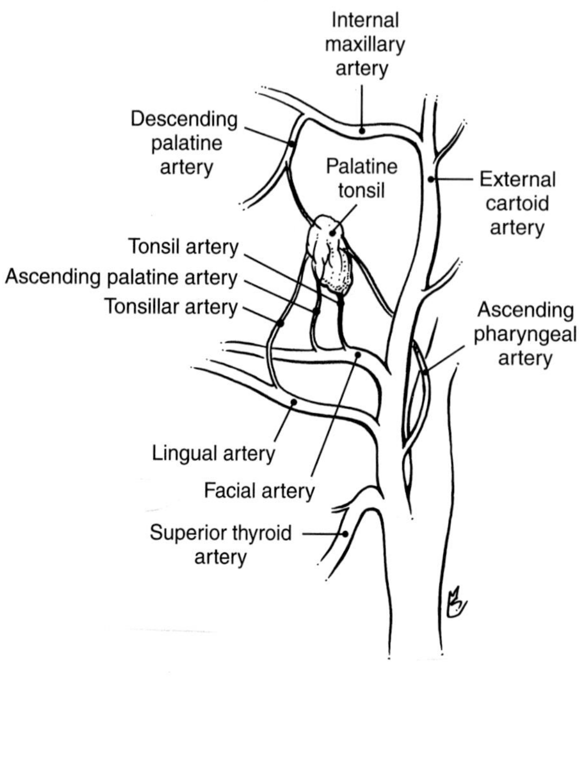

Figure 21–9. The blood supply to the tonsil involves many branches of the external carotid artery.

entity has not been established, a busy tertiary pediatric medical center treats between two and five children for retropharyngeal abscess each year. Choi and colleagues identified 24 children with features of retropharyngeal abscess formation in a 10-year review period.[48]

The retropharyngeal spaces of the young children contain two paramedian chains of lymph nodes that drain the paranasal sinuses, nasal cavity, nasopharynx, and soft palate. Thus, a variety of upper respiratory infections may lead to retropharyngeal adenitis and subsequent abscess formation. About one half of the children diagnosed with retropharyngeal abscesses have histories of recent upper respiratory illnesses. The retropharyngeal lymph nodes atrophy at puberty.[49] The retropharyngeal space extends from the skull base to the mediastinum at the level of the 1st and 2nd thoracic vertebrae.[50] Spread of retropharyngeal infection may lead to mediastinitis, and increasing mass in the hypopharynx or spontaneous rupture of the abscess into the pharynx can cause airway compromise.

Pharyngeal trauma may cause retropharyngeal abscess formation. Penetrating hypopharyngeal foreign bodies can create a focus of retropharyngeal suppuration.[47, 51] Pharyngeal trauma during instrumentation (endoscopy, endotracheal intubation, nasogastric tube placement, and so forth) has also been associated with retropharyngeal abscess formation.

Presentation

The most common symptoms of retropharyngeal abscess are sore throat and dysphagia. The most common signs are fever, drooling, and torticollis. Infants and young children may have drooling as the prominent feature of this infection. Neck swelling is apparent in about two thirds of children with retropharyngeal infection, and they classically display unusual head positions and difficulty in turning the head from side to side. Unilateral posterior pharyngeal wall bulging has been reported as a common feature in many published series, but this finding may be difficult to assess in ill children with excessive oral secretions, large tonsils, or other problems. Indeed, Thompson and associates found this sign in only 43% of confirmed retropharyngeal abscesses.[46] Trismus is an unusual finding with isolated retropharyngeal infection, as the pterygoid muscles are not involved. The presence of trismus suggests an infection in the peritonsillar or parapharyngeal spaces.

Airway signs and symptoms, including stridor, are unusual in early retropharyngeal abscesses, as the swelling in the hypopharynx is posterior and away from the laryngeal inlet. However, in cases of very large abscesses, late presentations, or retained oral secretions, children may exhibit signs of airway obstruction. Stridor was noted in 25% of 65 children treated for retropharyngeal abscess at the Children's Hospital of Los Angeles over a 36-year period.[46] Children with symptoms of airway obstruction require careful monitoring and more urgent evaluation and treatment.

Evaluation

A general examination must establish the severity of illness and assess the likelihood of airway compromise. The first diagnostic test for suspected retropharyngeal abscess is a lateral neck radiograph. A proper lateral neck radiograph is performed with the neck slightly extended, in the true lateral orientation, and on full inspiration. Oblique views, flexion of the neck, and crying and swallowing may artifactually increase the thickness of the retropharyngeal soft tissue.[52] Several components of the lateral neck radiograph should be evaluated to diagnose a retropharyngeal abscess. The presence of air (or air-fluid levels) in the soft tissues of the retropharyngeal space (Fig. 21–10) or the appearance of a radiopaque foreign body is highly suggestive of a retropharyngeal abscess. Such findings usually preclude the need for confirmatory studies, and operative intervention (surgical drainage or foreign body removal) is indicated. The normal lordotic curvature of the cervical spine may be absent on lateral neck radiographs because of muscle spasm secondary to adjacent inflammation.

The thickness of the retropharyngeal soft tissues must be evaluated on the lateral neck radiographs of children with suspected retropharyngeal abscesses. The retropharyngeal space, when assessed anterior to C-2, should be no thicker than 7 mm in a child or adult, and the retrotracheal space should be 14 mm or less in a child.[20, 52, 53] Another common means of assessing retropharyngeal thickness is by comparing it with vertebral body width. In general, the normal thickness of the retropharyngeal soft tissue should be less than one half of the anteroposterior dimension of the C-4 vertebral body.[54] In children younger than 1 year of age, the retropharyngeal soft tissues are thicker, up to one and one half times the anteroposterior size of the C-4 vertebral body.

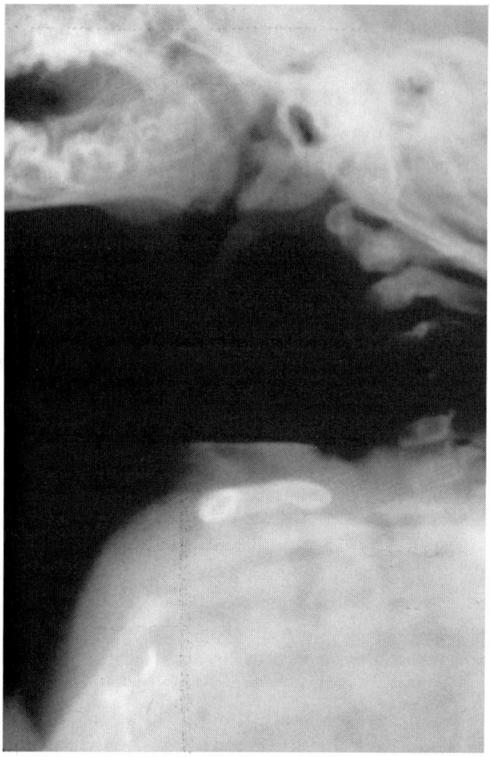

Figure 21–10. A lateral neck radiograph shows a large air collection in the retropharyngeal space. This toddler developed a retropharyngeal abscess from a penetrating hypopharyngeal foreign body.

If the retropharyngeal soft tissues are thickened on the lateral neck radiograph (Fig. 21–11), but the patient has no signs of airway compromise, confirmatory imaging studies are used to document the presence and location of a retropharyngeal abscess. Such imaging is necessary to rule out the possibility that the thickening of the retropharyngeal tissues on the radiograph is an artifact and to distinguish between cellulitis and an abscess. Fluoroscopy of the retropharyngeal profile during awake respiration is a useful technique to exclude retropharyngeal abscess when clinical suspicion is low. Fluoroscopic images are obtained during all phases of respiration and swallowing and in lateral and oblique projections; if the retropharyngeal profile shows normal thickness at any time, it is unlikely that an abscess or mass lesion is present.

A CT scan using intravenous contrast is the most useful test for establishing the presence and defining the anatomy of a retropharyngeal abscess (Fig. 21–12). A CT scan can assess the size of the abscess cavity and can help to determine the need for surgical drainage and the surgical approach to be used (transoral vs. transcervical). Some large retropharyngeal collections may extend outside the confines of this space and into adjacent lateral neck spaces (Fig. 21–13). Such abscesses may require an external approach for drainage.[48] CT scans are over 90% sensitive for the detection of neck abscesses, but specificity may be as low as 60%, with patients who have apparent abscesses on CT scan undergoing negative surgical exploration.[44]

Children with suspected retropharyngeal abscesses who cannot be safely sedated for CT scans and children in whom airway concerns have arisen should be taken to the operating room for examination of the pharynx under anesthesia. Needle aspiration of the retropharyngeal space is performed. If a retropharyngeal abscess is found, it should be drained definitively.

Priorities

Children with suspected retropharyngeal abscesses must be clinically evaluated to assess airway stability, and then radiographic confirmation of the diagnosis must be made. A careful history must be obtained to exclude the possibilities of pharyngeal trauma or retained pene-

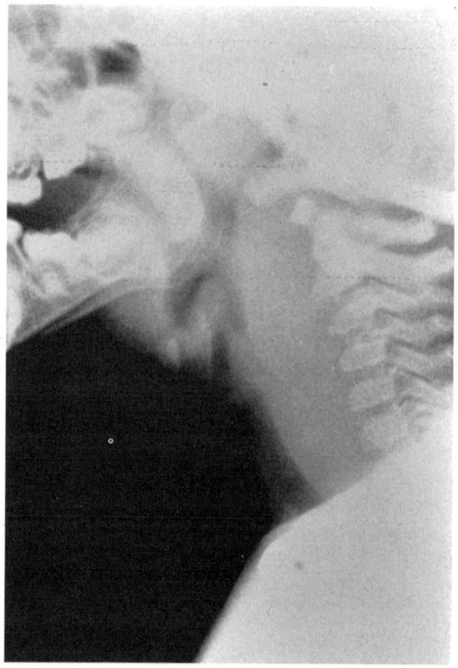

Figure 21–11. A lateral neck radiograph shows thickened retropharyngeal tissues caused by a retropharyngeal abscess.

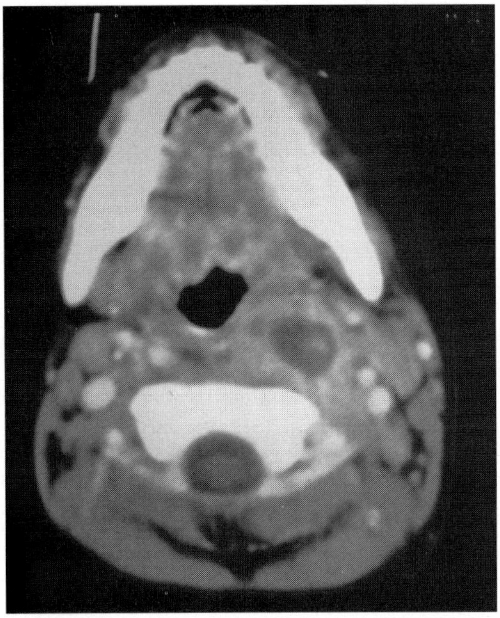

Figure 21–12. An axial CT scan of the neck, with intravenous contrast showing a retropharyngeal abscess. Note the ring enhancing, low-density mass in a paramedian position.

trating foreign bodies. Small abscess cavities may be successfully treated without surgical intervention by administering broad-spectrum intravenous antibiotics.[46, 47] Patients with systemic signs of infection, large abscess cavities, or airway issues require surgical management.

Operative intervention includes controlled induction of general anesthesia and strict attention to avoiding instrumentation of the posterior pharyngeal wall. Spontaneous rupture is unusual, as the abscess cavity and pharyngeal constrictor muscles are thick, but suction should be available to evacuate purulent material. The anesthesiologist should be aware that any laryngeal obstruction, if present, would arise from the posterior pharyngeal wall. In this way, laryngeal exposure for endotracheal intubation is usually uneventful.

Drainage is usually performed transorally using a Crowe-Davis mouth gag for exposure. Needle aspiration is performed to locate the abscess prior to drainage. If there is concern about the possible presence of retained penetrating foreign body, laryngoscopy and esophagoscopy are performed before the abscess is drained so that any mucosal lacerations of the pharynx or upper esophagus can be identified. The abscess is usually unilateral, well off the midline, and evident because of pharyngeal bulging. The tonsil may have to be retracted laterally to allow aspiration and drainage of the cavity.

The position of the abscess in relation to the carotid sheath vessels should be determined on the preoperative CT scan. If the abscess extends into the spaces lateral to these vessels, a transcervical drainage approach should be considered.[48]

When pharyngeal and laryngeal swelling is considerable, patients may be kept intubated for 24 hours after drainage. Most children can be extubated in the operating room. A liquid diet can be started shortly after surgery, depending on the size of the abscess cavity and pharyngeal incision. Placement of oropharyngeal drains into the abscess cavity has been described but is not always necessary.

Intravenous antibiotics are directed against the variety of organisms that have been isolated from retropharyngeal abscesses. Asmar reported polymicrobial infections in 88% of children with retropharyngeal abscesses, and 53% of these infections involved anaerobic organisms.[49] Clindamycin is usually included as part of the initial broad coverage because of its activity against oral anaerobic organisms (*Bacteriodes* species, and *Peptostreptococcus* species), *Streptococcus* species, and *Staphylococcus aureus.*

Outcomes

Early recognition and treatment of retropharyngeal abscesses enables the infection and

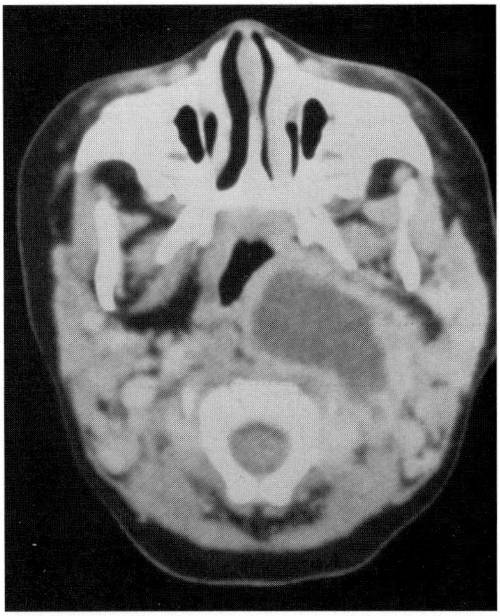

Figure 21–13. An axial CT scan of an infant with a large retropharyngeal abscess extending laterally into the parapharyngeal space.

symptoms to resolve within several days. Undiagnosed retropharyngeal abscesses and late presentation for treatment have been reported to cause complications, including jugular vein thrombosis, mediastinitis, and airway obstruction (see Chapter 19). Fortunately, these complications have become exceedingly rare since this condition has been recognized and treated aggressively with surgery and antibiotics.

SUPRAGLOTTITIS

Supraglottitis, also known as epiglottitis, is a rapidly progressing, life-threatening bacterial infection of the supraglottic larynx. This inflammation of the epiglottis and aryepiglottic folds, usually caused by *Hemophilus influenzae* type B (HIB), has an abrupt onset and rapid progression of symptoms. Management of this emergency requires suspicion of the disease followed by prompt diagnostic and treatment measures.

The annual incidence of supraglottitis is estimated to be 5 in 100,000 in the United States,[55] but the number of cases continues to fall as immunization becomes more widespread and as conjugate vaccines become more effective. Cases of supraglottitis have been seen in children who have received HIB polysaccharide vaccine, but immunization failure appears to be more unusual in children who have received the newer conjugate vaccines.[56] Senior and coworkers reviewed the epidemiologic patterns of supraglottitis in several children's hospitals and found a drop from a peak average of 32 cases per year in 1984–1986 to 5.7 cases per year in 1990–1992.[57]

Presentation

Supraglottitis usually occurs in children between 2 and 6 years of age,[56, 58] although it has been described in younger children and infants[59] as well as in adults.[60] Children with supraglottitis appear sick and generally have a high fever (> 38.5°C). Respiratory signs include inspiratory stridor, shallow respiration, and drooling. Children with supraglottitis classically assume a head-forward, sniffing position to facilitate respiration through a swollen laryngeal inlet. Symptoms usually progress over a relatively short time, with fever followed by respiratory symptoms and drooling within 4 to 8 hours.[58]

The differential diagnosis of supraglottitis includes viral laryngotracheobronchitis ("croup"), bacterial tracheitis, foreign body aspiration, and other disorders that cause airway obstruction. Laryngotracheobronchitis is usually a less dramatic illness that affects infants and young children, in which inflammation of the subglottic larynx is caused by a viral infection. Croup presents with a more gradual onset of symptoms (1 to 3 days) and lower-grade fevers than are found in supraglottitis.[58] A barky cough accompanies biphasic or inspiratory stridor, and the characteristic drooling and positioning seen in supraglottitis is usually absent.[61] More severe croup may require aggressive treatment with aerosolized epinephrine nebulizations and steroids.[58] Some infants with croup develop airway compromise that requires endoscopic evaluation and intubation for diagnosis and airway support.[62] When croup cannot be distinguished clinically from supraglottitis, neck radiographs or endoscopy can differentiate between these two entities.

Bacterial tracheitis is a bacterial infection of the subglottic larynx and trachea that is commonly caused by *Staphylococcus aureus*, although other bacterial pathogens have been isolated in these patients too. This disease is seen in children older than those affected with croup; one study reported a mean age of 54 months for patients with tracheitis with some patients as old as 13 years.[63] Patients with tracheitis often appear toxic and have marked cough, stridor, and fever. These patients require aggressive airway management with intubation, bronchoscopy, tracheal suctioning and, occasionally, tracheotomy.[64] The supraglottic larynx is not involved in such cases, but the severity of airway compromise and the need to suction tracheal secretions often requires an epiglottitis-type approach to diagnose and treat these patients.

Foreign body aspiration usually can be distinguished from supraglottitis and other airway infections by history (although history is often lacking), by absence of symptoms and signs of infection or by radiographic or endoscopic findings (Fig. 21–14). Nevertheless, an aspirated or swallowed foreign body may mimic inflammatory airway obstruction.

Evaluation

The evaluation for supraglottitis relies on appropriate suspicion of the disease, recognition of its clinical appearance, and initiation of an airway protocol. A multidisciplinary team includes otolaryngologists, anesthesiologists, intensivists, and emergency physicians experi-

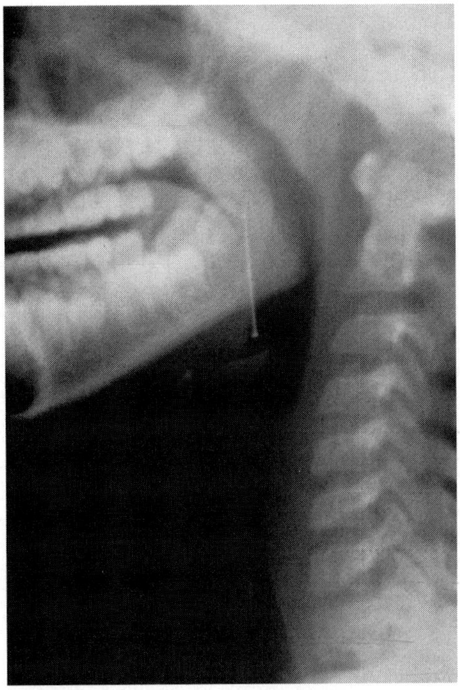

Figure 21–14. A lateral neck radiograph of a child with "supraglottitis-type" symptoms shows a straight pin in the oropharynx.

enced in the care of children with airway compromise. Protocols have been used to ensure appropriate staffing to care for a child with epiglottitis and to outline the best sequence of diagnostic tests and airway management.

If a child presents with severe airway compromise that is suspected to result from supraglottitis, the patient should be immediately transported to the surgical suite by the airway team without any preliminary tests. In the operating room, slow inhalation induction of general anesthesia is performed to allow examination of the larynx and trachea and subsequent endotracheal intubation. The team should be prepared for rigid endoscopy (laryngoscopy, bronchoscopy, or both) and tracheotomy, should laryngoscopy and intubation prove difficult. In a child with respiratory distress, the airway is secured with intubation when simultaneous direct laryngoscopy shows an inflamed swollen supraglottis. If the supraglottis appears normal, the entire upper airway should be examined to determine the cause of stridor. Intraoral examinations, flexible laryngoscopy, intravenous line placement, and radiographic assessments are usually deferred in such a case until the airway is stabilized, as agitation of a child in these circumstances may cause precipitous airway obstruction.

If a child with suspected supraglottitis appears stable, neck radiographs are performed to assess the supraglottic anatomy. The lateral neck radiograph of a child with supraglottitis shows characteristic thickening of the epiglottic profile (Fig. 21–15), the so-called thumbprint sign. If the lateral neck radiograph shows a normal epiglottis, the anteroposterior neck radiograph is examined for subglottic narrowing which is suggestive of laryngotracheobronchitis. If the radiograph shows a thickened epiglottis, the child is transported to the operating room for direct laryngoscopy to confirm the diagnosis and intubate the larynx.

Once the airway has been secured, blood and laryngeal cultures are obtained, and intravenous antibiotics directed against *Hemophilus influenzae* type B are administered. Ampicillin and chloramphenicol were historical antibiotic choices, but second- and third-generation cephalosporins effective against β-lactamase–producing *Hemophilus influenzae*, such as cefuroxime or ceftriaxone, are now used. Endotracheal intubation is maintained until systemic signs of infection abate and evidence of resolution of supraglottic swelling is seen. A patient with supraglottitis can usually be extubated when afebrile and after 24 hours of treatment, although some clinicians advocate direct inspection of the epiglottis before extubation.[65]

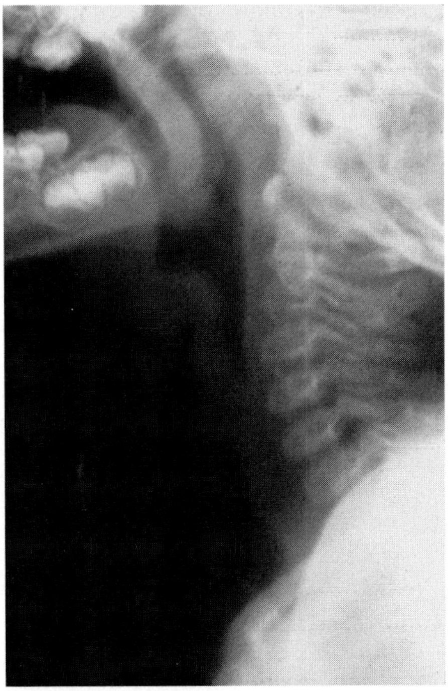

Figure 21–15. A lateral neck radiograph of a child with supraglottitis shows a thickening of the epiglottic profile.

Priorities

When supraglottitis is suspected, signs of airway compromise must be assessed. The child should be observed at all times. If respiratory distress is present, the pediatric airway team should be assembled and the operating room prepared. If respiratory distress is not present, neck radiographs are obtained to assess epiglottic size and shape. In the operating room, a well-coordinated induction of inhalation general anesthesia is achieved. Intravenous access is achieved, blood cultures are drawn, and parenteral antibiotics are administered. Direct laryngoscopy and intubation should be attempted when a deep level of anesthesia is achieved. The surgical team should be prepared to establish the airway by rigid endoscopy or tracheotomy. If the epiglottis is red or swollen, supraglottic cultures are performed. If the epiglottis is normal, a complete airway endoscopy is performed to look for an aspirated foreign body, laryngotracheobronchitis, or bacterial tracheitis. The patient should remain intubated until signs of systemic infection abate and supraglottic swelling decreases. Intensive care unit monitoring is necessary to avoid premature accidental extubation.

Outcomes

The mortality rate of children with supraglottitis used to be estimated to be as high as 6%, but figures from Sweden suggest a mortality rate of less than 1% if intensive treatment is provided.[55] The serious nature of this disease is emphasized by the report of Butt and colleagues, who noted that 8 of 349 (2.3%) children admitted with acute supraglottitis between 1979 and 1986 had experienced cardiopulmonary arrest.[65]

Rapid recognition of this serious airway infection, institution of protocols that allow access to a team experienced with endoscopic and surgical airway equipment, and modern expertise in the care of intubated patients have all but ensured recovery for children with acute supraglottitis. This approach recognizes that some children with airway obstruction resulting from other causes may undergo operative endoscopy to rule out supraglottitis, but such endoscopy allows rapid diagnosis and airway stabilization regardless of the cause of airway compromise.

CAUSTIC INGESTION

Ingestion of caustic or corrosive substances occurs approximately 26,000 times each year.[66] Of these ingestions, 53% occur in children age 6 years and under, but only 2.8% of the deaths that result from caustic ingestion occur in this age group.[67] Ingestions in older patients are more likely to be fatal, as they often occur as suicide attempts or suicidal gestures.

The number of caustic ingestions in children decreased when laws mandating poison warnings and antidote information on toxic substances were enacted in 1927.[66] In 1970 and 1971, legislation was passed that required childproof containers and appropriate labeling for caustic materials, further reducing the frequency of these injuries.[68] Also, the concentration of sodium hydroxide in liquid products was limited to 10%.

Alkaline solutions, such as lye (drain cleaners), soaps, and ammonia, cause injury by means of liquefaction necrosis, which causes progressive tissue damage until dilution of the caustic agent occurs, and deep esophageal injuries may occur. Acidic substances cause injury by means of coagulative necrosis, and the coagulum may limit the spread of injury and spare the deeper esophageal layers. Acidic substances have been associated with gastric burns as well. Solid caustic substances can cause deep focal burns that progress until the granules are removed. Fortunately, ingestions of solids involve small amounts, and distal esophageal and gastrointestinal injuries are uncommon. Ingestion of caustic liquids can involve considerable quantities that spread distally with a single swallow, causing severe esophageal and more distal injuries.

Ingestion of household bleach (sodium hypochlorite) usually results in minor mucosal irritation without significant burns, as bleach solutions (in the United States) usually contain less than 5.25% sodium hypochlorite.[69] Similar mild injuries have been reported with ingestion of hair relaxer, an alkaline substance.[70] Because significant esophageal mucosal burns have not been seen in patients after bleach or hair relaxer ingestions, these patients are usually observed without operative endoscopy unless airway or swallowing symptoms occur or mucosal injury in seen on preliminary examinations.

Presentation

A child with a recent caustic ingestion may present with rapid or progressive airway difficulties caused by pharyngeal or laryngeal edema. Swallowing difficulties may be prominent, with drooling and odynophagia. A history of a caustic ingestion may be available from caregivers. Perioral skin burns may be seen and there may be sloughing or burns of the oral and pharyngeal mucosa. Edema of the lips and tongue may be present.

The absence of oral or pharyngeal injury in the face of a history of caustic ingestion does not preclude the need for thorough evaluation. Between 10% and 20% of children with significant esophageal injury after caustic ingestion have no signs of oral or pharyngeal burns on routine examination.[68, 71]

Other symptoms and signs associated with caustic ingestions include abdominal pain, nausea and vomiting, hoarseness, tachypnea, fever, hemoptysis, refusal of food, and substernal pain.[67]

Evaluation

The initial evaluation should include a rapid assessment of airway patency and respiratory status. In a child with signs of airway compromise, endotracheal intubation should be performed before mucosal injury and airway edema worsen. Emergency tracheotomy may be necessary in severe injuries.

The parents or caretakers should be interviewed to determine the type of caustic substance involved, the amount ingested, and the timing of the ingestion. Emesis should not be induced, nasogastric tubes should not be passed blindly, and charcoal gastric lavage is contraindicated.

In a stable child with a history of caustic ingestion, examination of the oral cavity may help to indicate the severity of mucosal injury. Flexible fiberoptic laryngoscopy provides a view of the hypopharynx and larynx in an awake child and may help predict the need for airway stabilization. The skin of the entire body should be assessed for associated chemical burns resulting from spilled caustic substances. The chest and abdomen are examined for signs of injury, and a baseline chest radiograph is obtained.

Endoscopic evaluation of the pharynx, larynx, trachea, and esophagus should be considered for any child who has ingested a caustic substance (other than bleach). If the child is in stable condition, such endoscopy should be performed within 48 hours of injury. Controversy over the timing of endoscopy exists, as later examination (after 72 hours) may allow evaluation of fully evolved mucosal burns. However, it is unlikely that examination at 12 hours or more after injury would miss significant mucosal injuries.

Both rigid and flexible techniques of esophagoscopy have been advocated for examination after a caustic ingestion. Flexible endoscopes can be passed into the stomach and duodenum to look for more distal injuries. Air insufflation, which is required for this technique, may be hazardous if full-thickness injuries are present. Rigid esophagoscopy allows examination from the esophageal inlet to the gastroesophageal junction. At the time of esophagoscopy, laryngoscopy and bronchoscopy can be performed to look for airway injuries. The esophagoscope should be passed only through areas of the esophagus that have visible, patent lumens. Traditionally, the examination is terminated at the site of the full-thickness or circumferential burns.[66–68] Esophageal burns are graded as follows: first-degree burns, a superficial mucosal injury with erythema and punctate hemorrhages; second-degree burn, a partial-thickness mucosal injury with ulcerations and exudative pseudomembranes; third-degree burn, a full-thickness mucosal injury with pallor, eschar, and perforation into or through the muscular layer. If severe esophageal injury is displayed on endoscopy, a feeding tube should be placed under direct vision for gastric decompression and enteral feeding.

Staging laparotomy has been recommended for patients with severe esophageal injury to assess the extent of distal gastrointestinal injury and to place a gastrostomy or jejunostomy tube for enteral feeding.[72]

Antibiotics are administered, usually intravenous ampicillin or clindamycin, until a serious esophageal injury has been excluded. Medical therapy to prevent gastroesophageal reflux has been suggested for children with significant esophageal mucosal injury.[67]

Steroid administration has been studied in attempts to prevent the late stricture formation associated with deep esophageal injury. Anderson and associates found no reduction in stricture formation with steroid administration.[73] Stricture formation was related only to the severity of injury seen on initial endoscopy. Bautista and colleagues reduced esophageal stricture formation by treating children who had esophageal alkali burns with dexamethasone (1 mg/kg/day) instead of prednisolone (2 mg/kg/day).[74]

Steroids are usually given to patients with partial-thickness mucosal esophageal injury resulting from caustic ingestion,[67, 68] but they are not given when full-thickness mucosal injuries

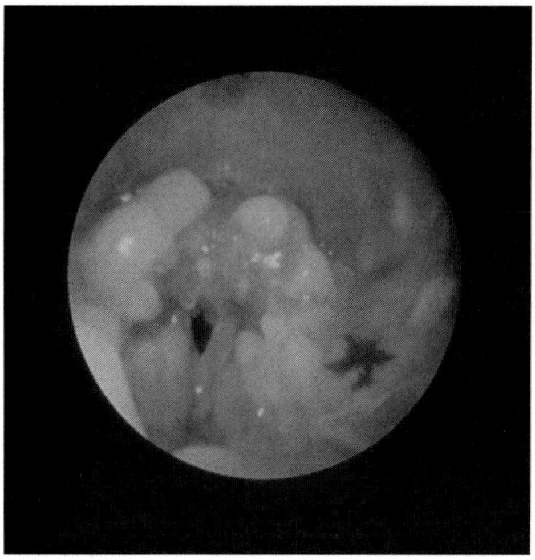

Figure 21–16. Severe destruction of the supraglottic and glottic laryngeal structures 3 weeks after ingestion of a concentrated acid solution. The patient also had severe esophageal and gastric injuries.

are seen, as they may mask the signs and symptoms of perforation.

Priorities

The airway must be assessed and secured if compromise is noted. The identity and quantity of the ingested substance should be determined. Esophagoscopy should be considered during the first 48 hours after injury to assess extent and severity of mucosal injury. Steroids are usually administered for partial-thickness burns, and antibiotics are given as well. Patients are monitored for signs of esophageal perforation if severe mucosal injuries are seen endoscopically.

Esophageal stricture may develop as a late complication of caustic ingestion. Follow-up endoscopy or contrast esophagography should be performed 3 weeks after a significant caustic ingestion to detect early stricture formation.

Outcomes

Partial-thickness esophageal burns caused by caustic ingestion usually heal without sequelae. Severe mucosal esophageal injuries, particularly transmural or circumferential burns, may lead to strictures in up to 33% of patients.[68] Such strictures may require dilation or, in severe cases, esophageal replacement. Laryngeal burns that result from caustic substances can cause progressive glottic and supraglottic stenosis, and there are few options for restoration of a patent and functional laryngeal airway (Fig. 21–16).

CONCLUSION

Pediatric head and neck emergencies require prompt recognition and treatment if serious complications are to be avoided. A multidisciplinary, coordinated approach to airway management that includes protocols that establish primary and back-up plans is necessary to treat critically ill children with emergencies of the head and neck. Basic management principles, emphasizing critical airway, breathing, and circulation issues and treatment of severe infection, apply to the wide variety of head and neck emergencies that can affect children.

REFERENCES

1. Holinger LD. Evaluation of stridor and wheezing. In Holinger LD, Lusk RP, Green CG, eds. Pediatric Laryngology and Bronchoesophagology. Philadelphia, Lippincott-Raven, 1997, pp. 41–48.
2. Tunkel DE, Zalzal GH. Stridor in infants and children: ambulatory evaluation and operative diagnosis. Clin Pediatr 1992; 31:48–55.
3. Tobias JD. Heliox in children with airway obstruction. Pediatr Emerg Care 1997; 13:29–32.
4. Grundfast KM, Harley E. Vocal cord paralysis. Otolaryngol Clin North Am 1989; 22:569–597.
5. Berkowitz RG. Laryngeal electromyography findings in idiopathic congenital bilateral vocal cord paralysis. Ann Otol Rhinol Laryngol 1996; 105:207–212.
6. Bower CM, Choi SS, Cotton RT. Arytenoidectomy in children. Ann Otol Rhinol Laryngol 1994; 103:271–278.
7. Narcy P. Arytenoidopexy for laryngeal paralysis in children. Int J Pediatr Otorhinolaryngol 1995; 32:101–102.
8. Zbar RIS, Smith RJH. Vocal fold paralysis in infants twelve months of age and younger. Otolaryngol Head Neck Surg 1996; 114:18–21.
9. Tunkel DE, Kosko JR. Vocal cord paralysis in children. Curr Opin Otolaryngol Head Neck Surg 1996; 4:419–423.
10. Benjamin B, Walker P. Management of airway obstruction in the Pierre Robin sequence. Int J Pediatr Otorhinolaryngol 1991; 22:29–37.
11. Andrews TM. Airway obstruction in craniofacial anomalies. In Meyers CM, ed. Pediatric Airway. Philadelphia, JB Lippincott, 1995, pp. 247–261.
12. Perkins et al. Airway management in children with craniofacial anomalies. Cleft Palate Craniofac J 1997; 34:135–140.
13. Jacobs IN, Gray RF, Todd NW. Upper airway obstruction in children with Down syndrome. Arch Otolaryngol Head Neck Surg 1996; 122:945–950.
14. Sterni L, Tunkel DE. Obstructive sleep apnea in children. Curr Opin Otolaryngol Head Neck Surg 1997; 5:367–372.
15. Kattwinkel J, Brooks J, Myerberg D. American academy of pediatrics task force on infant positioning and SIDS: summary statement. Pediatrics 1992; 89:1120–1126.
16. Tomaski SM, Zalzal GH, Saal HM. Airway obstruction

in the Pierre Robin sequence. 1995; Laryngoscope 105:111–114.
17. Handler SD, Keon TP. Difficult laryngoscopy/intubation: the child with mandibular hypoplasia. Ann Otol Rhinol Laryngol 1983; 92:401–404.
18. Markakis DA, Sayson SC, Schriener MS. Insertion of the laryngeal mask airway in awake infants with the Robin sequence. Anesth Analg 1992; 75:822–824.
19. Fisher QA, Tunkel DE. Lightwand intubation of infants and children. J Clin Anesth 1997; 9:275–279.
20. Tunkel DE et al. Polysomnography in the evaluation for readiness for decannulation in children. Arch Otolaryngol Head Neck Surg 1996; 122:721–724.
21. Burstein FD et al. Surgical therapy for severe refractory sleep apnea in infants and children: application of the airway zone concept. Plast Reconstr Surg 1995; 96:34–41.
22. James D, Ma L. Mandibular reconstruction in children with obstructive sleep apnea due to micrognathia. Plast Reconstr Surg 1997; 100:1131–1137.
23. Nunn DR et al. Tracheotomy removal after early mandibular advancement in patients with pediatric craniofacial syndrome. Otolaryngol Head Neck Surg 1997; 117:S187–S191.
24. Brown OE, Pownell P, Manning SC. Choanal atresia: a new anatomic classification and clinical management applications. Laryngoscope 1996; 106:97–101.
25. Rothman G, Wood RA, Naclerio RM. Unilateral choanal atresia masquerading as chronic sinusitis. Pediatrics 1994; 94:941–944.
26. Kaplan LC. The CHARGE association: choanal atresia and multiple congenital anomalies. Otolaryngol Clin North Am 1989; 22:661–672.
27. Richardson MA, Osguthorpe JD. Surgical management of choanal atresia. Laryngoscope 1988; 915–918.
28. Stankiewicz JA. The endoscopic repair of choanal atresia. Otolaryngol Head Neck Surg 1990; 103:931–937.
29. Lazar RH, Younis RT. Transnasal repair of choanal atresia using telescopes. Arch Otolaryngol Head Neck Surg 1995; 121:517–520.
30. April MM, Ward RF. Choanal atresia repair: the use of powered instrumentation. Operative Techniques Otolaryngol Head Neck Surg 1996; 7:248–251.
31. Randall DA, Hoffer ME. Complications of tonsillectomy and adenoidectomy. Otolaryngol Head Neck Surg 1998; 118:61–68.
32. Irani DB, Berkowitz RG. Management of secondary hemorrhage following pediatric adenotonsillectomy. Int J Pediatr Otorhinolaryngol 1997; 40:115–124.
33. April MM, Naclerio RM. Complications of tonsillectomy and adenoidectomy. In Eisele DW, ed. Complications in Head and Neck Surgery. St. Louis, Mosby, 1993, pp. 262–266.
34. Tami TA, Parker GS, Taylor RE. Post-tonsillectomy bleeding: an evaluation of risk factors. Laryngoscope 1987; 97:1307–1311.
35. Howells RC, Wax MK, Ramadan HH. Value of preoperative prothrombin time/partial thromboplastin time as a predictor of postoperative hemorrhage in pediatric patients undergoing tonsillectomy. Otolaryngol Head Neck Surg 1997; 117:628–632.
36. Cressman WR, Myer CM. Management of tonsillectomy hemorrhage: results of a survey of pediatric otolaryngology fellowship programs. Am J Otolaryngol 1995; 16:29–32.
37. Handler SD et al. Post-tonsillectomy hemorrhage: incidence, prevention, and management. Laryngoscope 1986; 96:1243–1247.
38. Close HL et al. Hemostatic assessment of patients before tonsillectomy: a prospective study. Otolaryngol Head Neck Surg 1994; 111:733–738.
39. Szeremeta W, Novelly NJ, Benninger M. Postoperative bleeding in tonsillectomy patients. Ear Nose Throat J 1996; 75:373–376.
40. Gallagher JE, Blauth J, Fornadley JA. Perioperative ketorolac promethamine and postoperative hemorrhage in cases of tonsillectomy and adenoidectomy. Laryngoscope 1995; 105:606–609.
41. Judkins JH, Dray TG, Hubbell RN. Intraoperative ketorolac and posttonsillectomy bleeding. Arch Otolaryngol Head Neck Surg 1996; 122:937–940.
42. Karas DE, Sawin RS, Sie KCY. Pseudoaneurysm of the external carotid artery after tonsillectomy: a rare complication. Arch Otolaryngol Head Neck Surg 1997; 123:345–347.
43. Mitchell RB et al. Pseudoaneurysm of the right lingual artery: an unusual cause of severe hemorrhage during tonsillectomy. Ear Nose Throat J 1997; 76:575–576.
44. Ungkanont K et al. Head and neck space infections in infants and children. Otolaryngol Head Neck Surg 1995; 112:375–382.
45. Pontell J, Har-El G, Lucente FE. Retropharyngeal abscess: clinical review. Ear Nose Throat J 1995; 74:701–704.
46. Thompson JW, Cohen SR, Reddix P. Retropharyngeal abscess in children: a retrospective and historical analysis. Laryngoscope 1988; 98:589–592.
47. Coulthard M, Isaacs D. Retropharyngeal abscess. Arch Dis Child 1991; 66:1227–1230.
48. Choi SS, Vezina LG, Grundfast KM. Relative incidence and alternative approaches for surgical drainage of different types of deep neck abscesses in children. Arch Otolaryngol Head Neck Surg 1997; 123:1271–1275.
49. Asmar BI. Bacteriology of retropharyngeal abscess in children. Pediatr Infect Dis J 1990; 9:595–597.
50. Goldenberg D, Golz A, Joachims HZ. Retropharyngeal abscess: a clinical review. J Laryngol Otol 1997; 111:546–550.
51. Ross MN, Janik JS. "Foil tab" aspiration and retropharyngeal abscess in a toddler. JAMA 1988; 260:3130.
52. Brechtelsbauer PB et al. Retropharyngeal abscess: pitfalls of plain films and computed tomography. Am J Otolaryngol 1997; 18:258–262.
53. Barratt GE, Koopman CF, Coulthard SW. Retropharyngeal abscess: a ten-year experience. Laryngoscope 1984; 94:455–463.
54. Hartmann RW. Recognition of retropharyngeal abscess in children. Am Fam Physician 1992; 46:193–196.
55. Takala AK, Peltola H, Eskola J. Disappearance of epiglottitis during large-scale vaccination with *Hemophilus influenzae* type B conjugate vaccine among children in Finland. Laryngoscope 1994; 104:731–735.
56. Valdapena HG et al. Epiglottitis and *Hemophilus influenzae* immunization: the Pittsburgh experience: a five-year review. Pediatrics 1995; 96:424–427.
57. Senior BA et al. Changing patterns in pediatric supraglottitis: a multi-institutional review, 1980 to 1992. Laryngoscope 1994; 104:1314–1322.
58. Bank DE, Krug SE. New approaches to upper airway disease. Emerg Med Clin North Am 1995; 13:473–487.
59. Blackstock D, Adderley RJ, Steward DJ. Epiglottitis in young infants. Anesthesiology 1987; 67:97–100.
60. Mayo-Smith MF et al. Acute epiglottitis in adults: an eight-year experience in the state of Rhode Island. N Engl J Med 1986; 314:1133–1139.
61. Mauro RD, Poole SR, Lockhart CH. Differentiation of epiglottitis from laryngotracheitis in the child with stridor. Am J Dis Child 1988; 142:679–682.

62. McEniery J et al. Review of intubation in severe laryngotracheobronchitis. Pediatrics 1991; 87:847–853.
63. Donnelly B, McMillan J, Winer L. Bacterial tracheitis: report of eight cases and review. Rev Infect Dis 1990; 12:729–735.
64. Fiedman EM et al. Bacterial tracheitis: a two-year experience. Laryngoscope 1995; 95:9–11.
65. Butt W et al. Acute epiglottitis: a different approach to management. Crit Care Med 1988; 16:43–47.
66. Forsen JW. Caustic ingestion. In Gates GA, ed. Current Therapy in Otolaryngology, Head and Neck Surgery. St Louis, Mosby, 1998, pp. 474–477.
67. Andrews TM, Cressman WR. Caustic ingestion in children. Curr Opin Otolaryngol Head Neck Surg 1997; 5:362–366.
68. Holinger LD. Caustic ingestion, esophageal injury, and stricture. In Holinger LD, Lusk RP, Green CG, eds. Pediatric laryngology and bronchoesophagology. Philadelphia, Lippincott-Raven, 1997, pp. 295–303.
69. Harley EH, Collins MD. Liquid household bleach ingestion in children: a retrospective review. Laryngoscope 1997; 107:122–125.
70. Forsen JW, Muntz HR. Hair relaxer ingestion: a new trend. Ann Otol Rhinol Laryngol 1993; 102:781–784.
71. Gaudreault P et al. Predictability of esophageal injury from signs and symptoms: a study of caustic ingestion in 378 children. Pediatrics 1983; 71:767–770.
72. Meredith JW, Kon ND, Thompson JN. Management of injuries from liquid lye ingestion. J Trauma 1988; 28:1173–1180.
73. Anderson KD, Rouse TM, Randolph JG. A controlled trial of corticosteroids in children with corrosive injury of the esophagus. N Engl J Med 1990; 323:637–640.
74. Bautista A et al. Effects of prednisolone and dexamethasone in children with alkali burns of the oesophagus. Eur J Pediatr Surg 1996; 6:198–203.

CHAPTER 22

Facial Nerve Emergencies

Howard W. Francis, MD

The facial nerve follows a complicated course through the temporal bone and parotid gland, two regions that are commonly involved in head and neck trauma and are frequently visited in the surgical treatment of head and neck pathology. Although the functional and aesthetic effects of facial nerve paralysis can be dramatic, treatment goals in the emergency management of a patient with acute facial dysfunction must be prioritized appropriately. The early assessment and close follow-up of facial nerve function is essential to timely and appropriate treatment as well as to determination of prognosis. This chapter discusses the diagnosis and treatment of paralysis in selected emergencies and describes the relevant facial nerve anatomy and pathophysiology that form the basis of clinical decision-making.

PARALYSIS OF THE FACIAL NERVE

Clinical Priorities

The urgent care of a patient with acute facial nerve paralysis should focus initially on the diagnosis and treatment of accompanying injuries that may result in permanent disability or death. The principles of basic life support should be closely observed, including access to and protection of the airway, establishment of ventilation, maintenance of hemostasis and perfusion, and immobilization of the cervical spine, especially in the setting of head trauma.[1] After these objectives have been achieved, a secondary survey of the patient's injuries should include a thorough examination of the head and neck, including an otoscopic examination, an assessment of cranial nerve function and mental status, and a radiologic assessment of the cervical spine and thorax. It is important to remember that the absence of external bleeding or hematoma formation does not rule out the presence of a life-threatening vascular injury at the skull base or in the thorax. A patient with penetrating trauma to the head or neck must be carefully assessed for vascular injuries by physical examination and arteriography, with surgical exploration indicated in selected cases (see Chapter 12). Any trauma to the head or neck that is associated with loss of consciousness or other neurologic abnormality and any penetrating trauma in proximity to the skull base should prompt an urgent brain scan to rule out intracranial injuries. There should also be a high level of suspicion for injuries to the upper aerodigestive tract, with clinical evaluation and repair being performed as described in Chapters 11 and 20.

The absence of global motor function due to severe neurologic impairment or the administration of muscle relaxants to facilitate airway access and ventilation may impede the recognition of immediate or evolving facial paralysis in a trauma patient. Facial nerve paralysis and other cranial nerve deficits should be documented, if possible, during the secondary survey and should be addressed in due course once the treatment of life-threatening injuries has been initiated. The primary objectives of early management of facial paralysis are (1) the preservation of corneal health and vision and (2) medical or surgical therapy to relieve nerve impingement, to slow the progression of nerve injury, or to reestablish the anatomic continuity of the nerve. In the rare event of bilateral facial nerve

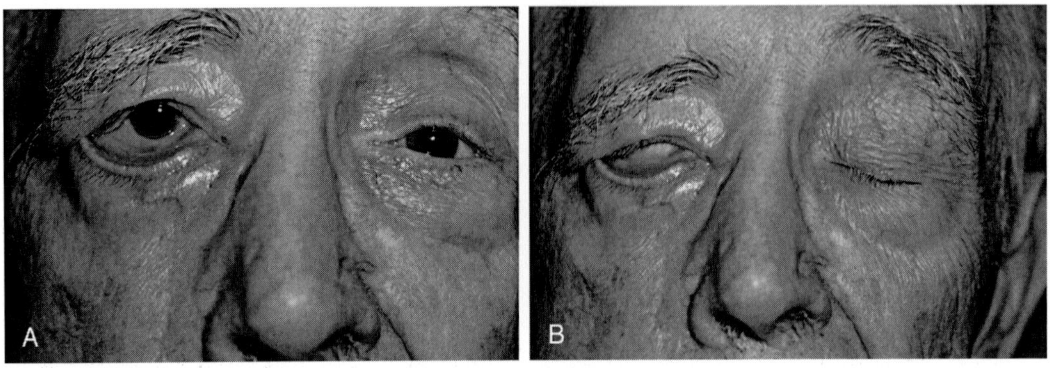

Figure 22–1. An elderly patient with unilateral right-sided facial paralysis resulting in lagophthalmos and severe ectropion and scleral show, with poor lubrication of the cornea. Note Bell's phenomenon of the right eye—corneal coverage upon eye closure due to upward rotation of globe. (Courtesy of John Frodel, M.D.)

paralysis, nutrition and orodental health are additional issues that may also have to be addressed.

Management of the Eye in Facial Nerve Paralysis

Facial nerve paralysis impairs the closure of the eyelids, leaving the eye susceptible to corneal desiccation and repeated trauma. The eye is therefore at risk for ocular complications ranging from corneal irritation and punctate keratopathy to ulceration, perforation, scarring, and blindness. The unprotected eye is most susceptible to abrasion caused by bedding and other objects during sleep. Corneal lubrication is impaired when blinking is no longer possible, and contact between the lower lid and the globe is lost because of decreased tone in the orbicularis oculi muscle (Fig. 22–1). When the facial nerve is injured at or proximal to the geniculate ganglion, xerophthalmia and the threat of keratopathy are further increased by the interruption of the preganglionic parasympathetic innervation of the lacrimal gland. The risk of corneal injury is further increased if the trigeminal nerve is also impaired, because of the diminution of sensitivity to touch and the decrease in the healing potential of the cornea.[2] (See Box 22–1.)

BOX 22-1

Indications for Early Surgical Treatment of the Eye in Facial Paralysis

- Patient is noncompliant or disabled
- Long-lasting paralysis is expected
- Bell's phenomenon is inadequate
- Cornea is insensate
- Xerophthalmia is present
- It is the only seeing eye

In collaboration with an ophthalmologist, the eye must be closely monitored for early signs of keratopathy. Complaints of soreness, the feeling that a foreign body is present, and excessive tearing are early indications of a dry eye and corneal irritation. Photophobia suggests corneal abrasion, whereas blurred vision is a harbinger of more severe corneal damage and early scarring. The adequacy of corneal protection and lubrication must be assessed during serial examinations. The extent of corneal coverage by the eyelid should be assessed during spontaneous blinking and voluntary eye closure, with and without effort. Increasing lagophthalmos and lower lid ectropion with scleral show should be anticipated even when they are minimal immediately after injury. The presence of Bell's phenomenon (upward rotation of the globe during attempted eye closure [see Fig. 22–1]) may initially allow sufficient protection and lubrication of the cornea. However, as muscle tone decreases, corneal exposure may gradually increase without the patient's realizing it, and progressive ocular injury and visual impairment may follow. A dry eye is often hyperemic due to associated inflammation. Disruption of the corneal epithelium can be detected using fluorescein dye under ultraviolet light. Clouding of the cornea is a worrisome sign that permanent changes are occurring in the cornea, including scarring.

Ocular lubrication and corneal protection are the mainstay of treatment for the exposed eye. Artificial tear preparations are usually applied to the eye every 2 to 4 hours during the day, and an ointment is applied prior to sleep. A variety of preparations of artificial tears that vary in viscosity and duration of efficacy are commercially available.[2] Cellulose-based products such as Celluvisc are preferred because of their long-lasting effects. A moisture chamber created by circumferentially taping a thin piece of plastic sheeting such as Saran wrap around the orbital rim so that it is not in contact with the globe or eyelid provides a barrier against trauma and desiccation, especially during sleep. Alternatively, the upper eyelid can be taped closed. However, this method has the potential to lead to corneal injury if the lid inadvertently opens during sleep. The moisture chamber is less likely to traumatize the cornea and can be used 24 hours a day because it permits binocular vision.

Unlike the methods described above, surgical management of a paretic eye may afford more reliable ocular protection, independent of patient abilities and compliance. The lateral tarsorrhaphy (Fig. 22–2A), the creation of a reversible adhesion between the upper and lower eyelids just lateral to the limbus, is an effective and time-honored method of providing eye protection and maintaining lubrication. This technique is not currently favored for long-standing paralysis because of the limitation of the field of vision and the potential for lower lid deformity due to scarring after separation. The subcutaneous placement of a gold weight in the upper eyelid (Fig. 22–2B) permits its passive closure while preserving levator function, so vision is unimpaired and cosmetic results are more favorable than those of tarsorrhaphy. The gold weight is, therefore, an increasingly popular method of eye protection in cases of facial paralysis. Although usually reserved for cases of long-term paralysis or delayed recovery, the early use of a gold weight in the management of facial paralysis is appropriate when patient reliability is in question, Bell's phenomenon is inadequate, the eye lacks sensation, lacrimation is impaired by perigeniculate injury, or for an only seeing eye.[3] The treatment of lower lid ectropion by shortening and suspending the lid and the tarsal plate further increases the protection and effective lubrication of the globe (Fig. 22–2C).

Relevant Anatomy of the Facial Nerve

Each segment of the facial nerve has unique anatomic features that render it susceptible to injury (Fig. 22–3). The bony fallopian canal provides a protective path for the facial nerve in the temporal bone but also plays an important role in the pathophysiology of injury. The narrow meatal foramen[4] and labyrinthine segment of the facial nerve canal[5] are sites where nerve edema due to inflammatory or traumatic causes leads to progressive compression, vascular compromise, and axonal injury. This narrow segment is also the site of termination of the vertebrobasilar arterial contribution via labyrinthine branches of the anterior inferior cerebellar artery and of the external carotid artery contributions via the petrosal branch of the middle meningeal artery and the stylomastoid artery that branches from the posterior auricular artery (see Fig. 22–3).[5,6] The labyrinthine segment of the facial nerve may therefore represent a watershed area that is predisposed to vascular compromise. It also lacks an epineurium, which provides a barrier to injury and a rich collateral blood supply to distal segments of the facial nerve.

The facial nerve is susceptible to injury in the region of the geniculate ganglion for three main reasons (see Fig. 22–3). First, the bone surrounding the geniculate ganglion is very thin and is dehiscent in approximately 20% of individuals (Fig. 22–4), so it is a weak site in the temporal bone through which fractures commonly travel.[7,8] In a case of dehiscence, the area of the geniculate ganglion is also vulnerable to injury during surgery of the middle fossa as the closely associated dura mater is being elevated (see Fig. 22–4). Second, the ganglion is separated from the supratubal recess of the middle ear by a thin layer of bone that may be eroded by pathology, leaving it susceptible to iatrogenic injury (see Fig. 22–3). Third, the greater superficial petrosal nerve (GSPN), which projects anteriorly, tethers the facial nerve at its hiatus and exerts intraneural traction and shearing forces that result from rapid accelerations and decelerations during head trauma. Any of these mechanisms may compromise facial nerve integrity by direct axonal injury or by producing edema and secondary compressive injury in the adjacent labyrinthine segment.

The tympanic segment, especially above the oval window, is the most common site of congenital dehiscence of the bony canal. Bony dehiscence by cholesteatoma is also common proximal to the second genu where the adjacent aditus ad antrum acts as a bottleneck through which disease must pass en route to the antrum, eroding structures in the posterior attic along the way. The dehiscent horizontal fallopian canal places the facial nerve at risk of injury by the unwary surgeon, especially when disease or

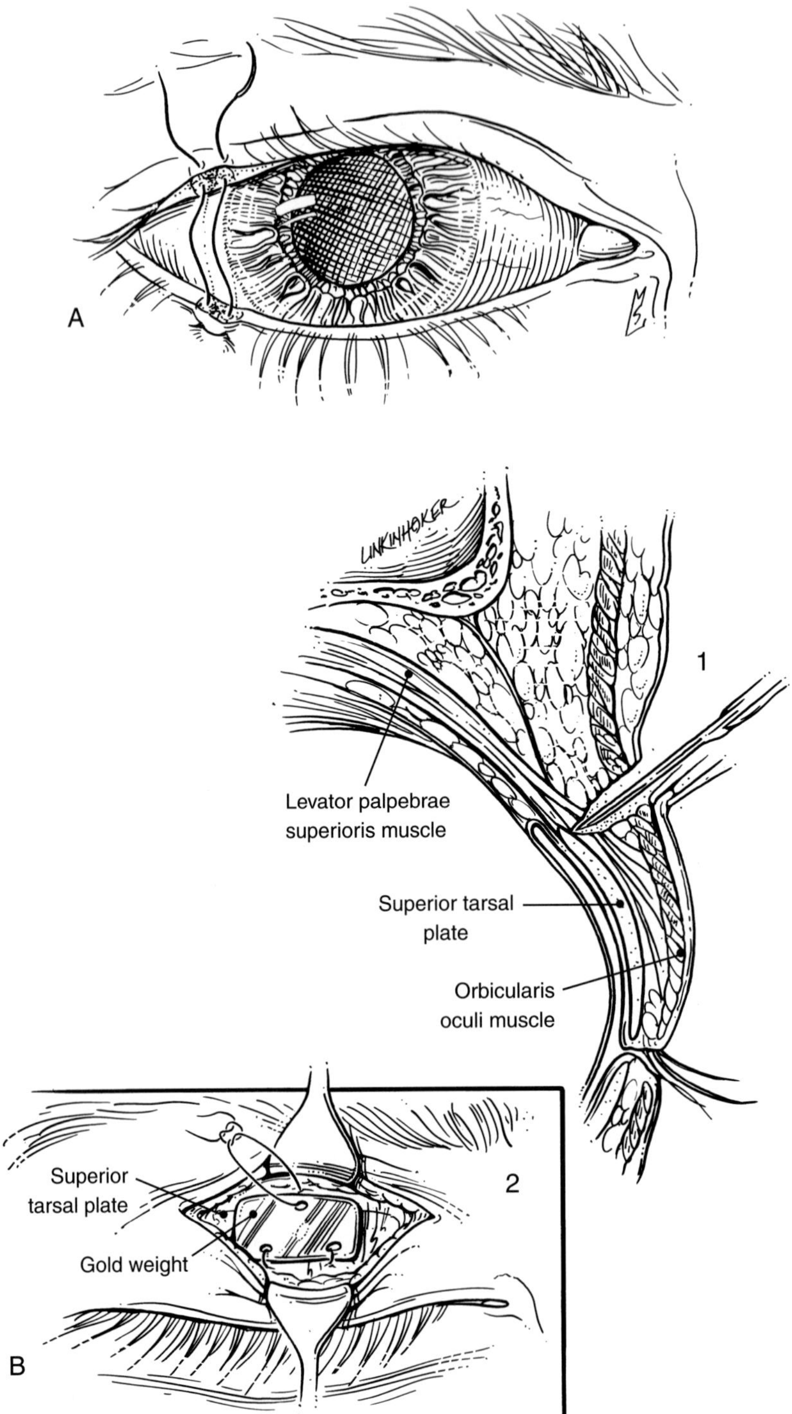

Figure 22–2. Preventative surgical management of the paralytic eye. A: Lateral tarsorrhaphy. A lateral adhesion between the upper and lower eyelids is created by first denuding the mucocutaneous junction 4 to 6 mm from the lateral canthus and then placing a horizontal mattress suture of 7-0 nylon to approximate these denuded surfaces. B: Gold weight. (1) After the appropriate weight is determined, an incision is made in the tarsal crease through the skin and orbicularis oculi muscle. (2) The anterior surface of the tarsal plate is exposed, and the implant is secured to it just lateral of midline of the lid, using permanent sutures.

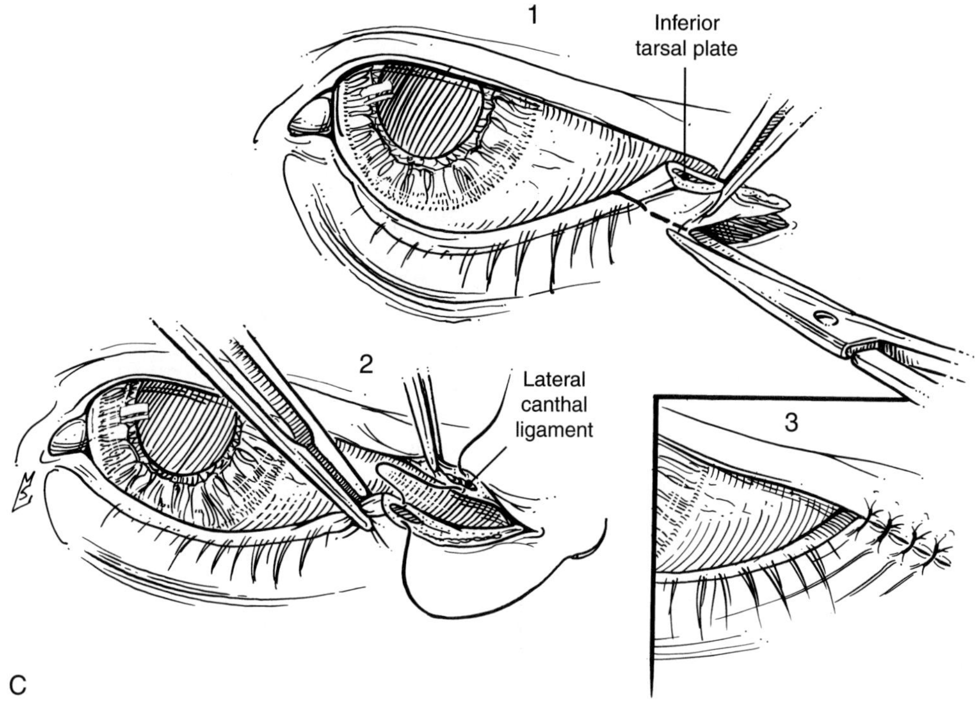

Figure 22–2 *Continued.* C: Lower lid shortening and canthoplasty. Full-thickness wedge resection of the lateral lower lid (1) followed by fixation of the cut margin of the tarsal plate to the lateral canthal tendon (canthoplasty) (2) provides effective functional and cosmetic management of paralytic ectropion of the lower lid.

previous surgery has altered the ear's anatomy. The vertical segment has the most variable path, especially in association with congenital malformations such as canal atresia. The nerve also courses lateral to the tympanic annulus as it approaches the stylomastoid foramen and can therefore be injured in transcanal procedures. In a newborn, the mastoid tip is underdeveloped, which places the styloid process and the adjacent facial nerve more superficially in the neck. The nerve is therefore susceptible to surgical injury in routine postauricular approaches and to compression injuries during forceps delivery. In its extratemporal course, the facial nerve is cushioned by the parotid gland through most of its course. However, the marginal mandibular branch is located in a relatively superficial position just deep to the platysma muscle and is susceptible to injury in trauma or surgery of the jaw and neck. Distortion by tumors of the parotid gland or neck places the extratemporal part of the facial nerve at increased risk of injury during surgery in this region.

Evaluation of Facial Nerve Injury

Facial nerve injury presents with a range of symptoms depending on the severity of dysfunction. In many cases, a patient has become aware of asymmetric movement of the face and a sense of heaviness of the paretic side. Facial dysfunction is visually confirmed by the patient in a mirror or by others. With progressive paresis, the patient notes increasing difficulty in carrying out tasks that depend on normal oral sphincter function, complaining of difficulty articulating plosives and other sounds formed at the lips, leakage of food from the mouth, and frequent biting of the paretic lip during deglutition. The patient is also frustrated by the inability to drink through a straw and may experience symptoms of xerophthalmia and progressive keratopathy, as described in the preceding section of this chapter. The assessment of facial function is nonquantitative and quite subjective. Loss of muscle tone is suggested by the drooping of the brow and oral commissure at rest and by less distinct rhytids, forehead furrows, and nasolabial fold on the paretic side. Muscle tone is particularly well preserved in the young to the degree that the paralyzed face may appear normal at rest. The loss of facial tone often follows the loss of voluntary motor function. Motor function is assessed by asking the patient to grimace, which demonstrates the function of all branches of the facial nerve. The House-

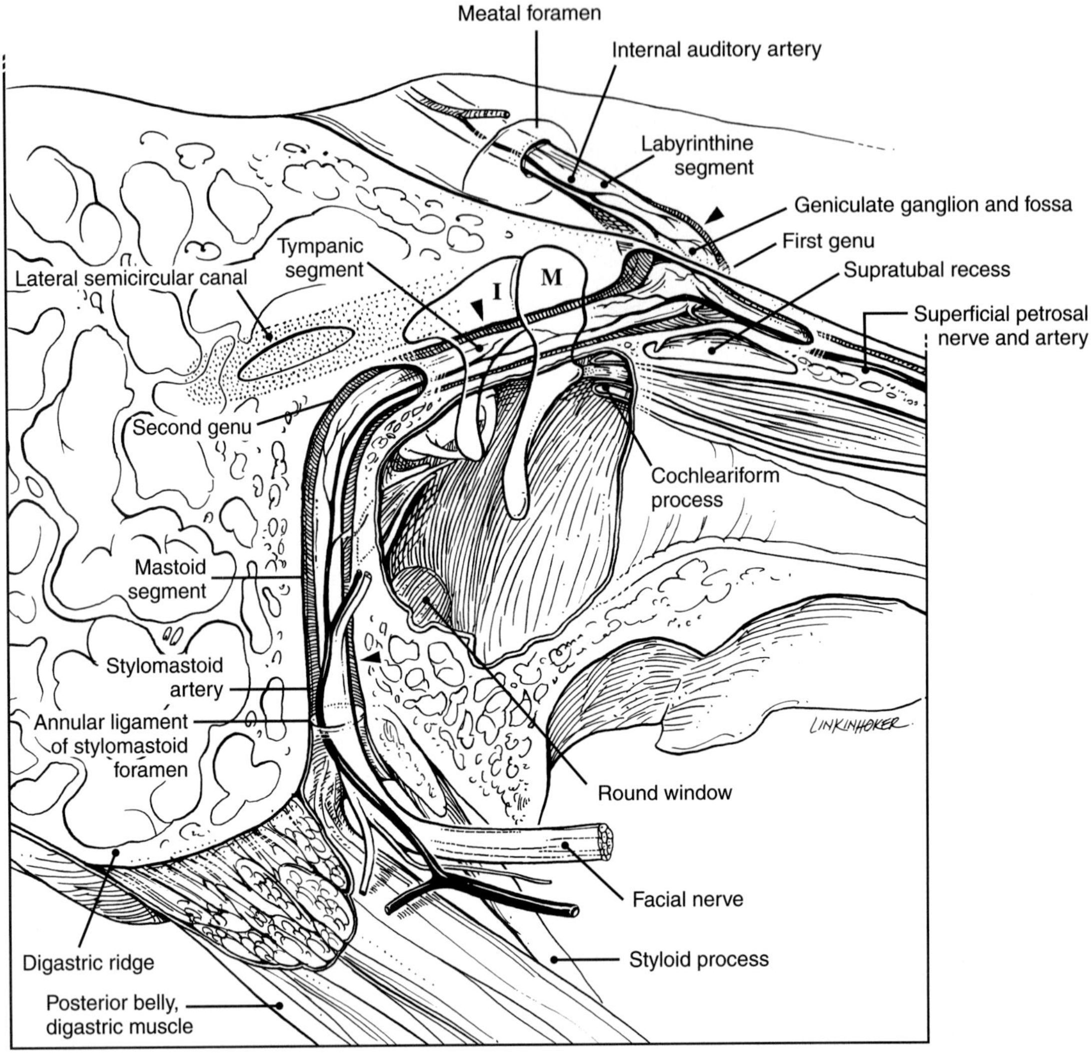

Figure 22–3. The anatomy of the intratemporal portion of the facial nerve and sites of vulnerability to injury (arrowheads). Perigeniculate region: Increased predilection of geniculate fossa to fracture, nerve is susceptible to compression, and ischemia in the narrow meatal foramen and labyrinthine segment. The first genu is tethered by the greater superficial petrosal nerve, increasing susceptibility to shearing injuries. It is also a vascular watershed area of the branches of the external carotid artery and posterior circulation. The geniculate ganglion is susceptible to injury during surgical dissection in the supratubal recess of the anterior epitympanum. Tympanic segment: The nerve is most commonly dehiscent above the oval window; the distal tympanic segment and second genu are susceptible to injury in cholesteatoma surgery as a result of pathological dehiscence or distorted anatomy and failure to identify important surgical landmarks. Mastoid segment: In the lower portion of its vertical course and just distal to the stylomastoid foramen, the nerve is positioned lateral to the tympanic annulus and is therefore susceptible to injury during surgery of the external auditory canal.

Brackmann system of grading facial nerve recovery attempts to standardize the description of facial nerve dysfunction in the nonacute setting (Table 22–1). This grading system is based on an assessment of facial symmetry at rest and in motion, including the ability to close the eye.

This grading system facilitates the monitoring of facial nerve recovery in individuals and the comparison of results across patient groups. However, the determination of prognosis and of appropriate treatment of facial paralysis in the acute setting is based on an estimation of the severity of nerve injury which is determined by history, physical examination, imaging, and electrophysiologic assessment.

Successful reinnervation of facial musculature by regenerating axons is limited by the integrity of the neural connective tissue at the

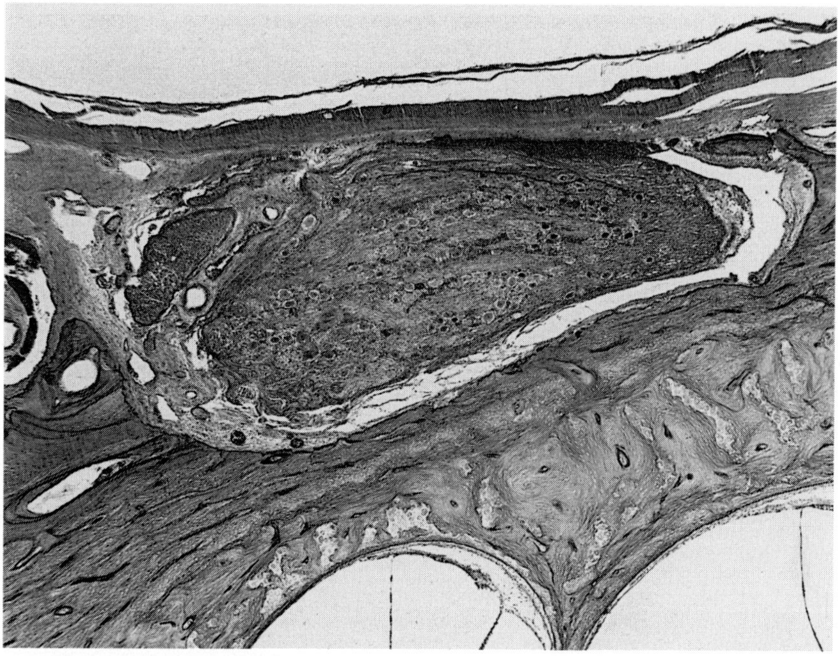

Figure 22–4. A paramodiolar vertical section through the right temporal bone at the level of the geniculate ganglion in an adult. The superior bony wall of the geniculate fossa is dehiscent, exposing the geniculate ganglion, which is firmly attached to the overlying dura mater of the middle cranial fossa (hematoxylin and eosin, original magnification × 50). (From Nager GT. Pathology of the Ear and Temporal Bone. Baltimore, Williams & Wilkins, 1993, p 153.)

site of injury.[9] This connective tissue consists of the endoneurium surrounding each axon, the perineurium surrounding the bundles, or funiculi, of axons providing tensile strength to the nerve, and the epineurium ensheathing the entire nerve trunk and providing collateral circulation to the nerve distal to the geniculate ganglion (Fig. 22–5A). The endoneurium is closely associated with the layer of Schwann cells surrounding each axon. The resulting endoneurial tubule provides passage for regenerating axons to target myocytes. Sunderland and Seddon have proposed grading systems for nerve injury based on the integrity of the axon's and nerve's connective tissue (Fig. 22–5B).[9, 10] According to Sunderland's scheme of neural injury,[9] first-degree injury is a reversible blockade of axoplasmic flow; second-degree injury is the degeneration of axons, with preservation of the endoneurium; third-degree injury occurs when both the endoneurium and the axons are disrupted, leaving the perineurium and epineurium intact. The preservation of endoneurium is most predictive of successful reinnervation of the face. As more of the connective tissue is disrupted, reinnervation becomes increasingly haphazard and compromised. In fourth-degree nerve injury, there is disruption of entire funiculi of nerve fibers, their endoneurial tubules, and the surrounding perineurium, and in fifth-degree injury, the entire nerve trunk, including the epineurium, is interrupted. An estimation of

Table 22–1. *The House-Brackmann Grading System of Facial Nerve Recovery*

	Symmetry at Rest	Eye Closure	Facial Motion
Grade I	Normal	Normal	Normal
Grade II	Symmetric, normal tone	Complete	Slight weakness
Grade III	Symmetric, normal tone	Complete with effort	Slight motion with effort; some synkinesis or spasm
Grade IV	Symmetric, normal tone	Incomplete	Minimal motion with effort
Grade V	Moderate asymmetry, low tone	Incomplete	Barely perceptible
Grade VI	Marked asymmetry, no facial tone	Incomplete	None

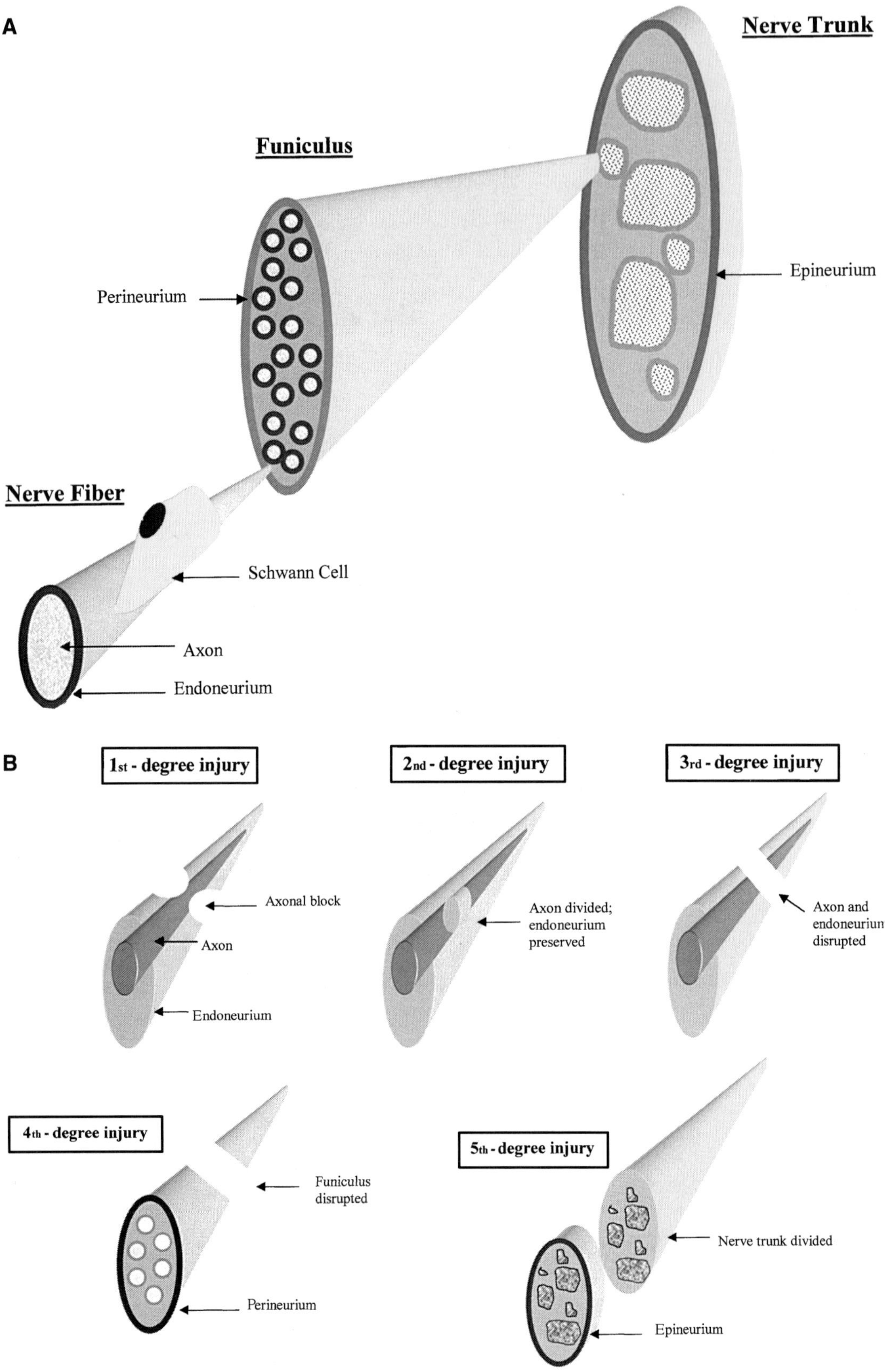

Figure 22–5. **A**: The architecture of the facial nerve and its connective tissue. **B**: The Sunderland grading system of nerve injury.

the extent of nerve injury by history, physical examination, radiologic assessment, and electrophysiologic measurements is also an attempt to determine the extent of connective tissue disruption and therefore the prognosis for effective spontaneous reinnervation of mimetic muscles.

Surgical exploration of the injured nerve is indicated when spontaneous reinnervation of the facial musculature is delayed or judged to be improbable, resulting in long-term abnormal facial movement. The determination of functional prognosis is based on the rate of degeneration and regeneration and on the extent of disruption of the surrounding temporal bone or soft tissue anatomy. Immediate paralysis, for example, is a poor prognostic sign for full spontaneous recovery. The history of posttraumatic facial nerve function from the patient, family, witnesses, and other health care professionals is crucial to clinical judgment in these cases. The physical examination should note the function of all the cranial nerves, signs of temporal bone trauma (including hemotympanum and ecchymoses of the mastoid area), and the nature of soft tissue injuries to the face. Radiologic assessment of the temporal bone can be useful in estimating the location and severity of facial nerve injury associated with temporal bone trauma. The course of the temporal bone fractures and whether or not they are displaced has clinical significance, as is discussed in the later section on temporal bone fractures. The audiologic assessment of the patient is important for the determination of disability and appropriate amplification. The hearing status may also influence the choice of surgical approach.

The degree of facial nerve dysfunction does not correlate well with the extent of nerve injury or distinguish conduction block and axonal disruption, so a variety of diagnostic tests have been proposed to more objectively assess nerve injury. Topognostic tests evaluate the function of motor, sensory, and autonomic branches of the facial nerve in an attempt to determine the site or level of injury. A battery of tests can be used, including Schirmer's test, which evaluates lacrimation and, therefore the function of the GSPN; taste and submandibular salivary flow, which assesses chorda tympani function; and stapedial reflex measurements. The site of injury of the nerve is presumed to be proximal to the dysfunctional nerve branch. However, because topognostic testing has been found to be inconsistent in predicting the site and severity of nerve injury, it has a limited diagnostic role.[11, 12] The serial assessment of muscle innervation using electrophysiology measurements provides some indication of the rate and extent of degeneration after facial movement can no longer be perceived. Unfortunately, the prognostic value of these measurements and their use in clinical decision-making are poorly tested, and the criteria reported in the literature for surgical exploration are highly variable, indicating the lack of agreement in the field. Rarely is surgical intervention needed in the acute phase of trauma. Watchful waiting is appropriate in many cases, with the option of surgical exploration being reserved for cases of obvious severe nerve injury or delayed recovery.

Electrophysiologic Assessment of the Facial Nerve

Electrophysiologic techniques that study the response of the facial muscles to electrical stimulation distal to the site of injury are used to monitor the rate and degree of Wallerian degeneration in the distal segment.[6, 12] These tests differentiate paralysis due to reversible axoplasmic blockade from that due to degeneration of the axon. The amount and rate of decline of the electrophysiologic response of the facial nerve is proportional to the magnitude of nerve disruption and has some prognostic value in the assessment of acute facial nerve paralysis. The nerve is electrically stimulated transcutaneously anterior to the stylomastoid foramen, and the facial muscle response is compared to that of the normal side. Because electrical stimulation of the nerve distal to the site of even the most severe injury elicits a muscle contraction until Wallerian degeneration is complete in 48 to 72 hours, electrical response tests are of limited use until after this time. The nerve excitability test (NET) determines the threshold current for facial movement on the involved as opposed to the normal side[13]; a difference of 3.5 milliamperes or more between the sides is associated with significant injury.[5] The maximal stimulation test (MST) grades the relative strength of contraction of the facial musculature in response to suprathreshold stimulation as being equal, slightly decreased, markedly decreased, or absent. Unlike the NET, the MST monitors denervation as it occurs in the entire nerve, so it has greater prognostic value.[14] Both the NET and the MST have been supplanted by electroneurography (ENoG), otherwise known as evoked electromyography, a modification of the MST that offers a more quantitative and objective assessment of facial denervation.[5, 12]

ENoG records the compound action potential (CAP) generated in mimetic muscles by a suprathreshold stimulus using surface electrodes placed in the nasolabial fold. The peak-to-peak amplitude of the CAP response on the involved side is reported as a percentage of that on the normal side. As the nerve degenerates, serial ENoG demonstrates a proportional decrease in the percent difference of the CAP amplitudes between both sides.[5] The use of the ENoG in clinical decision-making in trauma is based on observations by Fisch that after complete transection of the facial nerve in a human, there is a greater than 90% decrease in the CAP amplitude relative to the normal side within 3 to 5 days.[15, 16] This observation led Fisch to propose that a greater than 90% deterioration of the ENoG response within 6 days after the onset of paralysis is an indication of severe nerve injury that warrants surgical exploration and repair. Daily ENoG measurements are recommended between 3 days and 2 weeks after the onset of facial paralysis to detect the extent and rate of degeneration of the CAP amplitude. A weakness of EnoG is its sensitivity to the technique of test administration and the high variability among testers. ENoG reflects the extent of degeneration within the facial nerve only after Wallerian degeneration has been completed and before regeneration occurs (Fig. 22–6A and B). When facial paralysis occurs either at the time of trauma or in a delayed fashion, the differentiation of nerve blockade from degeneration becomes an important determinant of prognosis and treatment plan. When Wallerian degeneration is complete in a 2nd-degree or more severe injury, the ENoG should demonstrate a proportional decrease in CAP amplitude. The beginning of axonal regeneration is marked by changes in the metabolic status of neurons in the facial motor nucleus at about 3 weeks after injury (see Fig. 22–6A). As the axons of an injured nerve regenerate, their myelin sheaths mature at varying rates, which results in variable current-conducting properties. The absence of synchronous conduction in regenerating and deblocked axons 3 weeks after injury produces variable CAP amplitudes that are of neither diagnostic nor prognostic use.[17]

Electromyography (EMG) without extrinsic electrical stimulation is a useful tool for monitoring regeneration but it has very limited prog-

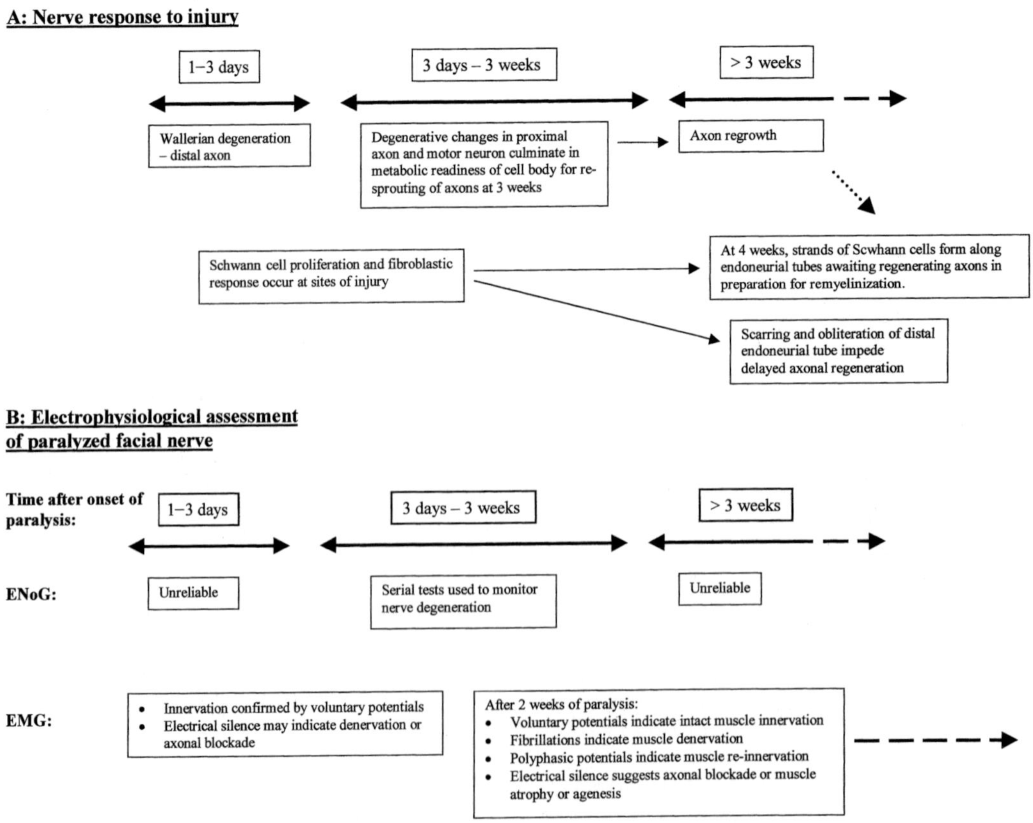

Figure 22–6. A: Nerve degeneration and recovery in response to injury. B: Appropriate timing of electrophysiologic testing during nerve degeneration and recovery.

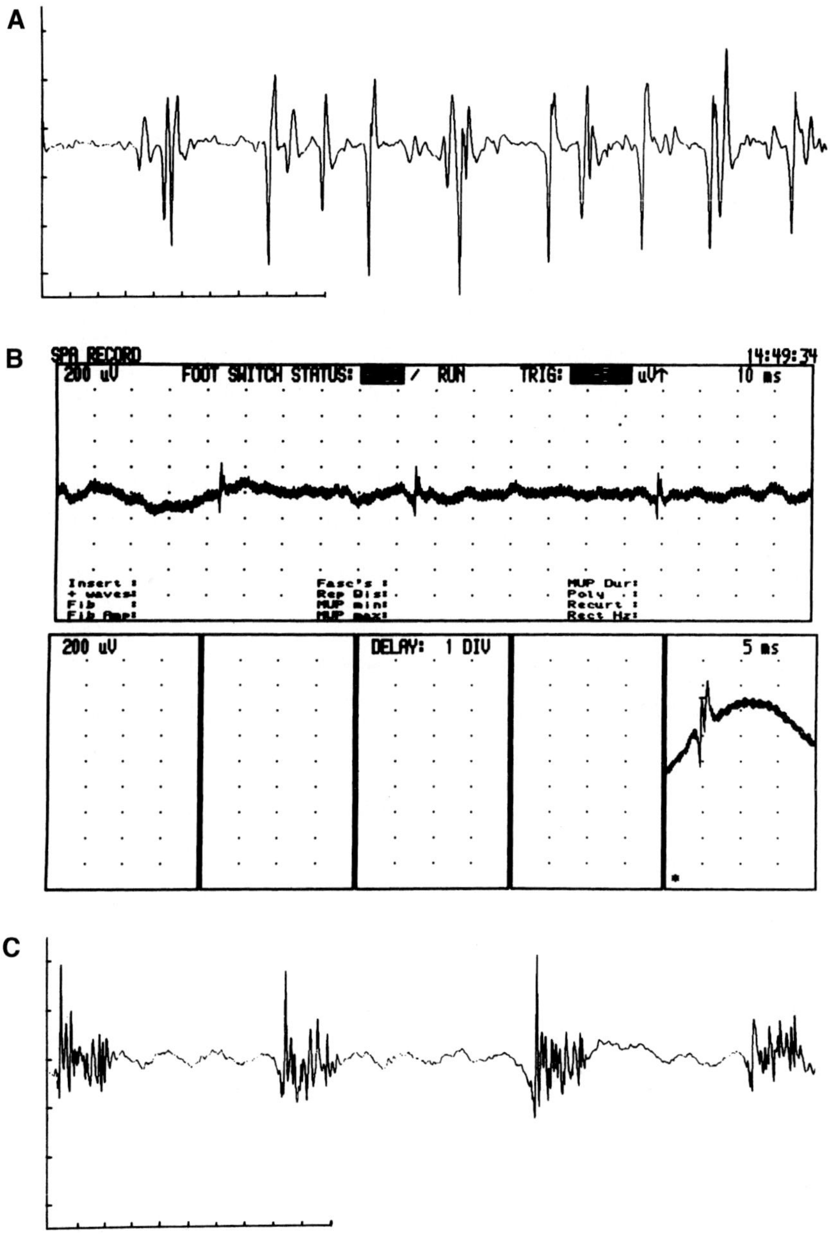

Figure 22–7. Myogenic responses in electromyography. A: Voluntary myogenic response. B: Fibrillation potentials in denervated skeletal muscle. C: Polyphasic potentials in muscle undergoing reinnervation. (From Kokesh J et al. Correlation between stroboscopy and electromyography in laryngeal paralysis. Ann Otol Rhinol Laryngol 1992; 102:852–857.)

nostic value.[6, 12] The EMG records the spontaneous postsynaptic membrane potentials initiated by effort or spontaneously generated in the muscle. These potentials are recorded by electrode needles that are inserted into the muscle. Persistent innervation of facial muscle produces myogenic potentials in response to voluntary effort (Fig. 22–7A). In a paralyzed muscle free of voluntary membrane potentials, nerve degeneration is distinguished from neurapraxia by the presence of low-amplitude, spontaneous potentials or fibrillation potentials in the former (Fig. 22–7B) and electrical silence in the latter. However, fibrillation potentials in a denervated muscle appear only 10 to 14 days after axonal injury (Fig. 22–7B).[9] Therefore, the presence of voluntary motor-unit potentials soon after injury is a good sign of intact innervation, but electrical silence on EMG within the first 10 to 14 days has limited clinical use, as axonal degeneration and nerve blockade cannot be distinguished. Muscle undergoing reinnervation initially demonstrates polyphasic spontaneous potentials (Fig. 22–7C) that eventually evolve into monophasic voluntary potentials. Although polyphasic potentials indicate reinnervation of muscle, the eventual quality of nerve function cannot be predicted. EMG most commonly influences treatment decisions when fibrillation potentials persist several months after injury, indicating severe injury and impaired regrowth of axons to the muscle. This situation may prompt surgical exploration and repair of the nerve or reanimation of the face by means of a variety of procedures.

Treatment

GLUCOCORTICOID THERAPY

Glucocorticoid steroids are used to treat a wide variety of inflammatory and traumatic disorders in the central and peripheral nervous system. They inhibit the inflammatory response in host tissues through their effects on immune cells, vascular tone and permeability, and mechanisms of free-radical injury. However, glucocorticoid steroids have not been shown to influence the functional outcome of peripheral nerve recovery. Despite the lack of convincing evidence for benefit, steroids are commonly used in the acute phase of facial paralysis, especially when injury is likely to exist intratemporally. By minimizing nerve edema, glucocorticoid steroids theoretically decrease axonal loss resulting from nerve compression by the bony canal. Glucocorticoid steroids are less likely to be beneficial in extracranial injuries of the nerve and are not indicated in the management of facial dysfunction resulting from acute suppurative infections of the temporal bone. Prednisone (1 mg/kg/day) is administered orally in two to three divided doses for 7 to 10 days, followed by a taper to zero over 10 days.[12] The use of steroids is contraindicated in a patient with a history of peptic ulcer disease or untreated tuberculosis and should be avoided during pregnancy. They should be given concurrently with H_2 blockers in all patients. Diabetes and hypertension may be exacerbated by steroid therapy. A patient with either or both of these disorders may therefore be a poor candidate for steroid therapy or may have to be hospitalized for close monitoring. Dexamethasone is a good alternative to prednisone because of its strong anti-inflammatory effects, low mineralocorticoid effects, and rapid onset.

SURGICAL THERAPY

The aim of surgical therapy is to decompress, assess, and repair the nerve. Unroofing the bony fallopian canal allows the nerve to be partially decompressed and directly examined. Impingements on nerve regeneration such as bone fragments and intraneural hematomas can be removed, and anatomic continuity can be reestablished by primary anastomosis or interposition grafting. Segments of the nerve may be examined selectively, or if the site of injury is unknown, the nerve may be explored from the meatal foramen to the terminal branches in the face. In the setting of nerve trauma, the nerve sheath should be opened to provide better visualization of the nerve and to provide maximal decompression. The transected or severely attenuated nerve should be prepared for neurorrhaphy using epineurial sutures. Tension at the anastomosis must be avoided to minimize fibrous ingrowth, which obstructs axon regeneration. After debridement of the cut ends of the nerve, mobilization of proximal and distal segments with and without rerouting decreases the resulting gap and may obviate the need for a nerve graft which may be associated with less effective regeneration than primary anastomosis. Nerve rerouting may provide as much as an additional centimeter of length.[18] A cable graft should be reserved for a case in which there is tension at the anastomotic site despite mobilization and rerouting of the nerve.

An interposition graft is usually needed if the gap between the endings of the unmobilized nerve exceeds 0.5 to 1.0 cm. The greater auricular nerve is the most convenient source of nerve graft. It provides up to 10 cm of nerve if harvested in its entirety from the cervical plexus deep to the posterior border of the sternocleidomastoid muscle at Erb's point to its terminal branches in the tail of the parotid and inferior to the auricle (Fig. 22–8A). The sural nerve provides as much as 30 cm of nerve length. It is found just posterior to the lateral malleolus of the ankle (Fig. 22–8B) and can be harvested by means of multiple small transverse incisions in the leg. Cable grafts should be reversed so that the distal end is sutured to the proximal segment of the transected nerve. This ensures that the regenerating axons are not diverted away from the distal segment of nerve by branches of the graft. However, branches can be advantageous when grafting the proximal trunk to multiple branches of the pes anserinus. The approximated nerve ends are stabilized with interrupted 9-0 nylon placed in the epineurium.

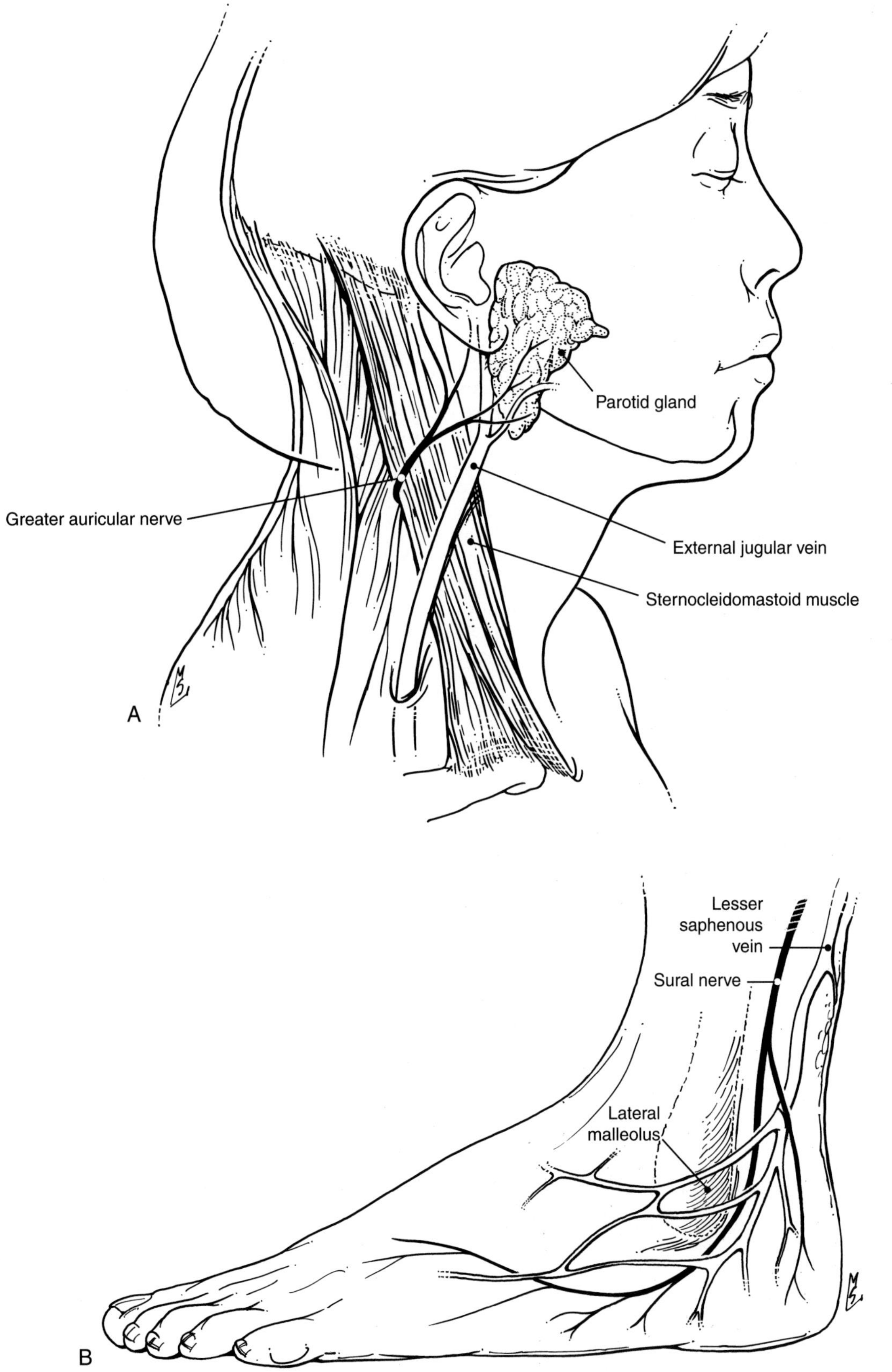

Figure 22–8. A: The greater auricular nerve emerges from the posterior border of the sternocleidomastoid muscle and courses toward the ear, sending branches to the parotid tail and the postauricular region. B: The sural nerve courses behind the lateral malleolus adjacent to the lesser saphenous vein and provides a lengthy graft for facial nerve repair.

The choice of surgical approach depends on the suspected sites of injury and the serviceability of residual hearing. Nerve injuries distal to the stylomastoid foramen (SMF) require the standard parotidectomy approach to the facial nerve.[19] The landmarks of the main trunk of the facial nerve just distal to the SMF include the posterior belly of the digastric muscle as it inserts into the tip of the mastoid, the tragal pointer, and the tympanomastoid suture line. The nerve is located just medial and anterior to the digastric muscle near its insertion into the mastoid tip. It can also be found approximately 1 cm inferior and medial to the cartilaginous tragal pointer, almost colinear with the tympanomastoid suture line.

If the anatomy is distorted by trauma such as a blast injury, the proximal end of the nerve can be found in the mastoid using standard landmarks (see the subsequent section), and the distal end can be identified by retrograde dissection of distal branches of the pes anserinus. If possible, it is advantageous to perform the surgical exploration within 3 days of injury when nerve branches distal to the site of injury still elicit muscle movement and action potentials on electrical stimulation. The marginal mandibular branch is usually the easiest branch to find. It can be found as it crosses the lateral surface of the posterior facial vein within the parotid gland.[20] The vein is found in the neck and followed cephalad into the parotid gland where it intersects with the nerve. The branch can then be followed proximally to the main trunk. The buccal branch can be found running parallel to and 1 cm below the zygomatic arch and just inferior to Stenson's duct.[19] Once identified and debrided, the cut ends of the nerve can be brought closer together by dissecting the proximal and distal segments from the surrounding parotid tissue. A superficial parotidectomy followed by dissection of the nerve from the deep lobe provides additional length to the distal nerve segment, possibly making an interposition graft unnecessary.[21] Additional length in the proximal segment may also be acquired by decompressing and rerouting the mastoid segment.

The intratemporal portion of the facial nerve distal to the geniculate ganglion is best approached by a canal-wall-intact mastoidectomy.[18] Access to the tympanic segment of the nerve can be optimized for nerve repair by enlarging the aditus ad antrum laterally and removing the incus to be replaced by a partial ossicular reconstruction prosthesis. Decompression and rerouting of the nerve distal to the geniculate ganglion also requires an extended facial recess. Extension of the facial recess into the tympanic bone inferior to the external auditory canal provides a shortcut for the facial nerve between the mastoid segment and the pes anserinus, bypassing the SMF. Up to 1 cm of additional length can be achieved by rerouting the facial nerve distal to the geniculate ganglion, bypassing both the second genu and the SMF.

The approach to the facial nerve proximal to the geniculate ganglion is dictated by hearing status.[18] If hearing is not serviceable, the translabyrinthine approach provides the most direct access to the nerve throughout its intratemporal course (Fig. 22–9).[22] Additional length can be

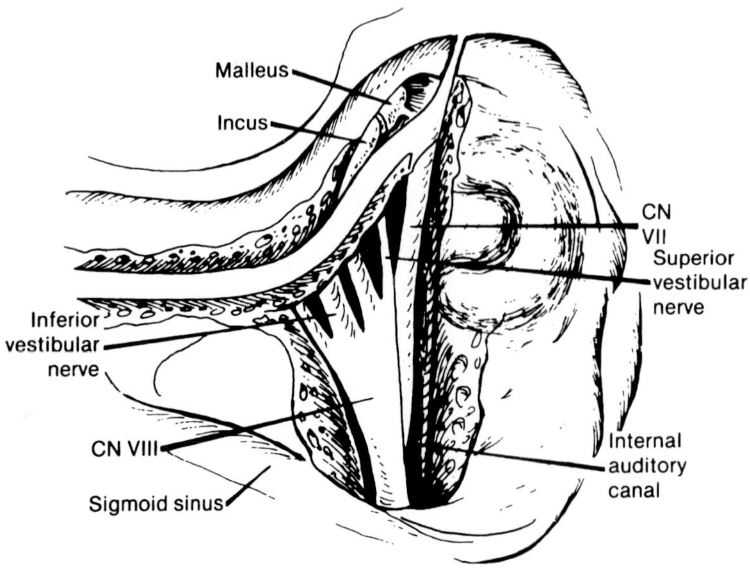

Figure 22–9. The translabyrinthine approach provides access to all intratemporal segments of the facial nerve. (From Cummings CW et al., eds. Otolaryngology Head and Neck Surgery, 3rd ed. St. Louis, Mosby, 1998, p 2796.)

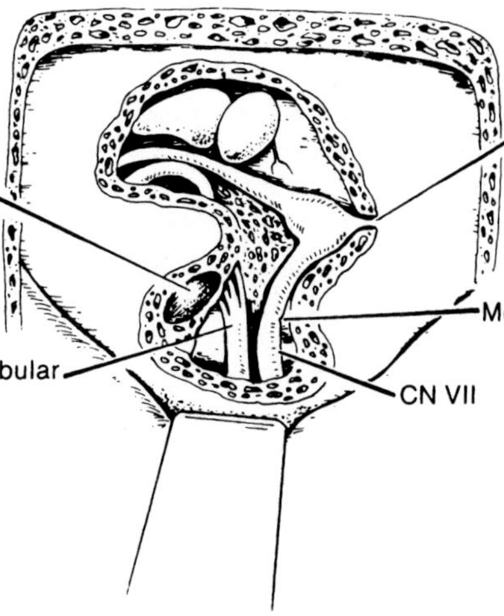

Figure 22–10. The middle fossa approach to the temporal bone spares hearing while providing access to the labyrinthine segment of the facial nerve. (From Cummings CW et al., eds. Otolaryngology Head and Neck Surgery, 3rd ed. St. Louis, Mosby, 1998, p 2792.)

obtained by sectioning the GSPN and rerouting the tympanic and labyrinthine segments posteriorly, bypassing the first genu. When hearing is to be preserved, a transmastoid extralabyrinthine approach or middle fossa craniotomy approach (Fig. 22–10)[23] can be used. In the transmastoid extralabyrinthine approach the vestibular labyrinth and, in particular, the ampulla of the superior semicircular canal obstruct access to the entire labyrinthine segment in many patients, which limits the utility of this approach in the repair of injuries proximal to the geniculate ganglion.[12, 19] The middle fossa approach provides better access to the facial nerve proximal to the geniculate ganglion. However, access to the tympanic and mastoid segments require a separate postauricular incision. To avoid nerve grafting, the labyrinthine segment can be rerouted posteriorly, after sectioning the GSPN or excising the geniculate ganglion, and anastomosed with the tympanic segment through an opening created in the tegmen mastoidium.[24]

TRAUMA OF THE INTRATEMPORAL PORTION OF THE FACIAL NERVE

Temporal Bone Fractures

A high-energy blow to the skull may fracture the temporal bone, injuring the ossicular chain, the inner ear, and the facial nerve. Whereas temporal bone fractures have traditionally been categorized as longitudinal or transverse, many fractures are a combination of both types. Most fractures are predominantly longitudinal, following the path of least resistance along the petrosquamous suture line from lateral to medial and then along the lateral and anterior margins of the otic capsule at the interface of dense and porous bone in the petrous apex. These fractures often involve the middle ear structures and result in conductive hearing loss due to ossicular chain disruption and hemotympanum. A forceful blow to the occiput may produce a transverse fracture that courses anteroposteriorly through the dense petrous bone, including the otic capsule and internal auditory canal. Transverse fractures occur about one third as often as longitudinal fractures. Because of the force required to produce them, there is a high incidence of associated intracranial complications. Profound unilateral sensorineural hearing loss, vestibular paresis, and facial nerve injury are prevalent sequelae of transverse fractures. Although approximately 50% of transverse fractures result in facial nerve dysfunction, as compared to 20% of longitudinal fractures, facial nerve injuries due to blunt trauma are more likely to be associated with longitudinal fractures because of their greater prevalence.

MECHANISMS OF NERVE INJURY

The geniculate ganglion and adjacent portions of the labyrinthine and tympanic segments are the predominant sites of injury in facial nerve paralysis associated with longitudinal fractures.[12, 25, 26] Perigeniculate injuries account for

80% to 100% of cases, whereas isolated injury to the mastoid segment is infrequent, accounting for less than 16% of cases.[26] The facial nerve is at increased risk in the geniculate region because of special anatomic features of the nerve and fallopian canal at the first genu. First, the thin and sometimes dehiscent bone that surrounds the geniculate ganglion stands in contrast to the hard bone of the adjacent otic capsule. Mechanical forces are readily deflected around the otic capsule and through the region of the geniculate ganglion along the path of least resistance (Fig. 22–11).[8, 15, 26, 27] A 20% incidence of dehiscence of the bony canal surrounding the geniculate ganglion further increases the susceptibility of this region to fracture (see Fig. 22–4).[7, 8] Traction injury often occurs in the region of the geniculate ganglion where the nerve is tethered anteriorly by the GSPN. Because of the transient distortions of the fallopian canal in this region during fracturing and the rapid acceleration-deceleration of the nerve, the nerve and its blood supply may be subject to disruptive shearing forces (Fig. 22–12).

Observations made during surgery provide some clues about the mechanisms of facial nerve injury associated with temporal bone fractures. Surgical decompression of the facial nerve in cases of longitudinal temporal bone fracture have revealed nerve edema, intraneural hematoma with and without associated fracture of the fallopian canal, impingement on the nerve by bone fragments, and nerve transection.[15, 25, 26] There are, therefore, at least two primary mechanisms by which the facial nerve is injured in the region of the geniculate ganglion: (1) distortion and comminution of the bony fallopian canal, which leads to direct injury, including contusion, impingement, or transection, and (2) traction injury at the second genu, which leads to the shearing of axons and disruption of the microvasculature. Immediate paralysis is most likely to occur in the setting of severe nerve injury associated with a displaced or comminuted fracture that compresses or transects the nerve. Progressive facial dysfunction may occur when nerve edema resulting from contusion or traction injuries extends to the adjacent labyrinthine segment where compression by the narrow bony canal incites a cycle of vascular compromise and increasing nerve impairment. Disruption of arterioles in the geniculate ganglion that originates from petrosal branches of the middle meningeal artery may lead to the gradual accumulation of an intraneural hematoma and delayed paralysis. Fisch has hypothesized that intraneural hematoma in the geniculate ganglion produces scarring at the facial hiatus that obstructs the path of regenerating motor fibers, diverting them instead along the GSPN.[15]

Surgical cases of facial nerve paralysis associated with transverse temporal bone fractures

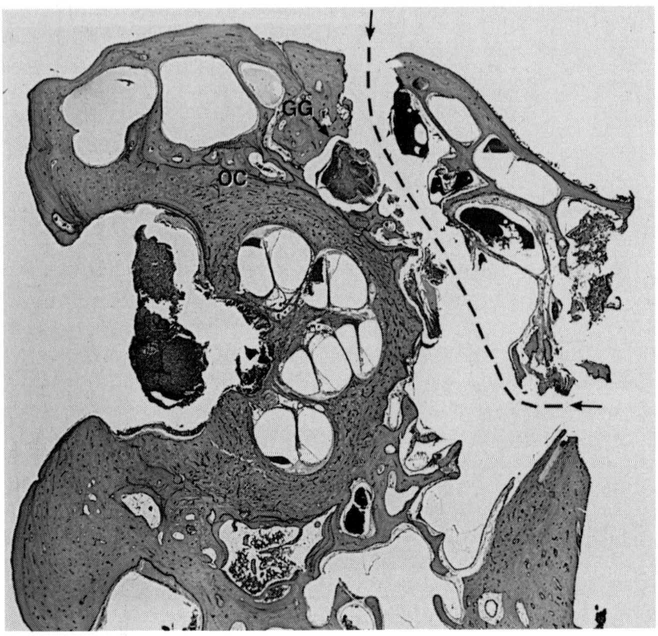

Figure 22–11. Vertical sections through the left temporal bone of an 18-year-old patient who suffered a longitudinal fracture. The fracture line (arrows) courses through the geniculate fossa, containing the geniculate ganglion (GG) and sparing the otic capsule (OC). (From Nager GT. Pathology of the Ear and Temporal Bone. Baltimore, Williams & Wilkins, 1993, p 1283.)

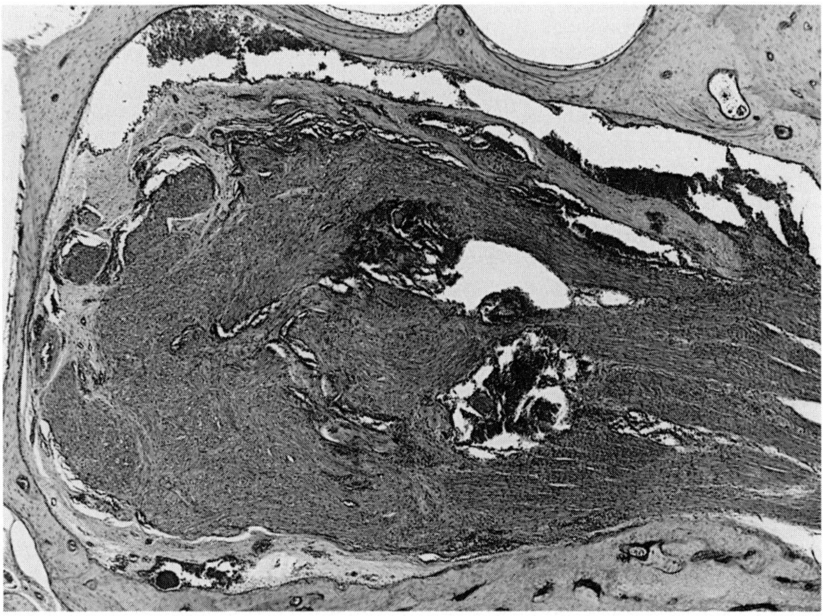

Figure 22–12. The right temporal bone in the same patient as in Figure 22–11. A vertical section through the geniculate ganglion shows many tears and intraneural hemorrhages despite an intact fallopian canal. (From Nager GT. Pathology of the Ear and Temporal Bone. Baltimore, Williams & Wilkins, 1993, p 1281.)

demonstrate transection of the facial nerve in its labyrinthine and meatal segments.[15] Because of the narrow diameter of the bony canal, even minimally displaced fractures are likely to cause severe injuries to the labyrinthine and meatal segments of the nerve. The fallopian canal in this region does not accommodate the edematous nerve as it enlarges, causing increasing compression and vascular compromise (see Fig. 22–3). The absence of an epineurium and its network of vessels also places the nerve at increased risk for injury from mechanical and ischemic insults. Terminal vessels that originate at the external carotid artery and vertebrobasilar systems interface in this region of the facial nerve, forming a vascular watershed that may further increase the risk for ischemia.

EVALUATION AND PRIORITIES

A fracture of the skull base should be suspected in any patient who has a history of severe head trauma and loss of consciousness or who presents with cranial nerve deficits, cerebrospinal fluid otorrhea or rhinorrhea, hemotympanum, or ecchymosis of the mastoid or periorbital regions. A temporal bone fracture, particularly the transverse type, indicates a high-energy impact to the head, which is likely to be associated with intracranial injuries. The identification of asymmetric facial function is therefore often delayed by the absence of spontaneous movements by these often unconscious patients and the immediate concerns of life-threatening injuries. When facial paralysis is noted, a concerted effort should be made to determine whether nerve dysfunction was immediate or delayed. This information can be garnered from medical records and interviews with the nurses and physicians involved in the care of the patient since admission as well as with any witnesses to the injury. Computed tomography (CT) scans of the brain and skull base are important studies in the evaluation of any patient who presents as described. The temporal bone CT scan is particularly helpful in determining the type and severity of the fracture and may influence the decision to explore the nerve when paralysis is associated with radiologic findings consistent with a transverse fracture. However, CT scans are of limited help in predicting the severity of nerve injury in longitudinal fractures. Topognostic testing such as Schirmer's test of lacrimation correlates poorly with the location of nerve injury in temporal bone trauma and is therefore rarely indicated. Auditory function, as measured by routine audiometry, is an important part of the overall assessment of disability resulting from head trauma and is a necessary component of the preoperative evaluation to determine whether a hearing-preservation approach to the labyrinthine and meatal segments of the nerve is indicated.

The clinical priorities in treating a patient with facial nerve paralysis due to temporal bone fracture were discussed at the beginning of the chapter. Because of the high prevalence of injury in the perigeniculate region, the risk of keratopathy is significantly greater because of decreased lacrimation resulting from compromise of the GSPN. The choice of treatment of the facial nerve injury depends on the severity of the injury. Corticosteroids decrease neural edema and theoretically slow the progression of vascular compromise that results from increasing compression of the swollen nerve by the fallopian canal in the labyrinthine segment. Although their impact on functional outcomes has not been adequately tested in cases of temporal bone fractures, corticosteroids are widely used in the immediate posttrauma period and tapered over days to weeks (see the earlier section that discusses glucocorticoid therapy).

In some cases, surgical intervention may significantly improve the functional outcome by retarding degeneration or by removing impedance to regeneration. Criteria for performing surgical intervention have been poorly tested, so they are useful only as guidelines to be applied on a case-by-case basis. Degeneration criteria for early surgical treatment are based on the premise that a patient with a severe injury such as nerve transection or impingement by a bone fragment presents with immediate paralysis and rapid decline in the amplitude of myogenic responses on ENoG testing.[15, 26] A patient with nerve injury resulting in delayed paralysis due to ongoing compromise such as intraneural hematoma or progressive nerve edema with strangulation may also show rapid deterioration of ENoG responses after the onset of paralysis, indicating the need for surgical treatment. The regeneration criterion for delayed exploration is simply the failure of reinnervation to take place within several months after trauma, as indicated by the persistence of fibrillation potentials and the absence of polyphasic potentials on EMG.[15, 26] The electrophysiologic criteria for surgical exploration of the nerve in temporal bone fractures were proposed by Fisch and were based on his observations that after surgical transection of the facial nerve, serial ENoGs reveal a 90% decline of the myogenic potential amplitudes within 3 to 5 days.[15, 16] He observed that in addition to the rate of decline, the endpoint of degeneration was also predictive of functional outcome. Independent of the rate of decline, when the amplitudes of the evoked responses fall more than 95% compared to the intact side, the outcome is universally poor, whereas a less than 90% fall in responses usually results in good function. Fisch has proposed that a greater than 90% decline in the EnoG response within 6 days of the onset of paralysis is evidence of severe nerve injury and is thus an indication for early surgical exploration of the nerve. The absence of regeneration within 6 months of injury has been proposed as an indication for delayed intervention.

The predictive value of these guidelines for the appropriate selection of cases amenable to surgical repair is inconsistent. In a surgical series of 40 patients with facial paralysis due to temporal bone fractures, who were selected using the degeneration and regeneration criteria described, Fisch reported a false-positive rate of 7%, the remaining 93% having significant nerve injuries, including intraneural hematoma (50%), nerve transection (26%), and impingement by bone fragments (17%).[15] Lambert and Brackmann reported a retrospective series of 26 patients with facial paralysis associated with longitudinal temporal bone fractures who were selected using the same regeneration criteria. However, their degeneration criteria were limited to the absence of response on MST testing or a greater than 90% decline in response amplitudes on ENoG testing over an unspecified period of time.[26] In patients who underwent surgery based on these degeneration criteria, findings included impingement by bone fragments (45%), perigeniculate edema without fallopian canal fracture (36%), transection (9%), and intraneural hematoma (9%). In all four patients with delayed regeneration, the nerve was found to have been transected. Coker and colleagues explored patients who demonstrated an increase in NET threshold of 3.5 mA or greater, or more than a 90% decline in myogenic responses on EnoG testing over an unspecified period of time.[25] Findings included intraneural hemorrhage (40%), bony fragment impingement (33%), and neural edema (93%). Because of the retrospective nature of these series and the lack of long-term results, the influence of early surgical intervention on the final functional outcome cannot easily be separated from the natural history of the disease process.

Stringent criteria for surgical exploration of the facial nerve in temporal bone fractures should be observed to ensure that the surgical risks of further nerve injury are outweighed by the benefit of improved nerve function. The absence of regeneration, and persistent fibrillation potentials on EMG after 6 or more months of paralysis, and the presence of a transverse fracture, as viewed on a CT scan, are predictive of severe nerve injury that may benefit from surgical treatment.[15, 16] Both the rate and the magnitude of decline of the ENoG response should be taken into consideration, as false-positive rates appear to be higher when only the magnitude or only the quality of the response is considered. Serial EnoG testing should begin on the third day of paralysis even when it has a delayed onset. A degeneration of more than 90% of the EnoG response within 6 days of onset of paralysis is likely to yield the lowest false-positive rate.[15] However, further clinical studies are needed to confirm the soundness of this criterion and its clinical outcomes.

The timing of intervention is controversial.[26] Early surgery avoids troublesome bleeding associated with granulation tissue, which is greatest at 2 to 4 weeks posttrauma. However, delayed surgery allows granulation tissue to resolve and may increase the chance of successful regeneration by coinciding nerve repair with the peak of metabolic readiness of neurons in the facial nerve nucleus for regeneration.[28] However, there appears to be a finite window of opportunity beyond which surgical repair is ineffective. The diminishing effectiveness of repair that is observed after 1 to 2 years of paralysis may result from the progressive scarring and obliteration of endoneural tubules distal to the site of injury (see Fig. 22–6A).[29]

Because of the prevalence of perigeniculate injury in temporal bone fractures, this region must be decompressed, examined, and repaired in all such cases. However, the coincidence of injuries to the perigeniculate and mastoid segments in up to 20% of cases and the occasional isolated injury at sites other than the geniculate region necessitate the exploration of the entire intratemporal course of the facial nerve.[26] The facial nerve can be decompressed from the SMF to the geniculate ganglion using a transmastoid approach with facial recess. The surgical approach to the labyrinthine and meatal segments depends on hearing status. A translabyrinthine approach (see Fig. 22–9) is ideal in patients with nonserviceable hearing, as it provides access to the facial nerve from the internal auditory canal to the SMF. The middle fossa approach (see Fig. 22–10) provides access to the geniculate ganglion and labyrinthine segment while preserving inner ear function in hearing individuals.

The nerve sheath should be incised from the meatal foramen to the tympanic segment, as well as proximal and distal to any other site where the fallopian canal is fractured or the nerve appears to be traumatized. If the nerve is intact and free of hematoma, nothing further need be done. Bone fragments impinging on the nerve should be removed. Intraneural hematomas at the geniculate ganglion should be evacuated. The transected nerve must be reanastomosed by first mobilizing the cut ends of the nerve. When transection occurs in the perigeniculate area, the second genu can be mobilized posteriorly by sectioning the GSPN and excising the geniculate ganglion, and the tympanic segment can be mobilized superiorly to permit a primary end-to-end anastomosis (see the earlier section that discusses surgical therapy).[15] Varying degrees of mobilization may be performed to decrease the tension of the anastomosis at more distal sites. When the distance between the ends of viable residual nerve is greater than 1 cm, interposition nerve grafting is likely to be necessary.

Blast Injuries of the Temporal Bone

The petrous portion of the temporal bone is very effective in shielding the central nervous system against high-velocity missiles. Bullets directed at the infraorbital region anteriorly and the infratemporal region laterally are most likely to encounter the temporal bone to which most of the kinetic energy is transferred.[30] Labyrinthine, middle ear, and facial nerve injuries and local wound complications are common sequelae. Involvement of the external auditory canal and mastoid are common, leading to canal stenosis, cholesteatoma, and chronic infection. Cases of tympanic membrane perforation and ossicular chain trauma frequently result in conductive hearing loss, and otic capsule fracture and transmission of blast energy to the cochlea produce permanent sensorineural deafness. Significant morbidity and mortality may also result from internal carotid artery injuries (Fig. 22–13), dural injuries complicated by leakage of cerebrospinal fluid, meningitis, and brain trauma.[30] Mechanisms of injury include disruption as a result of direct impact of the missile and its fragments and the transmission of a high-energy blast wave that causes fractures, ossiclar disarticulation, and soft tissue disruption beyond the site of penetration by the missile.[31]

As many as half of victims of temporal bone blast injuries experience facial nerve paralysis.[30]

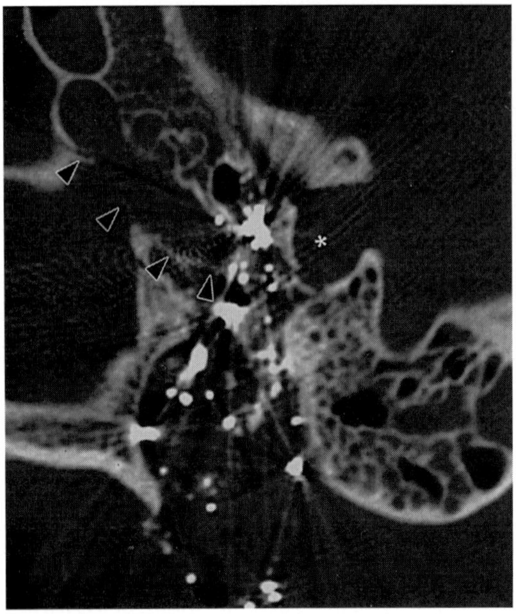

Figure 22–13. Axial CT scan of the right temporal bone in a gunshot victim. The petrous portion of the internal carotid artery is outlined by arrowheads, and the jugular bulb is indicated by an asterisk. A vascular injury is suggested by the proximity of bullet fragments to both structures.

In most cases, facial nerve dysfunction has an immediate onset. The tympanic and mastoid segments are common sites of injury (Fig. 22–14). The extent of nerve injury may include contusions due to blast wave effects, partial or complete transection associated with temporal bone fracture involving the fallopian canal, and avulsion of segments of the nerve due to violation of the canal by the missile.

The victim of a gun blast must be systematically evaluated and treated as proposed by the Advanced Trauma Life Support guidelines.[1] Other sites of injury must be sought, especially on the posterior surfaces of the body, as a delay in their identification and treatment can be life threatening. A thorough neurologic evaluation is an essential part of the workup. Vascular and central nervous system injuries must be ruled out using arteriography and CT scans of the head that encompass the brain, skull base, and neck. Eye care and prevention of corneal injury is a priority. Emergent surgery of the temporal bone is indicated only when the internal carotid artery is injured in its intratemporal course and skull base disruption results in brain herniation or injury. Other sequelae of blast trauma, including leakage of cerebrospinal fluid, conductive hearing loss, and facial nerve injury, can be treated conservatively at first, followed by elective surgical repair. CT scans are of limited use in demonstrating the site or severity of facial nerve injury except when a transverse fracture is identified, indicating the need to extend a planned exploration of the facial nerve to include the labyrinthine segment, a probable site of injury. CT scans are also useful in assessing the integrity of the tegmen and posterior fossa dural plate, the external auditory canal, and the mastoid air cells so that the simultaneous repair of other injuries can be planned.

Immediate paralysis is an indication of severe facial nerve injury in need of surgical repair. Early surgical intervention may be prompted by a high index of suspicion and the desire to use electrical stimulation to find the distal extratemporal branches. The tendency of blast injuries to produce Sunderland's grade 2 to grade 4 injuries along extended segments of nerve often leads to a rapid deterioration of the EnoG signal that mimics nerve transection, or grade 5 injury.[31] Therefore, the value of ENoG testing in monitoring nerve degeneration resulting from gun blasts is in question. Multiple sites of facial nerve injury should be anticipated and require decompression and exploration of the nerve from the geniculate ganglion to the pes anserinus. A cable nerve graft is likely to be necessary because blast injuries usually devitalize long segments of nerve. Standard transmastoid surgery usually provides sufficient access to the nerve in these cases. In the absence of temporal bone fractures, nerve injury proximal to the geniculate ganglion is unlikely. However, the labyrinthine segment should be explored when CT scans demonstrate a transverse fracture or a severe comminution or displaced longitudinal fracture. Audiometric assessment is an important determinant of the appropriate surgical approach to the labyrinthine segment, as previously noted.

By opening the bony canal and incising the nerve sheath, the facial nerve is maximally decompressed. Once exposed in this way, the nerve can also be carefully examined for partial or complete transection and intraneural hematoma. The presence of an intact nerve sheath after a blast injury to the temporal bone does not exclude the possibility of a disrupted nerve trunk within it as a result of the effects of the high-energy blast wave.[31] However, indications for excision and repair of severely contused but anatomically intact segments of blast-injured nerve have not been established, nor have the outcomes of such interventions been compared to spontaneous recovery.

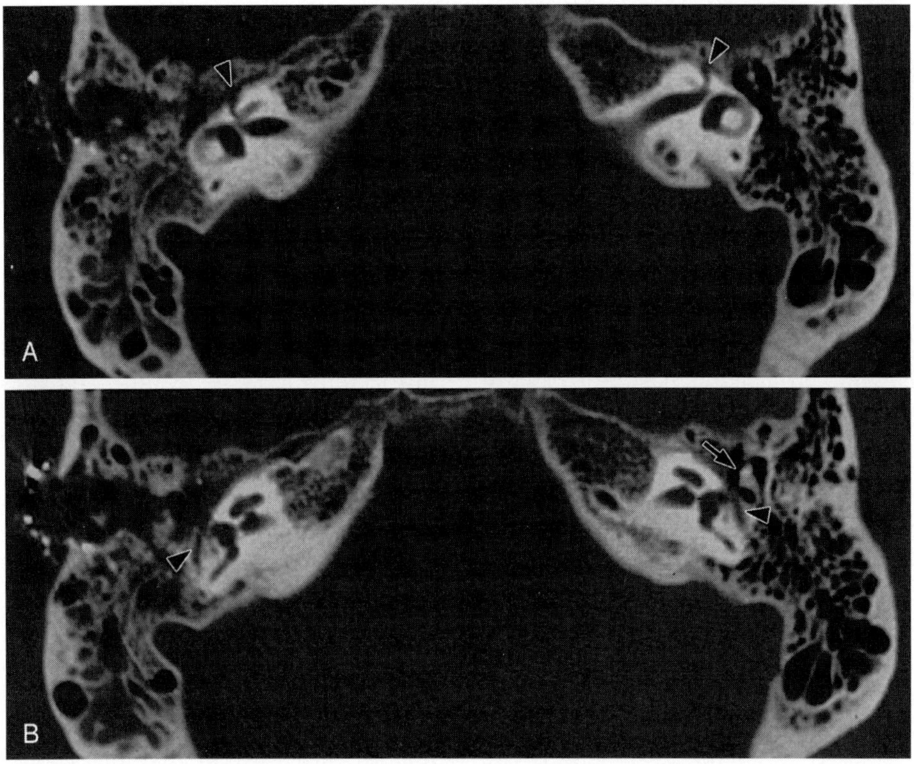

Figure 22–14. Axial CT scan of the temporal bone in a gunshot victim with right facial paralysis. A: The loss of bone separating the geniculate fossa (arrowhead) from the anterior attic in the right ear corresponds to the site of facial nerve injury identified at surgery. B: In this more inferior section ossicles are seen in the attic on the left side (arrow) but not on the right. The distal horizontal segment of the facial canal (arrowhead) appears to be intact.

TRAUMA TO THE EXTRATEMPORAL PORTION OF THE FACIAL NERVE

Significant and permanent facial nerve dysfunction resulting from blunt trauma is less frequent when the extratemporal portion of the nerve is affected. However, the nerve is much less well protected from penetrating trauma distal to the SMF. Nerve transection associated with stab wounds in the face produce immediate paralysis of the corresponding facial muscles. Whereas injuries to the proximal nerve trunk result in complete hemiparesis of the face and increased synkinesis, more distal sites of injury tend to produce segmental paralysis and better functional outcome. When the nerve is injured at or medial to the lateral canthus and the oral commissure, the results of surgical repair and spontaneous recovery are equivalent, and surgery is not indicated. However, it should be noted that nerve trauma sustained in a blast injury to the face is more complicated than that resulting from a knife injury. In addition to disruption of the nerve by the bullet and its fragments, the high-energy blast wave that spreads through the tissue produces thermal and mechanical trauma that extends beyond the path of penetration by the missile.[31] Significant nerve injury may therefore exist despite anatomic continuity and may produce immediate paralysis and diminished electrical responses.

A high index of clinical suspicion is an important determinant of whether to surgically explore a facial wound for nerve injury. Electrophysiologic monitoring of nerve degeneration is not as reliable in the evaluation of extratemporal injuries because nerve stimulation occurs proximal to the site of nerve injury. The immediate onset of complete facial palsy after a penetrating injury is very suggestive of nerve transection. Within the first 3 days after injury, before Wallerian degeneration is complete, the electrical stimulation of the nerve distal to the site of injury elicits facial movement or a response on EMG, which can facilitate its identification in surgery. Timely exploration therefore increases the likelihood that the transected ends can be found and reapproximated. Anastomosis should be tension-free and stabilized with epineurial sutures. The surgical management of the nerve is discussed in the section on surgical therapy. In summary, the main trunk can be identified using the following landmarks: (1) it emerges from the stylomastoid foramen within 1 cm medial and inferior to the cartilaginous pointer of the tragus; (2) it emerges from the stylomastoid foramen in line with the tympanomastoid suture line but 6 to 8 mm medial to it; (3) it exits the stylomastoid foramen just superior to and in the same plane as the posterior belly of the digastric muscle, where it inserts in the digastric groove; and (4) the nerve in the mastoid cavity may be identified and followed into the neck. Major nerve branches can be found distally and followed retrograde to their cut ends or to the main trunk. The marginal mandibular branch is located in the tail of the parotid where the nerve crosses the posterior facial vein, and the buccal branch runs parallel and 1 cm inferior to the zygomatic arch adjacent to Stenson's duct. Length can be gained by performing a superficial parotidectomy and mobilizing the nerve from the deep lobe or by rerouting the nerve in the mastoid cavity.

Facial nerve concerns are often accompanied by other challenges, including loss of soft tissue and injuries to Stenson's duct. The assessment of these injuries, including hemostasis of the facial wound, should be conducted in the controlled environment of the operating room where adequate exposure, lighting, and magnification can be obtained to minimize injury to intact portions of the nerve. The loss of facial soft tissue and skin and the need to debride nonvital tissue may prevent primary closure of the wound. Wound healing by secondary intention and multiple-stage reconstruction do not provide ideal circumstances for stable nerve anastomosis and regeneration. Under these circumstances, nerve repair should be delayed until skin closure has been achieved. However, identification and tagging of the cut ends of the transected nerve within the first 3 days after injury facilitates the eventual repair of the nerve. Stenson's duct can be repaired over a Silastic tube or a new ostium can be created in the buccal mucosa in cases of distal injury.

SURGICAL TRAUMA OF THE FACIAL NERVE

Iatrogenic injury of the facial nerve is a difficult event for both the patient and responsible surgeon. Early recognition and timely repair with the assistance of an otologist are appropriate responses to this problem. The most effective strategy is to prevent injury in the first place by identifying the facial nerve through the use of established landmarks.

Iatrogenic Injury During Otologic Surgery

A great deal of effort is spent in otologic training learning how to identify and preserve the facial nerve during temporal bone surgery. In many cases the injury is not identified at surgery and is suspected only when the patient awakes with facial paralysis.[32] The variable anatomy of the temporal bone and facial nerve requires the use of a few reliable anatomic relationships for the identification of the nerve. The nerve is most often injured in transmastoid surgery and not infrequently in transcanal procedures.[32, 33] The most common site of injury is the lower tympanic segment and second genu, followed by the vertical mastoid segment.[32, 33] Synchronous injuries may exist in multiple segments. The severity of nerve injury ranges from violation of the epineurium and contusion of otherwise intact neural tissue to partial or complete disruption of nerve continuity.[32, 33]

The propensity of the distal horizontal segment and the second genu of the facial nerve to be injured results from distortions of antral relationships by a low-lying tegmen or absent canal wall, and congenital or acquired dehiscence of the nerve. If it has not been recognized, a low-lying tegmen in a sclerotic mastoid will cause the surgeon to enter the contracted antrum too inferiorly, leading to injury of the nerve at the second genu as anterior dissection to the aditus ad antrum is attempted.[33] Concurrent injury to the lateral semicircular canal may occur for the same reason and was found in almost half the cases of iatrogenic facial nerve injury reported by Green and associates.[32] Absence of the posterior wall of the external auditory canal in a radical cavity can be very disorienting, especially when granulation tissue further distorts the anatomy. As the prominence of the lateral semicircular canal is variable and may be diminished by previous surgery or disease, there may be no landmarks for the second genu in the radical cavity. The distal horizontal segment of the fallopian canal is often eroded at the inlet to the aditus ad antrum where cholesteatomas remain for long periods of time before extending through this aperture into the antrum.[32] Difficult visualization of the distal tympanic segment because of adjacent disease, especially in intact canal wall surgery, may lead to injury of the unprotected nerve during blind dissection in this area. Finally, the dehiscence of the horizontal segment of the facial nerve, especially above the oval window, is the most common congenital anomaly of the facial nerve, occurring in as many as 55% of temporal bones.[7, 34] The exposed nerve is at increased risk during stapes surgery, especially if it slightly herniates from the bony canal and protrudes into the oval window.

The vertical segment of the facial nerve is vulnerable to injury in mastoid surgery because of its variable course, especially in association with congenital anomalies.[7] During surgery of the external auditory canal, the nerve may also be injured because of the lateral location of the inferior mastoid segment relative to the tympanic annulus and its location under the canal floor just distal to the stylomastoid foramen.[35] The removal of bone on the posterior and inferior surfaces of the external auditory canal during canalplasty or removal of exostoses should therefore be performed with care.

The geniculate ganglion is vulnerable during dissection in the supratubal recess (Fig. 22–3), from which the ganglion is separated by a thin wall of bone on the superior medial surface of the recess.[36, 37] Congenital dehiscence or the erosion of this bony partition by cholesteatoma in the anterior attic places the geniculate ganglion at risk for injury during blind dissection in this area. Visualization of this recess is normally impeded by the head of the malleus and "cog," requiring the removal of both structures to ensure the safe removal of cholesteatoma in the anterior attic. The facial nerve is also at risk during the surgical approach to and dissection within the internal auditory canal and cerebellopontine angle. In the middle fossa approach, the geniculate ganglion can be injured while elevating dura from the middle fossa floor if the bony roof of the geniculate fossa is dehiscent (see Fig. 22–4), as it is 20% of the time.[7, 8] If the facial nerve is displaced superiorly by an inferior vestibular schwannoma, it is at risk when opening the roof of the internal auditory canal and during tumor dissection. The intracannulicular segment of the nerve lacks an epineurium and the rich anastomosing network of vessels associated with it. Therefore, a nerve that is already attenuated by tumor compression is further susceptible to both mechanical and ischemic injury during tumor removal.

EVALUATION AND PRIORITIES

Surgical injury of the facial nerve may be recognized intraoperatively or deduced if the patient awakes with facial nerve dysfunction. The decision to surgically explore the nerve depends on how the facial nerve dysfunction presents and on whether the surgeon is confident that the nerve was identified and preserved (Table 22–2). Transient postoperative facial weakness may result from the effect of local anesthetic on a dehiscent nerve during surgery. This effect should resolve by 2 hours after surgery. Persistent facial nerve dysfunction strongly suggests that the nerve has been injured and mandates exploration of the nerve in a timely fashion.

The function of all branches of the facial nerve should be systematically evaluated as soon as the patient is able to follow directions after every otologic procedure. If normal function is confirmed initially but progressive dysfunction occurs after a delay, the nerve is likely to recover completely.[33] Immediate onset of facial paresis with perceptible but reduced facial movement may also be associated with good prognosis. However, there should be close follow-up by physical examination until recovery occurs while receiving steroid therapy. If paresis evolves to paralysis and the nerve was not identified during surgery, the nerve should be reexplored. However, if the nerve was identified and preserved, serial EnoG testing is recommended starting 3 days after the onset of paralysis, with exploration indicated if the amplitudes of the myogenic potential are diminished by more than 90% within 7 days.[38] When in doubt, early exploration to decompress the nerve and confirm its continuity is the safest option.

Because the facial nerve may be injured at multiple sites during otologic surgery, it should be decompressed from the stylomastoid foramen to the proximal horizontal segment. Signs of injury include a violated nerve sheath, with

Table 22–2. *Management of Iatrogenic Facial Nerve Injury*

Nature and Timing of Dysfunction	Action
Delayed onset paralysis	Follow,* steroid therapy
Immediate, persistent paralysis	Explore
Immediate paresis	Follow,† steroid therapy

*Follow with serial EnoG (see text); explore if amplitude falls by more than 90% compared to contralateral side.
†If progresses to paralysis, follow with serial EnoG (see text).

or without associated ecchymosis, granulation tissue, and edema. The nerve sheath should be incised proximally and distally from the site of injury until normal-appearing nerve is encountered. Injuries limited to the sheath require no further therapy, but violation of the nerve trunk may require the reestablishment of nerve continuity by primary anastomosis or grafting. The cut ends of the transected nerve should be freshened and the ends reapproximated without tension, using fine sutures through the epineurium. (Surgery of injured nerves is discussed in the earlier section on surgical therapy.) In summary, several millimeters can be gained by limited rerouting of the nerve to minimize tension at the anastomosis. As much as 10 mm in length can be gained by rerouting the nerve anteriorly between the parotid gland and the geniculate ganglion. However, because burr injuries are rarely discrete, and long segments of nerve may be involved, interposition grafting may be necessary. However, facial nerve function is thought to be better after primary anastomosis than after nerve grafting, with House-Brackmann grade III function prevalent in the former and grade IV function more commonly seen in the latter.[38]

The management of partial-thickness nerve injuries is more controversial because of the difficulty accurately assessing the extent of injury. The transection of more than 50% of the nerve's diameter has been proposed as an indication for the excision of the injured segment followed by primary anastomosis or cable grafting.[39] However, the margins of injury extend beyond the visible depth of nerve trauma, and inflammation and bleeding make accurate assessment of the depth of nerve injury difficult. A conservative approach is to decompress the partially transected nerve by incising the sheath, with excision and repair reserved for reexploration if recovery is very poor.[33] At the other extreme is the opinion of Green and coworkers: "When doubt exists as to depth of injury, it is preferable to err in [the direction of] repairing the nerve."[38] Unfortunately there are no well-controlled studies to test the efficacy of these disparate philosophies.

PREVENTION

The tenets of otologic surgery should be closely followed to reduce the risk of facial nerve and labyrinthine injuries associated with anatomic distortion due to disease and previous surgery. When approaching the antrum, attic, and facial nerves, bony and soft tissue dissection should proceed from superior and posterior to anterior and inferior. The mastoid cavity is saucerized to maximize visualization and increase the access of instrumentation. A thin bony tegmental plate is defined over the middle fossa dura laterally, and the sinodural angle is followed medially to enter the antrum superiorly and posteriorly while hugging the tegmen. This approach is particularly important in sclerotic mastoids and should prevent inadvertent injury of the second genu and lateral semicircular canal when the tegmen is low-lying. Visualization of middle-ear disease and anatomy, and access of instrumentation, should be maximized prior to dissection in the attic and posterior mesotympanum by removing the canal wall or by opening the facial recess. An exposed nerve is very susceptible to injury and should be suspected in revision surgery or in the presence of large cholesteatomas. Dissection should be performed carefully with blunt instruments in a direction that is parallel to the anticipated path of the nerve rather than perpendicular to it. Facial nerve monitoring is useful in this setting to warn of stretching or compression of the exposed nerve.[40] A nerve stimulator set at low current levels may also be used to confirm the location of the nerve.

The cochleariform process is a useful landmark of the horizontal segment of the facial nerve (see Fig. 22–3), as it is invariably located just inferior and posterior to the geniculate ganglion and its dense otic bone is resistant to erosion by middle-ear pathology. This landmark is most safely found by dissecting anteriorly along the tegmen mastoideum and tegmen tympanum until the cochleariform process is identified just medial to the neck of the malleus. The tympanic segment of the facial nerve can then be located superiorly and followed posteriorly toward the second genu. Other landmarks that may be used to identify the tympanic segment include the oval window located just inferior to the distal horizontal segment, the pyramidal eminence from which the stapedial tendon originates, located just anterior to the second genu, and the prominence of the lateral semicircular canal, which is located slightly lateral, posterior, and superior to the second genu (see Fig. 22–3).

Landmarks that assist in the safe identification of the vertical segment of the facial nerve include the short process of the incus and the mastoid insertion of the posterior digastric muscle. The short process of the incus is oriented approximately co-linear with the facial recess just anterior to the vertical segment of the facial nerve. At its anterior limit, the cephalic edge of the posterior digastric muscle forms a fibrous sleeve around the nerve at the stylomastoid foramen. As this fibrous sleeve is followed superiorly, the nerve will be encountered. When drilling the posterior or inferior walls of the external auditory canal during canalplasty and removal of canal exostoses, the postauricular approach should be used for maximum visualization. Canal patency should be maximized by removing bone from the anterior and superior walls of the external auditory canal where facial nerve injury is unlikely to occur. Dissection in the posterior and inferior walls should be performed carefully and to a limited extent.[32]

Iatrogenic Injury of the Facial Nerve During Surgery of the Face and Neck

The extratemporal portion of the facial nerve is most commonly injured in parotid surgery or during the excision of neck lesions originating from or adjacent to the parotid gland. Preservation of the facial nerve first requires the identification of the main trunk and its branches in the vicinity of the surgical procedure. Recall that the main trunk can be identified by using the following landmarks: (1) It emerges from the stylomastoid foramen approximately 1 cm medial and inferior to the cartilaginous pointer of the tragus; (2) it emerges from the stylomastoid foramen in line with the tympanomastoid suture line but 6 to 8 mm medial to it; (3) it exits the stylomastoid foramen just superior to and in the same plane as the posterior belly of the digastric muscle where it inserts into the digastric groove; (4) it can be identified by retrograde dissection from the marginal mandibular branch, which can be located on the masseter muscle or in the tail of the parotid where it crosses the posterior facial vein; and (5) it can be identified in the mastoid cavity, as described in the previous section, and followed into the neck.

Facial nerve dysfunction resulting from extratemporal surgery usually results from accidental transection of the unidentified nerve or from excessive traction or compression of the nerve during tissue dissection or wound retraction. Monopolar cautery can also cause thermal and electrical injury of the facial nerve when it is used in proximity to its branches. To prevent injury, the marginal branch should be identified as it crosses the body of the mandible superficial to the posterior facial vein in the posterior inferior parotid gland, or in its path on the superficial layer of the deep cervical fascia. Once identified, the associated fascia should be incised inferiorly and displaced cephalad, with the nerve out of harm's way. Avoiding retraction of the superior wound margin and the use of monopolar cautery in the lateral suprahyoid region can further minimize marginal mandibular branch injury. The frontal branch is also at risk for injury superior to the zygomatic arch where it runs within the superficial layer of the deep temporal fascia. Elevation of this fascial layer during a bicoronal flap procedure, for instance, may lead to transection or traction injury of the frontal branch and unilateral forehead and brow ptosis. This complication is avoided by dissecting into the deep temporal fat pad superior to the zygomatic arch, which establishes a plane deep to the nerve and allows safe elevation of the superficial temporal fascia.[41]

A patient with immediate facial paresis who develops delayed paralysis usually recovers fully. Such a patient should be observed, and the necessary eye care should be provided. The absence of a restrictive bony canal makes it unlikely that extratemporal nerve injury will progress because of compression. Therefore, steroid therapy has a limited role in the management of this kind of case. A patient who awakes from general anesthesia with complete paralysis should be suspected of having severe injury of the nerve. If the surgeon is confident that the nerve was identified and preserved and was intact at the end of the case, the patient should be followed without surgical intervention. ENoG testing does not reliably monitor the degeneration of the facial nerve in cases in which the nerve is injured distal to the stylomastoid foramen. EMG recordings can be performed starting 10 days to 2 weeks after surgery to monitor regeneration of the facial muscles. If there are no signs of regeneration on EMG after 3 to 6 months, the nerve should be explored. If the anatomic integrity of the nerve is unknown and the facial paralysis is present immediately after surgery, the nerve should be explored and repaired as soon as possible. Within the first 3 days after injury, before Wallerian degeneration is complete, identification of the distal nerve segments can be facilitated by the use of electrical stimulation. Timely exploration therefore increases the likelihood that the transected ends can be found and reapproximated. Anastomosis should be tension-free and stabilized with epineurial sutures. Surgical repair of facial nerve injuries medial to the lateral canthus and the oral commissure does not provide a better outcome than spontaneous recovery.

NEONATAL FACIAL PARALYSIS

Asymmetric facial function in a newborn may be a congenital anomaly or may result from birth-related trauma. Whereas the majority of children with facial paralysis due to perinatal trauma recover normal function without associated morbidity, congenital facial paralysis is permanent and may be associated with other congenital abnormalities, some of which may be life threatening.[42] Congenital causes of asymmetric facial function include the agenesis of motor neurons in Möbius's syndrome, the anomalous development of the facial nerve in craniofacial anomalies such as Goldenhar's syndrome, and the abnormal development of facial muscles in hypoplasia of the depressor anguli oris muscle.[43] A child with a developmental cause of asymmetric facial function has an increased risk for congenital anomalies of the head and neck and other organ systems. Cardiac anomalies are of particular concern as they are associated with increased rates of mortality.[44] These anomalies tend to occur ipsilateral to the facial nerve dysfunction.[45] Hypoplasia of the depressor anguli oris muscle is associated with congenital anomalies at the rate of 62% in the series by Kumari and colleagues.[44] One third of these were cardiac anomalies predominantly associated with right-sided facial involvement.[44]

The incidence of facial nerve paralysis in the newborn ranges from 1 in 2,000 to 1 in 500, and the majority result from perinatal injury of the nerve (79% to 88%).[42, 43] A decrease in the use of forceps in obstetrical practice accompanied by an increase in cesarean births is thought to account for the fall in the incidence of neonatal facial dysfunction from a rate as high as 7.5 in 1,000 births reported in one earlier series.[46] As the facial nerve exits the fallopian canal into the neonate's face at the stylomastoid foramen, it is located in a lateral and superficial position relative to the mastoid process. The immature mastoid has not yet projected a tip that will eventually provide a bony and fibromuscular shield lateral to the nerve at the stylomastoid foramen. The nerve is therefore susceptible to various degrees of injury by compression against the styloid process medial to it by forceps during birth. Facial nerve dysfunction caused by forceps trauma ranges from paresis to paralysis involving some or all nerve branches. Orbicularis oculi function is often spared, suggesting that the nerve is compressed distal to the pes anserinus in many cases.[47] Rarely, severe birth trauma can lead to distortion or fractures of the temporal bone and injury to the nerve in its temporal course, which produces dysfunction in all branches.[42] Temporary paralysis in the neonate may also occur in routine spontaneous deliveries, accounting for as many as 30% of the cases of neonatal facial paralysis in one series.[46] Facial weakness associated with normal spontaneous vaginal delivery may result from nerve compression by the neonate's ipsilateral shoulder during uterine contractions or by the maternal pelvis during delivery.[42, 48] This mechanism of facial nerve injury most commonly occurs during the first pregnancy, presumably because of the smaller uterine space of the primipara mother.

Evaluation

A newborn with unilateral facial nerve dysfunction demonstrates an asymmetric face when crying; the face is commonly symmetric at rest. The presence of normal facial movement at birth followed by progressive facial weakness is suggestive of perinatal nerve trauma.[49] Paralysis noted at birth may result from trauma or congenital disease. The diagnostic evaluation of neonatal facial palsy should occur within the first 72 hours of life to afford the best chance for accurate diagnosis and determination of prognosis.

The clinical history should identify any details of the delivery that may suggest a facial paralysis due to perinatal trauma (Table 22–3). Forceps delivery is an important risk factor for

Table 22–3. *Differences Between Congenital and Traumatic Causes of Neonatal Facial Paralysis*

Congenital	Perinatal Trauma
History	History
Family history of craniofacial anomalies	Forceps delivery
	>3.5 kg Birth weight
	Primipara pregnancy
	Prolonged stage 2 vaginal delivery
Physical Examination	Physical Examination
Bilateral facial dysfunction	Bruising of lateral face and mastoid regions
Partial facial involvement	Other complications of birth trauma
Multiple cranial nerve deficits	Brachial plexus palsy
Craniofacial and other anomalies	Clavicular fractures
Minimal signs of trauma	Shoulder dystopia
	Hemotympanum
	Shoulder depression in mastoid region

***Table 22–4.** Signs of Birth Trauma*

	Intratemporal Injury	Extratemporal Injury
All branches affected	Yes	Usually (70%)*
Hemotympanum	Yes	Unlikely
Facial bruises	Yes, severe	Yes
CT findings	Fracture and/or fluid	Usually normal

*Smith JD, Crumley RL, Harker LA. Facial paralysis in the newborn. Otolaryngol Head Neck Surg 1981;89:1021–1024.

perinatal facial nerve trauma and is associated with the majority of these cases.[42, 43] An occiput-posterior position of the infant during delivery and the use of middle-level forceps are associated with increased risk for facial nerve injury.[50] Other risk factors for birth trauma include prolonged second-stage labor, infant birth weight over 3.5 kg, and first pregnancy.[43, 46] On physical examination, the presence of hemotympanum and of bruising and edema of the mastoid, pinnae, or face are very suggestive of birth trauma (Table 22–4). These stigmata may be absent, however, when facial nerve injury is associated with spontaneous delivery. In such a case, a depression in the ipsilateral jaw and mastoid region that has been molded by the ipsilateral shoulder suggests compression of the nerve during intrauterine life.[48] In the absence of the stigmata of trauma, the presence of bilateral facial nerve paralysis, unilateral facial weakness limited to the upper or lower face, or other cranial nerve deficits, including abnormal auditory brain-stem evoked responses, suggests a congenital cause, such as Möbius's syndrome.[49, 51, 52] The upper division is often spared in partial facial dysfunction associated with birth trauma, but the opposite is true in partial dysfunction associated with Möbius's syndrome.[51] In a case of multiple cranial nerve dysfunction in a newborn, intracranial injury due to birth trauma should be ruled out. Deformities of the chest wall and extremities should also be noted, as they too are associated with Möbius's syndrome. Craniofacial anomalies, including hemifacial microsomia and Goldenhar's syndrome, clefts and hypoplasia of the maxilla, and anomalies of the first and second brachial arches such as microtia and canal atresia, are sometimes associated with congenital facial paralysis and should be noted on physical examination.[42, 49, 52]

EMG testing within 72 hours of birth is an important component in the diagnostic workup of neonatal facial paralysis (Table 22–5). Voluntary action potentials on EMG indicate muscle innervation, whereas the presence of fibrillation potentials within the first 3 days after birth indicate that (1) facial muscles are present and were once innervated, and (2) denervation occurred prior to birth, possibly because of intrauterine nerve compression. EMG performed after 10 days of paralysis distinguishes traumatic from congenital causes by the presence of fibrillation or polyphasic potentials in the former and the absence of any electrical activity in the latter.[49] When ENoG responses on the affected side are present in the first 3 days of birth and subsequently diminish, birth trauma is the likely cause of facial dysfunction. However, because nerve injury due to birth trauma is likely to occur at or distal to the site of electrical stimulation in EnoG testing, the absence of these responses is, therefore, of limited diagnostic value.

Priorities

In addition to monitoring the eye and providing corneal protection and lubrication as needed, a neonate with facial nerve paralysis of any cause

***Table 22–5.** Interpretation of Electrophysiology in the Newborn with Facial Paralysis*

EnoG in First 3 Days/ Serial Tests	EMG Within 3 Days of Birth	EMG After 21 Days	Diagnosis
Initial response with diminishing amplitude	No voluntary potentials	Fibrillations	Birth trauma, muscle denervation
Initial response with diminishing amplitude	No voluntary potentials	Polyphasic action potentials	Birth trauma, regenerating nerve with reinnervation
No response to stimulation	No spontaneous electrical activity	No spontaneous electrical activity	Congenital absence of facial nerve or mimetic muscles
No response to stimulation	Fibrillations	Fibrillations or other myogenic potentials	Nerve injury occurred prior to birth

should be monitored for adequate nutritional intake, especially if paralysis is bilateral. A patient determined to have congenital dysfunction should undergo further tests to rule out anomalies of other organ systems. A neonate with traumatic injury to the facial nerve acquired during delivery should be carefully assessed for other trauma to the head and neck, including intracranial injury, Erb's paralysis of the brachial plexus, shoulder dystopia, and clavicular fractures.[43] Hemotympanum and bruising of the mastoid should prompt a CT scan of the temporal bone in search of fractures. The absence of signs of reinnervation on EMG after several weeks in an infant with temporal bone fractures is one of the rare cases in which surgical exploration of the temporal portion of the nerve may be indicated.[42] However, in the majority of cases, normal facial nerve function recovers spontaneously.

Outcomes

The incidence of full spontaneous recovery of facial nerve function ranges from 90% to 100%.[42, 44, 52, 53] In the series of Falco and Eriksson, only 10% of children had incomplete recovery after a mean of 34 months.[43] Of the children with full facial nerve recovery, 78% recovered within the first 2 weeks of life, whereas the remaining 22% recovered after a mean of 4 months. All 22 patients in Kumari's series showed signs of early recovery within 4 to 7 days of birth, with full recovery confirmed in all 16 patients for whom follow-up was available.[44] Surgery is therefore rarely indicated, as the majority of injuries are crush injuries distal to the stylomastoid foramen. Only in cases of temporal bone fracture, especially transverse fractures or displaced longitudinal fractures, is surgical exploration of the nerve likely to result in facial function that is better than that of spontaneous recovery. In such cases the entire intratemporal path of the nerve should be decompressed and examined, which requires a combined mastoid and middle fossa approach. Although exploration of the nerve guided by the results of serial electrophysiology testing and the persistence of fibrillation on EMG has been advocated,[42, 49, 52] there are insufficient published data on the clinical outcomes of the surgical treatment of perinatal facial nerve injury to support these recommendations.

FACIAL NERVE PARALYSIS IN ACUTE BACTERIAL INFECTIONS OF THE EAR

Acute suppurative otitis media complicated by facial paralysis more commonly occurs in children than in adults. The patient often presents with 2 to 3 days of progressive facial dysfunction associated with ipsilateral otalgia, fever, and otoscopic findings consistent with middle ear empyema.[54] Facial paralysis usually occurs in the absence of coalescence or other temporal bone or intracranial complications. Facial nerve dysfunction is thought to result from a toxic neuritis in response to byproducts of the suppurative process that gain access to the nerve through a dehiscence of the facial canal (Fig. 22–15). A temporal bone CT scan is required to rule out mastoid coalescence which, if present, should be treated with antibiotics and cortical mastoidectomy.[12] In the absence of coalescent mastoiditis, antibiotics and drainage of the middle ear with a wide myringotomy are appropriate initial measures. If fever persists for 24 hours or if facial paralysis remains for longer than 1 week, cortical mastoidectomy is required.[12] Nerve decompression is almost never required except when paralysis is prolonged.

In an adult, facial nerve dysfunction due to chronic suppurative otitis media is commonly associated with a longstanding history of cholesteatoma.[55] Mechanisms of nerve injury include toxic neuritis, bony canal erosion with external nerve compression by cholesteatoma, and intraneural extension of infection.[6, 12] The tympanic and mastoid segments are most often affected. Prior to complete paralysis, abnormal hyperkinetic facial movements may occur, including facial twitches and spasm.[54] The aim of surgical treatment is the removal of irreversible disease in the middle ear and mastoid and the decompression of the nerve without opening the nerve sheath.[12] In the case of longstanding paralysis, the nerve sheath should be opened to directly examine the nerve for evidence of necrosis, which would require debridement and nerve grafting.[6]

Malignant otitis externa is a deep-seated infection of the temporal bone and skull base that starts in the bony ear canal of the immune-compromised host, especially the diabetic. The offending organism is the gram-negative *Pseudomonas aeruginosa*. As the infection spreads along the vascular channels at the base of the skull, cranial nerves are compressed in their bony canals and foramina.[56] Facial nerve paralysis is the most commonly occurring cranial neu-

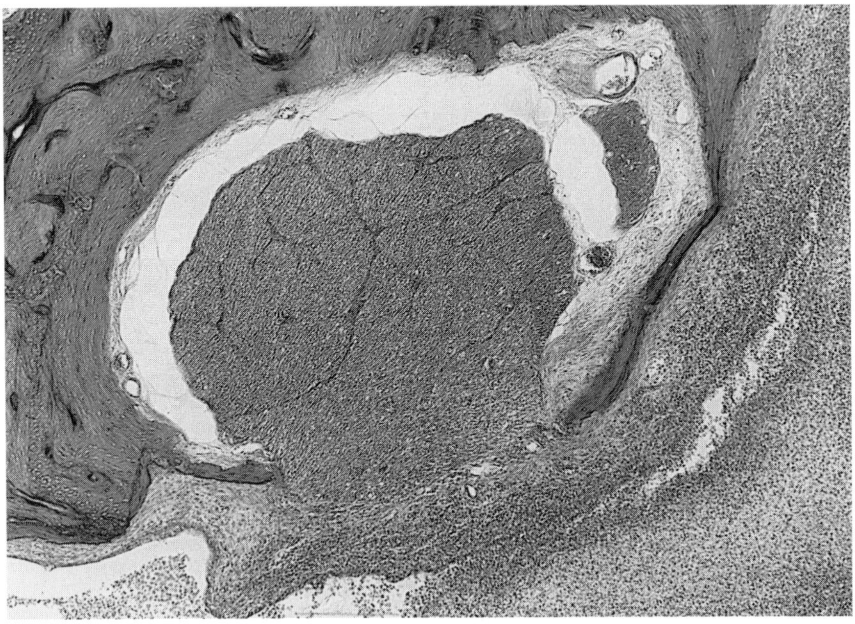

Figure 22–15. Dehiscence of the facial canal in its horizontal segment provides a pathway by which toxic byproducts of the adjacent suppurative otitis media may produce nerve dysfunction. (From Nager GT. Pathology of the Ear and Temporal Bone. Baltimore, Williams & Wilkins, 1993, p 260.)

ropathy in malignant otitis externa, and it is associated with a poor prognosis.[6] As the infection penetrates the skull base, lethal intracranial sepsis may result.

Malignant otitis externa presents with otalgia and otorrhea. Otoscopic findings include ulceration of the canal skin and granulation tissue at the bony-cartilagenous junction.[12] The differential diagnosis includes malignant neoplasm of the temporal bone, herpes zoster oticus, acute or chronic suppurative otitis media with otorrhea, and granulomatous diseases such as Wegener's granulomatosis and tuberculosis. Biopsy of the granulation tissue or other canal lesions for histopathologic evaluation is an important part of the workup to rule out malignancy. CT scans for bony erosion in malignancy or for osteopenia in osteomyelitis are also useful in the diagnostic evaluation. A technetium-Tc 99m-pertechnetate bone scan is useful to confirm the diagnosis of malignant otitis externa, and a gallium-67-citrate scan is used to monitor the response to therapy, the mainstay of which is a 6-week course of parenteral antipseudomonal antibiotics. Surgical therapy is reserved for advanced cases in which increasing cranial neuropathies occur despite antibiotics.[6]

REFERENCES

1. Committee on Trauma of the American College of Surgeons. Advanced Trauma Life Support course. Chicago, American College of Surgeons, 1988.
2. Levine RE. Ocular management and rehabilitation of the patient with facial paralysis. In Jackler RK, Brackmann DE, eds. Neurotology. St. Louis, Mosby-Year Book, 1994, pp. 1421–1433.
3. Maas CS et al. Primary surgical management for rehabilitation of the paralyzed eye. Otolaryngol Head Neck Surg 1994;110:288–295.
4. Proctor B, Nager GT. The facial canal: normal anatomy, variations and anomalies. Ann Otol Rhinol Laryngol 1982;97:33–61.
5. Esslen E. The Acute Facial Palsies. Berlin, Springer-Verlag, 1977.
6. Jackson CG. Facial nerve paralysis: diagnosis and treatment of lower motor neuron facial nerve lesions and facial paralysis. Washington, DC, American Academy of Otolaryngology-Head and Neck Surgery Foundation, 1986.
7. Nager GT, Proctor B. Anatomic variations and anomalies involving the facial canal. Otolaryngol Clin North Am 1991;24:531–553.
8. Nager GT. Pathology of the Ear and Temporal Bone. Baltimore, Williams & Wilkins, 1993.
9. Sunderland S. Nerves and Nerve Injuries, 2nd ed. Edinburgh, E & S Livingstone, 1978.
10. Seddon HJ. Three types of nerve injury. Brain 1943;66:237.
11. Ganz B, Gmur A, Fisch U. Intraoperative electromyography in Bell's palsy. Am J Otolaryngol 1982;3:273–278.
12. Niparko JK. The acute facial palsies. In Jackler RK, Brackmann DE, eds. Neurotology. St. Louis, Mosby-Year Book, 1994, pp. 1291–1319.
13. Hilger J. New instrument, facial nerve stimulator. Trans Am Acad Ophthalmol Otolaryngol 1964;68:74–76.
14. May M, Blumenthal F, Klein S. Acute Bell's palsy: prognostic value of evoked electromyography, max stimulation and other electrical tests. Am J Otol 1983;5:107.
15. Fisch U. Facial paralysis in fractures of the petrous bone. Laryngoscope 1974;84:2141–2154.

16. Fisch U. Prognostic value of electrical tests in acute facial paralysis. Am J Otol 1984;5:494–498.
17. Fisch U. Maximal nerve excitability testing vs. electroneuronography. Arch Otolaryngol 1980;106:352–357.
18. Gantz BJ, Rubinstein JT. Intratemporal facial nerve surgery. In Cummings CW et al., eds. Otolaryngology Head and Neck Surgery. St. Louis, Mosby, 1998:2785–2799.
19. Wetmore SJ. Surgical landmarks for the facial nerve. Otolaryngol Clin North Am 1991;24:505–530.
20. Patey DH, Ranger I. Some points in the surgical anatomy of parotid gland. Br J Surg 1958;45:250.
21. Adkins WY, Osguthorpe JD. Management of trauma of the facial nerve. Otolaryngol Clin North Am 1991;24:587–611.
22. May M. Total facial nerve exploration: transmastoid, extralabyrinthine, subtemporal: indications and results. Laryngoscope 1979;89:906.
23. House WF. Surgical exposure of the internal canal and its contents through the middle cranial fossa. Laryngoscope. 1961;71:1363–1385.
24. Fisch U, Lanser MJ. Facial nerve grafting. Otolaryngol Clin North Am 1991;24:691–708.
25. Coker NJ et al. Traumatic intratemporal facial nerve injury: management rationale for preservation of function. Otolaryngol Head Neck Surg 1987;97:262–269.
26. Lambert PR, Brackmann DE. Facial paralysis in longitudinal temporal bone fractures: a review of 26 cases. Laryngoscope 1984;94:1022–1026.
27. Ulrich K. Verletzungen des Gehöhrorgans bei Schädelbasisfrakturen. Acta Otolaryngol (Stockh) 1926;Suppl 6:1–150.
28. McCabe BF. Facial nerve grafting. J Plast Reconst Surg 1970;45:70–75.
29. May M. Surgical rehabilitation of facial palsy. In May M, ed. The Facial Nerve. New York, Thieme, 1986, pp. 681–777.
30. Duncan NO et al. Gunshot injuries of the temporal bone. Otolaryngol Head Neck Surg 1986;94:47–55.
31. Telischi FF, Patete ML. Blast injuries to the facial nerve. Otolaryngol Head Neck Surg 1994;111:446–449.
32. Green DJ Jr, Shelton C, Brackmann DE. Iatrogenic facial nerve injury during otologic surgery. Laryngoscope 1994;104:922–926.
33. Graham MD. Prevention and management of iatrogenic facial palsy. Am J Otol 1984;5:513.
34. Baxter A. Dehiscence of the fallopian canal. J Laryngol Otol 1971;85:587–594.
35. Litton WB et al. The relationship of the facial canal to the annular sulcus. Laryngoscope 1969;79:1584–1604.
36. Chu FWK, Jackler RK. Anterior epitympanic cholesteatoma with facial paralysis: a characteristic growth pattern. Laryngoscope 1998;98:274–279.
37. Horn KL et al. The supratubal recess in cholesteatoma surgery. Ann Otol Rhinol Laryngol 1986;95:12–15.
38. Green JDJ, Shelton C, Brackmann DE. Surgical management of iatrogenic facial nerve injuries. Otolaryngol Head Neck Surg 1994;111:606–610.
39. Kamerer DB. Intratemporal facial nerve injuries. Otolaryngol Head Neck Surg 1982;90:612–615.
40. Yingling CD. Intraoperative monitoring of cranial nerves in skull base surgery. In Jackler RK, Brackmann DE, eds. Neurotology. St. Louis, Mosby-Year Book, 1994:967–1002.
41. Frodel JL, Marentette LJ. The coronal approach: anatomic and technical considerations and morbidity. Arch Otolaryngol Head Neck Sur 1993;119:201–207.
42. Smith JD, Crumley RL, Harker LA. Facial paralysis in the newborn. Otolaryngol Head Neck Surg 1981;89:1021–1024.
43. Falco NA, Eriksson E. Facial nerve palsy in the newborn: incidence and outcome. Plast Reconstr Surg 1990;85:1–4.
44. Kumari S et al. Facial palsy in newborn: clinical profile and long-term follow-up. Indian Pediatr 1980;17:917–922.
45. Pape KE, Pickering D. Asymmetric crying facies: an index of other congenital anomalies. J Pediatrics 1972;81:21–30.
46. Levine MG et al. Birth trauma: incidence and predisposing factors. Obstet Gynecol 1984;63:792–795.
47. McLellan MS, Vautier T. Neonatal seventh nerve palsy in the absence of hemotympanum. Am J Obstet Gynecol 1973;117:572–574.
48. Parmelee AH. Molding due to intra-uterine posture. Am J Dis Child 1931;42:1155–1159.
49. May M et al. Facial paralysis in children: differential diagnosis. Otolaryngol Head Neck Surg 1981;89:841–848.
50. Pearl ML et al. Vaginal delivery from the persistent occiput posterior position: influence on maternal and neonatal morbidity. J Reprod Med 1993;38:955–961.
51. Rubin LR. The Möbius syndrome: bilateral facial diplegia. Clin Plast Surg 1976;3:625–636.
52. Bergman I et al. Management of facial palsy caused by birth trauma. Laryngoscope 1986;94:381–384.
53. Alberti PW, Biagioni E. Facial paralysis in children: a review of 150 cases. Laryngoscope 1972;82:1013–1020.
54. Pollock R, Brown L. Facial paralysis in otitis media. In Graham MD, House WF, eds. Disorders of the Facial Nerve: Anatomy, Diagnosis and Management. New York, Raven, 1982, pp. 221–228.
55. Sheehy JL, Brackmann DE, Graham MD. Complications of cholesteatoma: a report of 1,024 cases. In McCabe BF, Sade J, Abramson M, eds. Cholesteatoma, First International Conference. Birmingham, AL, Aesculapius, 1977 pp. 429.
56. Kohut RI. Necrotizing ("malignant") external otitis: histologic processes. Ann Otol Rhinol Laryngol 1979;88:714–720.
57. Kokesh J et al. Correlation between stroboscopy and electromyography in laryngeal paralysis. Ann Otol Rhinol Laryngol 1992;102:852–857.

CHAPTER **23**

Otologic and Skull Base Emergencies

Andrew J. McWhorter, MD,
Charles J. Limb, MD, and
John K. Niparko, MD

The subject of otologic and skull base emergencies encompasses a broad range of topics. Despite the large array of possible emergencies, few truly constitute life-and-death situations. In fact, otologic injuries commonly present in the context of systemic traumatic injury that requires immediate attention, prior to otologic management. Still, evaluation of otologic and skull base emergencies should take place as soon as medical circumstances permit. Therapy instituted within the first 24 hours after injury typically produces quicker and fuller recovery of function.

Traumatic injuries to the ear can be caused by a wide range of events, such as foreign-body entrapment, tympanic membrane perforation, temporal bone fracture, inner ear barotrauma, and lightning damage. In addition to trauma, infection may be the source of a problem that mandates urgent treatment. Immunocompromised patients are at particular risk for developing serious infections. Such infections are usually bacterial or fungal in nature and can involve the pinna, external auditory canal, middle and inner ear structures, mastoid bone, or brain. Nontraumatic, noninfectious causes of otologic emergencies, such as sudden sensorineural hearing loss, acute labyrinthine disorders, and surgical complications, which will be discussed only briefly, are other serious disorders that demand prompt attention. These subjects form the outline on which this chapter is based.

The symptoms associated with otologic and skull base emergencies are myriad. Hearing loss, dizziness, facial nerve dysfunction, otorrhea, cranial neuropathies, and pain may all be referable to the ear and the base of the skull. Given that these symptoms may also present in situations that are not necessarily life threatening, the physician should have a thorough grasp of the most common otologic emergencies so that they can be recognized early and the outcomes can be as positive as possible.

This chapter is intended to be helpful both in defining an otologic or a skull base emergency and in identifying the preliminary interventions required. The discussion of each category of injury or disease follows the same format—a brief introduction is followed by presenting symptoms, steps for evaluation, priorities in management, and outcomes. Although a considerable amount of literature exists regarding each entity and symptom complex described, this chapter aims to provide a synthesis of the material, with a focus on the aspects that genuinely warrant emergent diagnosis and treatment.

TRAUMA

Foreign Body

A foreign body in the ear can be one of a myriad of objects and such a case is commonplace in general medical practice. The pediatric population is at greatest risk, especially children under the age of 12 years.[1] The presence of a foreign body often does not constitute an emergency, but prompt attention can prevent infection and facilitate removal. Some foreign bodies such as insects and batteries do require acute intervention to prevent further injury. Of special concern are foreign bodies associated with trauma to the middle ear. These cases can lead to a variety of complications, including ossicular disruption, labyrinthitis with hearing loss and vertigo, and facial nerve injury. In all of these situations, there should be a high index of suspicion for the presence of multiple foreign bodies.

PRESENTATION

The anatomy of the ear must be kept in mind when considering the removal of a foreign body. The external auditory canal (EAC) extends from the concha of the auricle to the tympanic ring, angled anteroinferiorly. The outer third, or membranous portion, is composed of an incomplete cartilaginous cylinder that attaches to the bony portion of the canal. Inconsistent fissures (the fissures of Santorini) filled with connective tissue communicate with the parotid fascia and the superficial mastoid region. The squamous portion of the temporal bone completes the posterior and superior external canal, and the tympanic bone forms the anterior and inferior limits of the bony external auditory canal. The bony segment of the EAC is slightly concave posteriorly, resulting in the S-shaped canal in adults. The isthmus, the narrowest portion of the EAC, is roughly at the middle of the bony segment.[2]

Any object that is retained in the external auditory canal is considered a foreign body. In 212 pediatric emergency department visits, the items most commonly removed from ears were roaches, paper wads, toy parts, earring parts, hair beads, eraser tips, and food.[3] Insects in the canal may be very irritating and cause severe distress to the patient. Other frequently seen objects are biologic materials, such as cerumen, beans, and seeds that can be difficult to manage because of their hygroscopic nature.[4, 5] Adherent materials such as Superglue and hearing aid molds can be quite traumatic when the middle ear is invaded.[4, 6] Special cases include small batteries and slag.[4]

Most objects are lodged at the isthmus or the bony-cartilaginous junction. Foul-smelling otorrhea or purulent drainage may be the presenting symptom. Complete obstruction causes a conductive hearing loss. Penetrating foreign bodies commonly present with otalgia, otorrhagia, and decreased hearing. More significant injury involving the middle ear can present with facial nerve weakness and vertigo.

EVALUATION

The goals of foreign-body management are safe removal and the prevention of granuloma formation.[4, 7] A thorough history usually reveals the time course and the type of material. The physician should always inquire about a history of tympanic membrane perforation and the patient's premorbid level of hearing. A foreign body in the only hearing ear poses a threat of profound deafness that should be addressed by an experienced otologist. The pediatric population may present with signs of unilateral otitis media, including a draining ear and decreased hearing. A full head and neck examination should be completed to rule out foreign bodies in multiple sites.

Otoscopy is the cornerstone of physical examination. Microscopic otoscopy is indicated when there is incomplete visualization, contact of the foreign body with the tympanic membrane (TM), perforation, or trauma to the middle ear.

Exudate should first be removed with suction. The ball-end right-angle hook is the instrument of choice for most objects, particularly if the object's surface is smooth. Forceps are a good alternative when an edge is accessible. Irrigation with room-temperature water works well if the TM is intact. Irrigation is contraindicated if the foreign body is hygroscopic, because it can lead to swelling and further impaction, and if there is preexisting hearing loss. Irrigation should be directed to the space between the object and the posterosuperior aspect of the canal, if possible. This technique works well for hard, small objects like sand and cerumen and to mobilize posteriorly positioned objects anteriorly.[4, 8, 9]

Complete inspection of the ear canal after removal of debris is important to exclude more significant injury to the canal skin, tympanic membrane, or ossicles caused by the foreign body or its extraction. These injuries are discussed in the section on tympanic perforations and penetrating injury. Small areas of skin violation heal spontaneously; minor bleeding is best managed with epinephrine-soaked cotton balls. Topical antibiotics serve to reduce moisture and bacterial counts, which expedites reepithelialization.[4] Systemic antibiotics are used when there is concomitant otitis media, otitis externa, or chondritis. Removal of tenacious cerumen is facilitated by 5 to 7 days of softening with otic drops.[4]

PRIORITIES

Foreign-body removal is generally not an emergency, although it is important to remove it in a reasonable period of time, as a chronic foreign body may lead to complications such as acute otitis media or otitis externa, which require prompt attention. Insects, destructive agents, and objects associated with penetrating trauma should be removed as soon as possible. A child often requires sedation or general anesthesia for safe extraction of a foreign body located medial to the bony isthmus. Canal skin is very thin and sensitive, and the more medially the object is located, the more difficult it is to remove. Medial positioning of the object also increases the likelihood of associated middle ear trauma. Inspection after removal is crucial in order to exclude more significant injury; evaluation of hearing should be pursued as indicated.

An insect in the ear is extremely irritating. A live insect should be drowned in lidocaine solution, which both paralyzes the bug and topically anesthetizes the canal.[4, 10] The insect can then be removed in the standard fashion under direct visualization, with care being taken to remove the entire insect.

A hearing aid battery is sometimes found in the ear of a child or of a geriatric patient who has trouble manipulating and inserting the aid.[11] These batteries typically range in diameter from 0.5 to 1.5 cm and can deliver 1.5 volts.[4] Immediate removal of the battery is mandatory to prevent local destruction of tissue. Batteries cause tissue damage through a combination of three mechanisms: direct corrosive action by the battery's electrolytes, low-voltage burn, and pressure necrosis.[4, 12–14] A moist environment allows alkaline electrolyte leakage, which induces liquefactive necrosis.[15] Injuries due to liquefactive necrosis include bone necrosis, chondritis, tympanic membrane perforation, ossicular damage, and facial nerve paralysis.[15, 16] After removal of the battery, necrotic tissue should be debrided and steroid otic drops applied. Deep injury and circumferential injury should be handled as discussed under penetrating injuries. Using drops prior to removal of the battery has been shown to increase the depth of the burn.[16]

Slag injuries are caused by sparks and molten metal generated by welding and grinding machinery. Slag in the ear causes significant thermal injury to the canal skin and bone which may extend to the tympanic membrane and middle ear. Devascularization of the skin and mucosa results in chronic otorrhea and persistent tympanic membrane perforation.[17] Facial nerve injury, peripheral vestibular injury, and hearing loss are thought to be secondary to thermal damage. Temperatures of these foreign bodies can approach 1,000°C. On exploration, neural structures are usually found to be intact but demonstrate evidence of severe edema and, unfortunately, rarely recover normal function.[17] Frequent debridement and topical antibiotics are the early treatments of choice; steroids should be considered so as to reduce edema.

OUTCOMES

The majority of foreign bodies are relatively easily removed and do not cause long-term morbidity. Removal in the operating room may be necessary to reduce the risks to the tympanic membrane or middle ear structures. Circumferential injuries can produce canal stenosis and are discussed in the next section.

Excessive prescription of and prolonged use of otic drops can lead to fungal overgrowth in the canal. Neomycin-containing compounds can cause a hypersensitivity reaction with erythema and vesicle formation.[4] These changes resolve with discontinuation of the offending agent.

Injuries by batteries and slag can be more problematic, as they can lead to chronic otorrhea and persistent tympanic membrane perforation. Full recovery from facial nerve and cochleovestibular injuries caused by slag is rare.[17]

Penetrating Injuries and Traumatic Perforations

Penetrating injuries and traumatic perforations can be caused by foreign bodies, elongated instruments introduced to remove cerumen, and stab and gunshot wounds. Perforations can also be caused by barotrauma, blunt blows, lightning, and exposure to loud noise. The extent of such injuries ranges from inconsequential to life threatening. In a series of 60 tympanic membrane perforations published by Lindeman and colleagues, 12 were caused by penetrating injury and 48 were caused by percussion or barotrauma.[18] Other series have reported varying incidences of traumatic perforations; Kristensen and coworkers reported an annual incidence of 1.4 perforations per 100,000 persons.[19]

Penetrating temporal bone injuries and temporal bone fractures are discussed in the next section. Laceration, avulsion, hematoma, thermal injury, and frostbite of the external ear are addressed in Chapters 7 and 13.

PRESENTATION

The extent of injury and level of acuity are assessed by a good history and physical examination. Stabilization of the patient and evaluation of the facial nerve are the first priorities. A cranial nerve examination, otoscopy, and an assessment of hearing and vestibular function are mandatory components of a complete evaluation and are described in greater detail in the section on temporal bone fractures. Circumferential injuries, otorrhagia, hemotympanum, cerebrospinal fluid otorrhea, diminished hearing, dizziness, and facial nerve injury are important findings that require more immediate intervention.

EVALUATION

The history and physical examination should place special emphasis on the mechanism of injury and on any preexisting deficits. Standard principles of trauma management should be observed, and the patient should be stabilized prior to examination. The severity of the injury dictates whether the operating room is required for management or whether the trauma is minor enough to be handled in an office setting.

Otoscopic examination, cranial nerve evaluation, and tuning fork tests are mandatory. Foreign material should be removed and the ear debrided and irrigated as necessary to permit a complete examination. Major penetrating injury should be assessed by means of a computed tomography scan (CT) to determine the medial extent of trauma and whether neurovascular injury has occurred.

Hearing loss associated with penetrating injury can be conductive, mixed, or sensorineural. The most commonly seen deficit is a mild conductive loss due to tympanic membrane perforation. The next most common cause of hearing loss is ossicular disruption, usually caused by incudostapedial subluxation.[20, 21] Figure 23–1 shows an incudostapedial injury and exposed oval window caused by a cotton tipped–swab injury. Stapes crural fracture occurs less commonly but can be missed if the response of the footplate to ossicular manipulation is not carefully observed. A stapes crura fracture should be suspected when there is a conductive loss combined with an intact stapedius reflex.[21] Every patient should have a complete audiogram, and if the hearing loss is significant, a CT scan should be obtained. Conductive loss is maximal at 60 dB, whereas damage to the inner ear may result in a dead ear. A patient with nystagmus or vestibular symptoms should also undergo electronystagmography testing to assess labyrinthine involvement.

PRIORITIES

The first priority in the case of a penetrating injury is to examine the full extent of the injury. Small lacerations of the ear canal and auricle in the presence of an intact tympanic membrane

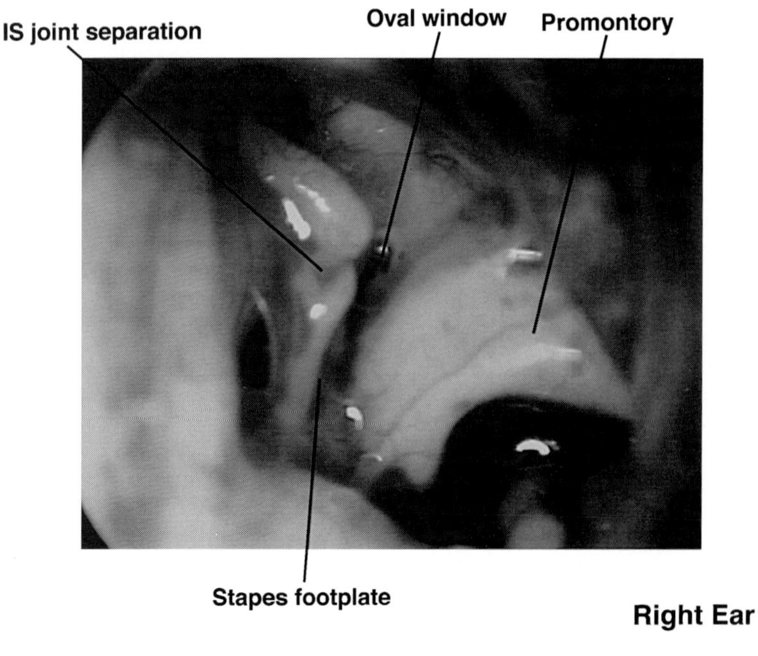

Figure 23–1. Intraoperative photo: Cotton tipped–swab injury with resultant incudostapedial (IS) joint separation and displacement of the stapes footplate. (Courtesy of H. Francis, M.D.)

do not constitute an emergency and can be handled expectantly. The ear should be suctioned clean. A postauricular anesthetic block may improve the patient's comfort and compliance. Lacerations should be cleaned, and skin and cartilage heal better if well reapproximated. Circumferential lacerations predispose the canal to stenosis, which is very difficult to repair. In such a case, the canal should be packed or stented open with Silastic, wicks, Gelfoam, or a red rubber catheter for 10 to 14 days.[4, 21] Standard principles of wound care should be observed, and antibiotic coverage should be instituted to prevent infection. It is important to keep in mind that superficial infections can spread to the parotid space and the upper neck via the fissures of Santorini. Fractures of the external canal also require stenting to prevent stenosis. A dislocated canal can be reduced with a nasal speculum and then packed.

A traumatic perforation in the posterosuperior quadrant of the TM with persistent, severe vertigo and nystagmus requires immediate intervention because this location and these symptoms suggest stapedial dislocation. Operative exploration is necessary to rule out stapes dislocation into the labyrinth and to repair the perilymph fistula. Failure to repair this traumatic rupture puts the patient at risk for complete hearing loss. An exploratory tympanotomy via a transcanal approach enables the removal of unstable segments of the stapes and the grafting of the oval window.[22] Some experts recommend placement of a stapes prosthesis at this time to stabilize the graft.[21]

Although posterosuperior quadrant perforation with symptoms requires urgent care, the majority of traumatic tympanic membrane perforations are located in the anteroinferior and pars tensa region of the TM.[21] An average of 45 dB of conductive hearing loss occurs in traumatic perforation, with an upper limit of 60 dB being the maximum conductive loss.[21] A tympanic membrane perforation should be examined under a microscope. Pneumatic otoscopy should be avoided, and the patient should be instructed to avoid nose blowing, sneezing, and exposure to water. If infection is present or if the perforation is contaminated, as occurs in injuries suffered during such activities as water skiing, antibiotic steroid drops should be used.

Inner ear concussion is one possible cause of sensorineural loss.[21] Concussion may occur after a hard blow to the head that damages the membranous cochlea. A high-frequency hearing loss carries a better prognosis than a low-frequency loss. The patient may experience nausea and vomiting as well as dizziness and vertigo. Treatment is bed rest and antiemetics.

Barotrauma and lightning are two causes of tympanic membrane and middle ear injury and are discussed independently later in the chapter.

Blast injury is another source of tympanic membrane and middle ear injury. Blast waves are pressure waves that travel faster than sound.[22] The most frequent injury is a slitlike TM perforation. Ossicular injury and delayed cholesteatoma have also been reported. The other common findings are sensorineural hearing loss and tinnitus that usually are self-limited but may be permanent. Complications of blast injuries are treated in the same way as any other traumatic middle ear injury.

Vestibular symptoms are generally treated with supportive, expectant care. They commonly present with acute, severe symptoms that gradually improve. Fluctuation of symptoms may indicate a perilymph fistula. This is often seen in a compressive injury. There can be dislocation of the ossicles and rupture of the round or oval window or both. These insults can be handled with supportive management, although persistent symptoms of fluctuating hearing loss or vertigo require exploration.[23] Exploratory tympanotomy under local anesthesia is adequate to examine the entire round and oval windows. Attention should also be focused on the annular ligament of the stapes and the fossula of the cochlear window. When a fistula is found, it is repaired by denuding the mucosa and placing a graft (usually cartilage or fascia) over the window. A stapedectomy may be required in order to effectively patch the oval window. Antibiotics are recommended as prophylaxis against labyrinthitis if the wound is contaminated.

OUTCOMES

A small and slitlike TM perforation can close in as little as 24 to 48 hours, and approximately 90% of such perforations heal spontaneously within 3 months.[18] Repositioning the membrane remnants to restore normal anatomic position can accelerate closure. Some experts recommend patching, but it does not facilitate a significantly higher rate of closure according to these series.[23a] When there is no complicating injury, such a perforation is best left to heal spontaneously. Factors that complicate the rate of spontaneous healing and lead to persistent perforation are associated otitis media, blast injury, and larger areas of perforation. One rare late complication is the delayed development of cholesteatoma. A patient should be reexamined at 3 and 12 months to determine the status of the healing and to test the hearing.

The natural history of a perilymph fistula is still a controversial subject, but it is usually believed to heal spontaneously. Glasscock and colleagues recommended surgical exploration and repair when symptoms persist for more than 2 weeks.[23] In this study, 8 fistulas were discovered in 34 patients. The authors reported difficulty in diagnosing posttraumatic fistulas, but the group of patients (25%) who had intraoperatively demonstrated fistulas had nearly complete resolution of vestibular complaints and improvement in hearing after repair. Although immediate exploration for a fistula is not warranted because of the inability to predict accurately whether a particular patient has a fistula, early exploration may increase the likelihood of preserving the hearing. Patients with symptoms of a fistula that persist for 1 to 2 weeks after trauma should have surgical exploration.

Temporal Bone Fracture

Temporal bone fractures are commonly associated with traumatic head injuries. Overall, between 14% and 22% of skull fractures involve injury of the temporal bone.[24–26] Blunt or penetrating trauma, often caused by a motor vehicle accident, frequently produces temporal bone fracture. If life-threatening injuries such as intracranial, cervical spine, or organ trauma are present, they should be assessed and stabilized prior to the investigation of a temporal bone injury. A temporal bone fracture constitutes an emergency because of its high rate of associated injuries, which range from hearing loss and facial nerve injury to cerebrospinal fluid (CSF) leakage and other intracranial complications.

Traditional classification of temporal bone fractures is based on the orientation of the fracture line in relation to the long axis of the petrous pyramid. This orientation is best assessed by means of a CT scan. The fracture line's orientation predicts the extent of labyrinth damage and the pattern of cranial nerve injury. To the astute observer, patterns of damage seen on examination can indicate the extent and orientation of the temporal bone fracture.[4]

PRESENTATION

A patient with a temporal bone fracture is the victim of severe traumatic head injury, either blunt or penetrating. Immediate systemic evaluation, stabilization, and resuscitation are mandatory. The mechanism of injury and the direction of impact determine the type of temporal bone fracture. Cranial nerve abnormalities may be present. Hearing loss and nystagmus may be present in the case of labyrinthine disruption. Battle's sign and raccoon eyes (mastoid and periorbital ecchymosis, respectively) are commonly associated with skull base injury. Otorrhagia and hemotympanum are often present and are helpful in determining the site of bleeding. Figures 23–2 and 23–3 demonstrate the orientation of fracture lines and the common symptoms that are the results of the fractures.

A longitudinal fracture is generated by forces directed laterally to the head at the temporal and parietal regions. The fracture extends along the long axis of the temporal bone and commonly spares the labyrinth. Laterally, the fracture extends into the external auditory canal and the middle ear. The medial extent of the fracture parallels the eustachian tube, often extending tangential to the internal auditory canal (IAC) and ending in the middle cranial fossa near the foramen spinosum and foramen lacerum.[27] This type of fracture frequently presents with otorrhagia or hemotympanum and a conductive hearing loss. Facial nerve paralysis and CSF leakage are less common, with an incidence of approximately 6% to 25%.[25, 26] Vestibular complaints can arise in an average of 30% to 50% of patients.[4]

The presence of hemotympanum and otorrhagia in a longitudinal fracture is attributable to the high incidence of external auditory canal fracture, canal skin laceration, and TM perforation, and all usually occur in the posterosuperior quadrant near the tympanosquamous suture line. The conductive hearing loss can be multifactorial, including such causes as TM perforation and annulus rupture, hemotympanum, an obstructed EAC, ossicular discontinuity (most commonly incudostapedial joint separation), and CSF leakage into the middle ear due to fracture of the tegmen. Facial nerve paralysis in a longitudinal fracture is almost always the result of the fracture's extension to the geniculate ganglion (the perigeniculate fallopian canal), and it frequently has a delayed onset corresponding to neural edema, compression, or ischemia.[4, 28] Traumatic causes of vertigo associated with longitudinal temporal bone fracture include benign positional vertigo, labyrinthine concussion, and brain-stem trauma.[4, 29]

Transverse fractures make up approximately 10% to 20% of temporal bone fractures and are generated by forces that come into contact with the frontal and occipital regions.[26, 30] Because

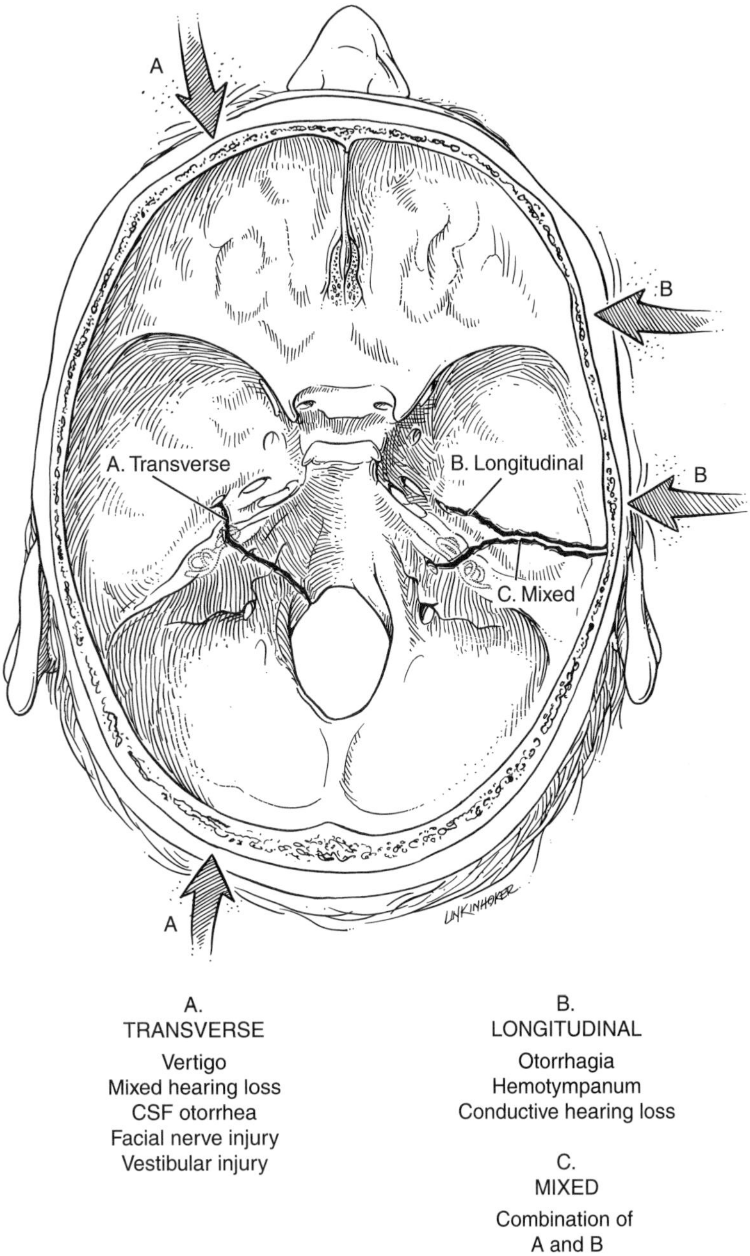

Figure 23–2. Fronto-occipital and temporoparietal forces with resultant transverse and longitudinal bone fractures, respectively, and their common fracture line orientations. Commonly resulting symptoms are listed.

the fracture line extends perpendicular to the petrous ridge, considerably more force is required to cause a fracture in this orientation. The fracture plane extends perpendicular to the long axis of the petrous pyramid, from the foramen magnum across the posterior cranial fossa, and transversely across the petrous pyramid to the middle fossa, ending in the foramina lacerum and spinosum (see Fig. 23–2).[27]

A transverse temporal bone fracture rarely produces otorrhagia or tympanic membrane perforation. Rather, there is a high incidence of vertigo and mixed hearing loss with a large sensorineural component. Hemotympanum is less common but CSF otorrhea is more common than in longitudinal fracture. Approximately 50% of cases have signs of both facial nerve and vestibular injury.[26] The higher incidence of sensorineural hearing loss and vertigo in transverse fractures is the result of damage to the cochlea and vestibular end-organs. This type of hearing loss is therefore less likely to be recovered, and the damage is commonly permanent.[31] Vestibular injury is usually caused by

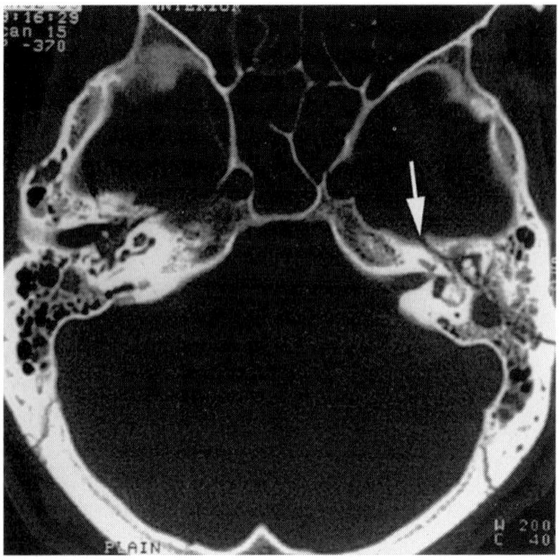

Figure 23–3. Axial CT image of a left longitudinal temporal bone fracture.

intralabyrinthine fracture, membrane disruption, or hemorrhage. Recovery of ipsilateral vestibular function is unlikely, but most patients compensate for fixed deficits within the first year after insult.[29] Delayed symptoms similar to those of Meniere's disease occur with fractures that go through the vestibular aqueduct.[32] Facial nerve paralysis is usually immediate and complete because of transection of the nerve (commonly between the IAC and the horizontal portion distal to the geniculate ganglion in the perigeniculate and tympanic segments of the fallopian canal).[28] Hemotympanum is attributable to fractures of the medial wall of the middle ear; rupture of the TM or EAC is rare.

An intracranial injury is not uncommon in a transverse fracture. It can vary from an open skull fracture to a subdural or, more frequently, an epidural hematoma. An intracranial hematoma is associated with injury to the transverse and sigmoid sinuses and the middle meningeal artery.

A mixed fracture has components of both a longitudinal and a transverse fracture. About 8% of fractures are mixed; they are usually caused by the most substantial injury forces.[33, 34] Symptoms and findings correlate with the presence or absence of otic capsule involvement. Trismus and otorrhagia are signs of condylar and temporal bone fracture.

The oblique fracture is a more recent classification of temporal bone fracture; it is diagnosed on the basis of CT scans with three-dimensional reconstruction.[33] In contrast to a longitudinal fracture that runs through the petrotympanic fissure, an oblique fracture crosses the fissure horizontally, extending superiorly and obliquely toward the middle fossa cranial plate. The otic capsule remains unaffected as the fracture extends to the petrous apex and the foramen lacerum.

The pattern of a temporal bone fracture in a child differs from that in an adult. An oblique temporal bone fracture is the most common presentation in children.[34a] Facial nerve injury and sensorineural hearing loss are less common, but conductive loss is more common than in the adult population. Peaks in incidence at 2 to 3 years of age and 13 to 16 years of age reflect a shift from automobile-pedestrian accidents to falls and motor vehicle accidents as children mature.

EVALUATION

Following trauma protocol, a systemic evaluation is performed and a focused history is obtained. The history should seek to determine the mechanism of injury and the direction (frontal/occipital vs. temporal/parietal) of the insult, as this indicates the type of fracture line to expect. It is also important to investigate any disability that existed prior to the injury, including the level of hearing and any balance dysfunction.

An efficient cranial nerve examination provides invaluable information when managing a patient who must be quickly intubated and paralyzed so life-sustaining measures can be performed. The physical examination focuses on otoscopy and neural function. Assessing the functional status of the facial nerve is of primary importance. Meticulous cleansing of the external ear canal with sterile instruments facilitates a complete determination of injuries. Abnormal neurologic findings should be thoroughly investigated and CSF otorrhea should be ruled out.

If the patient is stable and there is a possible temporal bone fracture, a CT scan is the definitive imaging study. Fine-cut images 1.5 to 2.0 mm apart should be acquired as soon as the patient is stable and cooperative. The scan should reveal both the orientation of the fracture and the structures involved in the injury. A CT scan can also reveal other, undiagnosed intracranial injuries. Air in the temporomandibular joint is an indirect sign of fracture.[35]

Hearing is initially assessed with a 512-Hz tuning fork; Weber's and Rinne's tests are useful for differentiating sensorineural and conductive losses. Full audiologic evaluation should be performed as soon as possible after the injury. Vestibular testing is performed by examining the direction of spontaneous and induced nystagmus.

PRIORITIES

The first priority following stabilization of the patient is assessment of the facial nerve. If a patient does not require operative intervention for vascular or brain injury, facial nerve decompression is the next most likely reason for operative intervention. Complete facial paralysis after injury often indicates severe contusion or total transection of the nerve. (Facial nerve evaluation and treatment interventions are discussed in Chapter 22.) After the vestibulocochlear and facial nerves, the abducens nerve and the trigeminal nerve in Meckel's cave are the cranial nerves most commonly injured.[4] If there is evidence of vagus injury, potential damage to nearby vascular structures such as the carotid bulb or jugular vein should be investigated.

Intracranial injuries are most commonly seen in transverse, mixed, and open fractures. Intracranial hematomas are associated with injury to the transverse and sigmoid sinuses and the middle meningeal artery. Other vascular injuries, such as carotid pseudoaneurysms, carotid-cavernous fistulas, and carotid lacerations, are seen in severe blunt head trauma.[36, 37] Intracranial injuries require immediate action and distinguish temporal bone fractures as true emergencies. Multidisciplinary care and early involvement of a neurosurgeon are crucial.

Gunshot and stab wounds are a unique subset of temporal bone fractures. As in cases of severe blunt trauma, vascular injuries (32% to 33%) and intracranial injuries (36% to 53%) are common and carry high mortality rates.[38, 39] Immediate intervention by a neurosurgeon is mandated. Most fractures are mixed and have multiple resultant injuries. Both conductive and sensorineural hearing loss are usually seen and there is a 50% incidence of facial nerve injury.[38, 39] Because of the highly destructive nature of these injuries the presence of other maxillofacial trauma is also common. Potential further complications include meningitis and cholesteatoma due to diffuse seeding of the middle ear with squamous tissue. Radical mastoidectomy is commonly required to adequately treat the significant destruction.[39]

Findings on early audiometry should be interpreted with caution, because debris and fluid in the middle ear can cause temporary conductive loss. An early audiogram is important, however, to document sensorineural function. If a conductive loss is present, a follow-up audiogram should be obtained in 2 to 3 months. This delay allows for resolution of hemotympanum and effusion and identifies persistent conductive losses. Middle ear exploration should be performed at least 3 months after injury to maximize results.[4]

Documentation of nystagmus is especially important in a patient with a transverse fracture. Balance function testing should be utilized as indicated by clinical findings. Rotary-chair testing can be of particular use in defining vestibular dysfunction in a patient with CSF otorrhea or a tympanic membrane perforation, both of which are contraindications to water irrigation for caloric testing.[4]

CSF leakage can be discovered by otoscopy or CSF rhinorrhea and symptoms such as a salty taste in the mouth or a postnasal drip. CSF leakage from an otologic source can present through the nose if the eustachian tube is patent, but it occurs more commonly through the EAC.[25] CSF otorrhea occurs in up to 21% of patients with fractures.[40] The β-2 transferrin assay is the most accurate method available to determine whether otorrhea consists of CSF. This CSF-specific protein can be detected in microliter quantities by using immunologic methods.[41] The traditional ring-sign test and the quantification of glucose lack specificity.

A fracture that does not have associated facial nerve injury or more serious injury can be handled conservatively. Cleaning and a follow-up audiogram are necessary. Antibiotic steroid drops should be used only in the presence of active infection or when wicks are used to stent the canal.

OUTCOMES

The majority of temporal bone and related injuries heal spontaneously with conservative management. However, temporal bone fractures are far from innocuous. Survival, particularly in the case of a transverse or mixed fracture, is low because of the mechanism of action and the propensity for associated vascular and intracranial injuries. Early detection and intervention by a multidisciplinary team is the key to limiting complications and increasing the likelihood of survival.

External canal injuries and tympanic membrane perforations generally do well on their own. Hemotympanum and associated conductive hearing loss usually improve spontaneously within 3 months. When conductive loss is persistent, exploratory tympanotomy is warranted to attempt closure of the air-bone gap.

Immediate sensorineural hearing loss is irreversible, but progressive loss may indicate a perilymph fistula or endolymphatic hydrops.[31, 32] Operative repair may be undertaken to attempt stabilization and possible improvement in hearing. Vertigo and nystagmus resulting from temporal bone fracture usually resolve in 2 to 3 weeks with bed rest and antiemetics. Most peripheral vestibular injuries are compensated for by the contralateral ear and the central vestibular system.[29]

A CSF leak usually closes spontaneously with bed rest and head elevation. A CSF leak that does not close spontaneously within 7 days is associated with a significantly higher rate of meningitis.[25] The use of prophylactic antibiotics is warranted in a patient who has a CSF leak that does not close within 3 days. If leakage persists beyond 7 days, serial lumbar punctures or a lumbar drain should be considered. (Chapter 24 discusses CSF leaks in greater detail.)

Long-term concerns include the seeding of the middle ear with squamous debris, which leads to the latent formation of cholesteatoma.[27, 39] A follow-up cleaning of the ear may help to prevent cholesteatoma. Lastly, encephaloceles and meningoceles can develop over time and can go unrecognized until they present with more serious sequelae such as meningitis.

Barotrauma

A variety of injuries are caused by barotrauma. Barotrauma to the ear is the most common injury to result from scuba diving and is one of the most common causes of tympanic membrane rupture.[18, 42] Barotrauma can also be related to air travel.[43] Most pressure-induced injuries are minor, but improper decompression can be an emergent event. The most common injury due to barotrauma is middle ear damage caused by inadequate pressure equalization during compression or descent in general or during scuba diving in particular. The eustachian tube is unable to equalize the surrounding and middle ear pressures, which results in pain and possible injury. Inner ear barotrauma is especially worrisome because it carries a risk of perilymphatic fistula.[44] A 1988 Norwegian study noted an incidence of 0.5% of inner ear barotrauma in 15,000 dives.[45, 46] Inner ear decompression sickness is the most significant of the barotrauma injuries and is a true otologic emergency. As in standard decompression sickness (the bends), nitrogen bubbles form in the inner ear secondary to inadequate decompression and can result in permanent hearing loss.

Surprisingly, very shallow depths are all that are required for injury to the ear when diving. Boyle's law describes the physics that determine pressure related to depth or altitude. The basic tenet is that with increasing atmospheric pressure, the volume of gases decreases. It takes only a few feet of water depth to produce significant differences, as opposed to the thousands of feet of altitude required. Farmer nicely correlates the level of descent and the pressure on the middle ear.[47] Starting at a depth of approximately 2.6 feet of seawater, a 60 mm Hg differential is generated between the pressures of the middle and inner ear, and the first otologic symptoms of fullness and dysequilibrium can be appreciated. As the depth increases to 4 feet, the differential increases to 90 mm Hg, causing eustachian tube occlusion that cannot be overcome voluntarily. Further descent without equalization and maneuvers at this level to clear the ears can lead to perforation, hemotympanum, and fistula.[42, 44, 46, 47, 47a]

PRESENTATION

Inner ear barotrauma occurs when middle ear pressure does not equilibrate completely. A number of mechanisms have been postulated to explain this kind of injury. The pressure difference alone, when transmitted to the inner ear, can cause damage, as can maneuvers used by divers (such as the Valsalva) to attempt equilibration. The most popular theory proposes that increased intracranial pressure is transmitted to the inner ear, causing subsequent damage to either Reissner's membrane or the basilar membrane or causing the formation of a perilymphatic fistula.

Many divers have otologic complaints and yet continue to dive. They may present with complaints of pain, aural fullness, vertigo or dysequilibrium, tinnitus, or hearing loss. The timing of onset of symptoms provides the best clues as to the cause of the problem. Nitrogen bubbles form when there is inadequate time for the gases to resolubilize during a rapid ascent without adequate decompression time. The bubbles form within the inner ear fluid spaces, microcirculation, and bony structures, causing damage as they expand and obstruct. Decompression sickness occurs on ascent or shortly thereafter, and not on descent. The importance of determining whether a patient has undergone barotrauma or decompression sickness is twofold: Inner ear decompression sickness requires immediate intervention for preservation of hearing; however, inner ear barotrauma is aggravated by the therapeutic intervention for decompression sickness.[47]

EVALUATION

The general workup for diving-related injuries is the same, regardless of the cause. A complete history with emphasis on the timing of the accident and the history of the dive is essential. A neuro-otologic examination should also be carried out with audiometry. Vestibular testing is necessary when there is nystagmus or dizziness.

The diagnosis of inner ear decompression sickness should be made based on history and physical examination. A physical examination does not always provide evidence of inner ear barotrauma. Systemic and neurologic symptoms caused by improper decompression are good clues to diagnosis. Specifically, the dive profile should be addressed and the depth of the dive, the gases used, and the decompression times recorded. The absence of systemic symptoms does not preclude a diagnosis of decompression sickness, as a patient can present with isolated otologic symptoms.[47]

PRIORITIES

The first priority is to determine whether inner ear decompression sickness has occurred. A patient is at risk for permanent hearing loss as well as many complications of systemic injuries that can be life threatening. It is imperative to distinguish such a patient from a patient with inner or middle ear barotrauma so that rapid recompression can be instituted. The degree of recompression by means of a hyperbaric oxygen chamber should be to three atmospheres of pressure greater or deeper than where the diver experienced the onset of symptoms.[47]

Middle ear barotrauma can be handled expectantly. Bed rest with head elevation and avoidance of pressure changes (no diving or airplane travel) are indicated. If symptoms worsen or do not improve, surgical exploration should be considered. Perilymph fistulas are not uncommon and present with fluctuating hearing loss and vestibular dysfunction. They should be treated conservatively unless there are persistent symptoms of longer than 1 week's duration, at which time they should be explored as discussed in the section on penetrating injury. Tympanic membrane perforation should be treated, as described earlier, with antibiotic steroid drops and careful observation to ensure proper healing. All patients who have suffered barotrauma should be instructed in methods of equalizing middle ear pressure, such as the Valsalva maneuver, before resuming diving or flying.

OUTCOMES

Middle ear barotrauma is commonly self-resolving. A patient with more serious sequelae, such as a perilymph fistula or TM perforation caused by barotrauma, generally does well, as already noted. Early recompression following decompression sickness is strongly linked to better outcomes, both systemically and in terms of vestibulocochlear function.[46, 47] A patient with delayed recompression often has permanent sensorineural hearing loss that can be profound. Even with proper recompression, a patient may have vestibular symptoms for 4 to 6 weeks after treatment. A patient with inner ear decompression sickness is encouraged to stop diving because of fibrosis and altered microcirculation in the inner ear. However, a study by Parell and Becker showed that a patient might have persistent hearing deficits but no further deterioration in vestibulocochlear function with continued diving.[42]

Lightning

Injury by lightning is a much more common occurrence than is generally suspected; there are thousands of strikes per year. In the United States, it is the most common cause of death resulting from natural disaster.[48] Data from the Centers for Disease Control report 1,318 deaths attributed to lightning in the United States between 1980 and 1995.[49] Of the individuals struck by lightning, approximately 10% suffer from otologic sequelae. Injury can result from direct strikes and also from charges of electricity that travel through telephone lines. A study conducted in Australia revealed an incidence of up to 60 cases per year of telephone-mediated lightning strike.[50]

Perforation of the TM is the most common otologic injury caused by lightning, followed by sensorineural hearing loss and vestibular injury.[51–53] A number of mechanisms have been proposed to explain lightning injuries, and there is more than one mechanism of injury in most cases. The most commonly accepted mechanism is direct transmission of electrical energy. Lightning carries an immense amount of energy—up to 100 million volts and 200,000 amps.[51] Electricity follows the path of least resistance through the body, with nerves and blood vessels having the highest conductance, and fat and bone the least. In telephone-related injuries, lightning can transmit sound pressure levels of 150 to 160 dB and it also conducts an electrical charge.[50, 54]

PRESENTATION

A patient who has been struck by lightning commonly has sustained significant systemic injury, and the standard principles of trauma management should be followed in evaluating and stabilizing the patient. However, otologic symptoms can be the only presenting complaint and a complete otologic workup should be performed for every lightning-strike victim. A patient requires thorough audiologic evaluation, as both sensorineural and conductive losses commonly occur. The need for a further vestibular workup can be ascertained through clinical assessments and the patient's reports of vestibular function.

EVALUATION

A complete history and physical examination is always the first step after stabilizing a patient who might be suffering from life-threatening injuries. Otoscopic examination should focus on possible burns to the ear canal and evaluation of the tympanic membrane for perforation. It is not uncommon for a patient to have uninjured canals and near total tympanic membrane perforations.[4] Debridement of the ear under direct microscopy is recommended. Weber's and Rinne's tests should be followed by formal audiometric evaluation as well as vestibular examination. Histologically, total rupture of Reissner's membrane and degeneration of the stria vascularis and organ of Corti can be seen, but many times, the cochlear nerve is spared.[55]

PRIORITIES

The first priority is stabilization of the patient, followed by complete examination. Burns to the external ear and canal are handled routinely, as described in Chapter 7, but the depth of burn can be greater than is initially apparent in lightning-injured ears. As a result, bony injury can occur and can lead to osteomyelitis and chronic otorrhea.[4] The usual treatment is conservative debridement of necrotic bone and application of topical antibiotics. Sensorineural hearing loss does have some potential for recovery, but the extent is variable.[52] Treatment should be expectant, as there is no strong evidence in favor of early middle ear exploration. Perilymphatic fistulas are reported and should be handled as discussed in the section on penetrating injuries. Conductive hearing loss and TM perforation should be followed expectantly.

OUTCOMES

The outcomes of injuries by lightning strikes are variable. The most common finding is a TM perforation that is complete, or holotympanic. This kind of perforation is unique in that despite its extent, it often heals completely. Bergstrom and others have noted that a perforation of this nature can take as long as 6 months to resolve spontaneously.[51–53, 55, 56] It is recommended that repair be delayed longer than 3 months to provide adequate opportunity for delayed healing, although operative intervention is sometimes required. Burns generally heal well with appropriate wound care, but chronically draining ears have been reported when there is associated bony injury.[4] Facial nerve injuries are reported and are discussed in Chapter 22. Sensorineural hearing loss and vestibular symptoms can occur in the presence and in the absence of tympanic membrane disruption. In fact, sensorineural loss has been reported as the only finding in an otherwise normal examination.[52] Unfortunately, there are no good predictors for recovery of hearing loss in this population, and the most common outcome is permanent loss below the premorbid level of hearing. Vestibular symptoms are often well compensated for after a period of adaptation.

INFECTION

Necrotizing Otitis Externa

Necrotizing otitis externa, also known as malignant otitis externa, is a severe infection of the outer ear that occurs in immunocompromised patients. It is a disease that can be locally aggressive and invasive and has life-threatening sequelae when left untreated. Although not all otitis externa is necrotizing, every case should be treated aggressively, especially in the diabetic or otherwise immunodeficient patient.

There is approximately a 10% incidence of otitis externa in the general population.[57] Only a small subset of these cases progress to necrotizing otitis externa. Otitis externa is common in the pediatric population, usually in association with swimming, instrumentation of the ear canal, or hearing aid use.[58] Necrotizing otitis externa is also associated with these risk factors but occurs only in the immunocompromised patient; the pathogen is usually *Pseudomonas aeruginosa*. Approximately 80% of necrotizing cases occur in diabetic patients.[59]

Other disease processes can lead to otitis externa or be confused with it. Chondritis, perichondritis, foreign bodies, furuncles, and carbuncles can all cause occlusion of the ear canal and the subsequent development of otitis externa.[60] Furuncles and carbuncles are infections of the skin appendages in the cartilaginous canal. They are usually caused by *Staphylococcus* species and should be incised and drained.

Herpes zoster oticus can also present as otitis externa. This disease is caused by reactivation of a dormant varicella zoster virus, usually in the glossopharyngeal nerve. Vesicles develop along the dermatome of the ear, resulting in subsequent swelling and debris. Treatment consists of local debridement and antivirals such as acyclovir, both enterally and topically. Involvement of the facial nerve constitutes the Ramsay Hunt syndrome, which is treated by adding steroids.

Otomycosis is a fungal external otitis commonly caused by *Aspergillus* and *Candida* species. Immunocompromised patients are at risk for invasion and subsequent skull base involvement. Early recognition and treatment with antifungals and acidification of the canal are important to prevent the development of advanced disease and the need for surgical intervention.

Benign necrotizing osteitis is a rare condition that can present like necrotizing otitis externa; it is characterized by persistent, but not progressive, necrosis of the external auditory meatus in healthy people.[61] It is felt to be caused by a compromise in the vascular supply to the bone, and surgical excision is necessary.

PRESENTATION

The moist ear, with its keratinacious buildup, is an ideal alkaline environment for bacterial growth. *Staphylococcus* species are the normal agents in routine otitis externa, but *Proteus* species and other anaerobes are also seen. *Pseudomonas* species are the causative organisms in diabetic patients and in chronic infections. Pre- and postauricular adenopathy is not uncommon, and erythema can extend to the surrounding soft tissues.

Otitis externa usually presents with otalgia, otorrhea, and swelling of the external auditory canal. A patient commonly describes pruritus and decreased hearing when the canal swelling causes occlusion. Tragal tenderness, erythema and edema of the external auditory canal, and keratinacious exudate are commonly found on examination. White blood cell counts are not necessarily elevated. Symptoms are usually progressive over 1 week, and a history of water exposure or local trauma is usually elicited. Water irrigation for cerumen removal is a very common cause.

Necrotizing otitis externa presents with otorrhea and severe otalgia that are usually worse at night. Trismus can be seen due to erosion into the temporomandibular joint. Necrotizing otitis externa can, however, present initially with signs of more advanced disease such as facial paralysis. Cranial nerve VII is by far the most common cranial nerve involved.[62] Facial nerve paralysis can occur because infection spreads through the fissures of Santorini and into the parotid fascia or because skull base osteomyelitis extends to the stylomastoid foramen. A diabetic patient, an immunocompromised patient, or a therapeutically immunosuppressed patient who has otitis externa does not necessarily have necrotizing otitis externa. The presence of granulation tissue at the bony-cartilaginous junction is required for a diagnosis of necrotizing otitis externa. Typically, the patient is an elderly, non-insulin–dependent diabetic with recalcitrant otitis externa.[63]

EVALUATION

Examination of the infected ear can be difficult because of pain. It is important to attempt visualization of the tympanic membrane, although this is frequently impossible because of swelling. Any debris and exudate in the canal should be suctioned away under direct microscopy. Debridement of the ear not only helps to clear the infection more quickly but is essential for evaluation of granulation tissue and necrosis. Palpation of the canal floor can demonstrate erosion. Identification of a necrotic process is extremely important, as significant complications can result from osteomyelitis and possible intracranial extension if it is left untreated. Meningitis and brain abscess are other serious sequelae of malignant otitis externa. A full cranial nerve examination should be completed in every patient. Weber's and Rinne's tests are adequate evaluations of hearing in a patient who denies trauma as the inciting event.

Nuclear medicine scans such as technetium-99m-pertechnetate Tc and gallium-67-citrate scans are frequently used to diagnose bone involvement and to follow the course of the disease. A positive technetium scan is the most sensitive test for bone involvement. The gallium scan is used to determine the endpoint of therapy; some experts recommend a scan every 3 weeks until resolution of disease.[59, 64] A high-resolution CT scan should be obtained in any patient with suspected osteomyelitis in order to define the extent of invasion and bony erosion. Audiograms and vestibular testing are rarely needed for evaluation of otitis externa.

PRIORITIES

Debridement of the ear and visualization of the tympanic membrane are the highest priorities. This helps to establish the diagnosis of necrotizing otitis externa. If there is no suspicion of necrosis, therapy with antibiotic drops should be implemented. Acetic acid solutions are usually not as effective as antibiotic preparations. A standard first line of therapy is the combination of neomycin, polymixin B sulfate, and hydrocortisone. Any patient who is allergic to neomycin, has a chronic infection, or is suspected of having a *Pseudomonas* species infection should receive a fluoroquinolone or aminoglycoside preparation. Drops should be administered 3 to 4 times per day. When the TM cannot be visualized, a wick should be placed to facilitate delivery of the antibiotic drops and to stent the canal open. Depending on the severity of the infection, the wick should be changed every 2 to 5 days. Repeated microscopic examination with cleansing hastens resolution of the infection. Simple infections should resolve within 2 weeks. The affected ear should be kept dry, and analgesics are often required for comfort. Antibiotics are indicated in cases of more severe infections that are evidenced by periauricular erythema and edema.

If the patient is at increased risk for necrotizing otitis externa, greater vigilance should be employed. A diabetic patient should be followed for blood glucose control. Sugar levels are often poorly controlled during the infection, and normalization of blood glucose does help resolution of the disease process. Routine otitis externa in an immunocompromised patient can be resistant to standard therapies and can evolve into necrotizing otitis externa over a 1- to 2-week period. Control of blood glucose during the infection may help to prevent the development of further disease. Persistent or deep pain should raise the suspicion of disease extension. When granulation tissue is present, a biopsy should be taken to rule out malignancy. Treatment with 750 mg of ciprofloxacin twice a day plus rifampin or metronidazole has been proven to be as efficacious as and considerably more cost-effective than the previous standard of extended hospitalization and intravenous antibiotics.[65] If the disease does not respond well to treatment, or if there is radiologic evidence of advanced disease, intravenous antibiotic therapy should be instituted with tobramycin and clindamycin for 6 to 8 weeks. Many times, a patient is treated with antibiotics at home. Treatment should be continued until resolution of the external ear findings. Failure to respond to intravenous antibiotics, advancement of disease, or evolution of cranial neuropathies necessitates surgical debridement of the affected tissue.[66] Hyperbaric oxygen is now being used in some centers as adjuvant therapy to speed resolution of osteomyelitis.[67]

OUTCOMES

Routine cases of otitis externa should clear in 1 to 2 weeks without any permanent sequelae. An individual who has had otitis externa once is at risk for recurrence. Chronic infection is likely to occur in a patient with stenotic canals and also in the setting of underlying allergic or dermatologic disease.

Necrotizing otitis externa is usually responsive to aggressive therapy and careful follow-up. However, long-term morbidity may be seen in a patient who presents with advanced symptoms. Fortunately, with modern antibiotics and the close monitoring of disease, complications such as brain abscess, meningitis, and death are rare. The mortality rate in those with necrotizing otitis externa has changed from 60% to 70% to accounts of 18% and lower.[68] Despite these advances, there is still significant morbidity associated with necrotizing otitis externa, and a high level of vigilance is required to prevent serious complications.

Bullous Myringitis

The cause of bullous myringitis is uncertain. Bullous myringitis was once thought to be caused by the influenza virus, *Mycoplasma* species, or bacterial infection, but the actual cause remains unknown.[69, 70] Bullous myringitis is an infection of the tympanic membrane in which the subepithelial surface, usually the lateral side, develops fluid-filled blebs. The external auditory canal may also be affected, although middle ear involvement is not common. It may be confused with otitis media and otitis externa. Although bullous myringitis is often self-resolving and without significant sequelae, a patient with this condition commonly seeks medical attention because of the painful nature of the process.

PRESENTATION

It is predominantly younger children who are susceptible to bullous myringitis. The outbreak of the disease is often epidemic in nature.[71] Although occasionally present, fever is not an essential feature of this disease.

Bullous myringitis is painful. In addition to pain localized in the ear, mastoid tenderness may be present.[72] Spontaneous rupture of the blebs, with discharge, has been known to occur, producing a slightly hemorrhagic otorrhea. Occasionally, the blebs may become secondarily infected with bacteria; the resultant condition may be difficult to separate from acute otitis media. A patient may or may not have associated hearing loss, depending upon when he or she presents during the course of the disease. Early disease tends not to show hearing loss, whereas later disease with effusion may produce a conductive hearing loss.[72] In addition to conductive hearing loss, sensorineural hearing loss has been reported to occur and has even remained permanent in several cases.[73, 74]

EVALUATION

The combination of a history of severe pain and physical findings of tympanic membrane vesicles is generally sufficient for diagnostic purposes. History may reveal an associated upper respiratory infection or a viral illness presumed to be influenza, although this is not always the case.[69] Examination of the TM reveals slight redness and the presence of several blebs that may be serous or serosanguinous. There may also be mildly bloody discharge from ruptured vesicles. The bullae may cover much of the area of the tympanic membrane and may vary in size. In some cases, the external auditory canal is affected.[71] As part of the evaluation, bedside tests of hearing loss should be performed, and the disease should be differentiated from otitis media, which usually has associated systemic symptoms and no discrete bullae.

PRIORITIES

Analgesia is the first step in the management of bullous myringitis. Oral analgesics, topical drops, and warm compresses may be helpful. Although incision of bullae and application of topical anesthesia may provide some pain relief, this is a measure designed primarily to reduce superinfection of the bullae and is unnecessary for the management of the disease.[72] Once analgesia has been achieved, treatment is directed at the prevention of secondary infection. The disease process itself generally lasts 2 to 3 days.[71] Broad-spectrum oral antibiotics and topical antibiotics are appropriate to prevent infection, especially if there is evidence of effusion. Bacterial cultures reveal pathogenic organisms in 65% of cases, and these are usually the same organisms responsible for otitis media. *Mycoplasma pneumoniae* is rarely recovered from culture fluid.[69] Hearing loss is of concern, and if there is clinical suspicion of conductive or sensorineural hearing loss, audiologic evaluation should be pursued.

OUTCOMES

Analgesia can usually be achieved through medication, although incision of bullae is attempted in some cases for analgesic purposes with marginal success.[72] As stated, bullous myringitis usually resolves within a few days. The majority of patients with hearing loss recover, although permanent hearing loss has been reported.[73, 74] Treatment with antibiotics is effective in preventing bacterial superinfection. Incision of bullae has been performed in the hope of preventing recurrence, but the data have not supported this as a useful measure.[71]

Perichondritis and Chondritis

Perichondritis and chondritis are two related entities that generally affect the external ear after trauma or other injury. Burns are the most common predisposing factor, with up to 25% of burned ears developing infection.[75] This category of injury merits acute intervention because of the risk of progression of disease and the loss of viable tissue when the injury is not treated aggressively. The disease process itself is aggressive and can lead to loss of the entire ear cartilage. Perichondritis has been reported in the literature to progress to necrotizing fasciitis, although this is unusual.[76]

PRESENTATION

A history of trauma in one form or another is essential to the diagnosis of either perichondritis or chondritis, because these two processes result from cartilaginous injury. Although burns and auricular hematoma are the two most common preceding injuries, any injury to the pinna puts the patient at risk. Recently there has been an increase in infections caused by the piercing of the cartilaginous ear.[77, 78] Perichondritis is a local infection of the perichondrium characterized by signs of local inflammation. Such a patient presents with complaints of pain, redness, and swelling. A diagnosis of chondritis implies the progression of perichondritis to abscess formation. Both require intravenous antibiotics, and incision and drainage are required for treatment of chondritis.

Relapsing polychondritis is an entity that presents in a similar fashion. It is a rare disease of unknown cause that is characterized by recurrent episodes of inflammation and destruction of cartilage. Although relapsing polychondritis is a systemic disease, it frequently presents with ear symptoms.[79] Up to 93% of cases demonstrate ear involvement and it is one of the diagnostic criteria set out by McAdam for making the diagnosis.[80, 81] Diagnosis is made clinically or by biopsy. The characteristic symptoms are sudden, bilateral onset without a history of trauma, in a pattern that occasionally spares the earlobes. Swelling, erythema, warmth, and pain are also present. Relapsing polychondritis requires accurate diagnosis, as its treatment involves oral steroid administration and systemic evaluation.

A second disease process that can mimic perichondritis is erysipelas. Erysipelas is an infection of the dermis by group A β-hemolytic streptococcus organisms that presents with pain, erythema, swelling, induration, and blistering. The erythema and swelling do not follow anatomic boundaries but are well demarcated. Constitutional symptoms of fever and malaise are also present. This infection is treated with oral penicillin; because of its progressive nature and life-threatening potential, prompt treatment is critical.

EVALUATION

Evaluation begins with a thorough history and physical examination, which reveals a warm, erythematous, and tender ear. Obstruction of the external canal is possible, and otitis externa must be ruled out. Edema and fluctuance can obscure normal anatomy and should raise suspicion for underlying cartilage necrosis. The infection can eventually cause the breakdown of the overlying skin.

Prevention of chondritis is the best treatment, including early identification and institution of therapy in burned ears. A study of 4,794 burned ears showed a reduction in the incidence of chondritis from 20% to 3% with the avoidance of pressure and the use of topical antipseudomonal agents.[82]

PRIORITIES

In order to save viable cartilage, therapy should be implemented promptly. The causative organism in 90% to 95% of cases is *Pseudomonas aeruginosa*. These infections can be polymicrobial, with *Staphylococcus aureus* being the second most common pathogen isolated. The treatment for perichondritis is intravenous antibiotics directed against these organisms; however, early perichondritis can be treated with oral fluoroquinolones.[83] Perichondritis is very painful and warrants the use of analgesics. Swelling can lead to stenosis of the canal and resultant otitis externa. Antipseudomonal otic drops are a good preventive measure.

If the disease progresses to chondritis, surgical intervention is necessary. In the past, wide excision of the cartilage was the standard, but this is no longer considered appropriate. The minimal acceptable intervention currently is incision, drainage, and culture of the abscess, along with debridement of the necrotic cartilage. An incision can usually be made posteriorly or hidden in the natural curves of the antihelix. A minimal incision includes the anterior wall of the abscess and a thin rim of normal cartilage.

A variety of new therapies have resulted in improvement in cartilage survival. The placement of multiperforate catheters in the plane between the perichondrium and the cartilage and subsequent irrigation with antipseudomonal antibiotics has been successful.[84, 85] A technique gaining in popularity is iontophoresis, which consists of submerging the ear in a bath of antibiotic solution to which direct-current power is applied such that positively charged antibiotics (e.g., gentamicin) are driven into the tissue during three to four treatments a day.[86, 87]

OUTCOMES

Chondritis is a deforming disease process. The goal, therefore, is to treat it rapidly and aggressively in order to achieve the best cosmetic outcome. Insufficiently treated infection causes rampant loss of cartilage and significant resultant deformity. Although reconstruction is possible with a variety of techniques, the best result is achieved by preventing the loss of normal cartilage. Pain subsides with adequate treatment. Prolonged hospital stays are not uncommon because of the need for parenteral antibiotics and the use of local antibiotic instillation or iontophoresis.

Otitis Media, Mastoiditis, and Complications

Otitis media is one of the most common reasons for a patient to see a physician; 24.5 million pediatric visits were recorded in 1990.[88] Most cases are managed by primary care physicians and are uneventful. However, complications can develop, and progression of the disease involves many potentially adverse effects. Acute and chronic otitis media are not otologic emergencies, but their complications and acute mastoiditis certainly represent disease processes that require acute intervention. Suppurative otitis media currently results in a 0.024% incidence of coalescent mastoiditis.[89]

Acute mastoiditis is usually a complication of otitis media but it can also be the first presentation of a middle ear infection. Immediate treatment is mandatory because of the potential for both intratemporal and intracranial complications. Figure 23–4 lists the most common intratemporal complications (coalescent mastoiditis, subperiosteal abscess, petrositis, labyrinthitis, facial nerve paralysis, hearing loss, cholesteatoma) and intracranial complications (meningitis, sigmoid/lateral sinus thrombosis, subdural/epidural abscess, brain abscess, otitic hydrocephalus).

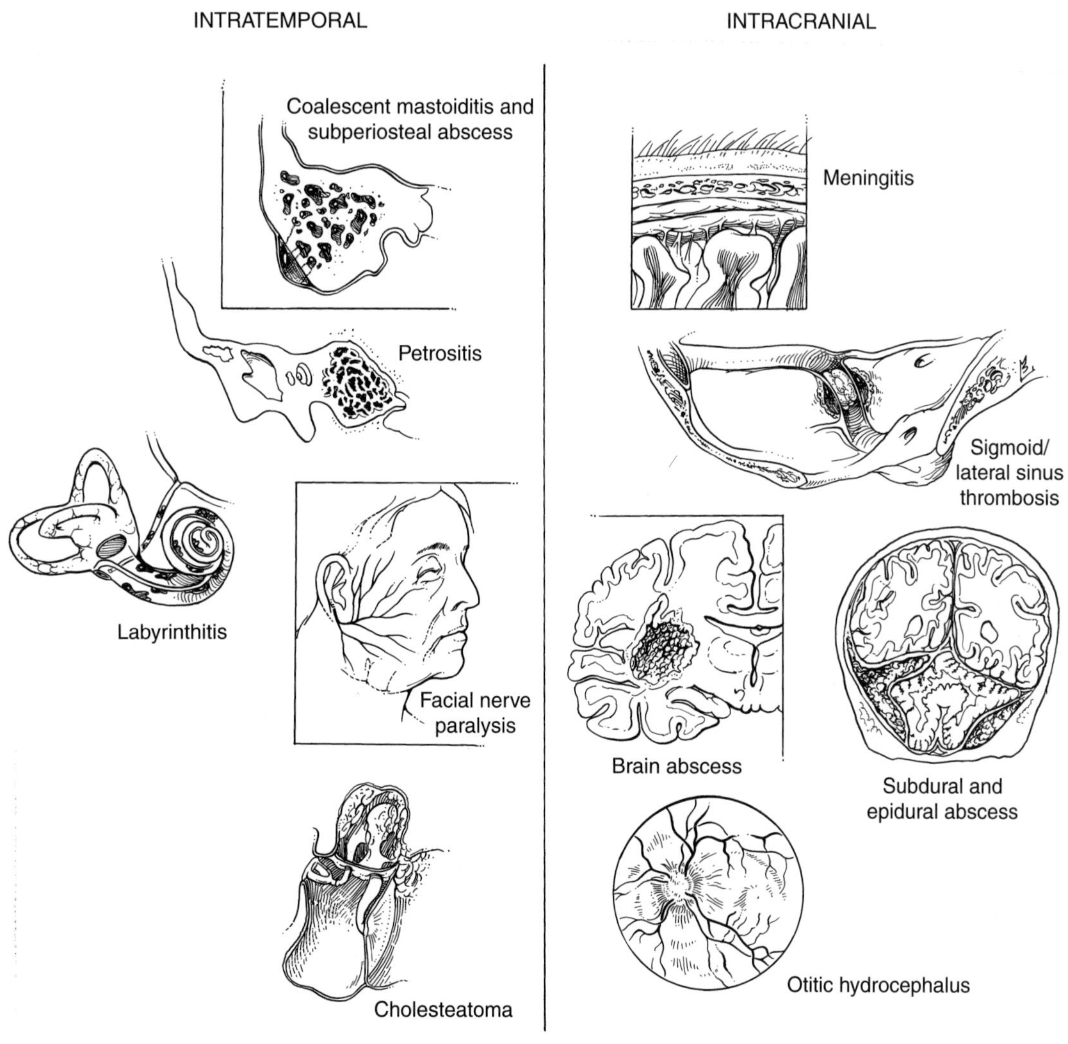

Figure 23–4. Intratemporal and intracranial complications of otitis media.

Acute mastoiditis can affect people of all ages, but there is a higher incidence in children because of the higher incidence of otitis media. The same pathogens that cause otitis media are responsible for acute mastoiditis: *Haemophilus influenzae*, *Streptococcus pneumoniae*, *Staphylococcus aureus*, and β-hemolytic streptococcus organisms. In patients with chronic ear disease, *Pseudomonas aeruginosa* is the most common offending agent. Cultures also frequently reveal *Proteus*, *Klebsiella*, *Escherichia coli*, and *Bacteroides* species. The infection spreads to the mastoid through the aditus; edema or chronic infection leads to obstruction and subsequent mastoiditis.

PRESENTATION

Acute otitis media and chronic otitis media may progress through the steps to mastoiditis or may present initially with advanced complications. Of the possible complications, acute otitis media more frequently presents with meningitis or isolated facial nerve palsy.[90, 91] Chronic otitis media has a higher rate of serious sequelae such as brain abscess.[92] Figure 23–5 shows an early serous mastoiditis. Infection in general takes approximately 2 weeks to develop into coalescent mastoiditis.

The patient presenting with acute mastoiditis usually appears systemically ill and may have a history of preceding otitis media. A Scottish study reported that approximately 1.5% of adults have active chronic otitis media.[93] Chronic otitis media with cholesteatoma may

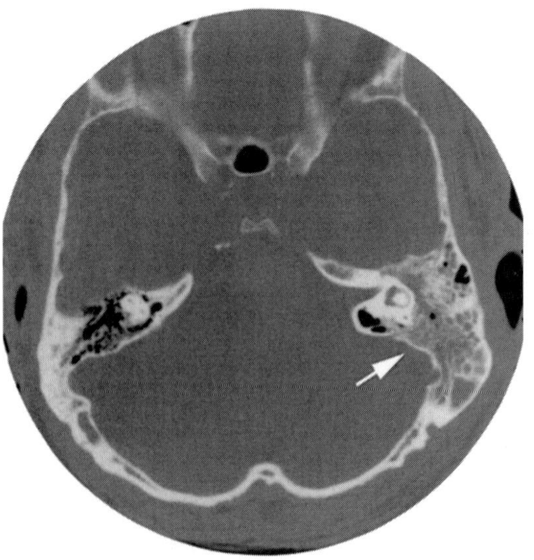

Figure 23–5. CT image showing serous mastoiditis of left ear.

also cause subsequent mastoiditis and is associated with the highest risk of complications.[94, 95] Whatever the cause, the infection presents with postauricular pain, tenderness, swelling, and erythema. Erosion of disease through the postauricular Macewan's triangle leads to subperiosteal abscess formation. An abscess may manifest over the zygoma or over the sternocleidomastoid muscle, which is known as Bezold's abscess. These findings are the sine qua non for a diagnosis of acute mastoiditis, but subperiosteal abscess, the most common of these abscesses, is seen in only 50% of cases.[89] There may be an increase in the auriculocephalic angle as well, with a protruding pinna. Otoscopic examination reveals signs of acute otitis media or perforation with foul-smelling otorrhea. Sagging of the canal skin in the posterosuperior quadrant is also a classic finding.[96]

A patient may present initially with signs of advanced disease. Cranial neuropathies such as facial nerve paralysis and abducens nerve palsy are seen.[95] Hearing loss is primarily conductive, but sensorineural loss may occur with cochlear or intracranial involvement. Vertigo, nystagmus, and dysequilibrium are uncommon as isolated findings, but in conjunction with hearing loss may indicate labyrinthitis, which can be a harbinger of impending intracranial complications. A change in mental status, stroke, and seizures are late complications of acute mastoiditis that are occasionally seen. A patient with a draining ear and subtle signs such as headache, fever, and nausea should be examined with a high index of suspicion of early presentation of possible intracranial complications.[97, 98]

EVALUATION

A good neurologic history and examination are required for proper evaluation. Cranial nerve testing as well as ophthalmoscopy may reveal early signs of advanced disease. Otologic examination should include periauricular palpation, otoscopy, Weber's and Rinne's tests, and vestibular evaluation. Clinical examination should be sufficient for diagnosis. A CT scan is unnecessary unless there are complications requiring definitive diagnosis or further evaluation. An abnormal neurologic examination mandates a temporal bone CT scan as well as a CT scan of the brain using intravenous contrast. Magnetic resonance imaging (MRI) with gadolinium is superior to a CT scan for the diagnosis of intracranial infectious processes and for sigmoid sinus thrombosis.

When the tympanic membrane is intact,

tympanocentesis with culture should be performed in order to direct antibiotic therapy.[99] Some surgeons believe that the placement of a pressure-equalization tube helps to resolve infection more quickly by providing drainage and access for local antibiotic delivery. A special indication for tympanocentesis that merits mention is that of an infant with sepsis.[100] Although acute mastoiditis is unlikely in such a case, otitis media is a cause of sepsis in this population and a potential source of meningitis. In the case of perforation, microscopic local debridement is warranted.

A patient with acute mastoiditis usually exhibits symptoms of systemic illness and commonly has an elevated white blood cell count. A state of immunocompromise may alter treatment course, and a diabetic patient should be followed closely for blood glucose control. After obtaining a CT scan to rule out any intracranial pathology, a patient exhibiting signs of meningitis should undergo lumbar puncture to direct more specific antibiotic therapy. If vestibular dysfunction is elicited, the patient should undergo audiometric testing to rule out cochlear involvement.

PRIORITIES

The first priority in the management of acute mastoiditis is to determine the extent of disease. Empiric intravenous antibiotics should be instituted, and broad coverage with ceftriaxone and clindamycin is recommended; there are a number of appropriate antibiotic regimens. A history of chronic ear disease merits coverage of *Pseudomonas* organisms, and intracranial complications require antibiotics with adequate penetration of the blood-brain barrier. Acute mastoiditis in the setting of chronic ear disease and cholesteatoma carries a significantly higher risk of intracranial complication.[94, 98] Early surgical intervention has been proven to be associated with decreased morbidity. Samuel and colleagues note that despite resolution of obvious middle ear infection, extension of disease and subsequent complications may still be seen.[101] Drainage of the subperiosteal abscess is generally deferred in favor of early simple mastoidectomy as the therapy of choice. Surgical intervention is warranted if there is any evidence of abscess or progression of disease. At the time of mastoidectomy, a pressure-equalization tube is recommended.[99] Culture-based intravenous antibiotics should be continued until there is clear resolution of disease. Figure 23–6 demonstrates a classic attic cholesteatoma.

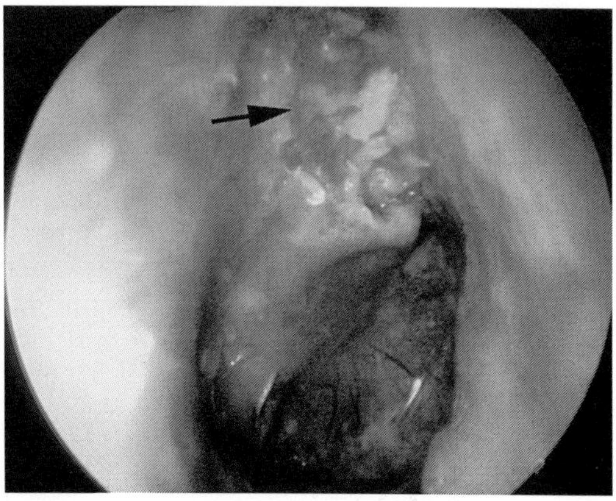

Figure 23–6. Transcanal photo of chronic otitis media with attic cholesteatoma perforating the tympanic membrane.

Petrositis, or petrous apicitis, is a rare complication of both acute and chronic mastoiditis. The classic syndrome described by Gradenigo in 1907 is composed of deep facial or retro-orbital pain, otitis media or mastoiditis, and abducens nerve palsy, although a patient does not necessarily present with all three components of this classic triad.[102] Persistent, recalcitrant mastoid disease with deep pain is more commonly seen, with inflammation of the petrous portion of the temporal bone. There are five tracts, or pathways, for disease to follow medial to the otic capsule and into the petrous apex, which is pneumatized in only one third of people.[103] A CT scan confirms the diagnosis, which should be treated with intravenous antibiotics. Close monitoring is necessary to prevent meningitis, brain abscess, or thrombophlebitis of the inferior petrosal sinus. Usually, a patient requires surgical drainage, which is accomplished via an extended transmastoid, middle cranial fossa, or transglenoid fossa approach. Occluded air cells can result in cholesterol granuloma formation (Fig. 23–7), which frequently involves the petrous apex, necessitating drainage.

Labyrinthitis is the most severe and worrisome intratemporal complication. It has the highest association with hearing loss and intracranial complications. Labyrinthitis due to otitis media or mastoiditis can be divided into three major categories.

1. A labyrinthine fistula is seen in about 6% of temporal bones in cases of chronic otitis media.[104] It is commonly caused by cholesteatoma and is usually located in the lateral semicircular canal (Fig. 23–8). It can be asymptomatic, have mild audioves-

tibular symptoms, or present as suppurative labyrinthitis.[105] Treatment of the penetrating cholesteatoma is best handled by leaving the cholesteatoma matrix in place.[104, 105]

2. Serous labyrinthitis is due to the diffusion of toxins from the local infection into the inner ear. Vestibular symptoms are more pronounced than audiologic symptoms. Treatment involves antibiotics and close observation for development of suppurative labyrinthitis.
3. Suppurative labyrinthitis is the development of purulence within the labyrinth and is characterized by sudden onset of severe vertigo and hearing loss. Meningitis can be the cause or the result of suppurative labyrinthitis. Cephalosporins are the treatment of choice, along with close observation for intracranial extension.[106]

Facial nerve paralysis is usually caused by a dehiscent facial nerve in the transtympanic segment, but it may also arise from direct invasion by infection or swelling into the fallopian canal. Cholesteatoma is found in 80% of cases of paralysis in the setting of chronic suppurative otitis media.[95] In acute otitis media, conservative treatment with broad-spectrum antibiotics may be sufficient intervention.[91] Mastoidectomy, however, is required in chronic disease and in mastoiditis for decompression of the nerve. (Facial nerve paralysis is covered in detail in Chapter 22.)

Cholesteatoma and tympanic membrane perforation are the most common complications of otitis media in children.[107] Hearing loss can be conductive, sensorineural, or mixed. The risk

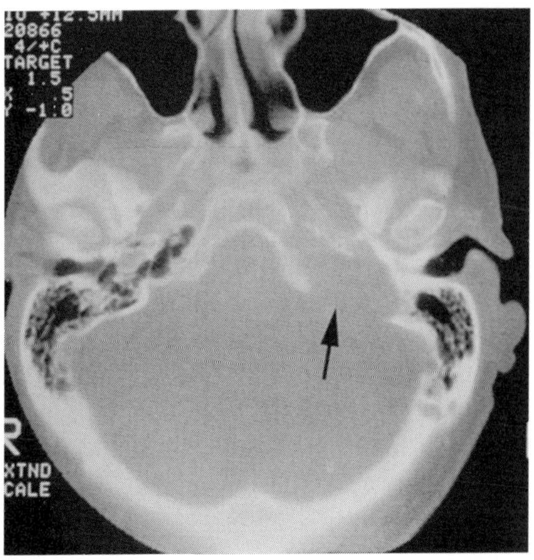

Figure 23–7. CT image of a large petrous apex cholesterol granuloma in the left ear.

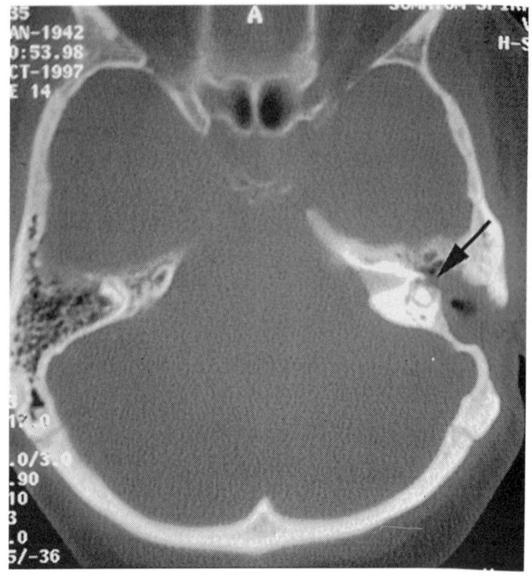

Figure 23–8. CT image demonstrating erosion into the left horizontal canal by recurrent cholesteatoma in a left ear. (Courtesy of H. Francis, M.D.)

of sensorineural hearing loss increases with the duration of chronic otitis media.[108]

Intratemporal complications are more common than intracranial complications. They usually present prior to intracranial complications and should raise the level of suspicion for possible further advancement of disease. In a study of 102 complications in 17,144 cases of otitis media, intratemporal and intracranial complications were seen at a rate of 0.45% and 0.24%, respectively.[109]

Intracranial complications of acute mastoiditis include meningitis, sigmoid sinus thrombosis, otitic hydrocephalus, intracranial abscess, and epidural and subdural abscesses. If history or physical examination suggests any evidence of such complications, neurosurgical involvement at an early stage is critical. Similarly, the patient should be carefully monitored for the development of any new neurologic findings, which may be an indication that the disease has progressed and that more aggressive therapy is necessary. As previously mentioned, the first signs of intracranial extension are fever and headache.[97, 98, 109, 110]

Meningitis is the most common of the intracranial complications; it presents approximately 77% of the time as the intracranial complication of otitis media.[94, 109, 111, 112] It can be isolated or it can occur in combination with one or more other complications. It is commonly seen in combination with brain abscesses and subdural empyemas.[111, 113] Meningitis is also the most common intracranial complication of acute otitis media; it accounted for 91% of the intracranial complications in a study of a pediatric population by Friedman and colleagues.[90]

Meningitis occurs as a result of otitis media by direct extension through the bone or by means of labyrinthitis. Figure 23–9 demonstrates a CT scan that shows mastoiditis with erosion through the posterior plate in a patient presenting with meningitis. It is caused by the same organisms that cause acute and chronic otitis media and that are the offending agent in that patient. However, the majority of cases are caused by *Haemophilus influenzae* B, *Streptococcus pneumoniae*, or *Proteus* species.[90, 109, 112] It is diagnosed by the characteristic signs of meningeal irritation, including headache, photophobia, and nuchal rigidity. Lumbar puncture with cell count, glucose, and culture is confirmatory. Imaging studies should be performed to rule out other intracranial complications. Treatment involves rapid introduction of broad-spectrum parenteral antibiotics and either myringotomy or mastoidectomy, as indicated, to remove the otologic source. (Meningitis and its treatment are more thoroughly addressed in Chapter 24.) Meningitis can still be fatal, despite modern antibiotics, as can the intracranial pathologies that are associated with it and the devastating consequences of those pathologies. Meningitis alone also carries the risk of hearing loss if there is involvement of the labyrinth, and an audiogram should be performed after the resolution of the disease.

Sigmoid sinus or lateral sinus thrombosis is a fairly uncommon intracranial complication of otitis media.[111, 112] However, it carries the second-highest mortality rate after brain abscess among the complications of otitis media. It occurs as a result of erosion of the bone overlying the sigmoid sinus in the mastoid or through the emissary veins to the sinus, allowing infection to spread and form a perisinus abscess. The abscess causes a thrombus to form within the sinus, which results in obstruction leading to subsequent infection, propagation, and emboli.

A high index of suspicion should be held in making this diagnosis, as early detection is key in preventing progression of symptoms and death.[114, 115] It presents with fever, headache, otalgia, and papilledema. Classically, picket-fence fevers (spiking fevers caused by septic emboli) were common but with current antibiotic regimens these are not characteristically seen.[116] Griesinger's sign, or tenderness and edema over the mastoid, is caused by obstruction by means of thrombophlebitis extension into the mastoid emissary vein. Further extension of the clot may result in torticollis and neck pain with involvement of the internal jugular vein or in abducens palsy with extension of the clot into the inferior petrosal sinus. Diagnosis is best confirmed with imaging. The Queckenstedt test, occlusion of the contralateral internal jugular vein and observation for signs of increased cerebrospinal fluid pressure, is now thought to be unreliable and possibly dangerous.[116] Both CT scans and MRI can be very helpful in making the diagnosis. The cord sign is a high-density clot seen in the sinus on noncontrast CT; it is uncommonly seen but is pathognomonic. Similarly, the empty delta sign is seen in about 35% of cases, on contrast CT or MRI with contrast, in the emissary veins around the clot.[116, 117] The combination of MRI and magnetic resonance angiography is believed to be helpful because it provides the advantages of angiography and of MRI without the risk that accompanies invasive procedures; it is becoming the imaging and diagnostic tool of choice.[115, 116]

The treatment of sigmoid sinus thrombosis is mastoidectomy with exposure of the sinus, followed by aspiration or venotomy and removal of the clot and infection. Parenteral antibiotics should be continued for 2 weeks after the primary intervention to avoid further chance of septicemia and septic emboli. Recently, with advances in interventional neuroradiology, the use of selective thrombolytic therapy has become another alternative.[118, 119] In cases in which septic emboli are persistent, ligation of the internal jugular vein may be warranted.[120, 121]

Otitic hydrocephalus is a complication that should be described along with sigmoid sinus

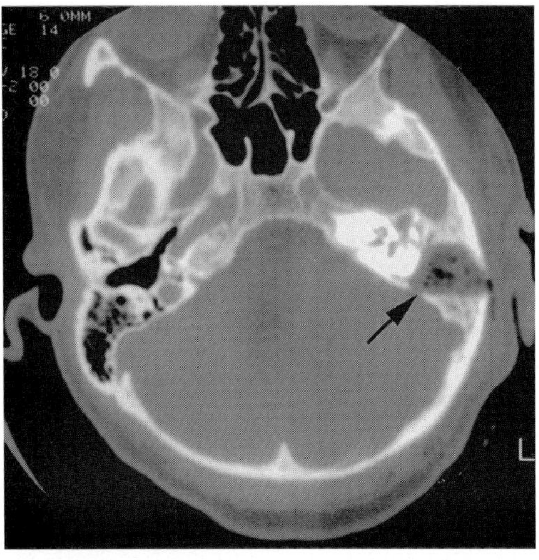

Figure 23–9. CT image of a patient with chronic ear disease presenting with meningitis. CT demonstrates source of infection via bone erosion into the posterior fossa from chronic otitis media of the left ear.

thrombosis. It is a rare complication that is of debated cause but is currently thought likely to be caused by thrombosis of the sigmoid or another venous sinus.[122] Otitic hydrocephalus is elevated intracranial pressure without an infectious intracranial process and without ventricular dilation. It is characterized by a high CSF opening pressure, commonly above 20 cm H_2O. A patient has the symptoms of headache, lethargy, nausea, and vomiting. Papilledema is a good diagnostic sign, and abducens palsy is not uncommon. Diagnosis is best made based on the combination of high CSF pressures on lumbar puncture and sigmoid sinus thrombosis on MRI.[123] Treatment is the same as that for sigmoid sinus thrombosis plus treatment of the otologic focus and evacuation of the clot.[124] The high CSF pressures are handled like pseudotumor cerebri—with serial lumbar punctures, acetazolamide, steroids, and mannitol.

The most worrisome of the intracranial complications of otitis media is brain abscess. It is most commonly associated with chronic ear disease and cholesteatoma but can be a result of acute otitis media.[92, 111] Cerebral or temporal lobe abscesses are the most common, followed by cerebellar abscess.[92, 111, 125] The combined mortality rate in patients with these types of abscesses is still between 10% and 40%.[92, 111] They occur through direct extension from the ear or by means of thrombophlebitis. Headache, fever, and vomiting are the most common symptoms. Meningitis and its findings are seen in up to 71% of abscesses.[111] Diagnosis of the abscess is made by CT or MRI. Treatment should be instituted immediately, with the cooperation of the neurosurgery team. Both the intracranial abscess and the otologic focus must be addressed. (Brain abscesses are more fully covered in Chapter 24.)

Epidural and subdural abscesses are very different from each other. Epidural abscesses are not that uncommon, as any perisinus abscess is, by definition, an epidural abscess. Subdural abscesses—or, more appropriately, subdural empyema—are the most uncommon of intracranial complications. Otorhinologic sources have dropped from being the primary source for both to causing only 29% of them.[113] Both are caused by erosion through the bone of the mastoid and by involvement of the dura mater. Epidural abscesses are usually contained, whereas subdural abscesses spread over the plane of the dura. Epidural abscesses may be silent or may present with headache or otalgia. Subdural abscesses, on the other hand, present with signs of meningeal irritation, focal neurologic findings, and seizures. Both CT scans and MRI show subdural abscesses well, but epidural abscesses may be missed on a CT scan.[113] Both entities are treated by means of neurosurgical decompression and subsequent removal of the otologic source. (These topics are more fully covered in Chapter 24.)

OUTCOMES

Management of otitis media and mastoiditis and their subsequent outcomes depend on early recognition of disease and early intervention. A high index of suspicion must be maintained in order to prevent extension of disease and resultant complications. A patient with mastoiditis who is handled conservatively must be followed closely for any change in symptoms. Fever and headache should not be ignored and may be early warning signs of progression of disease. Mastoiditis, in the setting of chronic ear disease and cholesteatoma, should be treated and evaluated more aggressively because of its propensity for intracranial complications.

Intratemporal and intracranial complications are uncommon but are seen every day nonetheless, and early recognition is vital for preventing long-term morbidity and mortality. Intracranial complications still carry an overall mortality rate of 18.6%.[109] With complication prevalences in suppurative otitis media of 0.45% (intratemporal) and 0.24% (intracranial) of cases when there are 24.5 million office visits for acute otitis media in the United States alone, it is clear that there is considerable potential for complications.[88, 109]

Sudden Sensorineural Hearing Loss

Sudden sensorineural hearing loss (SSNHL) is a challenging but incompletely understood symptom complex that most likely represents the end result of several distinct processes, including traumatic, infectious, vascular, autoimmune, neoplastic, neurologic, and other causes.[126] As such, SSNHL is difficult to manage. When no apparent cause may be identified for the hearing loss, the presentation is termed idiopathic sensorineural hearing loss.

PRESENTATION

Although the precise definition of SSNHL varies somewhat, an acceptable definition is this: a 30 dB or more loss across three contiguous frequencies that commonly occurs within a 12-hour period.[127, 128] The incidence of SSNHL is estimated to be 1 in 10,000 to 15,000 persons.[127] These figures are likely to underestimate the true incidence of SSNHL, as there are, no doubt, patients who experience self-limited SSNHL but never seek medical attention.

The predominant feature of SSNHL is loss of hearing that may affect all frequencies or only a small subset. The loss is commonly noticed by the patient while using the telephone, but its onset may not be immediately apparent to the patient. Other symptoms that may accompany SSNHL are vertigo, tinnitus, and aural fullness. In the event of an obvious cause for the SSNHL such as temporal bone fracture in a motor vehicle accident, additional symptoms may be present that are consistent with the history. Certain features of SSNHL such as a downsloping tympanogram and the presence of vertigo have been shown to be poor prognostic factors in the natural history of the disease, whereas tinnitus appears to have no relationship to prognosis.[129] SSNHL affects men and women equally, at a mean age of 46 years, and it is usually unilateral, with both sides being affected at equal rates.[130]

EVALUATION

The first step in evaluating SSNHL is to establish the diagnosis. Complete details about how the hearing loss began, according to the patient, should be obtained. Of particular importance is a popping sound heard by the patient at the onset of hearing loss or whether the onset awoke the patient from sleep, as these findings may suggest certain diagnoses such as intracochlear membrane rupture and may argue against others.[127, 129] Any medications that have known ototoxicity should be immediately discontinued and a suitable nonototoxic alternative selected. An audiogram is essential, as is a thorough physical examination to identify possible explanations for the hearing loss. Some authors consider MRI with gadolinium to be a mandatory part of the workup of idiopathic SSNHL so as to rule out a mass lesion.[128, 131] Given the importance of vertigo as a prognostic factor, it is crucial to establish definitively the presence or absence of this finding at the time of initial presentation.[131]

In most cases of SSNHL, the exact cause is not identified.[128] The full list of possible causes of SSNHL and the range of laboratory tests that address these causes is extensive. Table 23–1 is a list of some of the more common causes and their associated laboratory measures.

Table 23–1. *Causes and Diagnostic Measures of Sudden Sensorineural Hearing Loss*

Cause	Diagnostic Measure
Medications	Serum levels, dosage history
Aminoglycosides	
Furosemide	
Salicylate	
Viral cochleitis	Viral cultures and titers
Arterial occlusion	Coagulation studies
Inner ear fistula	Fistula test
Autoimmune disease	Antigen-specific serology Western blot
Cerebellopontine angle tumor	MRI
Temporal bone fracture	CT
Acoustic trauma	Audiogram
Meningitis	CSF studies
Meniere's disease	None; history

For some diagnoses, good, objective laboratory tests are not available, as is indicated in the table. Viral cultures, human immunodeficiency virus status, autoimmune serologies, sedimentation rate, CT scans, coagulation studies, and perilymphatic fistula tests may all be appropriate when the cause of hearing loss is not easily identified.

As a standard protocol for evaluation of patients with SSNHL, we recommend several steps. After an audiogram has been obtained and hearing loss established, an examination of the ear should be performed under the microscope. A history of the hearing loss and any previous ear surgery or trauma should be elicited. Signs of upper respiratory infection should be noted. As mentioned, vestibular symptoms should be clearly identified at the onset of symptoms. Blood work should include a complete blood count, a chemistry panel, thyroid function tests, tests for syphilis (Venereal Disease Research Laboratories and fluorescent treponemal antibody absorption) and rheumatoid factor, erythrocyte sedimentation rate, antineutrophil cytoplasmic antibodies (to evaluate Wegener's granulomatosis), and inner ear antigen serologies (69 kDa protein). MRI with gadolinium should be obtained to evaluate the cerebellopontine angle.

PRIORITIES

SSNHL constitutes an otologic emergency. The urgency does not, however, necessarily mean that prompt treatment always improves the course of the disease. Glasscock and associates argued in 1971 that sudden hearing loss was an emergency because the sooner the treatment is instituted, the better the prognosis for recovery, as was found in a number of cases.[129] This viewpoint has subsequently been corroborated.[127]

The priority of initial management is to identify treatable causes of the hearing loss and to take appropriate action. In some cases, such as when the patient is taking aminoglycosides, the response is obvious. In general, the discontinuation of offending ototoxic agents is of the utmost importance for recovery of hearing.[131] When a clear cause is found, a plan for treatment should be decided upon and treatment begun, preferably within the first 24 hours—for example, the prompt administration of antibiotics for suspected bacterial meningitis. As noted, the early obtainment of an audiogram is a priority in the management of SSNHL and should include pure tone, speech discrimination, and tympanometry testing.[127] If a diagnosis of perilymph fistula, neoplasm, or temporal bone trauma is made, early surgical exploration may be warranted.

Because the list of possible causes of SSNHL is vast, treatment is especially difficult when no clear explanation for the hearing loss can be established. The natural history of the disease is such that about two thirds of patients recover at least partial hearing without any treatment.[131, 132] Only 10% to 15% of cases result in identification of a cause, so empiric therapy is directed at improving the course of SSNHL despite the absence of clear cause.[131]

The empiric therapy advocated in the past has been referred to as "shotgun therapy," a battery of treatment agents and protocols aimed at the most likely causes.[129] This includes agents such as steroids, dextran, histamine, diuretics, carbogen (a mixture of 5% carbon dioxide in 95% oxygen), vasodilators (such as nicotinic acid), and heparin. Steroid treatment is based primarily on its anti-inflammatory effects in the event of viral cochleitis. Agents such as dextran aim to improve blood flow by decreasing viscosity. Histamine and carbogen cause vasodilation in an attempt to increase delivery of oxygen to the cochlea. Diuretics may be useful if endolymphatic hydrops is responsible for the hearing loss, as they decrease the extent of hydrops. Heparin is an anticoagulant that is directed at possible embolic causes of SSNHL. Most studies have shown questionable benefits of a shotgun approach, and there is no single accepted protocol. However, several authors advocate, at a minimum, the use of steroids (prednisone) and diuretics.[131] These two interventions should form the basis of initial therapy of SSNHL. A double-blind, randomized trial by Wilson and colleagues showed that steroid therapy was beneficial in the treatment of SSNHL.[133] The use of carbogen, a low-salt diet, and sometimes antivirals such as acyclovir are advocated by other authors, and although data to support these measures are lacking, they may be helpful in cases of persistent hearing loss.[128, 129, 131]

The mixed results of studies of the treatment of SSNHL and the various positions of authors on the subject reflect the heterogeneous array of causes that produce SSNHL. We recommend initial treatment with high-dose oral steroids administered over 2 weeks in a tapered dosage. Because their adverse effects are minimal, antivirals such as acyclovir or famciclovir may be instituted. We do not routinely use diuretics in the treatment of SSNHL unless it is clearly secondary to endolymphatic hydrops. Carbogen is also not routinely used in the initial management of SSNHL at our institution.

OUTCOMES

SSNHL resolves with treatment in about two thirds of cases, with one third of all cases attaining full recovery of hearing. Another third usually have a 40- to 60-dB speech reception threshold.[132] Recovery usually occurs within the first 2 weeks after presentation. In general, the worse the degree of hearing loss and the longer its duration, the less likely hearing is to return. Other prognostic variables are the shape of the audiogram (downsloping and flat losses indicate worse prognoses) and associated vertigo, which also carries an unfavorable prognosis.[128] Findings on electronystagmography, especially caloric testing, are often used to assess vertiginous symptoms. Causes of SSNHL presumed to be embolic in nature (on the basis of a history of risk factors for atherosclerotic disease) are also associated with poor prognoses. Last, the patient's age is important, with children and older adults faring worst.[127] Rehabilitation is especially important for children with permanent hearing loss and adults who do not regain hearing, and education about hearing aids and special schooling needs should be provided.

Acute Labyrinthine Disorders

The main feature of acute labyrinthine disorders is severe dizziness. The dizziness does not necessarily constitute true vertigo, which is defined as a false sense of motion either of self or of environment.[134] Vertigo may be caused by both central and peripheral vestibular disorders, some of which are urgent in nature and require prompt identification. Less emergent causes of dizziness include viral vestibular neuritis, benign positional vertigo, and Meniere's disease, whereas emergent sources include cerebellar infarction and intracranial hemorrhage. An accurate and thorough history forms the basis for the rapid assessment of acute labyrinthitis, and physicians should be familiar with the signs that indicate otologic emergencies.

PRESENTATION

Dizziness can arise from both vestibular and nonvestibular causes. According to Baloh, a sense of spinning almost always points to a vestibular cause of dizziness, whereas a patient with a nonvestibular cause of dizziness generally describes a stable external environment and exhibits no nystagmus.[135] In contrast to a patient who has vestibular causes of nausea as a result of the vertigo, a patient who has a nonvestibular disorder more commonly describes a feeling of lightheadedness. Although these descriptions are not sufficiently diagnostic, they help to guide the physician to the cause of dizziness. Nonvestibular causes of dizziness include a variety of medical abnormalities, such as vasovagal episodes, hypovolemia, hypoglycemia, and cardiac disorders, as well as medications such as phenytoin. These conditions are not discussed further here.

The differential diagnosis of acute spontaneous vertigo may be divided into peripheral and central causes, which dictate the specific details of a patient's presentation. Peripheral causes include benign positional vertigo, labyrinthitis, vestibular neuronitis, perilymphatic fistula, trauma, and Meniere's disease. Central causes include cerebellar infarct or hemorrhage, brainstem infarct, demyelinating disease, vertebrobasilar insufficiency, and tumors of the cerebellopontine angle.

A patient typically presents with vertiginous attacks that fall into one of three patterns: (1) prolonged spontaneous attacks that gradually improve over several days, (2) recurrent spontaneous attacks with full recovery in between, or (3) recurrent vertigo associated with position change.[136] The pattern of the vertiginous episodes helps greatly in determining the correct diagnosis. Nystagmus of central origin is generally vertical and persistent, unlike peripheral nystagmus, which is generally torsional and of short duration.[136] The combination of pattern and type of nystagmus provides a relatively quick method of identifying potentially life-threatening causes of vertigo. The life-threatening causes are acute bacterial mastoiditis, cerebellar or brain-stem infarct or hemorrhage, and neoplasms. The otologic but not life-threatening emergencies that may present with vertigo include labyrinthine ischemia and perilymphatic fistula.

EVALUATION

In the workup of an acute labyrinthine disorder, an accurate but efficiently acquired history is crucial. The history should be focused on the acute event that brings the patient to seek medical attention and on any medical or surgical history that may provide keys to the cause of vertigo. For example, a history of peripheral vascular disease or stroke would suggest an embolic or ischemic cause of dizziness. A careful description of symptoms is essential to ensure that the patient has a labyrinthine disorder; a description of lightheadedness or headaches is less likely to indicate a labyrinthine emergency. If the patient does appear to have true vertigo, subjective and objective evaluation for nystagmus should be performed. As part of the history, the nature of onset of symptoms (sudden or gradual) is an important piece of information, as peripheral labyrinthine disorders tend to involve a sudden onset of symptoms. In addition, a history of positionally related vertigo is extremely helpful in establishing a diagnosis.

Physical examination should be directed toward early identification of possible central causes of vertigo. Generally, a patient suffering from a peripheral vestibular disorder is able to ambulate somewhat, albeit with difficulty. In contrast, a patient with a central cause of vertigo usually has such severe symptoms that walking is impossible.[135] Evaluation of nystagmus should be similarly goal-directed. Nystagmus that is not suppressed by fixation and that often changes in direction is consistent with a central cause of vertigo. Peripheral nystagmus, on the other hand, is usually unidirectional and suppressed by fixation.[136]

Otoscopic examination should be performed as part of the initial workup for acute vertigo. Some peripheral causes such as cholesteatoma may be readily seen by otoscopy. Tuning fork tests, a fistula test, and bedside caloric tests should all be performed if the patient is stable; they will shed further light on the issue of whether a central or peripheral lesion is responsible.[137] Tuning fork tests point to either conductive or sensorineural hearing loss, if present; they suggest peripheral or retrocochlear pathology, respectively. A positive perilymphatic fistula test suggests a peripheral cause. Inability to suppress caloric nystagmus suggests a central disorder. A detailed neurologic examination should be performed to evaluate cranial nerve activity and the general level of cognition. Symptoms such as hemiparesis or poor mentation indicate more serious neurologic causes.[138] If an intracranial lesion is suspected or diagnosed, early involvement of a neurosurgeon is required.

If central pathology is unlikely, blood tests for evidence of infection (white blood cell count, syphilis screen) or autoimmune disease (erythrocyte sedimentation rate) can be carried out. If, however, history and physical examination are consistent with a possible central cause, imaging studies should be performed immediately to diagnose the problem and direct therapy. MRI with gadolinium is the test of choice to diagnose cerebellar or brain-stem infarcts as well as tumors. If the source is unclear, observation for 48 hours is an acceptable course of management. Symptoms that have resolved by then fall into the category of vestibular neuronitis, whereas symptoms that do not resolve can be assessed with MRI.[136]

PRIORITIES

As noted, the first priority is to identify life-threatening causes of vertigo as soon as possible. This is usually done by expediently taking a history and performing a focused physical examination and imaging studies. Central nervous system infarcts and hemorrhages are referred for neurosurgical management. Cerebellopontine-angle tumors can be managed using a combined approach involving both neurotology and neurosurgery teams. Neoplasms of the brain stem, such as gliomas and medulloblastomas, may cause rapid, progressive involvement of brain-stem centers, which will lead to death if untreated. Radiation therapy is the first line of treatment for brain-stem neoplasms.[139] Other tumors that may produce vertigo, such as tumors of cranial nerve VIII, may not require urgent surgical resection, but they should be carefully observed for progression over time.

The second priority is to identify an otologic emergency that may have caused the acute labyrinthine disorder. Labyrinthine ischemia, usually due to a vascular event, is the most worrisome diagnosis. It is based on a history of abrupt onset of vertigo, often with neurologic symptoms, and on evidence of brain-stem or cerebellar ischemia; hearing loss in this setting is generally profound.[140] Unfortunately, treatment of this condition is predominantly symptomatic, with a possible role for anticoagulation and antiplatelet therapy.[140] Perilymph fistula is also of significant concern, although intervention need not be immediate, as most fistulas heal spontaneously. Vertebrobasilar insufficiency, although not an otologic threat, may also be a cause of vertigo that is important but not life threatening. Treatment centers on anticoagulation, antiplatelet medication, and reduction of blood viscosity.[140]

Once these priorities have been addressed and emergent diagnoses have been excluded, a more thorough and systematic history and vestibular evaluation, including electronystagmography, rotational testing, and posturography, may be obtained in order to arrive at the correct diagnosis. Treatment for this group of diagnoses such as benign paroxysmal positional vertigo is nonemergent, and relief of symptoms becomes an important priority for patient management. A wide range of medications are useful for symptomatic relief, including antihistamines, anticholinergics, sympathomimetics, and sedatives, and a simple regimen of 25 to 50 mg of meclizine three times a day and diazepam dosed according to symptom severity provides relief for most cases of acute vertigo. If persistent nausea and vomiting prevent adequate oral intake despite medication, intravenous fluids should be administered to prevent dehydration.

OUTCOMES

The natural course and prognosis of an acute vertiginous disorder differ widely according to its cause. The life-threatening causes of vertigo generally indicate poor prognoses, especially if treatment is delayed. This outcome explains the emphasis placed on rapid identification of brain-stem infarcts or hemorrhage. Early treatment of these lesions is extremely important for improving outcomes, as delay can lead to mass effect, brain-stem compression, and death.[135]

Peripheral acute labyrinthine disorders have fairly good prognoses. The vestibular system is extraordinary in its capacity to compensate for peripheral deficits. In younger patients, adaptation may be complete as early as 1 week after onset of symptoms.[140] This unique ability is responsible in part for the good outcomes associated with acute peripheral vestibular disorders. The most common cause of acute peripheral vertigo is benign positional vertigo, in which repositioning maneuvers lead to resolution of symptoms in more than 90% of cases.[141] Other causes of acute vestibulopathy, such as Meniere's disease and vestibular neuronitis (which usually lasts several days, with progressive improvement), do not have definitive curative therapies.[141] However, symptomatic relief with antiemetics, vestibular suppressants, and sedatives is usually possible in the majority of cases. Acute perilymphatic fistulas tend to heal without surgical intervention, but a period of observation is warranted for fistula closure and resolution of symptoms. Labyrinthine ischemia, unfortunately, has no effective treatment. Rather, the measures described earlier attempt to restore blood flow to the labyrinth. Prognosis for this disease is poor, as ischemia is rarely limited to the labyrinth and often affects the brain stem.

In conclusion, vertigo due to acute labyrinthine disease is commonly self-limited, benign, and nonemergent. More serious causes of vertigo, usually originating in the central nervous system, constitute medical emergencies, and rapid treatment leads to the best possible outcomes.

Complications of Cochlear Implantation

Since the introduction in 1972 of the first commercially available device, cochlear implants have become an extraordinarily successful method of treating profound sensorineural deafness. Although differences in effectiveness are seen—postlingually deaf patients do better than prelingually deaf patients, and younger children do better than older children—cochlear implantation has been performed worldwide in approximately 20,000 individuals.[142] The electrode array has been shown to be very stable in a pediatric patient, with little migration after insertion.[143] The major complications of cochlear implantation involve cases that require revision surgery, including facial nerve paralysis and postauricular flap loss with device exposure.

PRESENTATION

Facial nerve paralysis as a result of cochlear implantation is rare because of the careful adherence to time-tested principles of otologic surgery. Furthermore, this complication is usually recognized by the surgeon during the procedure and therefore does not lead to permanent paralysis. Flap viability can be lost as a result of surgical technique, infection, or poor wound healing; the placement of the incision and preoperative control of infection are therefore important concerns.[144, 144a] The patient presents with infection of the incision or, if more severe, with frank dehiscence or pressure necrosis of the wound and with implant exposure or extrusion.[145, 146] Delay of extrusion until 21 months after implantation has been reported.[147] The incidence of such major complications is reported to be between 5% and 13%, according to various series.[142, 148, 149]

EVALUATION

Physical examination provides the key to diagnosis. Wound healing should be carefully followed, and evidence of systemic toxicity in the presence of wound infection is of significant concern. A detailed history regarding implant use and efficacy should be obtained. If electrode migration is suspected, imaging techniques have been shown to depict very clearly the location of the array within the cochlea.[143, 150] Management of abscess by incision and drainage plus antibiotic treatment can lead to implant salvage.[151] If the wound flap has lost viability, it is important to assess the degree of tissue loss and of implant exposure in order to determine the possibility of leaving the implant in place. In some cases, a rotational or transpositional flap may be required for wound closure and implant salvage.[140, 152] An important point that must be remembered is that the magnetic component of most cochlear implant devices precludes the use of MRI techniques, although newer technologies have been devised that permit removal of the implant's magnet.

PRIORITIES

The first priority is to assess the degree of infection, flap breakdown, and implant exposure. Wound infection or abscess formation should be aggressively treated with antibiotics and drainage. If diagnosed early, there is some chance that the implant will remain usable. Particular attention should be given to facial nerve function if the implant has been extruded. Surgical revision and removal of the implant may be necessary in cases of severe wound breakdown or total implant extrusion. Labyrinthitis must be prevented in order to maintain an implantable cochlea.

OUTCOMES

Major complications of cochlear implantation are uncommon; the incidence is between 5%

and 13%.[142] In some cases of wound infection, antibiotics may be sufficient to clear the disease. If flap breakdown has occurred, a revision flap may be employed.[146, 152] Facial paralysis as a result of cochlear implantation is exceedingly rare and has a good prognosis overall. In a series of 125 cochlear implant patients, Miyamoto reported no cases of facial nerve paralysis.[151] Although most complications of cochlear implantation are not immediately life threatening in nature, the otologic consequences of untreated implant extrusion are significant and should be promptly addressed.[151]

CONCLUSION

As this chapter has revealed, otologic emergencies are a diverse group of disorders whose management varies widely. We have discussed the most urgent otologic and skull base disorders, with an emphasis on traumatic injury, infection, hearing loss, and labyrinthine disease. In all of these conditions, the distinction between an emergent and an urgent presentation is largely semantic, and priority should be given to prompt identification and treatment rather than to classification of severity. Many of these diseases, most notably those of infectious origin, are progressive over a short period of time; during even a relatively brief interval, a patient's condition may deteriorate from a serious one to a fulminant one.

In contrast, most otologic emergencies are not necessarily life threatening, and their significance may be more subtle. Accordingly, a higher index of suspicion must be maintained when a patient presents to a physician and has otologic complaints. Within a particular diagnosis, the range of symptoms may span a broad spectrum, and only a portion of them indicate an otologic emergency. When a patient's condition appears urgent, the initial workup should be focused and efficient; if indicated, a more exhaustive workup can be completed once the patient is stable. By their nature, medical and surgical emergencies often produce a state of heightened tension during which clarity of thought and differential diagnostic ability are of paramount importance.

We hope this chapter has been helpful in highlighting the points toward which a focused workup should be directed. As outcomes are generally dependent upon rapid management, command of such essential points results in the best possible care for a patient with a serious otologic or skull base disorder.

REFERENCES

1. Bressler K, Shelton C. Ear foreign-body removal: a review of 98 consecutive cases. Laryngoscope 1993; 103:367–370.
2. Hollinshead WH. The ear. In Anatomy for Surgeons: The Head and Neck. Philadelphia, JB Lippincott, 1982, pp. 160–161.
3. Baker MD. Foreign bodies of the ears and nose in childhood. Pediatr Emerg Care 1987; 3:67–70.
4. Backous DB, Minor LB, Niparko JK. Trauma to the external auditory canal and temporal bone. Otolaryngol Clin North Am 1996; 29:853–866.
5. English GM. Common injuries to the ear. Prim Care 1976; 3:507–520.
6. Kiskaddon RM, Sasaki CT. Middle ear foreign body: a hearing aid complication. Arch Otolaryngol 1983; 109:778–779.
7. Jahn AF, Hawke M. Foreign body granulomas of the ear. J Otolaryngol 1976; 5:221–226.
8. Deguine C, Pulec JL. Beach sand in the ear. Ear Nose Throat J 1994; 73:719.
9. Peltola JL, Saarento R. Water used to visualize and remove hidden foreign bodies from the external ear canal. J Laryngol Otol 1992; 106:157–158.
10. Schittek A. Insect in the external auditory canal: a new way out. JAMA 1980; 243:331.
11. Strachan DR, Kenny H, Hope GA. The hearing-aid battery: a hazard to elderly patients. Age Aging 1994; 23:425–426.
12. Skinner DW, Chui P. The hazards of "button-sized" batteries as foreign bodies in the nose and ear. J Laryngol Otol 1986; 100:1315–1318.
13. Vottler TP, Nash JC, Rutledge JC. The hazards of ingested alkaline disc batteries in children. JAMA 1983; 249:2504–2506.
14. Capo JM, Lucente FE. Alkaline foreign bodies of the ear and nose. Arch Otolaryngol Head Neck Surg 1986; 112:562–563.
15. McRae D, Premachandra DJ, Gatland D. Button batteries in the ear, nose and cervical esophagus: a destructive foreign body. J Otol 1989; 18:317–319.
16. Kavanagh KT, Litovitz T. Miniature battery foreign bodies in auditory and nasal cavities. JAMA 1986; 255:1470–1472.
17. Panosian MS, Wayman JW, Dutcher PO. Facial nerve paralysis from slag injury to the ear. Arch Otolaryngol Head Neck Surg 1993; 119:548–550.
18. Lindeman P et al. Acute traumatic tympanic membrane perforations. Arch Otolaryngol Head Neck Surg 1987; 113:1285–1287.
19. Kristensen S et al. Traumatic tympanic membrane perforations: complications and management. Ear Nose Throat J 1989; 68:503–516.
20. Dommerby H, Tos M. Sensorineural hearing loss in posttraumatic incus dislocation. Arch Otolaryngol 1983; 109:257–261.
21. Belluci RJ. Traumatic injuries of the middle ear. Otolaryngol Clin North Am 1983; 16:633–650.
22. Garth RJN. Blast injury of the auditory system: a review of mechanisms and pathology. J Laryngol Otol 1994; 108:925–929.
23. Glasscock ME III, McKennan KX, Levine SC. Persistent traumatic perilymph fistulas. Laryngoscope 1987; 97:860–864.

23a. Kristensen S. Spontaneous healing of traumatic tympanic membrane perforations in man: a century of experience. J Laryngol Otol 1992; 106:1037–1050.

24. Cannon CR, Jahrsdoerfer RA. Temporal bone fractures: review of 90 cases. Arch Otolaryngol 1983; 109:285–289.

25. Brodie HA, Thompson TC. Management of complications from 820 temporal bone fractures. Am J Otol 1997; 18:188–197.
26. Nosan DK, Benecke JE Jr. Current perspective on temporal bone trauma. Otolaryngol Head Neck Surg 1997; 117:67–71.
27. Goodwin WJ. Temporal bone fractures. Otolaryngol Clin North Am 1983; 16:651–659.
28. Coker NJ. Management of traumatic injuries to the facial nerve. Otolaryngol Clin North Am 1991; 24:215–227.
29. Wennmo C, Sveensson C. Temporal bone fractures: vestibular and other related sequelae. Acta Otolaryngol Suppl (Stockh) 1989; 468:379–383.
30. Travis LW, Stalnaker RL, Melvin JW. Impact trauma of the human temporal bone. J Trauma 1977; 17:761–776.
31. Lyos AT et al. Progressive hearing loss after transverse temporal bone fracture. Arch Otolaryngol Head Neck Surg 1995; 121:795–799.
32. Shea JJ Jr, Ge X, Orchik DJ. Traumatic endolymphatic hydrops. Am J Otol 1995; 16:235–240.
33. Ghorayeb BY, Yeakley JW. Temporal bone fractures: longitudinal or oblique? The case for oblique temporal bone fractures. Laryngoscope 1992; 102:129–134.
34. Schubiger O et al. Temporal bone fractures and their complications: examination with high resolution CT. Neuroradiology 1986; 28:93–99.
34a. Williams WT, Ghorayeb BY, Yeakley JW. Pediatric temporal bone fractures. Laryngoscope 1992; 102:600–603.
35. Mercuri V, House RJ. Temporomandibular joint air in fractures of the skull base. Australas Radiol 1992; 36:129–130.
36. Goodwin JR, Johnson MH. Carotid injury secondary to blunt head trauma: case report. J Trauma 1994; 37:119–122.
37. Pollanen MS et al. Fracture of temporal bone with exsanguination: pathology and mechanism. Can J Neurol Sci 1992; 19:196–200.
38. Shindo ML et al. Gunshot wounds of the temporal bone: a rational approach to evaluation and management. Otolaryngol Head Neck Surg 1995; 112:530–533.
39. Duncan NO et al. Gunshot injuries of the temporal bone. Otolaryngol Head Neck Surg 1986; 94:47–55.
40. Ghorayeb BY, Rafie JJ. Fracture of the temporal bone: evaluation of 123 cases. J Radiol 1989; 70:703–710.
41. Oberascher G. Cerebrospinal fluid otorrhea: new trends in diagnosis. Am J Otol 1988; 9:102–108.
42. Parell GJ, Becker GD. Inner ear barotrauma in scuba divers: a long-term follow-up after continued diving. Arch Otolaryngol Head Neck Surg 1993; 119:455–457.
43. Hough JVD, McGee M. Otologic trauma. In Paparella MM et al., eds. Otolaryngology, vol. 2, 6th ed. Philadelphia, WB Saunders, 1991, pp. 1137–1160.
44. Pullen FW. Perilymphatic fistula induced by barotrauma. Am J Otol 1992; 13:270–272.
45. Molvaer OI, Eidsvik S, Kajen BK. Cochleovestibular barotrauma in diving. In Molvaer OI, ed. Effects of Diving on the Cochleovestibular System. Bergen, Norway, Norwegian Underwater Technology Centre, Report No. 29–88, 1988, pp. 3–48.
46. Shupak A et al. Diving-related inner ear injuries. Laryngoscope 1991; 101:173–179.
47. Farmer JC. Otologic barotrauma. In Britton BH, ed. Common Problems in Otology. St. Louis, Mosby-Year Book, 1991, pp. 342–353.
47a. Whinney DJD, Parikh AA, Brookes GB. Barotraumatic fracture of the stapes footplate. Am J Otol 1996; 17:697–699.
48. Lifschultz BD, Donoghue ER. Deaths caused by lightning. J Forensic Sci 1993; 38:353–358.
49. Lightning-associated deaths: United States, 1980–95. MMWR Morb Mortal Wkly Rep 1998; 47:391–394.
50. Andrews CJ, Darveniza M. Telephone-mediated lightning injury: an Australian survey. J Trauma 1989; 29:665–671.
51. Craig SR. When lightning strikes: pathophysiology and treatment of lightning injuries. Postgrad Med 1986; 79:109–123.
52. Jones DT et al. Lightning and its effects on the auditory system. Laryngoscope 1991; 101:830–834.
53. Ogren FP, Edmunds AL. Neuro-otologic findings in the lightning-injured patient. Semin Neurol 1995; 15:256–262.
54. Poulsen P, Knudstrup P. Lightning causes inner ear damage and intracranial hematoma. J Laryngol Otol 1986; 100:1067–1070.
55. Bergstrom L et al. The lightning-damaged ear. Arch Otolaryngol 1974; 100:117–121.
56. Redleaf MI, McCabe BF. Lightning injury of the tympanic membrane. Ann Otol Rhinol Laryngol 1993; 102:867–869.
57. Farrior JB. External otitis. In Gates GA, ed. Current Therapy in Otolaryngology-Head and Neck Surgery, 6th ed. St. Louis, Mosby-Year Book, 1998, pp. 1–4.
58. Russel JD et al. What causes acute otitis externa? J Laryngol Otol 1993; 107:898–901.
59. Strunk CL. Necrotizing otitis externa. In Gates GA, ed. Current Therapy in Otolaryngology-Head and Neck Surgery, 6th ed. St. Louis, Mosby–Year Book, 1998, pp. 8–9.
60. Bhisitkul DM, Dunham M. An unsuspected alkaline battery foreign body presenting as malignant otitis externa. Pediatr Emerg Care 1992; 8:141–142.
61. Kumar BN et al. Benign necrotizing osteitis of the external auditory meatus. J Laryngol Otol 1997; 111:269–270.
62. Hern JD et al. Malignant otitis externa in HIV and AIDS. J Laryngol Otol 1996; 110:770–775.
63. O'Sullivan TJ et al. The pathogenesis, differential diagnosis, and treatment of malignant otitis externa. J Otolaryngol 1978; 7:297–303.
64. Gips S et al. Quantitative bone and 67Ga scintigraphy in the differentiation of necrotizing external otitis from severe external otitis. Arch Otolaryngol Head Neck Surg 1991; 117:623–626.
65. Rubin J et al. Efficacy of oral ciprofloxacin plus rifampin for treatment of malignant otitis externa. Arch Otolaryngol Head Neck Surg 1989; 115:1063–1069.
66. Slattery WH, Brackmann DE. Skull base osteomyelitis. Otolaryngol Clin North Am 1996; 29:795–806.
67. Shupak A et al. Hyperbaric oxygenation for necrotizing (malignant) otitis externa. Arch Otolaryngol Head Neck Surg 1989; 115:1470–1475.
68. Rachidi-Alaoui F et al. Malignant otitis externa: apropos of 19 cases. Rev Laryngol Otol Rhinol (Bord) 1995; 116:315–319.
69. Marais J, Dale BAB. Bullous myringitis: a review. Clin Otolaryngol 1997; 22:497–499.
70. Roberts DB. The etiology of bullous myringitis and the role of mycoplasmas in ear disease: a review. Pediatrics 1980; 65:761–766.
71. Brown OE, Meyerhoff WL. Diseases of the tympanic membrane. In Paparella MM et al., eds. Otolaryngology, vol. 2, 3rd ed. Philadelphia, WB Saunders, 1991, pp. 1273–1275.

72. Mawson SR, Ludman H. Diseases of the Ear, 4th ed. Chicago, Year Book, 1979, pp. 272–273.
73. Schuknecht HF. Pathology of the Ear, 2nd ed. Philadelphia, Lea & Febiger, 1993, pp. 191–193.
74. Hariri MA. Sensorineural hearing loss in bullous myringitis: a prospective study of eighteen patients. Clin Otolaryngol 1990; 15:351–353.
75. Purdue GF, Hunt JL. Chondritis of the burned ear: a preventable complication. Am J Surg 1986; 152:257.
76. Skorina J, Kaufman D. Necrotizing fasciitis originating from pinna perichondritis. Otolaryngol Head Neck Surg 1995; 113:467–473.
77. Cumberworth VL, Hogarth TB. Hazards of ear-piercing procedures which traverse cartilage: a report of *Pseudomonas* perichondritis and review of other complications. Br J Clin Pract 1990; 44:512–513.
78. Urkeltaub SH, Habal MB. Acute *Pseudomonas* chondritis as a sequel to ear piercing. Ann Plast Surg 1990; 24:279–282.
79. Rampleburg O et al. ENT manifestations of relapsing polychondritis. Acta Otorhinolaryngol Belg 1997; 57:73–77.
80. Jung C, Muller-Hocker J, Rauh G. Relapsing poly(peri)chondritis diagnosed by biopsy during inflammatory free interval: destructive polychondritis versus fibrosing perichondritis. Eur J Med Res 1996; 1:554–558.
81. Zeuner M et al. Relapsing polychondritis: clinical and immunogenetic analysis of 62 patients. J Rheumatol 1997; 24:96–101.
82. Mills DC II et al. Suppurative chondritis: its incidence, prevention, and treatment in burn patients. Plast Reconstr Surg 1988; 82:267–276.
83. Noel SB et al. Treatment of *Pseudomonas aeruginosa* auricular perichondritis with oral ciprofloxacin. J Dermatol Surg Oncol 1989; 15:633–637.
84. Bassiouny A. Perichondritis of the auricle. Laryngoscope 1981; 91:422–431.
85. Stevenson EW. *Bacillus pyocyaneus* perichondritis of the ear. Laryngoscope 1964; 74:255.
86. Desai MH et al. The role of gentamicin iontophoresis in the treatment of burned ears. J Burn Care Rehabil 1991; 12:521–524.
87. Rigano W et al. Antibiotic iontophoresis in the management of burned ears. J Burn Care Rehabil 1992; 13:407–409.
88. Stool SE et al. Otitis media with effusion in young children, Clinical Practice Guideline No. 12. AHCPR publication no. 94-0622, Rockville, MD. 1994, pp. 1–8.
89. Spiegel JH et al. Contemporary presentation and management of a spectrum of mastoid abscesses. Laryngoscope 1998; 108:822–828.
90. Friedman EM, McGill TJ, Healy GB. Central nervous system complications associated with acute otitis media in children. Laryngoscope 1990; 100:149–151.
91. Henderson PE, Baldone SC. Facial nerve palsy secondary to acute otitis media. J Am Osteopath Assoc 1989; 89:207–210.
92. Szmcja Z et al. Otogenic brain abscesses in children. Otolaryngol Pol 1991; 45:405–410.
93. Nunez DA, Browning GG. Risks of developing an otogenic intracranial abscess. J Laryngol Otol 1990; 104:468–472.
94. Yaniv E, Pocock R. Complications of ear disease. Clin Otolaryngol 1988; 13:357–361.
95. Savic DL, Djeric DR. Facial paralysis in chronic suppurative otitis media. Clin Otolaryngol 1989; 14:515–517.
96. Nadal D et al. Acute mastoiditis: clinical, microbiological, and therapeutic aspects. Eur J Pediatr 1990; 149:56.
97. Munz M et al. Otitis media and CNS complications. J Otolaryngol 1992; 21:224–226.
98. Schwaber MK, Pensak ML, Bartels LJ. The early signs and symptoms of neurotologic complications of chronic suppurative otitis media. Laryngoscope 1989; 99:373–375.
99. Sie KCY. Acute mastoiditis. In Gates GA, ed. Current Therapy in Otolaryngology-Head and Neck Surgery, 6th ed. St. Louis, Mosby–Year Book, 1998, pp. 13–15.
100. Arriaga MA, Bluestone CD, Stool SE. The role of tympanocentesis in the management of infants with sepsis. Laryngoscope 1989; 99:1048–1051.
101. Samuel J, Fernandez CM, Steinberg JL. Intracranial otogenic complications: a persistent problem. Laryngoscope 1986; 96:36.
102. Chole RA, Donald PJ. Petrous apicitis: clinical considerations. Ann Otol Rhinol Laryngol 1983; 92:544–551.
103. Chole RA. Petrous apicitis: surgical anatomy. Ann Otol Rhinol Laryngol 1985; 94:251–257.
104. Jang CH, Merchant SN. Histopathology of labyrinthine fistulae in chronic otitis media with clinical implications. Am J Otol 1997; 18:15–25.
105. Vartiainen E. What is the best method of treatment for labyrinthine fistulae caused by cholesteatoma? Clin Otolaryngol 1992; 17:258–260.
106. Sun AH, Parnes LS, Freeman DJ. Comparative perilymph permeability of cephalosporins and its significance in the treatment and prevention of suppurative labyrinthitis. Ann Otol Rhinol Laryngol 1996; 105:54–57.
107. Farrior J. Complications of otitis media in children. South Med J 1990; 83:645–648.
108. Cusimano F, Cocita VC, D'Amico A. Sensorineural hearing loss in chronic otitis media. J Laryngol Otol 1989; 103:158–163.
109. Kangsanarak J et al. Extracranial and intracranial complications of suppurative otitis media. J Laryngol Otol 1993; 107:999–1004.
110. Albers FW. Neuro-otological complications of middle ear infections: the importance of early diagnosis. Ned Tijdschr Geneeskd 1996; 140:1726–1729.
111. Deric D, Arsovic N, Dordevic V. Pathogenesis and methods of treatment of otogenic brain abscess. Med Pregl 1998; 51:51–55.
112. Gower DJ, McGuirt WF, Kelly DL Jr. Intracranial complications of ear disease in a pediatric population with special emphasis on subdural effusion and empyema. South Med J 1985; 78:429–434.
113. Hlavin ML et al. Intracranial suppuration: a modern decade of postoperative subdural empyema and epidural abscess. Neurosurgery 1994; 34:974–980.
114. Debry C et al. Thrombophlebitis of the lateral sinus: apropos of a case. Rev Laryngol Otol Rhinol 1993; 114:355–358.
115. Fritsch MH, Miyamoto RT, Wood TL. Sigmoid sinus thrombosis diagnosis by contrasted MRI scanning. Otolaryngol Head Neck Surg 1990; 103:451–456.
116. Davison SP et al. Use of magnetic resonance imaging and magnetic resonance angiography in diagnosis of sigmoid sinus thrombosis. Ear Nose Throat J 1997; 76:436–441.
117. Kelly KE, Jackler RK, Dillon WP. Diagnosis of septic sigmoid sinus thrombosis with magnetic resonance imaging. Otolaryngol Head Neck Surg 1991; 105:617–624.

118. Gurley MB, King TS, Tsai FY. Sigmoid sinus thrombosis associated with internal jugular venous occlusion: direct thrombolytic treatment. J Endovasc Surg 1996; 3:306–314.
119. Tsai FY et al. Acute thrombosis of the intracranial dural sinus: direct thrombolytic treatment. Am J Neuroradiol 1992; 13:1137–1141.
120. Dallari S et al. Acute mastoiditis with complications: a report of two cases. Acta Otorhinolaryngol Belg 1997; 51:113–118.
121. Namyslowski G et al. Otogenic sigmoid sinus thrombosis in the course of chronic otitis media. Otolaryngol Pol 1995; 49:451–456.
122. Tomkinson A, Mills RG, Cantrell PJ. The pathophysiology of otitic hydrocephalus. J Laryngol Otol 1997; 111:757–759.
123. Sennaroglu L et al. Role of MRI in the diagnosis of otitic hydrocephalus. Am J Otol 1996; 17:784–786.
124. Isaacman DJ. Otitic hydrocephalus: an uncommon complication of a common condition. Ann Emerg Med 1989; 18:684–687.
125. Murthy PS et al. Otogenic brain abscess in childhood. Int Pediatr Otorhinolaryngol 1991; 22:9–17.
126. Kohut RI, Hinojosa R. Sudden sensory hearing loss. In Bailey BJ et al., eds. Head and Neck Surgery-Otolaryngology. Philadelphia, JB Lippincott, 1993, pp. 1820–1825.
127. Gulya AJ. Sudden sensorineural hearing loss: an otologic emergency. Compr Ther 1996; 22:217–221.
128. Arts HA. Differential diagnosis of sensorineural hearing loss. In Cummings CW et al., eds. Otolaryngology-Head and Neck Surgery, vol. 4, 3rd ed. St. Louis, Mosby-Year Book, 1998, pp. 2908–2933.
129. Glasscock ME III, Nechtman C, Altenau M. Sudden loss of hearing: a medical emergency. South Med J 1971; 64:1485–1489.
130. Mattox DE, Simmons FB. Natural history of sudden sensorineural hearing loss. Ann Otol Rhinol Laryngol 1977; 86:463–480.
131. Hughes GB. Sudden hearing loss. In Gates GA, ed. Current Therapy in Otolaryngology-Head and Neck Surgery, 6th ed. St. Louis, Mosby–Year Book, 1998, pp. 41–44.
132. Graham MD, Lee KJ, Goldsmith MM III. Noninfectious disorders of the ear. In Lee KJ, ed. Essential Otolaryngology, 6th ed. Norwalk, CT, Appleton & Lange, 1995, pp. 696–701.
133. Wilson WR, Byl FM, Laird N. Efficacy of steroids in the treatment of idiopathic sudden hearing loss: a double-blind clinical study. Arch Otolaryngol Head Neck Surg 1980; 106:772–776.
134. Minor LB, Zee DS. Evaluation of the patient with dizziness. In Cummings CW et al., eds. Otolaryngology-Head and Neck Surgery, vol. 4, 3rd ed. St. Louis, Mosby-Year Book, 1998, pp. 2623–2671.
135. Baloh RW. Dizziness: neurological emergencies. Neurol Clin North Am 1998; 16:305–321.
136. Baloh RW. Differentiating between peripheral and central causes of vertigo. Otolaryngol Head Neck Surg 1998; 119:55–59.
137. Singleton GT. Evaluation of the dizzy patient. In Bailey BJ et al., eds. Head and Neck Surgery-Otolaryngology, vol. 2. Philadelphia, JB Lippincott, 1993, pp. 1870–1876.
138. Lindeman RC. Acute labyrinthine disorders. Otolaryngol Clin North Am 1979; 12:375–387.
139. Baloh RW, Harker LA. Central vestibular disorders. In Cummings CW et al., eds. Otolaryngology-Head and Neck Surgery, vol. 4, 3rd ed. St. Louis, Mosby-Year Book, 1998, pp. 2706–2727.
140. Caplan LR. Management of acute peripheral vestibular disorders. Eur Neurol 1993; 33:337–344.
141. Schessel DA, Minor LB, Nedzelski J. Meniere's disease and other peripheral vestibular disorders. In Cummings CW et al., eds. Otolaryngology-Head and Neck Surgery, vol. 4, 3rd ed. St. Louis, Mosby–Year Book, 1998, pp. 2672–2705.
142. Niparko JK. Cochlear implants. In Cummings CW et al., eds. Otolaryngology-Head and Neck Surgery, vol. 4, 3rd ed. St. Louis, Mosby–Year Book, 1998, pp. 2934–2962.
143. Roland JT Jr et al. Stability of the cochlear implant array in children. Laryngoscope 1998; 108:1119–1123.
144. Axon PR et al. Cochlear implantation in the presence of chronic suppurative otitis media. J Laryngol Otol 1997; 111:228–232.
144a. Gibson WP, Harrison HC, Prowse C. A new incision for placement of cochlear implants. J Larngol Otol 1995; 109:821–825.
145. Hoffman RA et al. Delayed extrusion of the nucleus multichannel cochlear implant. Otolaryngol Head Neck Surg 1991; 105:117–119.
146. Harrison HC, Gibson WP, Thompson PG. Cochlear implant extrusion in a young child: a preventive procedure. J Laryngol Otol 1995; 109:425–428.
147. el-Naggar M, Hawthorne M. Delayed extrusion of a cochlear implant: a case report of an implant extruding 21 months after the original operation. J Laryngol Otol 1995; 109:56–57.
148. Wang RC, Parisier SC, Weiss MH, et al. Cochlear implant flap complications. Ann Otol Rhinol Laryngol 1990; 99:791–795.
149. Ito J et al. Surgical difficulties and postoperative problems associated with cochlear implants. Ann Otol Rhinol Laryngol Suppl 1995; 166:425–426.
150. Czerny C et al. Postoperative radiographic assessment of the Combi 40 cochlear implant. Am J Roentgenol 1997; 169:1689–1694.
151. Miyamoto RT. Cochlear implants. In Bailey BJ et al., eds. Head & Neck Surgery-Otolaryngology, vol. 2. Philadelphia, JB Lippincott, 1993, pp. 1850–1858.
152. Hampton SM, Toner JG, Small J. Cochlear implant extrusion in a child with keratitis, ichthyosis and deafness syndrome. J Laryngol Otol 1997; 111:465–467.

CHAPTER **24**

Intracranial Emergencies

Richard E. Clatterbuck, MD, PhD
Rafael J. Tamargo, MD

This chapter covers emergencies of the cranial base, vault, and contents, with emphasis on emergency conditions and postoperative complications in which appropriate management often includes a neurosurgeon and other head and neck surgical specialists. Topics include closed head injury, cerebrospinal fluid (CSF) leaks, central nervous system (CNS) infections (particularly as they relate to trauma), and postoperative pneumocephalus and intracranial hematoma.

Closed head injuries and penetrating cranial injuries are important public health issues. Patients with these diagnoses present commonly in most hospital emergency departments. It was recognized that care rendered to such patients lacked a certain degree of standardization outside of that offered by the American College of Surgeons' Advanced Trauma Life Support (ATLS) manual; this need was met and the care of the head-injured patient standardized by the *Guidelines for the Management of Severe Head Injury* published in 1995 by the American Association of Neurological Surgeons. The management of such patients is discussed in this chapter.

Leakage of CSF and CNS infections often present both diagnostic and management dilemmas for surgeons. This chapter focuses on these entities as emergencies that arise in the postoperative period and occur as a result of head injury. The current appropriate antibiotic and surgical management are discussed.

Finally, this chapter addresses the diagnosis and management of postoperative hematomas and pneumocephalus. In the immediate postoperative period, patients recovering from surgery at the base of the skull are typically admitted to intensive care units that specialize in the observation of neurosurgical patients. Patients who fail to regain appropriate levels of consciousness postoperatively should be considered to be experiencing life-threatening emergencies until proven otherwise. In addition, such patients must be carefully observed for the onset of new or progressive neurologic signs and symptoms not directly attributable to the procedures involved.

The first step to be taken in the case of a hemodynamically stable patient with such presentation includes ensuring a secure airway and obtaining an emergent computed tomography (CT) scan. Such scans fail to be informative about a patient simply slow to recover from anesthesia or a victim of a seizure, but they are the quickest method of uncovering life-threatening intracranial complications that require a return to the operating room. Postoperative CT scans reveal pathologies amenable to operative intervention such as mass lesions, intra- and extra-axial hematomas, and, less commonly, extra-axial collections of air under pressure, so-called tension pneumocephalus. Malignant cerebral or cerebellar edema requiring decompressive lobectomy is not discussed in this setting, as it is a strictly neurosurgical emergency.

HEAD INJURY

The American Association of Neurological Surgeons and the Joint Section on Neurotrauma and Critical Care have published a comprehensive treatise on this topic.[1] The following discussion of the management of closed head injury and intracranial hypertension is based on these guidelines. The number of fatal closed head injuries that occur each year is about 75,000, and the number of fatal gunshot wounds to the head is about 6,000 per year in the United States, statistics that underscore the importance of familiarity with these conditions.[2] The number of people in the United States who are living with disabilities as a result of neurotrauma is estimated to be 200,000.[1] Head injuries causing fracture of the skull base and frontal sinuses create circumstances in which otolaryngologists and neurosurgeons routinely interface. Basilar skull fractures are discussed in Chapter 23. The appropriate management of frontal sinus fractures is discussed here briefly and is discussed extensively in Chapter 18.

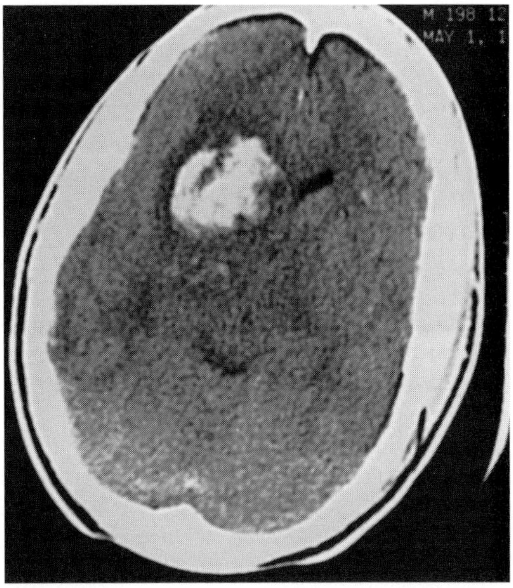

Figure 24–1. A CT image of a patient with a closed head injury shows a deep right frontal contusion. Blood appears white (hyperdense) in a CT image. Note the ring of hypodensity representing edema in the surrounding tissue.

Presentation, Evaluation, and Priorities

A patient who presents with a post-resuscitation Glasgow Coma Scale (GCS) score of less than 8 has suffered a severe head injury by definition and should be treated accordingly. Any patient presenting for care as a result of trauma must first undergo an ATLS evaluation. Any life-threatening visceral injuries should be treated as indicated. In the absence of life-threatening thoracic or abdominal injuries, a patient with a GCS of 8 or less should be intubated and ventilated to a $PaCO_2$ of 35 mm Hg while fluid resuscitation continues. Sedatives and short-acting paralytics are used as necessary. If clinical evidence of herniation is present or if the patient declines neurologically without extracranial cause, then hyperventilation and the administration of mannitol (1 g/kg) and diuretics should be initiated empirically prior to CT scanning. If imaging reveals a mass lesion amenable to surgery, the patient should be taken directly to the operating room. Epidural and subdural hematomas with mass effect causing midline shift fall into this category. In the absence of such a lesion, the patient should be transported to a critical care unit for the placement of an intracranial pressure (ICP) monitoring device and treatment for ongoing intracranial hypertension. Figure 24–1 is an example of a deep post-traumatic contusion/intracerebral hematoma not amenable to surgical intervention.

In the critical care setting, the management of intracranial hypertension mandates ongoing measurement of the ICP with a subarachnoid bolt or intraventricular catheter as a guide to therapy. Management should be aimed at maintaining an adequate cerebral perfusion pressure (CPP), which is the difference between mean arterial blood pressure and ICP. Once an ICP monitor has been placed, CPP should be maintained at 70 mm Hg or greater. If CPP is less than 70 mm Hg, initial therapy is drainage of CSF via a ventricular catheter. This device, rather than a subarachnoid bolt, should be placed whenever possible. The next line of therapy is the administration of mannitol in repeated 0.25 to 1.0 g/kg boluses while maintaining euvolemia. The endpoint of this intervention is a serum osmolarity of 320 mOsm/L. Hyperventilation to a $PaCO_2$ of 30 to 35 mm Hg is the next therapeutic maneuver. Intracranial hypertension refractory to all these interventions may require short periods of hyperventilation to $PaCO_2$ values less than 30 mm Hg, barbiturate coma, or surgical decompression. It should be kept in mind that a patient with refractory intracranial hypertension requires repeat CT scanning to rule out the development of a surgical mass lesion not evident on imaging at admission.

Fractures involving only the anterior table of the frontal sinus are elevated and closed for cosmetic reasons. When the fracture involves the posterior table, however, a neurosurgeon is commonly involved, as complete repair may require bicoronal craniotomy with cranialization of the sinus and dural repair, which is accomplished with an attached pericranial flap after removal of the mucosa. Although lesser procedures are advocated and may be appropriate for minor injuries to the posterior table, these fractures should be considered open skull fractures.[3]

The *Guidelines for the Management of Severe Head Injury* also recommend 1 week of seizure prophylaxis for any patient with a head injury that puts him or her at an increased risk for early post-traumatic seizures. This category includes any patient with a penetrating injury, a hematoma (intracerebral or extra-axial), a depressed skull fracture, a cortical contusion, a GCS of less than 10, or evidence of a seizure. There is no evidence that seizure prophylaxis should continue for longer than 1 week as protection against late post-traumatic seizures. The patient should be loaded with 20 mg/kg of phenytoin at a rate of 50 mg/min. As this drug can cause hypotension and arrythmia it should be given only after cardiovascular stabilization. Witnessed seizure activity prior to loading with phenytoin can be treated with 1- to 2-mg injections of lorazepam. Ongoing seizure activity refractory to initial management efforts (status epilepticus) may require induction of general anesthesia.

The treatment of penetrating cerebral trauma has not been formalized in the same way as treatment for closed head injury has been. Previously, few patients survived these injuries. Several studies have examined the treatment of gunshot wounds to the head during the Lebanese conflict[2, 4, 5] and during the Iran-Iraq War[6] and support limited debridement as a reasonable option. Some procedures consisted only of debridement and closure of the superficial wound.[4] In most cases, no effort was made to remove deep bone and metal fragments. Infections in these studies were related to CSF leaks.[5, 6] Several recent reports, however, support aggressive management in such a patient.[7–9] A patient with a GCS of 3 to 7 was taken to the operating room for craniotomy and debridement if pupillary responses were present and the patient was hemodynamically stable. The degree of surgical debridement varied from conservative tissue removal and closure to formal lobectomy. Bone flaps were not replaced in the setting of severe edema. A patient with a GCS of 8 to 15 was taken to the operating room for removal of intracranial bone fragments or clots with significant mass effect.

Outcomes

In 1991, data from the Traumatic Coma Data Bank were published.[10] This information was collected prior to the implementation of the *Guidelines for the Management of Severe Head Injury*. The data bank found the overall mortality rate to be 36%. Patients with postresuscitation GCS scores of 3 had the highest mortality rate, 76%; patients with GCS scores of 6 to 8 had an 18% mortality rate. One study of civilian gunshot wounds to the head reported a similar overall mortality rate of 34%.[9] This study demonstrated modest improvements in outcome and an increased survival rate of several percent; however, this and similar series supported previous results suggesting that bihemispheric/biventricular injuries (excluding bifrontal), multiple lobe injuries, intra-axial and extra-axial hematomas, and subarachnoid hemorrhage on initial CT are all indicators of poor prognosis.

The management of closed and penetrating head injuries continues to be an area of active research. Trials with various neuroprotectant compounds such as glutamate antagonists and calcium channel blockers are ongoing in academic centers. As the molecular mechanisms leading to neuronal injury become better understood, treatment continues to improve, leading to better outcomes.

CEREBROSPINAL FLUID LEAK

Leakage of CSF was first described in 1826 by Miller; he noted a nontraumatic leak in the setting of hydrocephalus, although traumatic leak is more common. Grant, in 1923, and Dandy, in 1926, first proposed neurosurgical approaches for the treatment of CSF leaks, and in 1927, Cushing reported surgical treatment in three cases of traumatic leakage. In 1948, Dohlman reported the first intranasal approach to anterior skull base CSF leaks.[11] Despite much ongoing interest in the diagnosis and treatment of CSF leaks, they continue to provide a source of frustration for surgeons because they are often refractory to efforts to correct them.

CSF leaks can be classified as traumatic, when they arise as a result of injury or surgery, or as nontraumatic or spontaneous.[11] The spontaneous leaks can be further classified as occurring in the setting of increased intracranial pressure (such as that caused by hydrocephalus) or occurring in the setting of normal intracranial pressure (as in congenital defects or bony erosion).

In one series of 41 patients, 27% of leaks resulted from skull fractures, 10% from congenital defects, 37% as a result of a brain tumors, and 47% as a result of neurosurgical or otolaryngologic procedures.[12] In this series, 24% of patients had associated meningitis and 7% required CSF shunting procedures to stop the leak. In this study, 27% of patients who underwent surgical repair required additional procedures for recurrent leakage. The sites of CSF leakage are varied; they include the frontal sinus, lamina cribrosa, sphenoidal roof, and petrous air cells via the eustachian tube. In the same series of 41 patients, 39% of the leaks came from the region of the cribriform plate and ethmoids, 15% from the frontal sinus, and 15% through the sella turcica via the sphenoid sinus. Three patients in this series had leaks originating in the mastoid air cells and 22% had no verified site. Because iatrogenic injury is common, local surgical practice may determine the most common site of leakage for any one institution.

Presentation

A torrent of clear fluid leaves little doubt as to the nature of the problem, but lesser amounts of rhinorrhea or otorrhea can be more difficult to identify definitively. A patient may present with identifiable fluid leaking from the nose or the ear; however, it is also possible to present with a complaint of postnasal discharge, postural headache, or a history of recurrent meningitis. To further complicate matters, a syndrome of pseudocerebrospinal rhinorrhea has been described after skull base surgery in which pericarotid sympathetic fibers have been disrupted.[13] In this case, a patient has facial flushing, decreased lacrimation, and nasal hypersecretion ipsilateral to the surgical procedure.

Evaluation

It is not always easy to establish that the fluid present at the nares or external auditory meatus is indeed CSF. Early tests to establish the nature of clear drainage were based on glucose determinations. Glucose oxidase test strips were known to be unreliable; absolute glucose determinations are somewhat more accurate, a glucose level of 30 mg/100 mL being diagnostic.[11] More recently, detection of β-2 transferrin by agarose gel electrophoresis and immunoblotting has proven to be more sensitive and specific.[14, 15] In practice, however, fluid is not often identified as CSF by means of laboratory findings because the diagnosis in suspected cases typically depends on imaging studies aimed at directly identifying the location of the leak. The halo, or double ring sign, is of little value in the formal evaluation of CSF leakage.

Imaging studies used in diagnosing CSF leaks have undergone a series of evolutions, but they all attempt to pinpoint the site of egress of CSF. The earliest efforts used plain radiographs and pluridirectional tomography in an attempt to visualize a bony defect. Various dyes have been used in attempted intraoperative identification of a leakage site. Radionuclides have been used, with and without the intranasal placement of cotton pledgets at specific locations, with subsequent nuclear scanning and scintillation counting of pledgets. The radio-iodinated serum albumin scan is still in use.[11] These methods are unsatisfactory because they are difficult to interpret and they fail to reveal a specific anatomic locus. With the advent of later-generation CT scanners and better reconstruction capabilities, as well as the use of water-soluble contrast agents, metrizamide CT cisternography has become the study of choice for localizing the site of skull base CSF leakage.[16, 17] This technique enjoys a high success rate in locating dural and osseous defects in the skull base that are responsible for CSF leaks. Figure 24–2 shows a coronal CT image in which an osseous defect in the cribriform plate is evident. Reports are now appearing in the literature describing the use of magnetic resonance imaging (MRI) in localizing CSF fistulas, but its use is not yet widespread and its value is still being debated.[18–20]

Priorities

Management of CSF leaks is as varied as their sites and causes. The literature contains little information regarding the timing of surgical repair of CSF leaks (traumatic or nontraumatic) or the role of conservative management. The management and timing of intervention depend on the presentation, symptomatology, and history of episodes of meningitis in a particular patient. At our institution, the first line of therapy for CSF leaks is bed rest, with the head of the bed elevated. If the leak persists for 24 hours, large-volume (30 mL), daily lumbar punctures are initiated. In the setting of persistent postoperative leak, a lumbar drain is often inserted for several days of controlled drainage

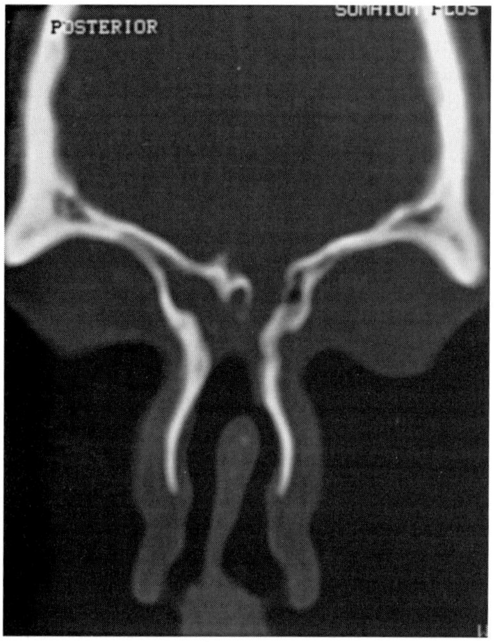

Figure 24–2. The bone windows of this coronal CT image demonstrate an obvious bony defect in the left cribriform plate.

of 5 to 10 mL/h (provided pneumocephalus is not an issue) prior to returning to the operating room, if necessary. At our institution, spontaneous and nontraumatic leaks are scheduled for elective surgical repair.

A topic of debate in the management of a patient with a CSF fistula, traumatic or nontraumatic, is the use of prophylactic antibiotics to prevent meningitis. The concern is the generation of antibiotic-resistant strains in the patient's flora which results in more virulent meningitis if infection occurs. In 1975, Ignelzi and colleagues reported on 129 patients with basilar skull fractures (43 had definite CSF leaks) and found no benefit in chemoprophylaxis.[21] In 1976, Klastersky and colleagues studied 52 patients (all with CSF leaks) in a controlled, double-blind fashion and also found no benefit in prophylactic antibiotics.[22] In 1976, another report appeared, this one by MacGee and associates, in which 58 patients were studied retrospectively and a meta-analysis was performed of 402 cases in the literature; all of the patients had traumatic CSF leaks, and again, no benefit was found in prophylactic use of antibiotics.[23] In 1993, Eljamel made a retrospective study of 253 patients with CSF leaks, almost all traumatic, and found no statistically significant benefit in antibiotic prophylaxis.[24] Of note is that the highest rate of CNS infection in any group in all of these studies was 14%.[23] In a 1981 report by Meirowsky and coworkers on Vietnam War casualties with CSF fistulas as a result of missile wounds, the CNS infection rate was 49.5%,[25] which suggests that when CSF fistulas include foreign bodies, prophylactic antibiotics may be indicated. In summary, prophylactic antibiotics have never been demonstrated to be of benefit.

Several methodologies for the surgical repair of CSF fistulas are currently in use. Leaks that can be visualized endoscopically may be amenable to endoscopic closure.[26] The advantage in this approach is its minimally invasive nature and associated low morbidity. External, extracranial approaches involving free and pedicled mucosal flaps may be necessary for leaks not amenable to endoscopic repair.[27] Leaks refractory to such treatment—those in unknown locations and those involving large bony defects—require more aggressive treatment.

Spetzler and Wilson have proposed a reasonable scheme of management of recurrent rhinorrhea.[28] After clinical diagnosis of a CSF leak, an assessment is made of the patient's intracranial pressure. In a patient with elevated intracranial pressure and a low-flow fistula, the first line of therapy is permanent CSF diversion by means of lumboperitoneal or ventriculoperitoneal shunting. A patient with elevated intracranial pressure and a high-flow fistula undergoes direct repair guided by information in imaging studies, with subsequent shunting as necessary. A patient with normal intracranial pressure proceeds to direct repair. Direct repair involves a transsphenoidal procedure for a sphenoid leak; intracranial repair of a leak in the cribriform plate, frontal sinus, or mastoid; and a bicoronal craniotomy for a leak of unknown origin. Direct repair is made if a site is seen; cribriform and sphenoid packing is performed if no site is identified. Of 39 patients, 10 required more than one operative procedure, and 10 required shunting; in the 10 requiring multiple procedures, 7 leaks were ultimately controlled by shunting.

Outcomes

Literature concerning outcomes of patients treated for CSF leaks is scarce. Many reports on the treatment of leaks are case series involving a limited number of patients with iatrogenic disease and are therefore of limited value in understanding the natural history of traumatic spinal fluid leaks. Some larger studies do exist, however. In a recent series of 820 temporal bone fractures in 699 patients, 122 CSF leaks were noted (in 15% of fractures), and 15 cases of meningitis were seen (in 12% of the CSF leaks and 2% of the fractures).[29] In this series, 95 of the 122 leaks (78%) closed spontaneously in a period of less than 7 days. Those that failed to close after 7 days involved a significantly higher risk of meningitis (23%) as compared to the leaks that closed spontaneously within 1 week (3%). A patient with concurrent infection was at higher risk, and prophylactic antibiotics in such a setting are advocated by the authors of that series.

INFECTION IN THE CENTRAL NERVOUS SYSTEM

Infection in the CNS, a potentially fatal complication of head trauma, neurosurgery, or systemic illness, is often discussed in a compartmentalized fashion. Although CNS infection is a continuum of disease in which spread from one compartment to the next is possible, it is useful to consider these entities as distinct from each other. The categories of CNS infection include meningitis, epidural and subdural abscess, cerebritis, and cerebral abscess.

Meningitis

Meningitis is inflammation and infection in the CSF and connective tissues surrounding the parenchyma of the brain and spinal cord. This diffuse process may become suppurative but does not form large, localized collections of purulent material (i.e., epidural or subdural abscesses). Although meningitis can present de novo in both immunocompetent and immunocompromised hosts, this discussion centers on meningitis in a patient with a head injury and on meningitis in a postoperative patient. It is important to note that meningitis, like epidural and subdural infection, can arise from preexisting sinusitis or otitis. This discussion does not address community-acquired meningitis.

PRESENTATION AND EVALUATION

The classic signs and symptoms of meningitis include fever, stiff neck, photophobia, headache, and an elevated white blood cell count in both blood and CSF samples.[30] Other clinical findings include rash, seizures, a decreased GCS score, and focal neurologic findings.[30] In one prospective series, the incidence of seizures was almost 25% and the incidence of focal neurologic deficits was almost 28%.[30] Common organisms include *Streptococcus pneumoniae*, *Neisseria meningitidis*, and *Hemophilus influenzae*. Post-traumatic meningitis, which is often associated with CSF leakage, has a similar presentation. As discussed by Baltas and colleagues in one large series of 860 patients with head injuries, 12 patients (1.39%) developed meningitis.[31] These 12 patients ranged from 17 to 59 years of age, with a mean of 27. Of the 12 patients, 9 (75%) had basilar skull fractures and 7 of the 9 had obvious CSF leaks. GCS scores ranged from 4 to 11 (a mean of 8) at the time of presentation. The period between injury and the onset of infection ranged from 6 days to 6 months (a mean of 27 days). Clinical infection in these patients was diagnosed by the criteria of fever, meningismus, a CSF cell count higher than 10/mm^3, and a glucose level below 40 mg/dL. In this same series, 5 patients had gram-positive infections by *Staphylococcal* and *Streptococcal* species, 6 had gram-negative infections by *Escherichia*, *Klebsiella* and *Acinetobacter* species, and 1 patient's cultures remained negative. The gram-positive organisms were uniformly sensitive only to rifampin and vancomycin, although several were also sensitive to ciprofloxacin and ceftriaxone. The gram-negative organisms were all sensitive to imipenem and most were sensitive to ciprofloxacin, whereas all 6 were resistant to ampicillin, 4 were resistant to ceftriaxone, 4 to amikacin, 4 to gentamicin, and 5 to aztreonam.

PRIORITIES

In a patient who presents with fever and meningismus after head trauma or surgery in or around the cranial vault, even months after the injury or procedure, meningitis must be ruled out as the cause. After history and pertinent physical examination, blood work should be performed, including a white blood cell count and blood cultures. Lumbar puncture should be performed urgently unless the patient has a focal neurologic finding, in which case an emergency CT scan of the head should be performed first to rule out the presence of a significant mass lesion that would make lumbar puncture dangerous—that is, where the possibility of herniation exists. Standard CSF evaluation for cell count and differential, glucose and protein determinations, and gram stain and culture should be performed as should latex agglutination assays for common agents. In an appropriate host, an India ink preparation and a serum cryptococcal antigen test should also be ordered. As soon as CSF samples have been obtained, appropriate antibiotic coverage should be initiated.

The study by Baltas and colleagues strongly suggests treating post-traumatic meningitis with vancomycin and ciprofloxacin or imipenem until culture data with sensitivities are available.[31] Previous recommendations from various sources have suggested vancomycin and a third-generation cephalosporin, but growing resistance to cephalosporins makes this combination suboptimal. The organisms found in post neurosurgical meningitis are, to a large degree, the same as those found in post-traumatic meningitis.[32, 33] Previous treatment recommendations have advocated vancomycin combined with a third-generation cephalosporin, but the caveats regarding emerging resistance profiles are likely to be important in this setting as well. Aminoglycosides have fair to poor CSF penetration, do not achieve adequate levels over the convexities when introduced via lumbar puncture, and have well-established systemic toxicities that require the measurement of serum levels, making them less than optimal for treating meningitis.[32] In addition, there have been reports of hydrocephalus following the intrathecal delivery of amikacin.[31] The use of steroids as adjunctive treatment in meningitis has proven effective in preventing deafness in infants with meningitis, but its value in treating adult patients is unproven.[34]

OUTCOMES

The outcomes of meningitis vary with the causes and circumstances of the infection. In the study of post-traumatic meningitis by Baltas and colleagues, all patients survived.[31] This suggests that post-traumatic meningitis is nonfatal if treatment is rendered.

The GCS outcome scores of those patients ranged from 2 to 5, with a mean of 4, which indicates an independent but disabled patient. In studies of patients with meningitis of various causes, overall mortality rates vary from 10% to 30%.[30]

Subdural Empyema and Epidural Abscess

Subdural empyema and epidural abscess are considered together here as intracranial, extra-axial suppurative disease. Reports consistent with intracranial suppurative disease can be found as early as the time of Galen.[35] The first recorded and published account of subdural empyema, however, is credited to Ceci and Onetti in 1889. MacEwen followed with a monograph on the topic in 1893 and subdural empyema became a recognized clinical entity.[36] Several informative case studies have discussed the modern imaging that forms the basis of current management of this neurosurgical emergency.

PRESENTATION

Weisberg published a 1986 study of 15 patients with subdural empyema—7 children and 8 adults.[37] The children, 6 months to 5 years of age, all developed this condition as the result of preexisting meningitis, 5 to 23 days after the onset of systemic illness. All were diagnosed following the onset of seizures or the discovery of focal neurologic findings. The 8 adults, 16 to 33 years of age, in this series presented with fever, headache, meningismus, and altered level of consciousness. Of the 8 patients, 7 had sinusitis, and no predisposing condition was found in 1. Seizures or focal neurologic deficits occurred in 2 patients, and 3 had papilledema.

Another series of 41 patients, almost all adults, with epidural abscess and subdural empyema that occurred over an 11-year period found that only 29% of patients had a focus of sinusitis or otitis as the cause of infection.[35] In this series, 66% (27 patients) had undergone previous craniotomy, which indicates that neurosurgery is the greatest risk factor for extra-axial suppuration. The study then focused on these 27 patients. Of them, 14 had an epidural abscess, 3 had a subdural empyema, and 7 had both. The remainder had some combination of extra-axial and intraparenchymal infection. Few patients presented with seizure or focal deficits. Fever and headache were slightly more prevalent, however, and wound infection and encephalopathy were the most common presentations in this population. The mean time between the causative procedure and presentation was nearly 33 months. Cancer, radiation therapy, and diabetes were the most common comorbidities in this series.

One of the largest studies treated 90 patients with extra-axial suppuration.[39] These patients presented with fever, headache, meningismus, and seizures. Definitive diagnosis was made by contrast-enhanced CT in all cases. Of the 90 patients, 53 had sinusitis and 19 had otitis. In a similar series of 32 patients, 56% of cases arose from sinusitis and the remainder from trauma or neurosurgery.[38] No cases in this series arose as a result of otitis.

EVALUATION

The evaluation of extra-axial suppurative disease consists of obtaining contrast-enhanced CT scans of patients suspected of harboring this CNS infection. The 1986 Weisberg series concentrated on the diagnosis by CT of subdural empyema.[37] Contrast-enhanced CT scans in children consistently demonstrated hypodense extra-axial lesions with medially enhancing membranes. One child also had an intraparenchymal lesion by direct extension. CT scans in adults performed 6 to 28 days after onset of neurologic symptoms demonstrated thin, hypodense extra-axial lesions with enhancement along the medial border. More striking was diffuse unilateral edema and mass effect underlying these subdural collections. The one case of subdural empyema that arose without preexisting sinusitis demonstrated a larger extra-axial collection and less mass effect. The five adult patients without papilledema in this series underwent lumbar puncture, which revealed polymorphonuclear pleocytosis with elevated protein and normal glucose. All cultures remained negative, underscoring the limited value of lumbar puncture in this setting.

In another study of these patients, 17 had elevated white blood cell counts, and of the 10 patients from whom CSF was obtained, 4 were completely normal, 4 suggested a parameningeal reaction, and 2 had counts consistent with meningitis.[35] Wound site culture, however, was highly successful in yielding a causative agent, whereas blood and CSF were positive in less than one third of cases. The most common organisms were gram-negative aerobes, *Staphylococcus* species, gram-positive anaerobes, and *Streptococcus* species. In a similar series, the organisms isolated were largely anaerobes and streptococci.[38]

PRIORITIES

In evaluating patients with sinusitis, otitis, or craniotomy wound infection who present with headache, fever, meningismus, or seizure, the diagnosis of extra-axial infection (epidural abscess or subdural empyema) must be considered. As white blood cell count and CSF findings are inconstant, the diagnostic procedure of choice is a contrast CT scan; however, case reports are now appearing that suggest that MRI is superior. Treatment consists of broad-spectrum antibiotics (tailored according to cultures), emergent craniotomy for debridement, and drainage of related sinus infections. Studies suggest that limited burr-hole procedures are efficacious in the appropriate settings.[39, 40]

OUTCOMES

Several of the case studies reported outcomes in patients treated for extra-axial suppurative disease. Overall mortality in these series ranged from 8% to 18.5%.[35, 38, 39] In general, the outcome correlated with the level of consciousness at presentation and the rapidity with which drainage was accomplished. Therefore, prompt diagnosis and rapid evacuation in conjunction with appropriate antibiotics are the crucial elements in the care of these patients.

Cerebral Abscess

Cerebral abscess, which occurs in 1,500 to 2,500 people per year in the United States, is one extreme of the spectrum of intracranial suppurative diseases, with meningitis on the other end of the spectrum.[41] Cerebral abscesses may be solitary or multiple. Multiple intracranial abscesses are the result of systemic illness and hematogenous spread, whereas solitary intracranial abscesses are the result of direct extension, often from a parameningeal focus of infection.[42] The most common sources of a solitary abscess are the cranial (mastoid and paranasal) sinuses at the base of the skull.[42] The management of brain abscesses, however, is similar regardless of cause, and general management is addressed here. Modern diagnosis and treatment of brain abscesses have had dramatic effects on this disease.

PRESENTATION

In the study by Mamelak and coworkers, 16 patients with multiple brain abscesses were studied.[41] These patients presented with alteration of consciousness (100%), headache (94%), focal neurologic deficit (75%), fever (44%), nausea and vomiting (31%), meningismus (25%), and seizures (19%). The most common sources of infection in this study were pulmonary (39%) and tooth abscesses (13%); however, in 44% of patients, no source was identified. Interestingly, 63% of patients in this study had no known risk factors.

EVALUATION

The mainstay of diagnosis is contrast-enhanced CT or MRI. Much has been published about the use of CT scans in diagnosing this disease, but no direct comparison of CT and MRI has been undertaken to determine whether one imaging modality is superior. Figure 24–3 is a contrast-enhanced CT scan of a cerebral abscess. The evolution in appearance of cerebral abscesses on contrast-enhanced CT has been studied, and a clinical staging system based on CT has been suggested.[45] In the early stages, abscess formation or cerebritis appears as an irregular, low-density area that may or may not enhance. Ring enhancement first becomes evident in late cerebritis and takes on its typical appearance in the capsule stage, with the enhancing ring on the ventricular surface being thinner than on the cortical surface. It may take more than 2 weeks for capsule formation. Some enhancement may persist in the healed abscess for up to 10 weeks after the completion of antibiotics.

A diagnostic dilemma may arise in the radiographic differentiation of cerebral abscess and glioblastoma, and more specific adjuncts to diagnosis have been sought. Serologic testing for C-reactive protein is reasonably sensitive and specific as long as the patient does not have another site of active inflammation.[46] Labeled white blood cell scans with technetium (Tc^{99m}) are also useful to distinguish cerebral abscess from glioblastoma, but steroids must be discontinued for 48 hours prior to testing.[46]

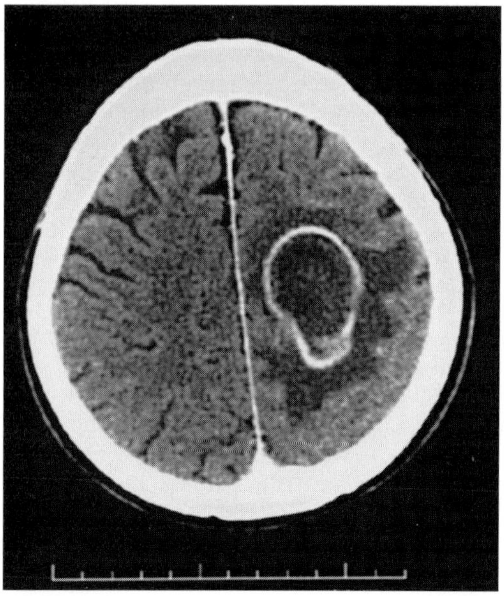

Figure 24–3. A contrast-enhanced CT image shows the typical appearance of a cerebral abscess with a ring of enhancement and surrounding edema.

Material for culture is obtained at the time of drainage. Although similar organism profiles are seen in general, the particular population under study may determine the percentage of patients with a given presentation or cause. In the Mamelek study, the most common organisms were *Staphylococcus* species (31%) and *Streptococcus* species (44%).[41] In this study, however, 19% of cultures were negative. One interesting observation from the literature is a suggested trend toward an increase in gram-negative and anaerobic infections with a concomitant decrease in staphylococcal infection.[42] In children, the predominant organisms are aerobic and anaerobic *Streptococcus* species, which have an isolation frequency of 60% to 70%, gram-negative anaerobic rods (20% to 50%), *Enterobacteriacaea* species (20% to 30%), *Staphylococcus aureus* (10% to 15%), and fungi (10% to 15%).[44] In immunocompromised patients, fungi and parasites play a more significant role.[42] Obviously, the organisms found in a solitary abscess are different from those found in multiple abscesses, as they are more likely to represent a direct extension from a chronic otitis or sinusitis.

PRIORITIES

The modern management of cerebral abscesses was initiated in the 18th century with the surgical drainage of an otitic abscess by the French surgeon Morand.[47] Mamelak and colleagues have presented an algorithm for the treatment of multiple brain abscesses that can also be applied to the treatment of a solitary cerebral abscess.[41] In this scheme, radiologic imaging is undertaken and the largest or most symptomatic lesion suspicious for abscess is aspirated stereotactically or drained by craniotomy. If purulent material is obtained, all lesions larger than 2.5 cm are drained. High-dose, broad-spectrum antibiotics are started only after cultures have been obtained, and they are narrowed when culture results are available. Intravenous antibiotics are continued for at least 6 to 8 weeks. Corticosteroids are used as needed to reduce the mass effect of vasogenic edema but are tapered as soon as possible. Repeat imaging should be performed weekly as long as the patient remains clinically stable. Any lesion that remains stable or increases in size on subsequent imaging should be drained or aspirated. We recommend consideration of craniotomy and excision of any lesion refractory to two aspirations. Following the completion of antibiotics, the patient is imaged monthly for 6 months or until all lesions resolve. If *Nocardia asteroides* is isolated, these authors recommended excision over aspiration, given the refractory nature of this particular organism. It should be noted that there is precedence in the literature for nonoperative management in a small group of patients.[48] In the modern era, outcome appears to correlate best with the patient's condition at the time of presentation.

The treatment for intracranial mycotic disease has traditionally been conservative because of the dismal outcomes in patients with fungal abscesses. Reports have been published, however, that suggest that aggressive surgical debridement and interstitial or intrathecal amphotericin B may lead to cure of these conditions.[42] Although the studies published have been case reports, more aggressive management should be considered for these patients on a case-by-case basis.

OUTCOMES

Since CT scans have been in use, mortality rates have decreased from estimates as high as 50% to generally quoted rates of less than 10%.[42, 43]

TENSION PNEUMOCEPHALUS

Pneumocephalus, or cranial aerocele, was first described by a Parisian named Lecat in 1741, although credit for the first description of intracranial pneumatocele is often given to Chiari in 1884.[49] Numerous authors have reviewed this topic extensively, including Dandy,[50] but the most comprehensive review during the pre-CT era was published in 1967 by Markham, who reported 11 cases and reviewed 284 cases dating back to 1884.[49] In all 295 cases, only 11 were the result of a surgical procedure; trauma was the most common cause. Among the 11 cases of postoperative pneumocephalus, the most common symptom was headache, and all the patients for whom an outcome was stated recovered. Lethargy or collapse was seen in 3 of these 11 and only 1 had seizure activity and a focal neurologic finding (hemiparesis). Time from onset to diagnosis ranged from hours to months. Of the procedures listed as causative, three were lumbar punctures for spontaneous CSF leaks, four were sinus procedures, one was a craniotomy for a sphenoid wing meningioma, and one was a transphenoidal hypophysectomy. Diagnostic x-rays of the skull were performed in all cases and all demonstrated the presence of air.

In the era of modern imaging, numerous reports of postoperative tension pneumocephalus have appeared in the literature, although no good general review has been published.[51–57] At our institution, Toung and associates reported four cases of postoperative tension pneumocephalus that were diagnosed with CT scans, and they reviewed the literature from the early years of CT use and found 11 additional cases.[54] Of these 15 cases, 12 involved posterior fossa or high cervical procedures, and 11 were performed in the sitting position. Twelve of the patients received nitrous oxide. Most of the patients were diagnosed in the immediate postoperative period, and the longest delay in diagnosis was 2 hours. The presentations of tension pneumocephalus in the 4 cases reported included failure to regain consciousness, increasing lethargy and confusion, hemiplegia, and seizure activity. Treatment in the 15 cases consisted of observation and slow recovery in 2 cases and some form of evacuation in the remainder. Evacuation methods included externalization of a ventriculostomy catheter, needle aspiration, twist-drill hole placement, burr-hole placement, and surgical exploration. All patients appeared to recover without recollecting significant amounts of air. In discussing these findings, Toung and colleagues believed that these cases had in common early postoperative onset, procedures performed in the sitting position, removal of large brain masses or hydrocephalus, nitrous anesthesia, and good prognosis with rapid evacuation.

Several larger series of patients with postoperative pneumocephalus have been reported since that time. In 1986, Toung and coworkers reported a retrospective series of 100 cases in which patients undergoing posterior fossa or high cervical procedures also underwent immediate postoperative skull radiographs.[56] When surgery was performed in the sitting position, 100% of patients showed the presence of air in postoperative radiographs. Approximately 73% of patients undergoing surgery in the park-bench position and 57% of those in the prone position also had postoperative pneumocephalus. Air in the ventricular system was less common but was still more likely to occur when the sitting position was used (78% of patients). Not a single patient in this report, however, was symptomatic—that is, none experienced tension pneumocephalus. In the same year, Di Lorenzo and associates published a similar series in which 30 patients underwent posterior fossa surgery in the sitting position, and although 100% had intracranial air, none developed tension pneumocephalus. They concluded that temperature and the use of nitrous oxide played no role.[55]

Although the role of nitrous oxide anesthesia in the development of tension pneumocephalus has been carefully examined, the association remains unclear. The increased solubility in blood and higher partial pressures of nitrous oxide can lead to rapid diffusion into air-filled spaces that outstrips the diffusion of nitrogen exiting these collections and thereby generates rapid and marked increases in pressure.[53] Nitrous oxide, however, should diffuse out just as rapidly. This agent is clearly not the sole factor to generate clinically significant pneumocephalus, but it is reasonable to discontinue nitrous oxide prior to dural closure. Tension pneumocephalus probably arises from a complex interplay of a myriad of factors, such as normalization of the partial pressure of carbon dioxide, collection of postoperative epidural and subdural blood, evolving brain edema, and rebound from osmotic diuretics, all leading to increased volume in the cranial vault.[56]

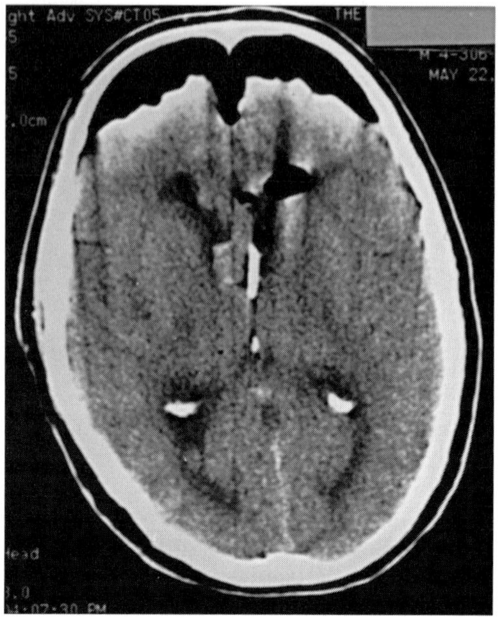

Figure 24–4. Pneumocephalus is seen in this postoperative CT image. The patient experienced a seizure after surgery and was scanned. Air appears black and can also be seen in the frontal horns.

Presentation

Although the incidence of postoperative intracranial air in patients undergoing craniotomy (particularly posterior fossa procedures) is quite high, the occurrence of tension pneumocephalus is quite rare. Patients with symptoms of trapped intracranial air under tension present, in the immediate postoperative period (within minutes to hours) or after trauma, with failure to awaken appropriately or with decline in level of consciousness after awakening. They may also manifest focal findings, particularly hemiparesis, and may have seizures.

Evaluation

To evaluate these patients, CT scans of the head are obtained. Air has a characteristic appearance: extremely low attenuation surrounded by a white halo that represents a reconstruction artifact, not blood.[58] It has a Hounsfield number of −1000. Air under pressure intracranially must be differentiated from postoperative pneumocephalus, which is extremely common. The shift of brain parenchyma and the overt mass effect can differentiate benign collections from those under tension. Figure 24–4 is a CT scan of a patient with postoperative tension pneumocephalus.

Priorities

Treatment of tension pneumocephalus involves stopping all drainage of CSF through externalized ventriculostomies or lumbar drains, as they may be generating pressure gradients and encouraging further ingress of air, and evacuating the existing collection of air that is under pressure.[59] The method of evacuation depends on the location of the air collection. Air can be evacuated using a needle or catheter if an existing burr hole overlies it; however, collections at a distance from the surgical site may require that twist-drill holes or burr holes be placed for access. Reexploration and placement of indwelling catheters for ongoing drainage can generally be avoided. These same diagnoses and treatment principles apply in situations in which tension pneumocephalus evolves in unoperated patients who are undergoing ventricular or lumbar drainage for diagnostic purposes, for treatment of infected shunts, or for treatment of CSF fistulas. Finally, patients whose operations have not involved craniotomy per se, such as those who have undergone transphenoidal approaches,[60] limited craniofacial procedures,[57, 61] or endoscopic sinus procedures[62] are also at risk. Patients with skull base trauma, especially if sinus compromise is involved, also fall into this category. In these patients, an appropriate index of suspicion must be maintained to avoid delayed or missed diagnoses.

Outcomes

With rapid evacuation, the prognoses for patients with tension pneumocephalus are excellent, and recurrence is extremely rare. Permanent sequelae of tension pneumocephalus seldom occur.

POSTOPERATIVE HEMATOMA

It is interesting to note that although much literature discusses tension pneumocephalus, the available literature concerning postoperative hematomas is sparse.[63–66] The cases that are presented and discussed in the literature center on hemorrhages in the infratentorial compartment after supratentorial surgery and hemorrhages in the supratentorial compartment after posterior fossa surgery. The four cases in the literature of cerebellar hemorrhage following supratentorial craniotomy were attributed to intracranial hypotension and disturbed blood coagulation (all four received low-dose heparin postoperatively).[66] This rare complication is managed as any other posterior fossa hemorrhage, with evacuation, which is always indicated unless the patient has a small hemorrhage and no neurologic symptoms of posterior fossa compression.

Perhaps more relevant to combined neurosurgical and head and neck surgical procedures are cases of supratentorial intracerebral hemorrhage after posterior fossa surgery.[63–65] Haines and colleagues reported in 1978 an incidence of 0.6% (5 in 825) in patients undergoing posterior fossa operations.[63] All 5 patients underwent retromastoid craniectomies and all 5 were elderly women, but no common cause could be determined. Modest intra- and postoperative elevations of blood pressure were observed; 1 patient experienced significant elevations of systolic blood pressure to 200 mm Hg. Of the 5 procedures, 4 were performed in the sitting position; 2 patients died and the other 3 were left with residual neurologic deficits. In 1985, Harders and colleagues reported 7 supratentorial hemorrhages that complicated 187 infratentorial procedures, an incidence of 3.7% (3 were intracerebral, 3 were subdural, and 1 was epidural).[64] Of the 3 patients with intracerebral hematomas, 2 were hypertensive elderly females.

In 1986 Seiler and Zurbrugg reported three similar cases and reviewed nine others from the literature.[65] All but one of these patients were also elderly females, and all but one of these procedures was performed in the sitting position. The authors concluded that this complication was a result of intracranial dynamics involving the shearing of subcortical veins. Hypertension was not apparent in these patients. Three patients died and the remainder were left with deficits. Of the above cases, roughly half underwent evacuation. The authors of these reports all emphasize the importance of head positioning to prevent compromise of arterial inflow and venous outflow, which can lead to ischemia-reperfusion or venous infarction. All authors also discuss the potential role of preexisting brain atrophy.

Much more common than the above hemorrhagic complications is bleeding at the operative site, either in the resection bed or extra-axially. Very little exists in the literature regarding this topic. This type of postoperative hematoma underscores the importance of meticulous hemostasis.

Presentation, Evaluation, and Priorities

Regardless of the location or cause, a postoperative hematoma should always be considered in a patient with the evolution of new neurologic findings or a decreasing level of consciousness. Diagnosis is made based on a CT scan. Figure 24–5 shows a postoperative hematoma after resection of a brain tumor. Management of this complication, whether medical observation or surgical evacuation, depends in a more complex way on the patient's status and the location of the hemorrhage. Extra-axial lesions in symptomatic patients should be promptly evacuated, whereas the decision to evacuate deep intracerebral lesions must be tempered by caution.

Outcomes

The literature regarding postoperative hematomas is scarce and consists of the small studies already discussed.[63–66] These studies almost uniformly report dismal outcomes. Mortality is as high as 50%, and most patients (in some reports 100%) are left with neurologic deficits.

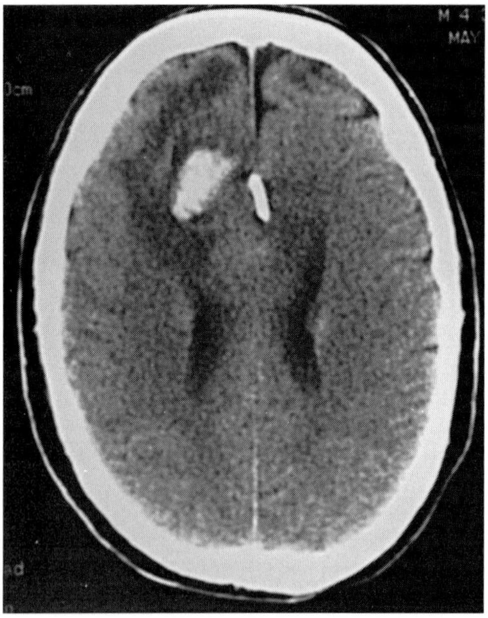

Figure 24–5. A postoperative CT scan shows a small hematoma in the resection bed of a brain tumor. The white linear structure in the midline is an intaventricular catheter placed at the time of surgery.

CONCLUSIONS

This chapter has reviewed the presentation, diagnosis, and management of head injuries, CSF leaks, CNS infections, tension pneumocephalus, and intracranial hematomas. Closed and penetrating head injuries are treated with a combination of careful management of elevated intracranial pressure and surgery when necessary to relieve significant mass lesions or debride and close open skull fractures. CSF leaks arise from a number of causes, and although diagnosis is straightforward, localization of persistent leaks can be difficult. The gold standard for diagnosis is CT cisternography. Once localized, persistent leaks may ultimately require intracranial surgery for repair. Infection of the CNS involves a spectrum of diseases, including meningitis, epidural abscess, subdural empyema, cerebritis, and cerebral abscess. Fever, headache, and change in mental status are the hallmarks of these infectious processes. Diagnoses are generally made by CSF culture or contrast-enhanced imaging. Treatment involves the drainage of infected collections and the provision of antibiotics. Tension pneumocephalus and postoperative intracranial hematoma present with decreased levels of consciousness and focal neurologic findings related to mass effect. Diagnosis is made by CT scanning, and treatment for life-threatening brain compression is evacuation of air or blood, accordingly.

REFERENCES

1. Bullock R et al. Guidelines for the management of severe head injury. Brain Trauma Foundation, 1995.
2. Brandvold B et al. Penetrating craniocerebral injuries in the Israeli involvement in the Lebanese conflict, 1982–1985: analysis of a less aggressive surgical approach. J Neurosurg 1990;72:15–21.
3. Brunner FX, Schwab U. Surgical management of trauma involving the skull base and paranasal sinuses. In Schmidek HH, Sweet WH, eds. Operative Neurosurgical Techniques, 3rd ed. Philadelphia, WB Saunders, 1995, p. 27.
4. Taha JM, Saba MI, Brown JA. Missile injuries to the brain treated by simple wound closure: results of a protocol during the Lebanese conflict. Neurosurgery 1991; 29:380–384.
5. Taha JM, Haddad FS, Brown JA. Intracranial infection after missile injuries to the brain: report of 30 cases from the Lebanese conflict. Neurosurgery 1991;29:864–868.
6. Aarabi B. Causes of infection in penetrating head wounds in the Iran-Iraq War. Neurosurgery 1989;25:923–926.
7. Kaufman HH et al. Patients with Glasgow Coma Scale scores 3, 4, 5 after gunshot wounds to the brain. Neurosurg Clin North Am 1995;6:701–714.
8. Levy ML et al. Outcome prediction after penetrating cranio-cerebral injury in a civilian population: aggressive surgical management in patients with admission Glasgow Coma Scale scores of 3, 4, 5. Neurosurgery 1994;35:77–85.
9. Stone JL, Lichtor T, Fitzgerald LF. Gunshot wounds to the head in civilian practice. Neurosurgery 1995;37:1104–1112.
10. Marshall LF et al. The outcome of severe closed head injury. J Neurosurg (suppl) 1991;75:S28–S36.
11. Ommaya AK. Spinal fluid fistulae. Clin Neurosurg 1976;23:363–392.
12. Ray BS, Bergland RM. Cerebrospinal fluid fistula: clinical aspects, techniques of localization, and methods of closure. J Neurosurg 1969;30:399–405.
13. Cusimano MD, Sekhar LN. Pseudo-cerebrospinal fluid rhinorrhea. J Neurosurg 1994;80:26–30.
14. Fransen P et al. Highly sensitive detection of beta-2 transferrin in rhinorrhea and otorrhea as a marker for cerebrospinal fluid leakage. Acta Neurochir (Wien) 1991;109:98–101.
15. Ryall RG, Peacock MK, Simpson DA. Usefullness of beta-2 transferrin assay in the detection of cerebrospinal fluid leaks following head injury. J Neurosurg 1992;77:737–739.
16. Naidich TP, Moran CJ. Precise anatomic localization of atraumatic sphenoethmoidal cerebrospinal fluid rhinorrhea by metrizamide CT cisternography. J Neurosurg 1980;53:222–228.
17. Ahmadi J et al. Evaluation of cerebrospinal fluid rhinorrhea by metrizamide computed tomographic cisternography. Neurosurgery 1985;16:54–60.
18. Eljamel MS et al. MRI cisternography and the localization of CSF fistulae. Br J Neurosurg 1994;8:433–437.
19. Eljamel MS, Pidgeon CN. Localization of inactive cerebrospinal fluid fistulas. J Neurosurg 1995; 83:795–798.
20. Hegarty SE, Millar JS. MRI in the localization of CSF fistulae: is it of any value? Clin Radiol 1997;52:768–770.

21. Ignelzi RJ, VanderArk GD. Analysis of the treatment of basilar skull fractures with and without antibiotics. J Neurosurg 1975;43:721–726.
22. Klastersky J, Sadeghi M, Brihaye J. Antimicrobial prophylaxis in patients with rhinorrhea or otorrhea: a double-blind study. Surg Neurol 1976;6:111–114.
23. MacGee EE, Cauthen JC, Brackett CF. Meningitis following acute traumatic cerebrospinal fluid fistula. J Neurosurg 1970;33:312–316.
24. Eljamel MS. Antibiotic prophylaxis in unrepaired CSF fistula. Br J Neurosurg 1993;7:501–506.
25. Meirowsky AM et al. Cerebrospinal fluid fistula complicating missile wounds of the brain. J Neurosurg 1981;54:44–48.
26. Kelley TF et al. Endoscopic closure of postsurgical anterior cranial fossa cerebrospinal fluid leaks. Neurosurgery 1996;39:743–746.
27. Wax MK et al. Contemporary management of cerebrospinal fluid rhinorrhea. Otolaryngol Head Neck Surg 1997;116:442–449.
28. Spetzler RF, Wilson CB. Management of recurrent CSF rhinorrhea of the middle and posterior fossa. J Neurosurg 1978;49:393–397.
29. Brodie HA, Thompson TC. Management of complications from 820 temporal bone fractures. Am J Otol 1997;18:188–197.
30. Pfister HW, Feiden W, Einhäupl KM. Spectrum of complications during bacterial meningitis in adults: results of a prospective clinical study. Arch Neurol 1993;50:575–581.
31. Baltas I et al. Posttraumatic meningitis: bacteriology, hydrocephalus, and outcome. Neurosurgery 1994; 35:422–427.
32. Garvey G. Current concepts of bacterial infections of the central nervous system: bacterial meningitis and bacterial brain abscess. J Neurosurg 1993;59:735–744.
33. Korinek A et al. Risk factors for neurosurgical site infections after craniotomy: a prospective multicenter study of 2944 patients. Neurosurgery 1997;41:1073–1081.
34. Lebel MH et al. Dexamethasone therapy for bacterial meningitis: results of two double-blind, placebo-controlled trials. N Engl J Med 1988;319:964–971.
35. Hlavin ML et al. Intracranial suppuration: a modern decade of postoperative subdural empyema and epidural abscess. Neurosurgery 1994;34:974–981.
36. Kubik CS, Adams RD. Subdural empyema. Brain 1943;66:18–42.
37. Weisberg L. Subdural empyema: clinical and computed tomographic correlations. Arch Neurol 1986;43:497–500.
38. Dill SR, Cobbs CG. McDonald CK. Subdural empyema: analysis of 32 cases and review. Clin Infect Dis 1995;20:372–386.
39. Bok APL, Peter JC. Subdural empyema: burr holes or craniotomy? J Neurosurg 1993;78:574–578.
40. de Falco R et al. Surgical treatment of subdural empyema: a critical review. J Neurosurg Sci 1996;40:53–58.
41. Mamelak AN et al. Improved management of multiple brain abscesses: a combined surgical and medical approach. Neurosurgery 1995;36:76–86.
42. Levy RM. Brain abscess and subdural empyema. Curr Opin Neurol 1994;7:223–228.
43. Rosenblum ML et al. Decreased mortality from brain abscesses since advent of computerized tomography. J Neurosurg 1978;49:658–668.
44. Brook I. Brain abscess in children: microbiology and management. J Child Neurol 1995;10:283–288.
45. Britt RH, Enzmann DR. Clinical stages of human brain abscesses on serial CT scans after contrast infusion: computerized tomographic, neuropathological, and clinical correlations. J Neurosurg 1983;59:972–989.
46. Grimstad IA, Hirschberg H, Rootwelt K. ^{99m}Tc-hexamethylpropyleneamine oxime leukocyte scintigraphy and C-reactive protein levels in the differential diagnosis of brain abscess. J Neurosurg 1992;77:732–736.
47. Stephanov S. Surgical treatment of brain abscess. Neurosurgery 1988;22:724–730.
48. Rosenblum ML et al. Nonoperative treatment of brain abscesses in selected high-risk patients. J Neurosurg 1980;52:217–225.
49. Markham JW. The clinical features of pneumocephalus based upon a survey of 284 cases with report of 11 additional cases. Acta Neurochir 1967;16:1–78.
50. Dandy WE. Pneumocephalus (intracranial pneumatocele or aerocele). Arch Surg 1926;12:949–982.
51. Lundsford DL et al. Subdural tension pneumocephalus: report of two cases. J Neurosurg 1979;50:525–527.
52. Black PM et al. Tension pneumocephalus of the cranial subdural space: a case report. Neurosurgery 1979; 5:368–370.
53. Pandit UA et al. Pneumocephalus after posterior fossa exploration in the sitting position. Anaesthesia 1982;37:996–1001.
54. Toung T et al. Tension pneumocephalus after posterior fossa craniotomy: report of four additional cases and review of postoperative pneumocephalus. Neurosurgery 1983;12:164–168.
55. Di Lorenzo N et al. Pneumocephalus and tension pneumocephalus after posterior fossa surgery in the sitting position: a prospective study. Acta Neurochir (Wien) 1986;83:112–115.
56. Toung TJK et al. Pneumocephalus: effects of patient position on the incidence and location of aerocele after posterior fossa and upper cervical surgery. Anesth Analag 1986;65:65–70.
57. Yates H et al. Incidence and perioperative management of tension pneumocephalus following craniofacial resection. J Neurosurg Anesth 1994;6:15–20.
58. Osborn AG et al. Intracranial air on computerized tomography. J Neurosurg 1978;48:355–359.
59. Grundy BL, Spetzler RF. Subdural pneumocephalus resulting from drainage of cerebrospinal fluid during craniotomy. Anesth 1980;52:269–271.
60. Yuceer N et al. Tension pneumocephalus after transsphenoidal surgery: two case reports. Acta Neurochir (Wien) 1995;137:58–61.
61. Wanamaker JR et al. Tension pneumocephalus following craniofacial resection. Head Neck 1995;17:152–156.
62. Clevens RA, Bradford CR, Wolf GT. Tension pneumocephalus after endoscopic sinus surgery. Ann Otol Rhinol Laryngol 1994;103:235–237.
63. Haines SJ, Maroon JC, Jannetta PJ. Supratentorial intracerebral hemorrhage following posterior fossa surgery. J Neurosurg 1978;49:881–886.
64. Harders A, Gilsbach J, Weigel K. Supratentorial space occupying lesions following infratentorial surgery: early diagnosis and treatment. Acta Neurochirurgica 1985;74:57–60.
65. Seiler RW, Zurbrugg HR. Supratentorial intracerebral hemorrhage after posterior fossa operation. Neurosugery 1986;18:472–474.
66. Konig A, Laas R, Herrmann HD. Cerebellar haemorrhage as a complication after supratentorial craniotomy. Acta Neurochir (Wien) 1987;88:104–108.

CHAPTER 25

Ophthalmologic Emergencies

Hilary A. Beaver, MD
Andrew G. Lee, MD

The periocular region composes only 0.27% of the total body surface area and 0.10% of the frontal silhouette, but it incurs 10% of all traumatic injuries. Trauma to this area may be associated with other facial, airway, and central nervous system injuries that can cause immediate threat to life.[1] Most ocular emergencies may be addressed after life-threatening injuries have been stabilized. One notable exception is ocular chemical injuries, which must be irrigated concurrent with other emergent interventions.

The history and examination should focus on the ophthalmologic system. The history should include the patient's premorbid visual acuity, subjective prior visual function such as the ability to read newsprint, any history of amblyopia, or "lazy eye," and any previous eye disease, eye surgery, or trauma. Detailed information should be obtained about the mechanism of the traumatic injury from the patient and witnesses. Penetrating injuries in the periorbital region may appear minor yet be associated with intracranial foreign bodies or neurologic injury. Cognitive disturbance in ophthalmic trauma patients should, therefore, prompt appropriate neuroimaging and consultation with neurology or neurosurgery. Blunt orbital trauma may cause direct ocular contusion if small objects are involved or indirect ocular injury if larger objects are deflected by the orbital rim, transferring kinetic energy to the orbit, facial bones, and sinuses.

Penetrating injuries to the eye can involve small foreign bodies that may be invisible on casual inspection. A patient presenting with a complaint about the presence of a foreign body should be specifically questioned regarding a history of hammering on hard surfaces such as metal or stone or using a grinding wheel. Fragments of the hammer, grindstone, or object being manipulated can travel at high velocities, passing through a self-sealing corneal wound into the anterior chamber, lens, or posterior segment. Intraocular foreign bodies may result in direct toxicity or intraocular inflammation that is related to their composition. Iron toxicity (siderosis) and copper toxicity (chalcosis) may cause glaucoma by damaging the delicate trabecular meshwork or may result in visual loss due to toxicity of the neural retina. Vegetative debris may lead to secondary bacterial and fungal intraocular infection (endophthalmitis). Other intraocular foreign bodies such as glass and porcelain are inert and may not require surgical excision.

EXAMINATION

An examination of the eye includes eight basic elements: visual acuity, external examination, pupil examination, anterior segment examination, extraocular motility assessment, intraocular pressure measurement, visual field examination, and ophthalmoscopy of the posterior segment. The patient's initial visual acuity must be documented, as it is an important indicator of visual prognosis. The vision may be tested for distance or near acuity, preferably using the patient's spectacle correction. If the patient is unable to read the acuity chart or vision card, a qualitative estimation of vision should be made, for example, finger counting at 1 foot, hand motion, and light perception. If the patient is unable to perceive light, this should be noted and the light source documented.

The external examination of the ocular adnexa should include drawings or photographs of all periocular abnormalities. The location, depth, and size of all lacerations should be documented. The extent and location of periocular ecchymosis and edema, symmetry of facial sensation, and stability of the facial skeleton should be noted. The patient should be evaluated for subconjunctival hemorrhage, periocular crepitus, orbital rim step-off fractures, proptosis, and enophthalmos. Asymmetry in globe position after trauma may occur as a result of orbital soft tissue edema, orbital fracture, or a traumatic carotid-cavernous fistula. A bird's-eye view from above looking down on the patient, or a worm's-eye view from below looking up at the patient, may demonstrate subtle proptosis or enophthalmos when formal exophthalmometry is not available.

The pupil examination should include assessment of the pupil's size and shape, its direct response to light, and the presence or absence of an afferent pupillary defect (APD). Pupil asymmetry (anisocoria) is caused by damage to the efferent (motor) pupillary pathway. Anisocoria may be due to traumatic miosis (small pupil) or mydriasis (large pupil). Traumatic miosis may result from direct trauma to the iris sphincter, causing spasm, or from concomitant Horner's syndrome with damage to the ipsilateral oculosympathetic pathways. Traumatic mydriasis may be caused by a tear in the iris sphincter or by damage to the parasympathetic fibers in the ciliary ganglion or in cranial nerve III. Injury to the afferent or sensory visual pathways causes an APD. The afferent pupillary pathway includes the ipsilateral retina, optic nerve, and optic tract. The swinging flashlight test for an APD involves three steps: (1) a light source illuminates one pupil (the ipsilateral direct response), and both pupils should constrict to light (the contralateral consensual response); (2) the light source is moved to the fellow eye (both pupils should constrict, again symmetrically); and (3) the light source is swung back to the first pupil (the pupils should remain constricted). In a patient with an APD, the direct response in the eye with the afferent defect is diminished when compared with the direct response in the fellow eye. When directly illuminating the normal eye, the consensual response in the affected eye is greater than its own direct response. Thus, when the light source is swung from the normal to the affected eye (the eye with the APD), the affected pupil dilates as it changes from a consensual to a direct response, rather than constricting or remaining unchanged. This indicates that the affected eye is sensing less light than the fellow eye, even though the light source remains the same. Pharmacologic dilation should be deferred until the swinging flashlight test has been performed, and any pupillary abnormality should be confirmed by ophthalmologic evaluation.

The anterior segment examination may be performed with a penlight, a direct ophthalmoscope, or a slit lamp biomicroscope. The conjunctiva, the vascular membrane overlying the tough scleral tissue, should be inspected for conjunctival injection, chemosis (edema), or laceration. The cornea should be clear and should be inspected for infiltration, opacity, penetrating injury, foreign body, or laceration. The anterior chamber of the eye should be formed and should not contain red blood cells (hyphema) or white blood cells (hypopyon). Loss of the normal formation of the anterior chamber may indicate an occult penetrating or perforating injury to the globe. The iris should be symmetric and should be inspected for iris sphincter damage and signs of penetrating injury. The lens is located behind the iris and can be seen through the pupil. The lens may be absent (aphakia) or present as a native lens (phakia) or an implanted intraocular lens (pseudophakia). The lens should be clear and should be inspected for foreign body penetration and cataract.

If there is suspicion of an open (penetrating or perforating) globe injury, a Fox shield or modified Styrofoam cup should be placed over the affected eye and ophthalmology consultation should be obtained immediately. Pressure on the globe and attempts at further ocular examination should be avoided, as they may result in the extrusion of the intraocular contents. The motility and intraocular pressure assessments should be performed only after an open globe has been ruled out, as these maneuvers may also prolapse ocular tissues.

The extraocular motility examination includes assessment of the movement of the eyes in the nine directions of gaze. Any subjective diplopia or objective ophthalmoparesis should be noted.

Intraocular pressure may be assessed by tactile tonometry, Schiøtz tonometry, or applanation at the slit lamp. Formal assessment of intraocular pressure is probably best determined by the ophthalmology consultant.

Visual field testing by confrontation should be performed in all patients. The patient is seated directly across from the examiner. Each eye is tested under monocular conditions with the fellow eye occluded. Finger counting in the various areas of the visual field of each eye is probably sufficient in the setting of an emergency department. The examiner's visual field serves as a control.

An examination of the fundus, with specific attention to the optic nerve, retinal vasculature, and retina, should be performed. Usually, the direct ophthalmoscope is a reasonable screening tool. The optic nerve should be examined for the presence or absence of optic disk edema or pallor. Retinal hemorrhages, exudates, or nerve fiber layer infarcts should be documented. In general, dilation should be left to the ophthalmologic consultant, as the pupil may be an important examination finding in a patient with a questionable neurologic status. Although there is a theoretic risk of precipitating angle-closure glaucoma in a patient who undergoes pharmacologic dilation, the Baltimore Eye Survey showed no attacks of acute angle closure in 4,870 patients and rated the risk in their population of occludable angles to be less than 1%. Excluding any patient with a narrow angle by penlight examination or a history of glaucoma decreased this risk to 1 in 333.[2] A patient whose pupils have been dilated may be told to return for further evaluation in the case of worsening pain, redness, or vision after dilation. In most cases, even in the event of an acute angle-closure attack, the episode is likely to be treated appropriately when it occurs in a hospital setting.

CORNEAL ABRASIONS AND FOREIGN BODIES

Corneal abrasion is a common ocular injury. The superficial epithelial layer of the cornea is easily scratched or sloughed, even with minimal trauma. The cornea is richly endowed with sensory nerve fibers, and an abrasion may cause pain symptoms that appear to be out of proportion to the physical findings or the mechanism of injury. A patient suffering a corneal abrasion and using contact lenses should temporarily discontinue use of the lenses, as they may predispose the patient to a corneal infection (microbial keratitis).

Presentation

The clinical presentation of a corneal abrasion includes acute, severe eye pain with tearing, photophobia, and spasm of the orbicularis muscle (blepharospasm). The conjunctiva is usually injected and chemotic (edematous).

Evaluation

The diagnosis of corneal abrasion may be facilitated by instillation of topical fluorescein dye in the affected eye. When viewed under a cobalt blue light filter the abrasion stains apple green. A single application of topical anesthesia such as proparacaine diminishes pain and blepharospasm and improves the patient's cooperation. A patient should never be given a topical anesthetic agent to use at home, as it may result in dependence on the anesthetic and cause secondary corneal toxicity (Fig. 25–1).

The cornea and conjunctiva should be thoroughly inspected for foreign bodies. Self-sealing lacerations and retained intraocular foreign bodies may be missed unless specifically sought, and the clinician should be especially meticulous in cases involving grinding or the hammering of metal on metal.

Priorities

The upper eyelid should be everted and inspected and the upper tarsal conjunctiva and fornix should be swept for occult foreign debris in a patient suspected of harboring a foreign body. Lid eversion is performed with the eyes in downgaze and both eyes open and relaxed. The examiner pulls downward on the upper lashes while putting pressure behind the upper tarsal border with a finger or cotton tip. Traction is then placed in an upward fashion on the lashes, everting the lid. The upper tarsus is inspected and microscopic debris is removed using a cotton tip soaked in topical anesthetic. The upper and lower conjunctival fornices may be likewise swept clean. The lid will return to its normal position after several blinks.

Corneal and conjunctival foreign bodies can be removed with an anesthetic-soaked cotton tip and gentle debridement. If there is any question of full-thickness corneal or conjunctival penetration, the foreign body should be left in place until evaluation by an ophthalmologic consultant is complete. Foreign bodies that have been present for hours to days may become more firmly fixed and may require removal by an ophthalmologist at a slit lamp biomicroscope. Rust rings may develop around ferrous

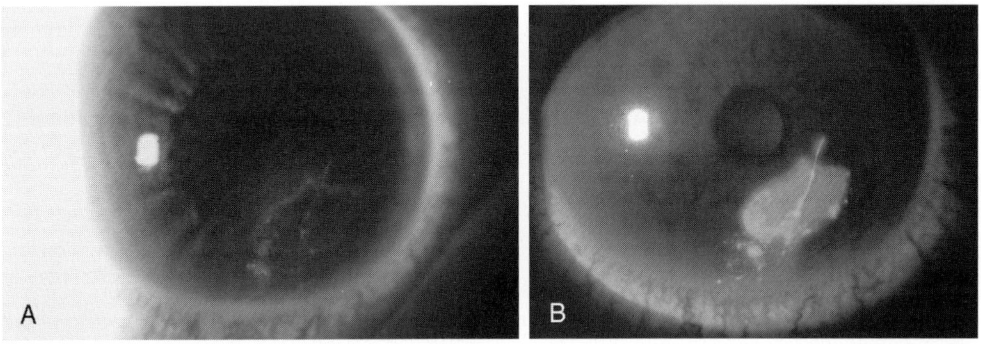

Figure 25–1. A: Corneal photograph demonstrates corneal epithelial abrasion. B: Apple-green fluorescence is seen using cobalt-blue lighting. This black and white figure demonstrates the corneal epithelial abrasion. (Courtesy of M. Bowes Hamill, M.D.)

particles; they are removed with a corneal burr by an ophthalmologist (Fig. 25–2).

The treatment of a corneal abrasion, in most cases, includes topical pharmacologic mydriasis and tight patching for comfort. Topical nonsteroidal anti-inflammatory agents such as ketorolac (Acular) may sometimes be employed, with or without patching. The procedure for placement of a tight patch is as follows: (1) overlay a folded eye patch and an unfolded open patch; (2) secure the patch with several strips of tape, starting at the patient's brow and stretching the tape inferolaterally; (3) lift the cheek before securing the tape to the cheek. This allows the natural downward force of both gravity and the facial tissues to place posterior pressure on the globe, decreasing globe mobility and pain. Short-acting topical mydriatics such as tropicamide or cyclopentolate are used to decrease the ache of ciliary spasm. The need for prophylactic topical antibiotics is controversial.

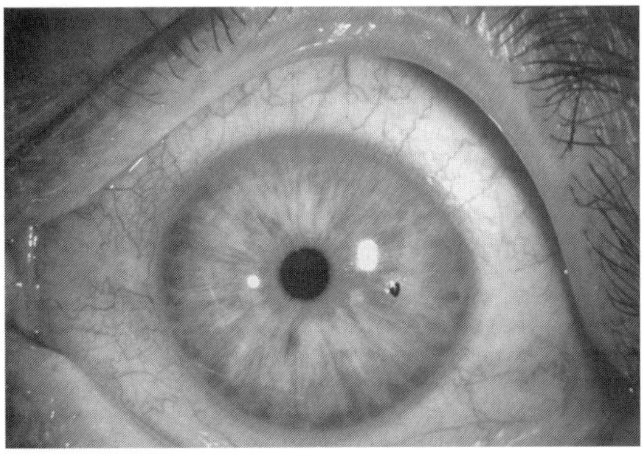

Figure 25–2. Corneal photograph demonstrates a metallic corneal foreign body. (Courtesy of M. Bowes Hamill, M.D.)

Outcomes

In most cases, a corneal abrasion heals within 1 to 2 days. Untreated corneal foreign bodies or corneal abrasions may lead to secondary infectious microbial keratitis and may cause irreversible scarring of the cornea. The patient should be seen by an ophthalmologist within 24 hours to confirm the healing of the abrasion.

PERIOCULAR LACERATIONS

Blunt or penetrating facial trauma may damage the lids and periocular tissues. As in any periocular injury, the presence of an open globe should be excluded before any further manipulation is performed.

Presentation

A patient may present with periocular lacerations that are superficial, partial-thickness skin abrasions or that involve deeper tissues. Superficial lacerations may not require closure and can heal by secondary intention. However, deeper lacerations involving full-thickness skin, orbicularis muscle, orbital septum penetration with fat herniation, or violation of the lid margin should be repaired (Fig. 25–3).

Evaluation

All lacerations should be explored prior to closure to ascertain the specific structures involved and to explore for retained foreign bodies. The herniation of orbital fat indicates a violation of

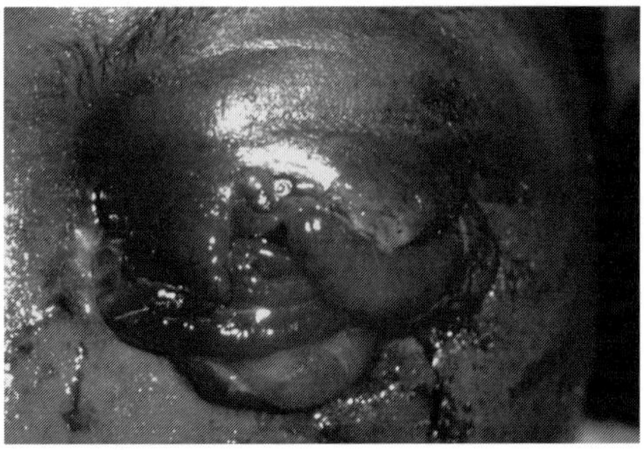

Figure 25–3. Complex upper and lower lid laceration. (Courtesy of James R. Patrinely, M.D.)

the orbital septum. The fat may be repositioned, but the septum should not be sutured during the repair as this can cause contracture and distortion of the lid structures. Lacerations of the levator muscle or aponeurosis compromise lid function, and the repair should be referred to an ophthalmic or plastic surgeon. Lacerations in the medial canthal area should likewise be approached with caution. Damage to the lacrimal drainage apparatus or the lacrimal puncta, canaliculi, or sac may risk persistent epiphora and should undergo meticulous closure.

Priorities

The repair of lid margin lacerations requires expertise, as incorrect technique may result in lid notching and corneal exposure, with secondary corneal scarring and visual loss. Correct lid margin repair requires a detailed understanding of eyelid anatomy. The layers of the lid are separated by the gray line of the lid margin. The anterior lamella is composed of skin and orbicularis muscle, and the posterior lamella is composed of the tarsal plate and conjunctiva. A corneal shield can be employed during repair to prevent inadvertent globe perforation. The lid margin is first reapproximated with interrupted 6-0 silk sutures anterior to, through, and posterior to the gray line along the lid margin. The suture ends should be left long to prevent corneal irritation; they will be incorporated into the subsequent skin closure. The tarsus itself is closed with 6-0 absorbable chromic or polyglactin (Vicryl) suture. Care should be taken during closure that no sutures pass through the conjunctiva, as they may abrade the corneal epithelium. Finally, the skin is closed with interrupted 6-0 Prolene sutures, with the lid margin silks incorporated to prevent corneal irritation. The skin sutures are removed after 5 days and the lid margin sutures after 10 to 14 days. The eye need not be patched during this time. Any lid laceration with evulsion of tissue should be referred to ophthalmology for closure (Fig. 25–4).

Outcomes

Incorrect closure of lid lacerations may compromise both function and cosmesis. Poor lid apposition may cause distortion of the lid and incorrect spreading of the tear film. The subsequent corneal desiccation can cause corneal thinning, scarring, infection, and even perforation.

CONJUNCTIVAL, CORNEAL, AND SCLERAL LACERATION

Conjunctival lacerations are often self-limited and generally do not require closure. Corneal and scleral lacerations have a more guarded prognosis, however, with risks of infection and autoimmune inflammation of both the injured eye and the fellow eye.

Presentation

Conjunctival lacerations present with disruption of the conjunctival membrane without disruption of the underlying sclera. There may or may not be an accompanying subconjunctival hemorrhage. The patient complains of pain, tearing, and the sensation of the presence of a foreign body. A patient presenting with corneal and scleral lacerations may have collapse of the anterior chamber, prolapse of brown uveal tissue or vitreous gel, or extensive chemotic subconjunctival hemorrhage.

Evaluation

The underlying tissues should be gently explored to rule out damage to the sclera or extraocular muscles, open globe injury, and foreign body. The conjunctiva may remain intact despite injury to the underlying structures. Bullous or chemotic subconjunctival hemorrhage may mask occult scleral rupture, so the presence of intact conjunctiva does not exclude an occult open globe. The tough fibrous coat of the eye, the sclera, is thinnest beneath the insertions of the extraocular muscles and along the corneal-scleral limbus. These areas are predisposed to

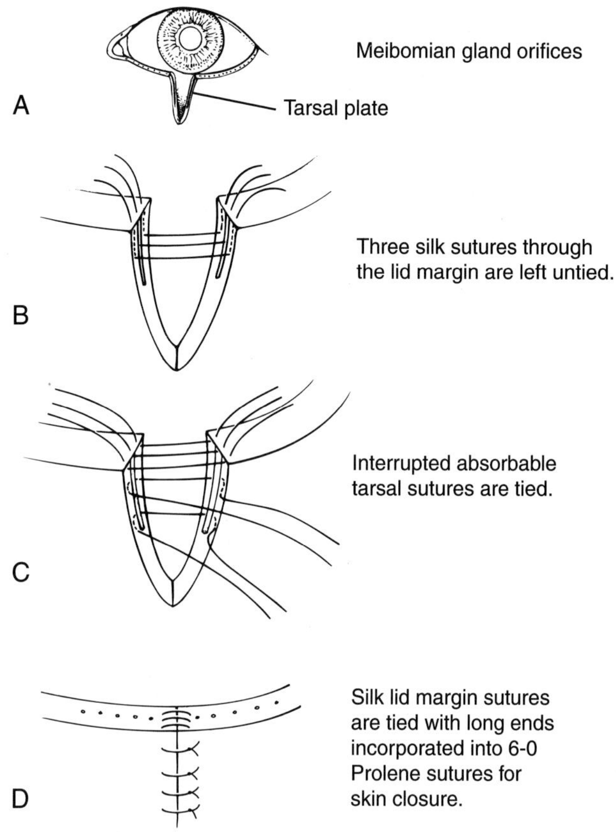

Figure 25–4. Steps in the repair of an eyelid laceration.

rupture with blunt trauma and should be inspected carefully for globe rupture.

As mentioned previously, an excessively shallow or deep anterior chamber depth may also indicate loss of aqueous humor or a posterior scleral rupture. Kylstra and colleagues found that a visual acuity level of light perception or worse, an intraocular pressure of 5 mm Hg, a deep or shallow anterior chamber, and severe intraocular hemorrhage or bullous subconjunctival hemorrhage were the strongest predictors of occult globe rupture. When accompanied by loss of retinal visualization by indirect ophthalmoscopy, these predictors had a sensitivity of 100% and a specificity of 98.5%. Of their patients, 25% of those with hyphema and 22% of those with hemorrhagic chemosis were found to have occult ruptures.[3] Werner and coworkers noted an afferent pupillary defect in 80% of ruptured eyes, as compared with 44% of controls, but did not find intraocular hemorrhage to be statistically higher in patients with open globes.[4]

Priorities

In cases of suspected occult rupture and in those with corneal or scleral lacerations, with or without uveal prolapse, further ocular examination should be halted. The eye should be protected with a Fox shield until emergent ophthalmologic consultation can be obtained (Fig. 25–5).

Outcomes

Recognition of open globe injuries is crucial, as modern microsurgical techniques have improved the salvage of eyes previously enucleated because of trauma. One early report of 280 eyes in consecutive patients of the Wilmer Eye Institute who presented before 1993 showed a 24% rate of enucleation. In a subsequent study of 476 eyes, there was a 6% decrease in enucleations, despite an increase in serious injuries in the later group.[5]

Prompt surgical repair may also decrease the risk of sympathetic ophthalmia, which occurs when the immunologically privileged intraocular contents are exposed to the host's immune system. The patient mounts an immunologic response to retinal and uveal antigens in the injured eye, which may result in an immune-mediated inflammatory response in the contralateral eye. Sympathetic ophthalmia has been

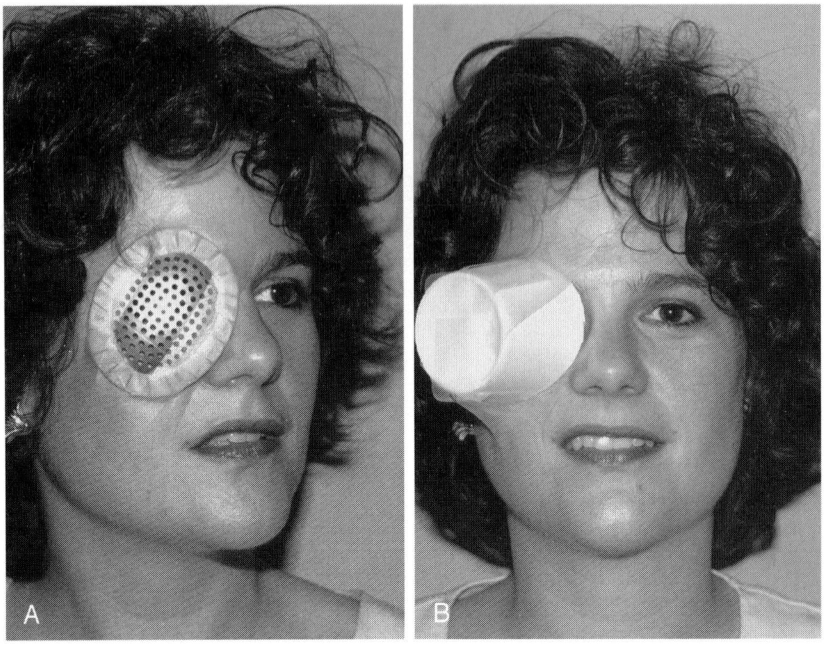

Figure 25–5. A: Fox shield covering the eye. B: Modified Styrofoam cup covering the eye. (Courtesy of Jim Shigley, ophthalmic photographer.)

documented to occur as early as 10 days and as late as many decades after injury. Risk may be lessened by prompt repair of an open globe or by enucleation in a blind eye within 2 weeks of injury.

Intraocular infection, endophthalmitis, may occur in up to 16.5% of patients with penetrating ocular trauma. The risk of endophthalmitis increases in cases that involve intraocular foreign bodies.[6] *Staphylococcus*, *Streptococcus*, and *Bacillus* species are the most common pathogens recovered in culture-proven cases.[6–8] Rapid recognition of open globe injuries and rapid institution of broad-spectrum, systemic antibiotics may decrease the risk of infectious endophthalmitis. Intravenous cefazolin and gentamicin are good empiric intravenous antibiotics for initial treatment in patients with open globes. Thompson and colleagues studied 13 cases of endophthalmitis after open globe injury; 54% of patients in this group retained visual acuity of at least 20/400.[6] The National Eye Trauma System Registry noted that 58% of 492 eyes with endophthalmitis after open globe injury attained visual acuity of 20/200 or better, with 23% reaching 20/40 or better.[8]

TRAUMATIC IRITIS AND GLAUCOMA

Trauma to the iris may cause either miosis (constriction) or mydriasis (dilation). In the setting of head trauma, a dilated pupil may be an ominous sign of transtentorial herniation. An isolated dilated pupil, however, is unlikely to represent herniation in an otherwise neurologically intact individual. Ophthalmology consultation should be obtained to evaluate for other signs of dysfunction of cranial nerve III. Iris sphincter damage and traumatic iritis are much more common causes of traumatic mydriasis than is palsy of nerve III.

Presentation

Inflammation of the anterior segment (iritis) is commonly seen in cases of concussive damage. A patient may complain of pain, photophobia, and tearing and may demonstrate injection of the conjunctiva.

Evaluation

Recognition of intraocular inflammation requires examination with a slit lamp biomicroscope to identify anterior chamber inflammatory cells and protein (flare).

Priorities

The treatment of traumatic iritis consists of topical steroids as well as mydriatics to prevent secondary iridolenticular adhesions and painful ciliary body spasm.

Outcomes

Treated iritis resolves without residual damage. Untreated, the patient may suffer intraocular scarring and risk for future glaucoma. Trauma severe enough to cause iritis may also damage the trabecular meshwork, placing the patient at an additional risk for glaucoma. Between 20% and 94% of patients with ocular trauma have angle recession, or damage to the aqueous outflow system. Between 5% and 20% of these patients may suffer acute or delayed increases in intraocular pressure, with the incidence of glaucoma increasing in proportion to the amount of angle recession. Of patients with 180 degrees of recession, 8% manifest glaucoma, although most traumatic glaucoma patients have 240 degrees or more of trabecular damage.[9, 10] Recognition of angle recession requires ophthalmologic consultation and specialized evaluation of the angle anatomy through gonioscopy. Intraocular pressure elevation and secondary glaucoma should be treated by an ophthalmologist.

HYPHEMA

Red blood cells in the anterior chamber, hyphema, may be present as a result of trauma. It occurs at an annual rate of 20 cases per 100,000. More than 70% of patients with traumatic hyphema are under age 20, and 75% to 85% are male.[11, 12]

Presentation

The cause of hyphema is most commonly a rapid, forceful blow to the periorbit. The direct compression in the axial length of the globe increases the intraocular pressure acutely, displaces the iridolenticular diaphragm posteriorly, and expands the equatorial circumference. The anterior ciliary body and peripheral iris tear and may disinsert from the scleral wall. Disinsertion of the ciliary body is known as cyclodialysis; evulsion of the iris is called iridodialysis. Intraocular bleeding arises most frequently from the splitting of the anterior ciliary body, with disruption of the vasculature of the iris and ciliary body. Hemostasis is eventually obtained through increased intraocular pressure, vasospasm, and platelet-fibrin clotting.[11–13] The patient may complain of pain, photophobia, red eye, and decreased vision (Fig. 25–6).

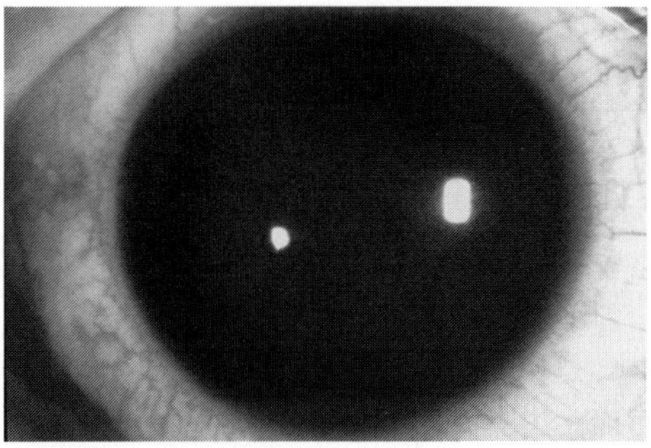

Figure 25–6. Grade I hyphema. (Courtesy of M. Bowes Hamill, M.D.)

Evaluation

Hyphemas are classified by the amount and type of hemorrhage present in the anterior chamber (Table 25–1).[11, 12]

A hyphema can be further described as layered blood or organized clot. As a hyphema ages, the blood clots, then retracts, which may reopen damaged vessels. A recurrent or secondary hemorrhage is commonly seen in the second to fifth days after injury, during the period of most active clot retraction. Rebleeding occurs more frequently in larger hyphemas and often results in a higher-grade hyphema than the initial bleed. The risk of rebleeding is higher (23% to 38%) in minority populations than in Caucasians (5% to 7%).[12, 13] Pediatric Caucasian patients were studied by Teboul and colleagues, who found a similar risk of rebleeding of 3.2%.[14] Other risk factors for secondary hemorrhage include presentation after 24 hours, visual acuity less than 20/200, grade II or higher hemorrhage, and elevated intraocular pressure. The presence of one risk factor increases the rate to 14%, and four risk factors increase the rate to 64%.[12] Berrios and Dreyer noted that increased risk is related to the severity of the initial hem-

Table 25–1. *Hyphema*

Microhyphema	Free-floating red blood cells only
Grade I	Less than ⅓ of the anterior chamber
Grade II	⅓ to ½ of the anterior chamber
Grade III	½ to ¾ of the anterior chamber
Grade IV	¾ to complete filling of the anterior chamber

orrhage; there is a risk of 66% in a patient with grade III hemorrhage or higher.[11]

Priorities

The treatment of hyphema remains controversial. Bed rest, hospitalization, topical mydriatics or steroids, and estrogens have not been proved effective[11, 12] and the benefit of oral steroids has remained inconclusive.[13] Elective surgery for orbital fractures should be delayed, however, to avoid eliciting a secondary hemorrhage. Miotics such as intraocular pressure–lowering agents should be avoided as they are known to increase intraocular inflammation. A patient's eye should be protected from further damage by the placing of a metal shield, and the blood should be encouraged to settle by elevating the head of the bed 30 degrees. Topical cycloplegics may be used to relieve painful ciliary body spasm. Topical prednisolone can be employed to treat the accompanying traumatic iritis. Aqueous suppressants, such as topical β-blockers and carbonic anhydrase inhibitors, are used to control elevated intraocular pressure. Aspirin and other anticoagulants should be discontinued. High-risk patients, including those with histories of aspirin use, bleeding diatheses, sickling hemoglobinopathies, or inability to comply with activity restrictions and follow-up, should be admitted for observation.

The increased incidence of rebleeding in minority populations has been shown to decrease significantly with use of aminocaproic acid (Amicar), from a high of 33% to as low as zero to 3%.[11, 12] This agent should be considered for patients who are members of minority populations because they are at greater risk as a result of higher natural histories of rebleeding. Aminocaproic acid was not found to decrease secondary hemorrhage in several large studies of Caucasian patients who were seen within 24 hours of trauma. Aminocaproic acid is contraindicated during pregnancy, in patients with hepatic or renal disease, in patients at risk for vaso-occlusive events, and in those on aspirin therapy or with underlying coagulopathies. Side effects include nausea, vomiting, diarrhea, hypotension, and thromboembolism. A baseline blood urea nitrogen and creatinine level should be drawn before instituting treatment.

Outcomes

The major complications of hyphema include acute or delayed glaucoma and corneal blood staining (CBS). Staining of the cornea by hemoglobin byproducts may cause complete corneal opacification, which may take months or years to clear. In a child, this can cause amblyopia and may necessitate a corneal transplant. Anterior chamber blood normally filters through the trabecular meshwork in the anterior chamber angle. Early glaucoma results from obstruction of aqueous outflow by erythrocytes, platelets, fibrin, and inflammatory debris as well as from direct concussive damage to the meshwork. The severity of the initial hyphema and the occurrence of secondary hemorrhage increase the risk of acute glaucoma. Rebleeding increases the risk of acute glaucoma to 50%.[11]

A patient with a hemoglobinopathy, specifically sickle cell anemia, is also at a high risk for glaucoma in hyphema, primarily as a result of obstruction of the trabecular meshwork. Sickled erythrocytes are inflexible and cannot slip between the trabecular pillars. The physical obstruction of the meshwork increases the intraocular pressure, decreasing the circulation through the intraocular structures. The anemia and decreased oxygen-carrying capacity that exist in a hemoglobinopathy further decrease the effective circulation in the eye, placing such a patient at risk for infarction of the optic nerve and central retinal artery occlusion. The carbonic anhydrase inhibitors used to treat increased intraocular pressure cause acidosis and hemoconcentration, both of which increase the likelihood of sickle crisis and ocular compromise, and thus are contraindicated. These potential complications should prompt testing in a patient at risk for a hemoglobinopathy who presents with hyphema.

Late glaucoma is caused by angle recession, concussive trabecular damage, and descemetization or scarring of the anterior chamber angle. Between 6% and 10% of hyphema patients develop delayed glaucoma, often years after injury.[11, 13] Late glaucoma is more common when half or more of the angle is recessed.[11]

CBS occurs in a patient with hyphema and increased intraocular pressure or compromised corneal endothelium. The overall risk of CBS in hyphema is 7%.[13] CBS decreases the ability of the physician to examine the eye and the ability of the patient to see and may take months to years to clear. A hyphema that is present for 6 days and is combined with intraocular pressures greater than 25 to 30 mm Hg is, therefore, considered for surgical drainage to decrease the risk of corneal blood staining.[11] Surgical intervention to remove the hyphema may be warranted in a patient with 5 days of intraocular pressure above 50 mm Hg, 1 week of pressure above 35 mm Hg, 10 days of total hyphema, or early signs of CBS.[11, 13]

The overall prognosis for a patient with hyphema depends on concurrent injuries and on the grade of hemorrhage. Between 25% and 50% of patients with grade IV hemorrhage and between 75% and 90% with grade I recover vision of 20/50 or better.

POSTERIOR SEGMENT CONTUSION INJURIES

Blunt trauma may damage the vitreous, retina, and choroid. As noted, anteroposterior compression of the globe causes expansion along the limbal equator. In a case of extreme blunt force, this equatorial expansion may evulse the anterior vitreous base from the anterior retina and pars plana. The peripheral retina is firmly attached at the vitreous base, and retinal traction caused by vitreous traction may cause retinal breaks. These breaks provide the liquid vitreous with access to the subretinal space. As vitreous fluid dissects into the potential space between the retina and choroid, the neurosensory retina may detach. If the retinal tear is bridged by a peripheral retinal vessel, the vessel may rupture and cause a vitreous hemorrhage. A patient with traumatic vitreous hemorrhage should be considered to have retinal tears and possible retinal detachments until proven otherwise by clinical examination or ultrasonography.

The expansile forces resulting from ocular compression may also rupture the choroid. Such traumatic breaks place the patient at lifelong risk for subretinal neovascular membranes, a potentially blinding condition if found in the macula (Fig. 25–7). Other injuries to the posterior pole include acute retinal contusion, or Berlin's edema, which is caused by a shearing injury to the photoreceptors (Fig. 25–8).

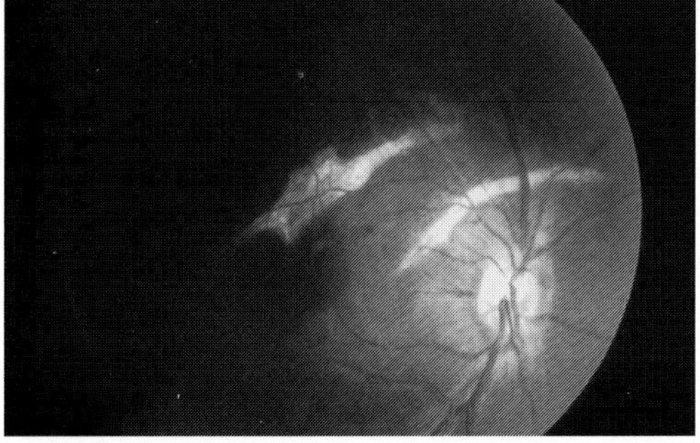

Figure 25–7. Fundus photograph demonstrates a choroidal rupture.

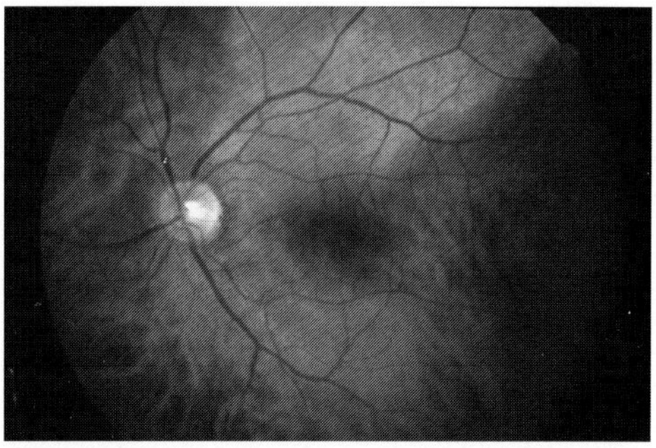

Figure 25–8. Fundus photograph demonstrates commotio retinae (Berlin's edema).

Presentation

The patient presents with a recent history of periocular trauma and may complain of photophobia, decreased vision, pain, or floaters. The patient may even be free of symptoms.

Evaluation

The evaluation of a patient for posterior segment injury requires a dilated fundus examination. Findings may include vitreous hemorrhage, retinal tears, hemorrhage, and opacification.

Priorities

Suspected retinal injury should be evaluated by an ophthalmologist, other ocular injuries should be ruled out, and the patient should be followed until resolution. Significant ocular trauma places a patient at lifelong risk for retinal detachment and merits close supervision by an ophthalmologist.

Outcome

Atmaca and colleagues reported 445 posttraumatic ocular injuries that were seen in an outpatient setting. The most common injuries were retinal detachment, chorioretinal atrophy, retinal contusion, choroidal rupture, optic atrophy, and vitreous hemorrhage. Industrial accidents were the most common cause of injury, followed by sporting accidents, home injuries, personal battery, and motor vehicle injuries. Of the eyes studied, 83% suffered visual loss below the ability to count fingers at 5 meters. This visual loss was permanent in the majority of the patients.[15]

TRAUMATIC OPTIC NEUROPATHY

Trauma to the orbit, forehead, or brow may result in traumatic optic neuropathy (TON). Injuries to these areas transmit force through the elastic sphenoid bone to the bony optic canal and optic nerve. The incidence of TON is 4 to 6 cases per 100,000 population annually.[16] As many as 0.5% to 5% of patients with closed head injuries and 2.5% of patients with midface fractures suffer TON.[16, 17] Of patients with TON, 40% to 72% experience loss of consciousness.[17] Various mechanisms contribute to TON, including the shearing of optic nerve fibers, intrasheath hemorrhage, neural edema, neural compression, vascular compromise, and direct optic nerve damage caused by bony fragments or optic canal fracture.[16–21]

Presentation

The patient may be unconscious at presentation and show evidence of only an afferent pupillary defect. A conscious patient may complain of visual loss, which may be sudden, delayed, or progressive and may occur after even seemingly minor trauma. The loss of vision may be mild, moderate, or severe, including no light perception.

Priorities

Each patient with TON should undergo a complete ophthalmologic examination. In a patient who is unresponsive or uncooperative with visual acuity testing, the presence of an unexplained afferent pupillary defect is indicative of TON. In a suspected bilateral case or in an unconscious or uncooperative patient, visual evoked potentials may demonstrate visual pathway impairment.[17] Thin-section axial and direct coronal computed tomography (CT) scanning with special attention to the optic nerve and optic canal should be considered in all cases. Neuroimaging may demonstrate bony canal or orbital fracture, and in some cases displaced bony fragments may be seen impinging upon the optic nerve (Fig. 25–9).

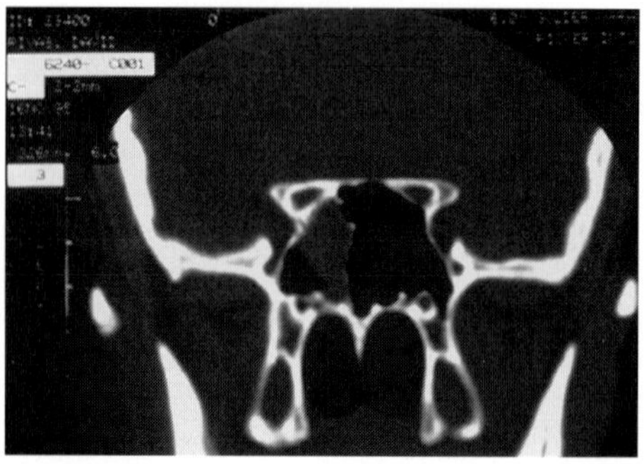

Figure 25–9. Coronal CT image of the orbit demonstrates a right optic canal fracture. (Courtesy of James R. Patrinely, M.D.)

The initial therapy for TON includes high-dose intravenous corticosteroids. The National Acute Spinal Cord Injury Studies (NASCIS II, NASCIS III) were multicenter, randomized clinical trials comparing the use of methylprednisolone to placebo in acute spinal cord injuries.[22, 23] A loading dose of intravenous methylprednisolone 30 mg/kg was followed with a 5.4 mg/kg/h infusion for 23 hours. The NASCIS data showed significant improvement in motor outcomes after spinal injury at the 6-month follow-up; the improvement was particularly apparent when steroids were instituted less than 8 hours after injury. Based on knowledge of the shared mechanism of response to cellular injury of the optic nerve and spinal cord, many practitioners employ a modified regimen of loading intravenous methylprednisolone 30 mg/kg followed by 15 mg/kg every 6 hours for 48 hours in cases of TON. There is evidence to suggest treatment can be started beyond the 8-hour time frame employed by NASCIS. The dose of steroids that is typically employed in a patient with head injuries to avoid cerebral edema does not, however, provide the protective antioxidant effect of the megadoses of methylprednisolone used in the NASCIS.[17]

A rapid oral taper may be instituted after 48 hours if the patient shows stable improvement on intravenous steroids. If improvement begins initially but the patient is steroid-dependent, or if no improvement is seen after 24 to 48 hours, extracranial optic canal decompression should be considered, even though risks include losing the improvement in vision already obtained.

Outcomes

Berestka and Rizzo reviewed seven studies of TON and found spontaneous improvement in

20% to 71% of patients.[16] In contrast, a review of four studies of patients treated with megadose steroids showed improvement in 36% to 100% of patients. Between 12% and 79% of patients improved with canal decompression.[17] Levin and colleagues performed a meta-analysis of 244 cases found in 46 journal articles to compare steroid treatment, surgical intervention, and a combination of the two. They found no difference among these treatment options in terms of visual outcome. These investigators found all forms of treatment to be superior to the natural history, however, and felt the visual prognosis was related to the severity of the initial injury.[27] The difficulty of obtaining a significant number of prospective cases limits the ability to conduct a randomized, prospective clinical trial of the various options available to treat this disease.

In contrast to the bony transmission of forces, rotary injuries involving the globe itself can directly damage the optic nerve. Such mechanisms may cause complete evulsion of the optic nerve from the posterior sclera (Fig. 25–10).[17,25] Portions of the nerve may be selectively damaged. If the nerve is not completely transected, megadose intravenous steroids should be considered.[17]

FACIAL FRACTURE

Facial trauma severe enough to cause bony fractures is often associated with ocular injuries.

Presentation

The patient presents with a history of periocular or facial trauma and facial fracture.

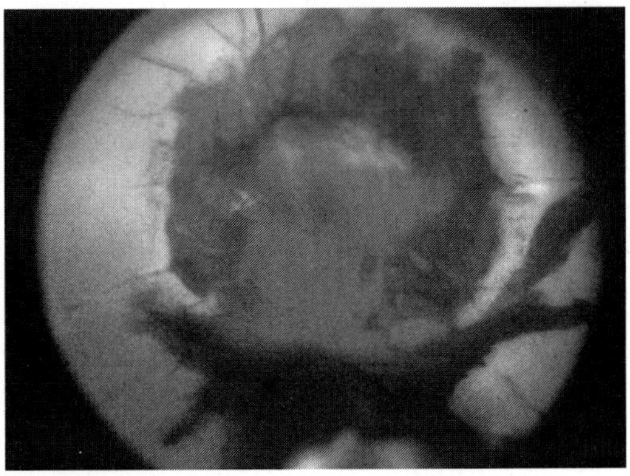

Figure 25–10. Fundus photograph demonstrates an optic nerve avulsion.

Evaluation

Every patient with a facial fracture should be considered for ophthalmologic consultation to exclude comorbid ocular conditions.[26,27]

Priorities

Holt and associates reviewed 1,436 patients with maxillofacial trauma, 55% of whom underwent complete ophthalmic examinations. They found ocular injuries in 29% of patients with mandibular fractures, 59% of patients with nasal fractures, 76% of patients with midface fractures, and 89% of patients with frontal fractures. The overall risk of eye injury was 67%.

Outcomes

Although the majority of ocular injuries in Holt's study were self-limited, 18% were severe, and 3% involved the loss of light perception or resulted in enucleation. The majority of severe eye injuries occurred in conjunction with midface, nasal, and frontal fractures.[27] Similar injury to the eye may occur in orbital fractures.[28–34]

ORBITAL FRACTURE

The periocular bony skeleton may transmit force through an intact orbital rim, allowing the orbital floor or medial wall to buckle. A fracture of the orbital rim may be palpable as a rim step-off, but a pure floor fracture leaves the rim intact.

Presentation

The patient may present complaining of recent facial trauma, diplopia, pain, or visual disturbance.

Evaluation

The clinical examination should include evaluation for proptosis from edema, hemorrhage, or orbital air and for enophthalmos resulting from floor or medial wall fracture. Orbital air may escape into the periocular tissues and may be palpated as subcutaneous crepitus. Either pure or combined floor fractures can create dysesthesia in the distribution of the infraorbital nerve.

A patient with an orbital fracture may complain of diplopia and may demonstrate difficulty in elevation, depression, abduction, or adduction of the eye. Extraocular motility may be restricted because of ocular motor nerve injury, orbital edema, or entrapment, hematoma, or contusion of the extraocular muscles. The motility should be recorded in the cardinal positions of gaze.

Priorities

A CT scan of the orbit, including fine axial and coronal sections, should be performed in cases of suspected fracture. An orbital fracture is not an emergency unless it is a rare case of extraocular muscle incarceration. An entrapped muscle may suffer a compartment syndrome with irreversible ischemia and loss of function (Fig. 25–11).

Outcomes

Late complications of orbital fractures include enophthalmos and diplopia.[18, 20, 28–43] Realistic goals of fracture repair are reduction of cosmetically disfiguring enophthalmos and resolution of diplopia in primary and reading gaze. The timing of and need for repair in orbital fractures to avoid these complications remain controversial. Some authors advocate early repair in all cases, others a delayed approach with late repair only in cases of persistent diplopia or cosmetically disfiguring enophthalmos. Supporters of early repair quote the relative ease of repair and good prognosis in surgeries performed within 2 weeks of injury. There is a progressive increase in scar tissue, as well as the possibility of persistent restriction in extraocular motility, with late repair.[28, 30, 31] However, the complications associated with repair may be severe, including persistent diplopia as well as loss of vision, including no light perception. Early repair should be reserved, therefore, for patients who are most likely to exhibit late enophthalmos or motility restriction resulting from muscle entrapment. Following these guidelines, Greenwald and coworkers studied patients with large fractures, enophthalmos on presentation, and positive forced duction testing. To test for restriction of the extraocular muscles by forced duction, the conjunctiva should be anesthetized with topical anesthesia and the limbal conjunctiva secured with 0.12 to 0.3 fine-toothed forceps. The eye is then rotated manually while the patient is instructed to look in the direction of rotation. A paralyzed muscle allows free rotation of the globe. A restricted muscle does not allow globe rotation. Although 91% of Greenwald's patients improved postoperatively, 33% of patients suffered surgical complications.[30] Jayamanne and colleagues performed early repair on six patients with diplopia in primary position, although half of these patients continued to complain of diplopia postoperatively. There was complete, spontaneous resolution of diplopia in the remaining 38 patients treated by observation alone. Jayamanne proposed that late enophthalmos was caused by enlargement of the orbital cavity due to orbital fracture and not fat atrophy. He recommended early repair of both the orbital floor and the medial wall in cosmetically significant early enophthalmos.[33] By restricting early repair to patients in whom more than one half of the orbital floor is fractured and to diplopic patients with tissue incarceration who show no improvement in the first 2 weeks, surgical complications can be minimized and symptomatic relief maximized (Fig. 25–12).[36, 39]

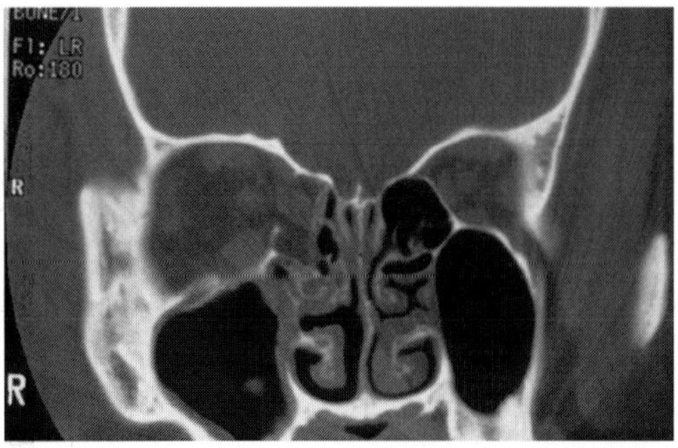

Figure 25–11. Coronal CT image of the head demonstrates medial rectus muscle entrapment on the right. (Courtesy of James R. Patrinely, M.D.)

Those advocating delayed orbital fracture repair note the high rate of spontaneous regression of diplopia with the resolution of orbital edema and the low rate of significant enophthalmos. Putterman and associates reviewed 57 patients with pure blow-out fractures of the orbital floor, with or without medial wall fractures; 28 patients were studied retrospectively, 29 prospectively. On initial examination, 72% of the retrospective patients and 65% of the prospective patients complained of diplopia in primary position and with vertical gaze. By the end of follow-up, only one patient complained of functional diplopia (this patient was in the retrospective group and was lost to follow-up after only 5 weeks); 21% and 27% of patients,

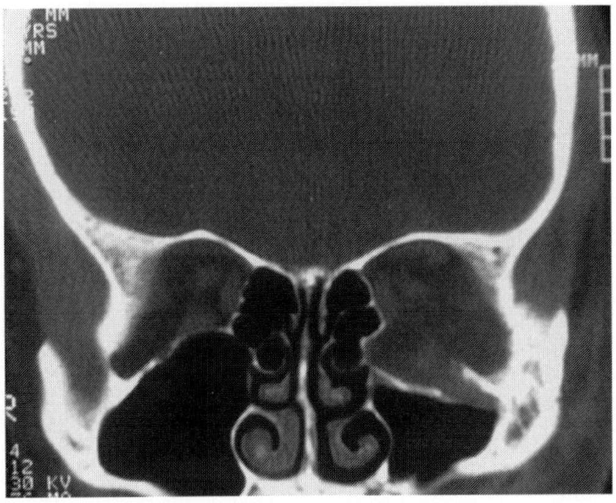

Figure 25–12. Coronal CT image of the orbit demonstrates a large left orbital floor fracture. (Courtesy of James R. Patrinely, M.D.)

respectively, had some diplopia in extreme gaze but were not bothered by it functionally. No patient desired correction for enophthalmos. These examiners believed the initial restrictions noted with forced duction were caused by hemorrhage within the orbital fat and herniated tissues and were not indications for repair.[43] This can now be confirmed by means of orbital imaging with special attention focused on the extraocular muscles. Emery and colleagues noted no difference in late enophthalmos in patients undergoing early repair as opposed to observation. Only 1 of 18 nonsurgical patients in their study complained of functional late diplopia when treated by observation alone.[29] In a separate study, Emery and colleagues confirmed complication rates of 10% to 38% with a variety of surgical approaches to fracture repair.[37]

Millman and colleagues prospectively randomized 38 patients with radiographically proven orbital fractures and diplopia to either steroid treatment or placebo to speed the determination of which patients would ultimately require surgery. All patients without muscle entrapment experienced resolution of their diplopia without surgery. The time to resolution was shortened, however, from 12.7 days in the nontreatment group to 4.4 days in the steroid treatment group. The patients with inferior rectus entrapment all suffered continued functional diplopia and required surgical repair at day 14 of the study. Of the steroid-treated patients undergoing surgical repair, 70% became clinically asymptomatic compared with 50% of the untreated group. Enophthalmos was stabilized within 1 week in the treated patients and within 5 months in the untreated patients, allowing an earlier determination of which patients would require orbital fracture repair. There were no complications of steroid treatment in this study.[41]

The only orbital fractures requiring emergent repair are those with rectus muscle entrapment, which, untreated, may cause muscle ischemia and infarction.

ORBITAL EMPHYSEMA

Orbital floor and medial wall fractures can be further complicated by orbital emphysema. Free air is noted within the orbit in up to 50% of orbital fractures, and in most cases it is a benign condition.[44–46] However, when air becomes trapped under high pressures, the circulation to the retina and optic nerve may become compromised. Orbital pressures have reached 50 to 120 mm Hg experimentally before rupture of the orbital septum occurs. However, the central retinal artery becomes occluded at pressures of 65 to 75 mm Hg.

Presentation

Orbital emphysema occurs most frequently in smaller fractures of the orbit, but it may present spontaneously. A forced expiration of air by sneezing or nose blowing increases the intranasal pressures to 190 to 290 mm Hg, forcing air into the orbit through a discontinuity in the bone and mucosa.[46, 47] Orbital fat covers and seals the fracture site, trapping the air by means of a ball-valve effect. Large fractures are unlikely to cause this entity, as entrapped orbital air has free access to the sinus cavities. The patient presents with a history of sudden painful proptosis, often with extraocular muscle dysfunction, ptosis, loss of vision, and an afferent pupillary defect.

Evaluation

The patient has proptosis as well as visual loss in the affected eye. The lids may be quite tense to palpation and the globe firm because of the transmission of orbital pressure. There may be palpable subcutaneous or subconjunctival crepitus. The syndrome may occur days after orbital trauma and after a history of recent forced expiration.

Priorities

Emergent orbital imaging may allow needle decompression of loculated orbital air, which has

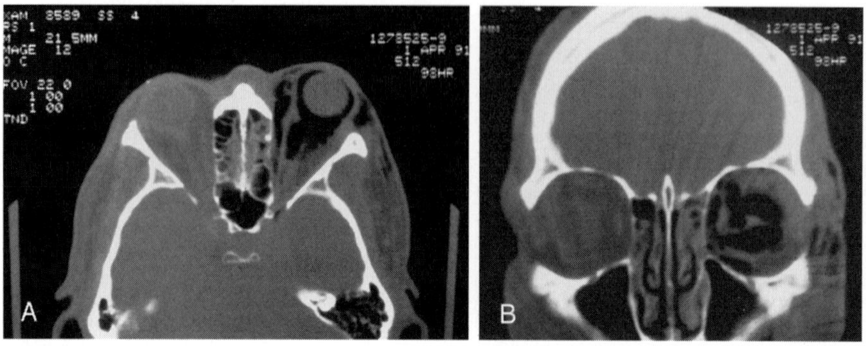

Figure 25–13. CT images of an orbit demonstrate left orbital emphysema. A: Axial image. B: Coronal image. (Courtesy of James R. Patrinely, M.D.)

been shown to prevent or reverse optic nerve and retinal ischemia (Fig. 25–13).[44–47] Hunts and colleagues described a four-stage rating system for orbital emphysema. Stage I is subclinical, with radiographic evidence of intraorbital air. Stage II includes proptosis, with normal vision. Stages III and IV include visual compromise, with a central retinal artery occlusion in stage IV. They recommend prophylactic oral antibiotics and decongestants and instructions against sneezing or nose blowing in stage I. Proptosis should be evaluated by means of a CT scan, and visual loss is treated with megadose intravenous steroids and drainage of loculated air. In a patient with evidence of severe visual loss or with retinal ischemia, the orbit should be immediately decompressed by lateral canthotomy and cantholysis. Emergent CT scanning is used to locate the loculated air for drainage. A syringe of saline coupled to a retrobulbar needle may then aid in the location and drainage of entrapped air.[45] This procedure should be performed by an ophthalmologist skilled in the techniques of retrobulbar injection.

Outcomes

The risks of air drainage include retrobulbar hemorrhage, laceration of the optic nerve, and inadvertent penetration of the globe. Untreated, however, stage III and stage IV orbital emphysema may cause ischemic infarction of the optic nerve and retina.

RETROBULBAR HEMORRHAGE

Fracture of the orbital floor may be associated with a laceration of the infraorbital artery or vein and a secondary retrobulbar hemorrhage. Increased venous pressure, anomalous vasculature, fragile atherosclerotic arteries, bleeding diathesis, and sinus disease may predispose to spontaneous hemorrhage or may worsen a traumatic hemorrhage.[48, 49] Regardless of the cause, a hematoma within the bony confines of the orbit may cause an orbital compartment syndrome with secondary vascular compromise and ischemic damage to the retina and optic nerve.

Presentation

The patient presents complaining of recent trauma or a forced Valsalva maneuver with subsequent hemorrhage, proptosis, pain, and visual loss.

Evaluation

The clinical findings in retrobulbar hemorrhage are pain, tense ecchymotic lids, proptosis, restricted ocular motility, and evidence of a compressive optic neuropathy. An optic neuropathy manifests with visual loss, sluggish pupillary reactions, and an afferent pupillary defect. Blood can track forward within the sub-Tenon and subconjunctival potential spacs, producing bloody conjunctival chemosis (Fig. 25–14).

Priorities

Immediate treatment should be initiated in a patient with a retrobulbar hemorrhage and severe retinal or optic nerve ischemia. A lateral canthotomy and cantholysis may allow a rapid decompression of the orbit. Fine-section axial and coronal CT scans may show the hemorrhage or nerve sheath hematoma. A patient who

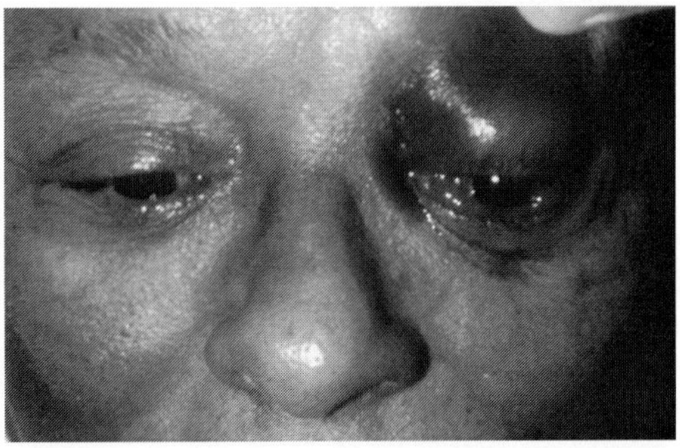

Figure 25–14. External photograph demonstrates left retrobulbar hemorrhage. (Courtesy of James R. Patrinely, M.D.)

does not respond to canthotomy should be considered for treatment with megadose steroids and referred for emergent orbital decompression. Needle drainage of subperiosteal hemorrhage may be successful.[50]

Outcomes

Recovery of vision with treatment may occur despite prolonged visual loss to the point of no light perception, and with the release of subperiosteal blood delayed by as many as 11 days.[47, 51–53] Untreated, the spontaneous recovery of vision is unlikely because of optic nerve and retinal ischemia.

IATROGENIC INJURY

Surgical procedures in the periocular region may have vision-threatening complications. Severe vision loss may occur following any orbital or periocular surgery, including orbital decompression, retrobulbar tumor excision, orbital biopsy, orbital floor fracture repair, and blepharoplasty.[54–57] The use of postoperative intermarginal sutures and the prolonged application of pressure patching have been suspected of compromising orbital blood flow.[55] Iatrogenic vision loss has been attributed to direct trauma to the optic nerve, vascular compromise, or orbital hemorrhage. Carter and colleagues reported several cases of vision loss associated with endoscopic sinus surgery, including inadvertent chiasmal biopsy with tension pneumocephalus, orbital hematoma with a compartment syndrome, and extraocular muscle damage or entrapment.[58]

Presentation

The patient presents postoperatively with a loss of vision and often with increased orbital tension.

Evaluation

Emergent evaluation should include the eight-point eye examination.

Priorities

Immediate canthotomy and cantholysis are indicated in cases of increased intraorbital pressure due to retrobulbar hemorrhage or edema. Emergent orbital decompression and high-dose intravenous steroids may improve vision in selected cases.[54, 56, 57]

Outcomes

Visual outcomes in orbital hemorrhage are similar to outcomes in cases of traumatic and spontaneous retrobulbar hemorrhages. However, direct optic nerve trauma indicates a more guarded prognosis. Untreated, the patient is unlikely to recover visual acuity spontaneously.

ORBITAL CELLULITIS

Facial trauma and sinusitis predispose a patient to orbital infection.[59, 60] The thin wall of the lamina papyracea, the lack of venous valves in the face and orbit, and the proximity of the sinuses and teeth may allow the spread of contiguous infection to the orbit.[59–61] The orbital veins drain posteriorly to the cavernous sinus and allow access of orbital infection to the central nervous system.

Presentation

It is important first to differentiate a patient with preseptal cellulitis from a patient with orbital cellulitis.[61, 62] Both patients present with tense lid edema and erythema. Orbital cellulitis, however, is characterized by the involvement of structures behind the orbital septum and can include proptosis, loss of vision, an afferent pupillary defect, ocular motility deficits, optic nerve edema, and retinal vascular compromise (Fig. 25–15).

Evaluation

The systematic evaluation of orbital cellulitis should include a complete blood count, blood cultures, and cultures of any orbital or sinus drainage. Nasal, conjunctival, and oropharyngeal cultures are unlikely to provide significant information.[60, 61] An ophthalmologic and otolaryngologic consultation should be obtained and the sinuses drained as necessary.

Treatment

The patient should be treated with broad-spectrum, systemic, intravenous antibiotics that include coverage for gram-positive and gram-negative pathogens, both aerobic and anaerobic. Common organisms include *Staphylococcus*, *Streptococcus*, and *Haemophilus* species (the latter being found especially in children). Polymicrobial infection is the rule. Antibiotic selections include metronidazole, clindamycin, aminoglycosides, penicillinase-resistant penicillins, cephalosporins, and vancomycin or chloramphenicol for penicillin-allergic patients.[59, 61] Topical and systemic decongestants should be started, and sinus drainage should be considered in a debilitated patient, in a patient with a poor response to antibiotics, and in a patient with multiple sinus involvement or other complications.[60] Debilitated patients and diabetics should be evaluated for mucormycosis and examined for evidence of primary intraocular infection and dental disease. Infectious disease consultation should be considered. Headache or a change in the level of consciousness may herald spread from the orbit to the central nervous system

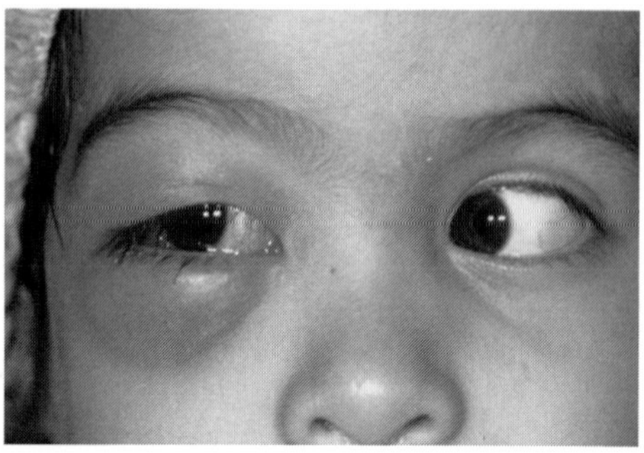

Figure 25–15. External photograph demonstrates restricted abduction due to right orbital cellulitis.

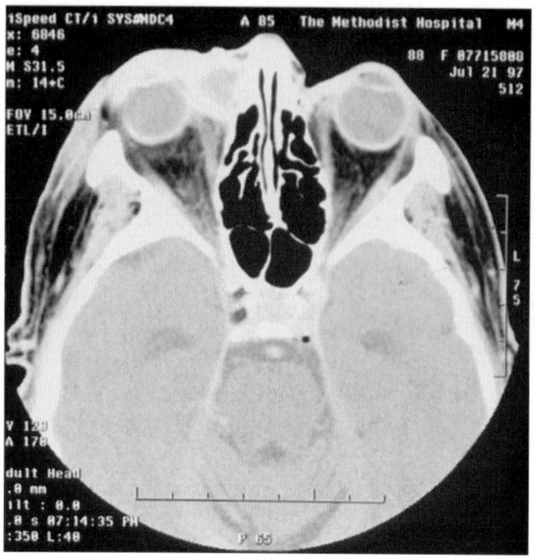

Figure 25–16. Axial CT image of an orbit demonstrates right dacryocystitis causing secondary orbital cellulitis and cavernous sinus thrombosis (not seen in this view). (Courtesy of Amy G. Coburn, M.D.)

and should prompt neuroimaging. CT scans of the head and orbits with thin-section axial and coronal cuts should be considered in any patient with orbital cellulitis. The patient should be followed closely, with repeat orbital and central nervous system imaging, if there is worsening or failure to improve after 48 hours (Fig. 25–16).

Outcomes

Orbital cellulitis should be considered an emergency and ophthalmologic consultation requested immediately. Untreated, mortality rates reach as high as 17%, with blindness in 25% of survivors.[61] Despite antibiotic treatment, patients may experience complications, including orbital, subperiosteal, or brain abscess, cavernous sinus thrombosis, and vision loss.

TUMORS THAT MIMIC CELLULITIS

Several types of tumor of the eye and orbit may present with signs that mimic orbital cellulitis.[60, 61, 63–66]

Presentation

Rapidly progressive proptosis, pain, and orbital inflammation have been seen in necrotic retinoblastoma. Shields and colleagues reported that

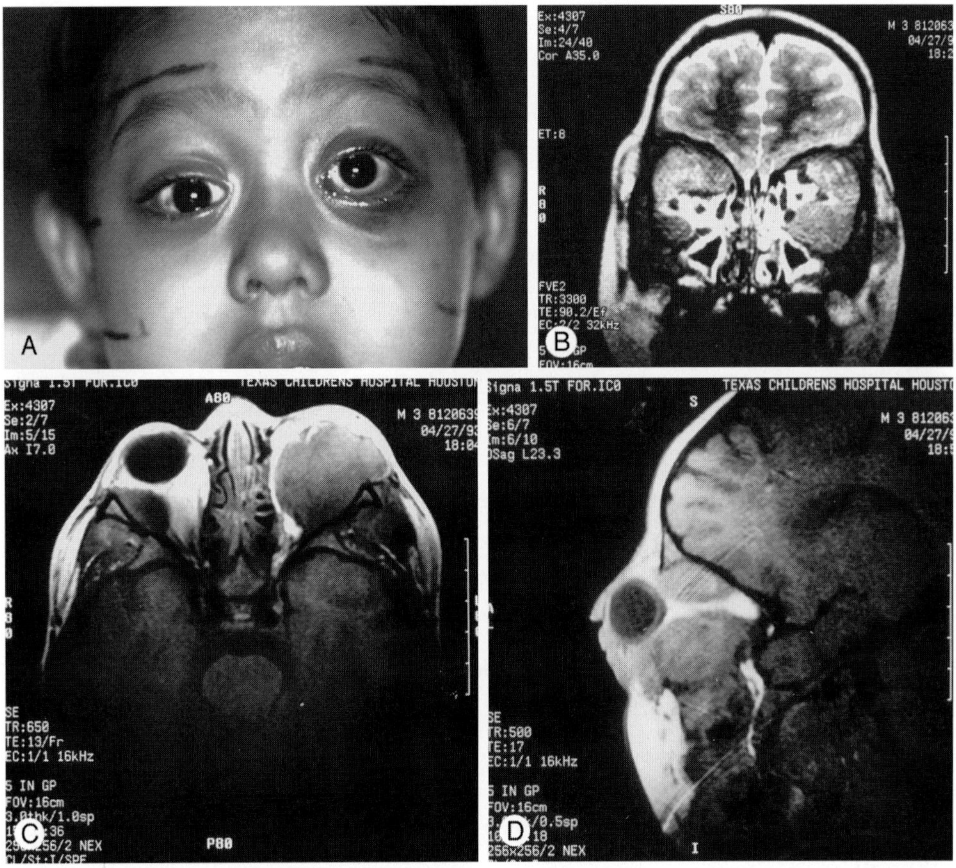

Figure 25–17. A: Photograph of a child with bilateral orbital infiltration due to acute myelogenous leukemia mimicking orbital cellulitis. MRI study demonstrates orbital soft-tissue leukemic infiltration. B: Coronal. C: Axial. D: Sagittal. (Courtesy of Jane E. Edmond, M.D.)

1.3% of 450 retinoblastoma patients presented as orbital cellulitis. Although these patients showed initial signs of soft tissue edema and inflammation, no patients were found to have extrascleral extension of tumor. Of patients with retinoblastomas seen at the Armed Forces Institute of Pathology, 7% presented originally as orbital cellulitis.[66] Other entities that mimic orbital cellulitis include rhabdomyosarcoma, invasive squamous cell carcinoma, leukemia, lymphoma, ruptured dermoid cyst, choroidal melanoma, orbital pseudotumor, orbital myositis, carotid-cavernous fistula, dural-cavernous fistula, metastatic disease, Wegener's granulomatosis, and systemic lupus erythematosus (Fig. 25–17).[60, 61, 63–66]

Evaluation

A patient with atypical signs of infection such as lack of infectious risk factor and failure to respond to antibiotics should undergo orbital imaging and neuroimaging to exclude orbital tumors and orbital pseudotumor. A patient with a mass lesion visible on imaging may require an orbital biopsy.

Priorities

If an orbital tumor is suspected, an ophthalmologist should be consulted immediately. Treatment requires coordinated care by an oncologist and possibly a radiation oncologist.

Outcomes

The outcome of an orbital mass lesion is in part dependent upon the tumor origin and metastatic status.

REFERENCES

1. Dunya IM, Rubin PAB, Shore JW. Penetrating orbital trauma. Int Ophthalmol Clin 1995; 35:1–35.

2. Patel KH et al. Incidence of acute angle-closure glaucoma after pharmacologic mydriasis. Am J Ophthalmol 1995; 120:709–717.
3. Kylstra JA, Lamkin JC, Runyan DK. Clinical predictors of scleral rupture after blunt ocular trauma. Am J Ophthalmol 1993; 115:530–535.
4. Werner MS et al. Predictors of occult scleral rupture. Ophthalmology 1994; 101:1941–1944.
5. Pieramici DJ et al. Open-globe injury. Ophthalmology 1996; 103:1798–1803.
6. Thompson WS et al. Endophthalmitis after penetrating trauma. Retina 1994; 102:1696–1701.
7. Alfaro DV, Roth D, Liggett PE. Posttraumatic endophthalmitis. Retina 1994; 14:206–211.
8. Thompson JT et al. Infectious endophthalmitis after penetrating injuries with retained intraocular foreign bodies. Ophthalmology 1993; 100:1468–1473.
9. Chi TSK, Netland PA. Angle-recession glaucoma. Int Ophthalmol Clin 1995; 35:117–126.
10. Salmon JF et al. The detection of post-traumatic angle recession by gonioscopy in a population-based glaucoma survey. Ophthalmology 1994; 101:1844–1850.
11. Berrios RR, Dreyer EB. Traumatic hyphema. Int Ophthalmol Clin 1995; 35:93–103.
12. Fong LP. Secondary hemorrhage in traumatic hyphema. Ophthalmology 1994; 101:1583–1588.
13. Endo EG, Mead MD. The management of traumatic hyphema. Int Ophthalmol Clin 1996; 14:757–761.
14. Teboul BK et al. Clinical evaluation of aminocaproic acid for managing traumatic hyphema in children. Ophthalmology 1995; 102:1646–1653.
15. Atmaca LS, Ylmaz M. Changes in the fundus caused by blunt ocular trauma. Ann Ophthalmol 1993; 25:447–452.
16. Berestka JS, Rizzo JF. Controversy in the management of traumatic optic neuropathy. Int Ophthalmol Clin 1994; 34:87–96.
17. Steinsapir KD, Goldberg RA. Traumatic optic neuropathy. Surv Ophthalmol 1994; 38:487–518.
18. Karesh JW et al. Orbital roof "blow-in" fractures. Ophthalmic Plast Reconstr Surg 1991; 7:77–83.
19. Krausen AS et al. Emergency orbital decompression: a reprieve from blindness. Otolaryngol Head Neck Surg 1981; 89:252–256.
20. Lipkin JF, Woodson GE, Miller RH. Visual loss due to orbital fracture. Arch Otolaryngol Head Neck Surg 1987; 113:81–83.
21. Warner JEA, Lessell S. Traumatic optic neuropathy. Int Ophthalmol Clin 1995; 35:57–61.
22. Bracken MB et al. A randomized, controlled trial of methylprednisolone or naloxone in the treatment of acute spinal cord injury. N Engl J Med 1990; 322:1405–1411.
23. Bracken MB et al. Administration of methylprednisolone for 24 or 48 hours or tirilazad mesylate for 48 hours in the treatment of acute spinal cord injury. JAMA 1997; 277:1597–1604.
24. Cook MV et al. Traumatic optic neuropathy. Arch Otolaryngol Head Neck Surg 1996; 122:389–392.
25. Park JH et al. Evulsion of the optic nerve. Am J Ophthalmol 1971; 72:969–971.
26. Freihofer HPM. Effectiveness of secondary post-traumatic periorbital reconstruction. J Craniomaxillofac Surg 1995; 23:150.
27. Holt JE, Holt GR, Blodgett JM. Ocular injuries sustained during blunt facial trauma. Ophthalmology 1983; 90:14–18.
28. Denny AD, Gonnering RS. Early repair of complex orbital fractures. Retina 1990; 10:S8–S19.
29. Emery JM, von Noorden GK, Schlernitzauer DA. Orbital floor fractures: long-term follow-up of cases with and without surgical repair. Trans Am Acad Ophthalmol Otolaryngol 1971; 75:802–812.
30. Greenwald HS, Keeney AH, Shannon GM. A review of 128 patients with orbital fractures. Am J Ophthalmol 1974; 78:655–664.
31. Jabaley ME, Lerman M, Sanders HJ. Ocular injuries in orbital fractures: a review of 119 cases. Plast Reconstr Surg 1975; 56:410–418.
32. Jayamanne DGR, Gillie RF. Orbital blow-out fractures: long-term visual outcome of associated ocular injuries. J Accid Emerg Med 1995; 12:273–275.
33. Jayamanne DGR, Gillie RF. Do patients with facial trauma to the orbito-zygomatic region also sustain significant ocular injuries? J R Coll Surg Edinb 1996; 41:200–203.
34. Tenzel RR. Complications of orbital fractures, their prevention and treatment. Eye Ear Nose Throat Mon 1975; 54:305–307.
35. Barr DR. Ocular muscle complications of orbital fractures. Ophthalmol Clin 1970; 10:153–160.
36. Crumley RL et al. Fractures of the orbital floor. Laryngoscope 1976; 934–947.
37. Emery JM, von Noorden GK, Schlernitzauer DA. Management of orbital floor fractures. Am J Ophthalmol 1972; 74:299–306.
38. Grove AS. Computed tomography in the management of orbital trauma. Am Acad Ophthalmol 1982; 89:433–440.
39. Hawes MJ, Dortzbach R. Surgery on orbital floor fractures. Am Acad Ophthalmol 1983; 90:1066–1070.
40. Iliff NT. The ophthalmic implications of the correction of late enophthalmos following severe midfacial trauma. Trans Am Ophthalmol Soc 1991; 89:477–548.
41. Millman AL et al. Steriods and orbital blowout fractures—a new systematic concept in medical management and surgical decision-making. Adv Ophthalmic Plast Reconstr Surg 1987; 6:291–300.
42. Paton D, Emery JM. Injuries of the eye, the lids and the orbit. In Zuidema G, Ballinger W, Rutherford R, eds. Trauma and the Surgeon, 2nd ed. Philadelphia, WB Saunders, 1973, pp. 219–254.
43. Putterman AM, Stevens T, Urist MJ. Nonsurgical management of blow-out fractures of the orbital floor. Am J Ophthalmol 1974; 77:232–239.
44. Fleishman JA, Beck RW, Hoffman RO. Orbital emphysema as an ophthalmologic emergency. Ophthalmology 1984; 91:1389–1391.
45. Hunts JH et al. Orbital emphysema. Ophthalmology 1994; 101:960–966.
46. Linberg JV. Orbital emphysema complicated by acute central retinal artery occlusion: case report and treatment. Ann Ophthalmol 1982; 14:747–749.
47. Linberg JV. Orbital compartment syndromes following trauma. Adv Ophthalmic Plast Reconstr Surg 1987; 6:51–62.
48. Choi S, Lawson W. Subperiosteal orbital hematoma. Arch Otolaryngol Head Neck Surg 1988; 114:1464–1466.
49. Krohel GB, Wright JE. Orbital hemorrhage. Am J Ophthalmol 1979; 88:254–258.
50. Markovits AS. Evacuation of orbital hematoma by continuous suction. Ann Ophthalmol 1977; 1255–1258.
51. Gillum WN, Anderson RL. Reversible visual loss in subperiosteal hematoma of the orbit. Ophthalmic Surg 1981; 12:203–209.
52. Katz B, Herschler J, Brick DC. Orbital haemorrhage

and prolonged blindness: a treatable posterior optic neuropathy. Br J Ophthalmol 1983; 67:549–553.
53. Kersten RC, Rice CD. Subperiosteal orbital hematoma: visual recovery following delayed drainage. Ophthalmic Surg 1987; 18:423–427.
54. Anderson RL. Bilateral visual loss after blepharoplasty. Arch Ophthalmol 1981; 99:2205.
55. Long JC, Ellis PP. Total unilateral visual loss following orbital surgery. Am J Ophthalmol 1971; 71 suppl:218–220.
56. McCartney DL, Char DH. Return of vision following orbital decompression after 36 hours of postoperative blindness. Am J Ophthalmol 1985; 100:602–604.
57. Nicholson, DH, Guzak SV. Visual loss complicating repair of orbital floor fractures. Arch Ophthalmol 1971; 86:369–375.
58. Carter K et al. Neuro-ophthalmologic complications of sinus surgery. Neuroophthalmol 1998; 19:75–82.
59. Goldfarb MS, Hoffman DS, Rosenberg S. Orbital cellulitis and orbital fractures. Ann Ophthalmol 1987; 19:97–99.
60. Rumelt S, Rubin PAD. Potential sources for orbital cellulitis. Int Ophthalmol Clin 1996; 36:207–221.
61. Lessner A, Stern GA. Preseptal and orbital cellulitis. Infect Dis Clin North Am 1992; 6:933–952.
62. Jackson K, Baker SR. Periorbital cellulitis. Head Neck Surg 1987; 9:227–234.
63. Bach MC, Knowland M, Schuyler WBJ. Acute orbital myositis mimicking orbital cellulitis. Ann Intern Med 1988; 109:243–245.
64. Grossniklaus HE, Wojno TH. Leukemic infiltrate appearing as periorbital cellulitis. Arch Ophthalmol 1990; 108:484.
65. Rootman J et al. Extensive squamous cell carcinoma of the conjunctiva presenting as orbital cellulitis: the hermit syndrome. Can J Ophthalmol 1987; 22:40–44.
66. Shields JA et al. Retinoblastoma manifesting as orbital cellulitis. Am J Ophthalmol 1991; 112:442–449.

Index

Note: Page numbers in *italics* refer to illustrations
Page numbers followed by the letter b refer to boxed material,
and those followed by the letter t refer to tables.

B

C

D

I

N

S

U

V

W

X

Z

ISBN 1-55664-470-1

90038

9 781556 644702